TRAUMA CARE

TRAUMA CARE

Beyond the resuscitation room

Edited by

Peter A. Driscoll
Senior Lecturer and Honorary Consultant in Emergency Medicine
Hope Hospital, Salford, UK

and

David V. Skinner
Consultant and Clinical Director
Accident and Emergency Department, John Radcliffe Hospital, Headington, Oxford, UK

© BMJ Books 1998
BMJ Books is an imprint of the BMJ Publishing Group

First published in 1998
by BMJ Books, BMA House, Tavistock Square,
London WC1H 9JR

British Library Cataloguing in Publication Data

A catalogue record for this book is available from the British Library

ISBN 0-7279-0933-9

Typeset by Latimer Trend, Plymouth
Printed and bound by Craft Print Pte Ltd, Singapore

Contents

Contributors

David J. Coleman
Consultant Plastic Surgeon, The Radcliffe Infirmary, Oxford

Martin P. Deahl
Consultant and Senior Lecturer in Psychological Medicine, St Bartholomew's Hospital, West Smithfield, London
Consultant Psychiatrist, 256 (L) Field Hospital, RAMC (V)

John H. Dempster
Consultant Otolaryngologist, Crosshouse Hospital, Kilmarnock

John S. Elston
Consultant Ophthalmologist, Oxford Eye Hospital

Richard J. Fairhurst
Past Chairman British Association for Immediate Care, Consultant in Accident and Emergency Medicine,
Chorley and South Ribble District General Hospital

Douglas Gentleman
Honorary Consultant Neurosurgeon, Ninewells Hospital, Dundee
Consultant, Centre for Brain Injury Rehabilitation, Royal Victoria Hospital, Dundee

Timothy R. Graham
Cardiothoracic Consultant, Queen Elizabeth Hospital, Birmingham

Carl L. Gwinnutt
Consultant Anaesthetist, Hope Hospital, Salford

Tim Hodgetts
Consultant in Accident and Emergency Medicine, Frimley Park Hospital NHS Trust, Frimley, Camberley, Surrey

Simon A. V. Holmes
Consultant Urologist, St Marys Hospital, Portsmouth

Michael A. Horan
Professor of Geriatric Medicine, Hope Hospital, Salford

Iain Hutchison
Consultant Oral and Maxillofacial Surgeon, St Bartholomew's Hospital and The Royal London Hospitals

Jonathan A. J. Hyde
Cardiothoracic Registrar, Queen Elizabeth Hospital, Birmingham

Sir Miles H. Irving
Professor of Surgery, University of Manchester, Department of Surgery, Hope Hospital, Salford

David J. Jones
Consultant Surgeon, Department of Surgery, Wythenshawe Hospital, Manchester

Keith Judkins
Medical Director for Burn Centre, Consultant in Anaesthesia and Intensive Care, Yorkshire Regional Burn Centre,
Pinderfields Hospital, Wakefield

Roger S. Kirby
Consultant Urologist, St George's Hospital, London

James R. S. Leggate
Consultant Neurosurgeon, Hope Hospital, Salford

Anthony McCluskey
Consultant in Anaesthesia and Intensive Care, Stepping Hill Hospital, Stockport

Fergal P. Monsell
Consultant Orthopaedic Surgeon, Great Ormond Street Hospital for Children NHS Trust, London

Julie Nancarrow
Royal Preston Hospital, Fulwood, Preston

Peter Nightingale
Consultant in Anaesthesia and Intensive Care, Withington Hospital, Manchester

Ken K. Nischal
Senior Registrar, Oxford Eye Hospital

Alan Phipps
Consultant Burns and Plastic Surgeon, Yorkshire Regional Burn Centre, Pinderfields Hospital, Wakefield

E. Raymond S. Ross
Consultant Orthopaedic Surgeon, Salford Royal Hospitals NHS Trust, Salford, Manchester

Jim Ryan
Leonard Cheshire Professor of Conflict Recovery, University College, London

Ashok Shetty
Cardiothoracic Registrar, Queen Elizabeth Hospital, Birmingham

Anthony D. Simcock
Consultant Anaesthetist, Royal Cornwall Hospital, Truro, Cornwall

Malcolm Smith
Consultant Trauma and Orthopaedic Surgeon, St James' University Hospital, Leeds

Iain R. C. Swan
Senior Lecturer, Department of Otolaryngology, Royal Infirmary, Glasgow

Catherine A. Sweby
Senior Physiotherapist, Hope Hospital, Salford

Jenny Walker
Consultant Paediatric Surgeon, Paediatric Surgical Unit, Sheffield Children's Hospital NHS Trust

T. D. Wardle
Consultant Physician, Countess of Chester Health Park, Chester

Stewart Watson
Consultant Plastic, Hand and Microsurgeon, Withington Hospital, Manchester

Robin Wood
UKAEA, Harwell, Didcot, Oxon

Introduction

Peter A. Driscoll and David V. Skinner

Trauma is the commonest cause of death between the first and fortieth years of life in most developed countries. The mechanism varies but the vast majority are victims of blunt trauma with road traffic accidents being the commonest cause. For each fatality one must also take into account two permanently disabled victims and many others who will have to endure significant periods of rehabilitation. Consequently the financial cost for this trauma epidemic is enormous, amounting to at least 1% of the gross national product for each country. The human cost is, however, incalculable.

The most effective way of reducing the human misery, and financial cost, is by accident prevention. There have been various initiatives in several countries which have had encouraging results. Legislation has been introduced with regard to drink–driving, the wearing of seatbelts for car occupants and the use of head protection by cyclists. To this must be added engineering initiatives with regard to more "pedestrian-friendly" cars and better urban planning. Health and Safety initiatives in the workplace have also helped to reduce the number of fatal and disabling injuries. It therefore behoves all healthcare professionals involved in trauma care to support any of these or similar initiatives.

Tragically, however, fatalities due to trauma still occur. We therefore must also be able to provide optimal treatment at the scene of the incident right through to the patient's eventual discharge from rehabilitation. As there are many components to this "chain of trauma care", the patient's chances of survival will only increase if personnel involved with each link provide optimal care.

In North America, the United Kingdom, and Australia, deficiencies in the chain of care have been identified. These have concentrated particularly on prehospital care and the management of the patient in the resuscitation room. Since these reports, educational programmes in "Prehospital Care", "Advanced Trauma Life Support" and more efficient organisation in the resuscitation room have all led to an improvement in the early recognition of significantly injured patients and their optimal resuscitation.

With better early treatment, however, problems in managing these patients once they leave the Emergency Department have become more evident. Critically injured patients are surviving longer and this puts greater pressure on anaesthetists, surgeons and emergency physicians who have to look after them in either their own hospital or a specialist centre before expert care can be provided. A team approach is essential in these circumstances. In addition it is important that all clinicians involved in this early stage of a patient's care are aware of the priorities of optimal trauma management. They can then recognise, initially treat, and subsequently communicate with the appropriate specialists in a timely fashion.

This book has therefore been written for all clinicians who will have to look after trauma patients. It gives the reader an in-depth insight into the specialist management of these patients and endeavours to be exhaustive in its scope from resuscitation to rehabilitation. Both "he" and "she" have been used as a pronoun for "the patient".

1 Initial assessment and management of the trauma patient

Peter A. Driscoll
Senior Lecturer and Honorary Consultant in Emergency Medicine, Hope Hospital, Salford

David V. Skinner
Consultant and Clinical Director, Accident and Emergency Department, John Radcliffe Hospital, Headington, Oxford

---

OBJECTIVES

■ To understand the structure and function of a trauma team.

■ To gain an overview of the management of the patient in the resuscitation room.

■ To see how care in the resuscitation room can extend into definitive care in the hospital.

To manage trauma victims appropriately, both immediately and potentially life-threatening conditions must be identified and treated before early and limb-threatening injuries. These in turn, should be dealt with before other, less severe, problems. Nevertheless, the latter must not be ignored because injuries, in particular to the wrist, hand, ankle, and foot, can give rise to prolonged morbidity and rehabilitation problems if not identified and managed correctly in the resuscitation room [1]. It follows that the same diligence applied to serious injuries must be extended, at the appropriate time, to those that appear to be less significant.

Prehospital information and communication

Direct communication from prehospital personnel enables essential information to be transmitted to the receiving hospital (see box). Without such a system the trauma team has to either rely on details relayed from the ambulance control centre or wait until the paramedics arrive with the patient.

Essential prehospital information

- The mechanism of injury
- Number, age and sex of the casualties
- Each patient's complaints, priorities, and injuries
- Airway, ventilatory, and circulatory status
- The conscious level
- Initial prehospital management
- Estimated time of arrival

It is crucial to determine the mechanism of injury as this gives invaluable information about the forces the patient was subjected to and the direction of impact. Further help comes from a description of the damage to the car (Figure 1.1) or the weapon used (see Chapters 10, 11 and 22).

Patterns of injuries occur following certain accidents. For example, a frontal impact can result in damage to the head, face, airway, neck, heart, lungs, thoracic aorta, main bronchi, liver, spleen, knee, shaft of femur, and hips (Figure 1.2). Where

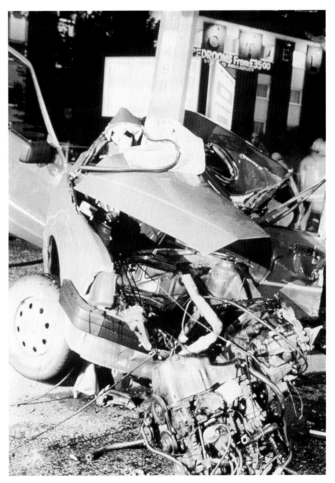

Figure 1.1 Prehospital personnel can provide invaluable information regarding the scene, mechanism of injury, and the state of the patients.

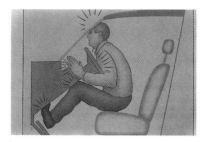

Figure 1.2 Frontal road traffic accident.

an occupant of a car is ejected following a collision, the victim has a 300% greater chance of a sustaining a serious injury. Fatalities at the scene following road traffic accident imply that considerable forces have been generated. Consequently, any survivors of such an accident should be considered to have serious injuries until proved otherwise.

Trauma team

The nurses and doctors who make up the trauma team need to be summoned once it has been decided that the patient requires resuscitation room facilities. As any time delay can be important, these people must be immediately available and preorganised to ensure that the right person gets to the right place at the right time.

They should assemble in the resuscitation room prior to the patient's arrival and be briefed on the prehospital information available by the trauma team leader. This person must also ensure that all personnel are familiar with their respective roles. In this way tasks can be performed simultaneously for the maximum benefit of the patient in the shortest possible time (Figure 1.3) [2,3]. It is also essential that each member of

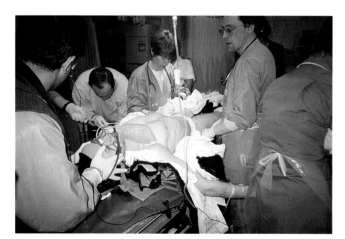

Figure 1.3 Trauma team in action with individual members carrying out tasks simultaneously.

the team is immunised against hepatitis and wearing protective clothing. Ideally universal precautions should be taken but, failing this, latex gloves, aprons, and goggles must be worn because all blood and body fluids should be assumed to carry HIV and hepatitis viruses [4].

Whilst protective clothing is being put on, a final check of the equipment by the appropriate team members can then take place.

Objectives

The team has the following objectives:

- Resuscitate and stabilize the patient.
- Determine the nature and extent of the injuries.
- Categorize the injuries in order of priority.
- Prepare for transport of the patient to a place of definitive care.

Personnel

The trauma team should comprise the following nursing, medical, and radiological staff:

Medical staff

- Medical team leader
- "Airway" doctor
- Two "circulation" doctors*

Nursing staff

- Nursing team leader
- "Airway nurse"
- Two "circulation nurses"
- "Relatives" nurse

In all cases, the nursing and medical personnel chosen for the respective roles must be appropriately trained. Seniority *per se* is no guarantee of competence.

Radiographer*

- At least one radiographer must be a member of the trauma team (Figure 1.4).

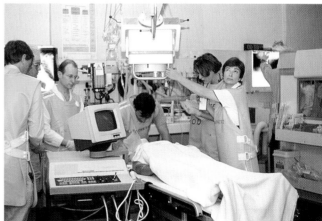

Figure 1.4 Radiographers are important members of the trauma team (courtesy of Mr A. Wilson, Royal London Hospital Trust.)

The aim of this initially large team is to achieve an efficient and rapid correction of all immediately life-threatening conditions. Once this has been completed, only the core personnel need remain and those marked with an asterisk can return to their normal duties.

Roles

Each member has to be thoroughly familiar with his/her respective duties so that tasks can be performed simultaneously for the maximum benefit of the patient in the shortest possible time. It is also essential that problems are anticipated rather than reacted to once they develop.

When nurses and doctors work in pairs, the efficiency of the team improves. Examples of paired roles and tasks are listed below. However, assignments may vary between units depending on the resources available.

Team leaders

Medical team leader

- Coordinates the specific tasks of the individual team members.
- Assimilates the clinical findings.
- Lists the investigations in order of priority.
- Liaises with specialists who have been called.
- Questions the ambulance personnel.
- Depending on the skill of the rest of the team members, carries out particular procedures, such as pericardiocentesis and thoracotomy.

Nursing team leader

- Coordinates the nursing team.
- Prepares sterile packs for procedures.
- Assists the circulation nurses and brings extra equipment as necessary.
- Records clinical findings, laboratory results, intravenous and drug infusion, and the vital signs as called out by the circulation nurse.

Airway personnel

Airway nurse

- Assists in securing and stabilising the cervical spine.
- Establishes a rapport with the patient giving psychological support throughout his/her management in the resuscitation room.

Airway doctor

- Clears and secures the airway whilst taking appropriate cervical spine precautions.
- Inserts central and arterial lines if required.

Circulation personnel

Circulation doctors

- Assist in the removal of the patient's clothes.
- Establish peripheral intravenous infusions and take blood for investigations.
- Carry out certain procedures such as urinary catheterisation and chest drain insertion.
- Carry out other procedures depending on their skill level.

Circulation nurses

- Measure the vital signs and connect the patient to the monitors.
- Assist with the removal of the patient's clothing.
- Assist with starting intravenous infusions, chest drain insertion, and catheterisation.

- Assist in special procedures such as pericardiocentesis.
- Monitor the fluid balance.

Relative's personnel

Relative's nurse

- Cares for the patient's relatives when they arrive.
- Liaises with the trauma team to provide the relatives with appropriate information and support.

Radiological personnel

- Take two standard x-rays on all patients subjected to blunt trauma, that is chest, pelvis and lateral cervical spine.

To avoid confusion, there should be no more than six people physically touching the patient. The other team members must stand back.

Reception and transfer

As the trauma victim's arrival is being noted by the recorder nurse, the rest of this team can concentrate on transferring the patient safely to the hospital trolley (Figure 1.5). The patient

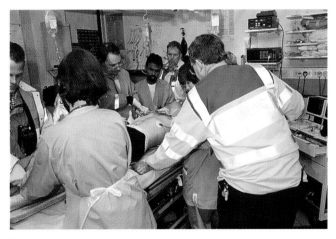

Figure 1.5 Trauma team completing the move of a patient on a long spinal board.

must be on a long spinal board, and five people will be required. This must be a well-drilled procedure in order to protect the spinal cord if it is intact and prevent further injury if it is already compromised. During this transfer the patient's head and neck must be stabilised by one member of the team, if not already appropriately immobilised, whilst three others lift from the side. This allows the fifth member to remove the ambulance trolley. The primary survey and resuscitation can then begin.

Primary survey and resuscitation

The objectives of this phase are to identify and correct any immediately life-threatening conditions. Consequently whilst the team leader is gaining information from the prehospital personnel, the activities listed in the box below are being performed simultaneously.

The primary survey
A Airway and cervical spine control
B Breathing
C Circulation with haemorrhage control
D Disability
E Exposure

Airway and cervical spine control

The airway personnel must initially assume the presence of an unstable cervical spine if the patient is a victim of blunt trauma or if the mechanism of injury indicates this region may have been damaged. Consequently, none of the activities described to clear and secure the airway must involve movement of the neck.

The airway nurse must manually immobilise the cervical spine at the same time as the airway doctor talks to the patient. Talking not only establishes supportive contact, but also can be used to assess the airway. If the patient replies with a normal voice, giving a logical answer, then the airway can be assumed to be patent and the brain adequately perfused.

An impaired or absent reply indicates that the airway could be obstructed, in which case the procedures described in Chapter 2 to clear and secure the airway should be carried out. The complications of alcohol ingestion and possible injuries of the chest and abdomen increase the chance of vomiting. Because it is impractical to nurse the trauma victim on his side, constant supervision in the supine position is required. If vomiting starts, no attempt should be made to turn the patient's head to one side unless a cervical spine injury has been ruled out radiologically and clinically. However, if a spinal board is in place, the whole patient can be turned. In the absence of this piece of equipment, the trolley should be tipped head down by 20° and the vomit sucked away as it appears in the mouth.

Once the airway has been cleared and secured, the patient should be given a high flow (12–15 l/min) of 100% oxygen and connected to a pulse oximeter (Figure 1.6). For those who

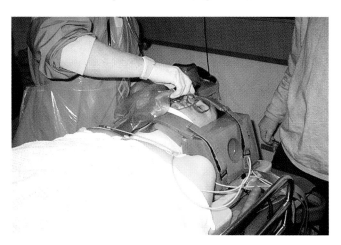

Figure 1.6 Once the airway has been secured all trauma victims should receive high flow oxygen. This picture also demonstrates the use of the commercially available cervical spine support.

are breathing adequately and spontaneously, oxygen should be provided by a mask with a reservoir bag attached. This will enable an inspired oxygen concentration of approximately 85% to be reached. When acceptable levels of oxygen cannot

be maintained, ventilatory support must be provided mechanically. In these cases an end-tidal CO_2 monitor must be fitted to confirm tracheal intubation and provide some indication of pulmonary perfusion (see Chapter 2).

The neck should then be inspected quickly for:

- Swellings and wounds which can indicate there is local injury, and damaged blood vessels.
- Subcutaneous emphysema from a pneumothorax or mediastinal emphysema.
- Tracheal deviation which may indicate a tension pneumothorax.
- Distended neck veins indicating there is a rise in the central venous pressure. This can result from a tension pneumothorax, cardiac tamponade or damage to the great vessels.
- Laryngeal crepitus indicating a fracture of the laryngeal cartilage.

To enable the airway nurse to safely release the patient's head and neck, the cervical spine must be secured by using either a semirigid collar, sand bags and tape, or a commercially available spine support (Figure 1.6) The only exception to this rule is the restless patient who will not keep still. In this case, the cervical spine can be damaged if the head and neck are immobilised whilst the rest of the patient's body keeps moving. A suboptimal level of immobilisation is therefore accepted, comprising a semirigid collar on its own.

Breathing

There are six immediately life-threatening thoracic conditions which must be searched for, and treated, during the primary survey and resuscitation phase (see box).

Immediately life-threatening thoracic conditions
- Airway obstruction
- Tension pneumothorax
- Cardiac tamponade
- Open chest wound
- Massive haemothorax
- Flail chest

To determine whether any of these conditions exist, the respiratory rate, effort, and symmetry needs to be monitored and recorded at frequent intervals by one of the circulation nurses. These are very sensitive indicators of underlying lung pathology. At the same time, the medical team leader should visually examine both sides of the chest. This is then followed by ausculation and percussion of the axillae to assess ventilation of the periphery. Listening over the anterior chest mainly detects air movement in the large airways which can submerge sounds of pulmonary ventilation. Consequently, differences between the two sides of the chest can be missed, especially if the patient is being artificially ventilated.

If there is no air entry to both sides, then there is either a complete obstruction of the upper airway, or an incomplete seal between face and mask if the patient is ventilated. The maintenance of an effective seal is by no means simple. Therefore the airway personnel need to be skilled in the use of a bag valve face mask device. Ideally a two-person technique should be used, with one holding the mask in place combined with jaw thrust, whilst the other squeezes the bag.

There is usually a local thoracic problem if there is a difference in air entry and percussion note between the right and left sides of the patient's chest. The immediately life-threatening conditions capable of producing this are a tension pneumothorax, an open chest wound, and a massive haemothorax. Their diagnosis and management discussed in detail in Chapter 3 (Figure 1.7).

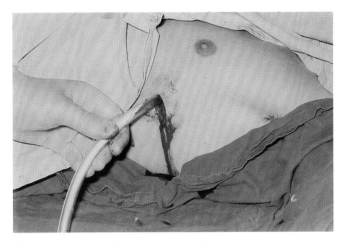

Figure 1.7 Patient with a tension pneumothorax having a chest drain inserted during the primary survey.

Circulation

The circulatory phase of the primary survey consists of stemming any overt bleeding, assessment of the cardiovascular state and gaining intravenous access.

Haemorrhage control

It is crucial during this phase that the trauma team identifies and controls any significant external haemorrhage. This bleeding can result from a compound long bone fracture, associated vascular injuries and soft tissue trauma (Figure 1.8).

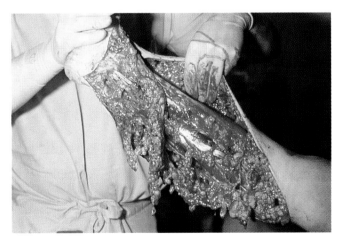

Figure 1.8 Limb trauma is often a source of external haemorrhage. A quick and effective way of gaining control is by direct pressure. In this case a tourniquet was also used because of the poor viability of the limb and clinical state of the patient.

When an artery is transected transversely, vasospasm owing to constriction of the muscle fibres in the tunica media will limit blood loss. In contrast, if there is a partial or longitudinal laceration, the vasospasm tends to keep the hole in the vessel open and blood loss continues. Veins have little muscle and therefore breeches in their walls will open or close depending upon the intraluminal pressure.

It is therefore preferable in the acute situation to control bleeding by direct pressure. Attempting to clamp vessels in the resuscitation room wastes time and may lead to further tissue damage. This applies also in cases of life-threatening haemorrhage because associated hypothermia, acidosis, and coagulopathy will enhance blood loss by preventing haemostatic control other than by direct pressure. These patients require further resuscitation, often in an intensive care environment, until they are in an optimum physiological state for surgery or embolisation of the bleeding vessels. It is therefore essential that these patients are identified early so that their appropriate management can be discussed by the surgeons, intensivists, and emergency medical personnel.

Because tourniquets increase intraluminal pressure, distal ischaemia, and tissue necrosis, they should be used only in cases where the limb is deemed unsalvageable. If this decision is taken, it is important to note the time the tourniquet was applied so that neighboring soft tissue is not jeopardised.

External fixation can be used in the resuscitation room to reduce and stabilise certain pelvic fractures. This controls life-threatening haemorrhage by reducing the pelvic and retroperitoneal volume. Therefore, the orthopaedic surgeon must review the patient and the radiographs to determine whether this procedure is appropriate and where it should be carried out (see Chapter 2). The pneumatic antishock garment (PASG), although controversial, can be considered if orthopaedic expertise is not rapidly available.

Assessment of blood loss

Blood loss from fractures (especially when open) and damaged adjacent vessels give rise to oedema in the surrounding tissues. These can be severe enough to cause hypovolaemic shock. Once any overt haemorrhage from any site has been stemmed, one of the circulation nurses should measure the blood pressure and note the rate, volume, and regularity of the pulse. An automatic blood pressure recorder and ECG monitor should also be connected to the patient at this time. Simultaneously the medical team leader should determine if the patient demonstrates any clinical evidence of shock (inadequate oxygen delivery to vital organs) (see Chapter 5). This requires the skin colour, clamminess, capillary refill time, heart rate, blood pressure, pulse pressure, and conscious level to be assessed.

It is important to be aware that patients have an altered cardiovascular response to haemorrhage after skeletal trauma [5–7]. The blood pressure and heart rate tends to be maintained even with significant blood loss but this is at a cost of increased tissue oxygen debt and higher incidences of multiple organ failure. Isolated vital signs are therefore unreliable for estimating the blood loss or the physiological impairment of the patient especially at the extremes of age [7,8]. They can be made more useful when they are combined as the shock index (heart rate/systolic blood pressure) [9]. Above 15% blood volume loss, the index rises over 0.8 in an almost linear fashion to reach 2.0–2.4 with losses of around 30%. With further losses the index plateaus and rises only a little [6].

Consequently, when blood loss is assessed in the early stages of the resuscitation, it is essential that the function of several crucial organs are taken into account. In this way reliance is not simply placed on a single vital sign such as blood pressure. Later on, depending upon the clinical situation, these clinical assessments can be augmented by recordings from invasive monitoring devices (see Chapter 11) (Figure 1.9).

Vascular cannulation

Immediate haemorrhage control and circulatory assessment should be accompanied by the insertion of two large-bore

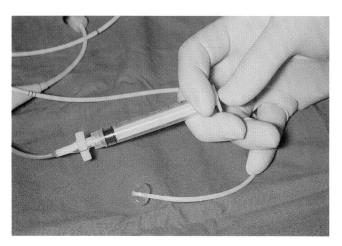

Figure 1.9 Invasive monitoring is sometimes required early on in the resuscitation when it is crucial that fluid replacement is accurately assessed. Examples include spinal injury, pulmonary contusion, and trauma victims with pre-existing cardiovascular disease.

intravenous lines. When the site for these cannulae is chosen, care must be taken to ensure that they are not placed distal to vascular or bony damage as this would allow the infused fluid to leak. Before infusion is started, 20 ml of blood must be taken from the cannula to allow grouping and cross-match, analysis of the the plasma electrolytes, and a full blood count. If it is not possible to gain peripheral intravascular access, either a venous cut down should be carried out or a short wide-bore central line inserted (see Chapter 5). The choice is dependent upon the clinical competence of the doctor carrying out the procedure. An arterial sample also needs to be obtained for blood gas and pH analysis (Figure 1.10). However, this can wait until the end of the primary survey.

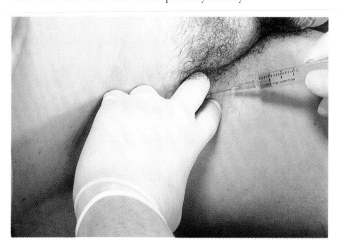

Figure 1.10 Arterial blood gas analysis provides useful information on both the adequacy of the resuscitation as well as the patient's respiratory state.

Intravenous fluid administration

The rate of fluid infusion needs to be appropriate to the clinical situation and therefore has to take into account the mechanism of injury. Evidence for this approach comes from clinical and animal studies [10–13]. Workers have shown an increase in survival when fluid resuscitation is limited, until surgery, in cases of unrepaired vascular injury following penetrating trauma. In contrast, infusing fluids to achieve a normal blood pressure in these cases increases blood loss. The reasons for this are not precisely known but it is probably due to a

combination of impaired thrombus formation and inhibition of the body's physiological compensatory response to blood loss. It follows that shocked patients from uncontrollable hemorrhage (for example penetrating trauma to the torso) need surgery rather than aggressive fluid resuscitation.

It is less clear how shocked patients should be managed if they are victims of blunt trauma. As the cardiovascular response to haemorrhage is altered after skeletal trauma, it can be anticipated that these patients will have lost a significant amount of their blood volume. Consequently they are at significant risk of developing multiple organ failure. Therefore, once any overt bleeding has been stemmed, our advice is to infuse enough warm crystalloid or colloid solution initially to maintain a radial pulse. Depending on the patient's response, warmed blood may also be needed. Following this preliminary approach, further clinical assessment is required along with more sophisticated monitoring devices (see Chapter 5). In this way the team can ensure adequate perfusion of the patient's vital organs until definitive care is underway (see later).

Disability

In the primary survey and resuscitation phase the conscious level of the patient, along with the pupillary response, must be recorded. These tests are then enhanced with the more detailed mini-neurological examination during the secondary survey.

If time permits the Glasgow coma score should be recorded at this stage. If this is not possible a rapid and gross assessment of the conscious level is made by asking the patient to put his or her tongue out, to wiggle the toes and to squeeze the clinician's fingers. In addition, conscious level can be assessed crudely by the AVPU system (see box). It is essential that these assessments are monitored frequently to detect any deterioration. There are many possible causes for this but the most common in the trauma patient are hypoxia, hypovolaemia, and raised intracranial pressure.

The AVPU system
A Alert
V Only responding to verbal stimulus
P Only responding to pain
U Unresponsive to any stimulus

Exposure

All clothing must be removed by the end of the primary survey so that the entire skin surface can be examined. Note, however, that trauma victims often have sharp objects such as glass and other debris in their clothing, hair, and on the skin. As ordinary surgical gloves give no protection against this, the personnel undressing the patient should initially wear more robust gloves.

The presence of injuries and the possibility of spinal instability means that garments must be cut along seams with large bandage scissors so that clothes can be removed with minimal patient movement. If the patient is conscious an explanation can be given and permission sought. Rings and other constricting jewellery should also be removed during this phase of the primary survey. Once stripped, trauma victims must be kept warm with blankets when not being examined.

In certain units, patients will arrive with a PASG applied and inflated. It is extremely important that this suit is deflated slowly and only after intravenous access has been gained to avoid circulatory collapse. Similarly, it is important to note that the rapid removal of tight trousers can precipitate sudden hypotension from the loss of the tamponade effect in the hypovolaemic patient. These garments should only be removed at the team leader's discretion and when two, large-bore peripheral intravenous lines are in place.

With practice the trauma team should complete the objectives of the primary survey and resuscitation phase within 10 minutes [2]. Prearrangement with the laboratory for rapid processing and reporting will facilitate the team leader's evaluation of the patient's state. The vital signs should be recorded every five minutes so that the patient's progress or deterioration can therefore be determined. An important question to ask is, "Is the patient getting better or worse?" This helps to determine if the team needs to move rapidly to definitive care. For example, the patient should be taken directly to theatre to gain control of a source of bleeding if there is a sudden deterioration following intravenous resuscitation.

> Only when all the ventilatory and hypovolaemic problems have been corrected can the team continue the more detailed secondary survey.

While the primary survey and resuscitation phase is under way, the relative's nurse should greet any of the patient's friends or relatives who arrive. The nurse can then take them to a private room which has all necessary facilities and stay with them (Figure 1.11). To be able to provide them with

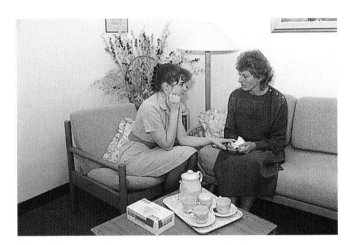

Figure 1.11 A sensitive nurse is a great asset after the news

support and information, the nurse will have to go periodically to the resuscitation room to receive an update from the team leaders. At the same time information can be given about the relatives and the patient's past medical history and current medication.

Once the primary survey has been completed, the leaders can disband the non-essential members of the team so that they can return to their normal activities in the hospital.

C-spine, chest, and pelvic x-rays can be taken at this stage, and it is crucial to note any actual or potentially life-threatening condition identified radiologically. These include unstable C-spine fracture, pneumothorax which will be made worse by ventilation, or severe pelvic fracture possibly leading to exsanguination.

Secondary survey

The objectives of this phase are listed in the box below. As with the primary survey, a well-coordinated team effort is required in which each member has a specific task. Procedures by individual team members are followed according to a precise protocol and again tasks are performed simultaneously rather than sequentially.

Objectives of the secondary survey
• Examine the whole patient to determine the full extent of the injuries
• Take a complete medical history
• Assimilate all clinical, laboratory and radiological information
• Formulate a management plan for the patient

The detailed assessment of the patient is usually carried out by the medical team leader who can call out his findings so that they can be recorded by the nursing team leader. The common error of being distracted before the whole body has been inspected must be avoided. This is because potentially serious injuries can be missed, especially in the unconscious patient. It is also important to note that should the patient deteriorate at any stage, the team leader must abandon the secondary survey and repeat the primary survey.

During the secondary survey the airway nurse must maintain verbal contact with the patient. At the same time, one of the circulation nurses should continue to measure the vital signs regularly and also take responsibility for monitoring the intravenous fluids.

Examination

Scalp

This must be examined for lacerations (Figure 1.12), swellings, or depressions. Its entire surface must be inspected but the

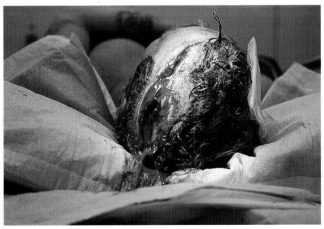

Figure 1.12 Significant scalp laceration. All scalp wounds need to be examined for bleeding points, soft tissue damage, and underlying fractures.

occiput will have to wait until the patient is turned or the cervical spine "cleared" both clinically and radiologically. Visual inspection may discover fractures in the base of lacerations. However, wounds should not be blindly probed as further damage to underlying structures can result. If there is major bleeding from the scalp, digital pressure or a self-retaining retractor should be used. It is important to remember that, in small children, scalp lacerations can bleed sufficiently to cause hypovolaemia; consequently haemostasis is crucial in these cases.

Neurological state

The medical team leader should now carry out a "mini-neurological" examination of the patient. This comprises an assessment of the conscious level (with the use of the Glasgow coma score), the pupillary response, and the presence of any lateralising signs (see Chapter 6). One of the circulation nurses should then continue to monitor these parameters. If there is any deterioration, hypoxia or hypovolaemia must be ruled out before an intracranial injury is considered.

Base of skull

Fractures to this structure will produce signs along a diagonal line demonstrated in Figure 1.13. Bruising can develop over

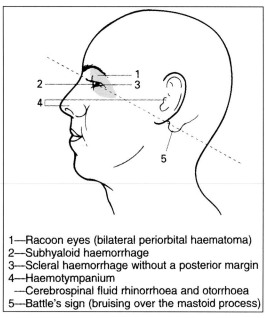

1—Racoon eyes (bilateral periorbital haematoma)
2—Subhyaloid haemorrhage
3—Scleral haemorrhage without a posterior margin
4—Haemotympanium
—Cerebrospinal fluid rhinorrhoea and otorrhoea
5—Battle's sign (bruising over the mastoid process)

Figure 1.13 Diagonal line demonstrating the level of the base of the skull.

the mastoid process (Battle's sign) but this usually takes 12–36 hours to appear (Figure 1.14). It is therefore of limited use in the resuscitation room. A cerebrospinal fluid (CSF) leak may be missed because it is invariably mixed with blood. Fortunately its presence in this bloody discharge can be detected by noting the delay in blood clotting and the double ring pattern when it is dropped onto an absorbent sheet. In this situation nothing, including an auroscope, should be inserted into the external auditory canal because of the risk of precipitating infection. As there is a small chance of a nasogastric tube passing into the cranium through the base of a skull fracture, these tubes should be passed orally when this type of injury is suspected.

Eyes

Inspection of the eyes must be carried out before significant orbital swelling makes examination too difficult. The assessor must look for haemorrhages, both inside and outside the globe, for foreign bodies under the lids (including contact lenses),

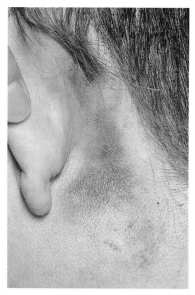

Figure 1.14 Battle's sign.

and for the presence of penetrating injuries. If the patient is conscious, the visual acuity can be tested by asking the patient to read a name badge or fluid label; if unconscious, the pupillary response and corneal reflexes are tested.

Face

This should be palpated symmetrically for deformities and tenderness. The assessor must also check for lost teeth and stability of the maxilla by pulling the latter forward to see if the middle third of the face is stable. Middle-third fractures can be associated with both an airway obstruction and base of skull fractures. However, only those injuries coexisting with an airway obstruction need to be treated immediately. Mandibular fractures can also cause airway obstruction because of the loss of stability of the tongue.

Neck

This must always be carefully examined if a cervical injury is suspected. Once the airway nurse has restored manual in-line stabilisation, the team leader can remove the sand bags, tape, and semirigid collar so that the neck can be assessed. It should be inspected for any deformity (rare), bruising, and lacerations. Each of the cervical spinous processes can then be palpated for tenderness or a "step-off" deformity. The posterior cervical muscles should also be palpated for tenderness or spasm. The conscious patient can assist in this examination by indicating if there is pain or tenderness in the neck and locating the site.

Lacerations should only be inspected and **never** be probed with metal instruments or fingers. If a laceration penetrates platysma, definitive radiological or surgical management will be needed, the choice depending upon the clinical state of the patient.

Thorax

The priority at this stage is to identify those thoracic conditions which are potentially life threatening, along with any remaining chest injuries (see Chapters 3 and 4).

The chest wall must be reinspected for bruising, signs of obstruction, asymmetry of movement, and wounds. Acceleration and deceleration forces can produce extensive thoracic injuries. However, these invariably leave marks on the chest wall which should lead the team to consider particular types of injury. For example, the diagonal seatbelt bruise may overlap a fractured clavicle, a thoracic aortic tear, pulmonary contusion, or pancreatic laceration (Figure 1.15). Good pre-hospital information is vital to determine the mechanism of injury.

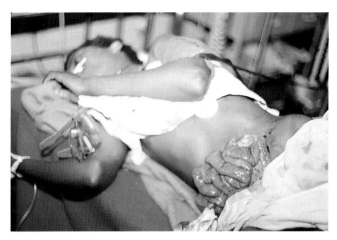

Figure 1.16 Exposed bowel needs to be covered with warm, saline soaked swabs.

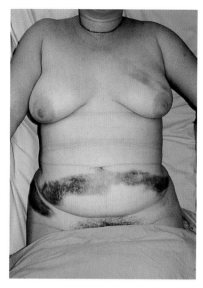

Figure 1.15 Seatbelt bruising following a road traffic accident. Bruising can take several hours to develop but abrasion in the same area should raise the possibility of underlying skeletal and visceral damage.

The clinician should palpate the sternum and then each rib, starting in the axillae and proceeding caudally and anteriorly. The presence of any crepitus, tenderness, and subcutaneous emphysema must be noted. Auscultation and percussion of the whole chest can then be carried out to determine if there is any asymmetry between the right and left sides of the chest.

Pulmonary and cardiac contusions are potentially life threatening and should be considered when the chest wall has received a significant direct blow. An example of this is the collision between a driver's thorax and a steering wheel following a road traffic accident. The intensive management that these patients require is discussed in detail in Chapter 4.

The thoracic aorta can be torn when the patient has been subjected to a rapid deceleration force, such as in a road traffic accident or a fall from a height. A high index of suspicion, along with a thorough examination and an erect chest x-ray are essential in these cases (see Chapter 4).

A ruptured diaphragm and a perforated oesophagus can follow both blunt and penetrating trauma. However, diagnosis is made usually on the appearance of the chest radiograph (see Chapter 3).

Abdomen

The objective of this part of the secondary survey is simply to determine whether the patient requires a laparotomy. A precise diagnosis of which particular viscus has been injured is both time consuming and of little relevance at this stage.

A thorough examination of the whole abdomen is required; therefore the pelvis and perineum must be assessed. All bruising, abnormal movement, and wounds must be noted and any exposed bowel covered with warm saline-soaked swabs (Figure 1.16). Lacerations should be inspected but not probed blindly as further damage can result. It is not possible to determine the actual depth of the wound if underlying muscle is penetrated; consequently these cases will require further investigations (see Chapter 11).

The abdomen needs to be palpated in a systematic manner so that areas of tenderness can be detected. Percussion is an ideal way of locating areas of tenderness without distressing the patient. The gross stability of the pelvis should then be evaluated and a rectal examination carried out. The latter provides five pieces of information:

- sphincter tone – this can be lost after spinal injuries;
- direct pelvis trauma;
- pelvic fractures;
- prostatic position – this can be disrupted after posterior urethral injury;
- blood in the lower alimentary canal.

The rate of urine output is an important indicator for assessing the shocked patient and therefore it should be measured in all trauma patients. In most cases this will require catheterisation. If there is no evidence of urethral injury, the catheter is passed transurethrally in the normal way. However, if urethral trauma is suspected (see box below), and the patient is unable to urinate, a suprapubic catheter may be necessary. The urine which is voided initially should be tested for blood and saved for microscopy and subsequent possible drug analysis.

Signs of urethral injury in a male patient
• Bruising around the scrotum
• Blood at the end of the urethral meatus
• High-riding prostate

Marked gastric distention is frequently found in crying children, adults with head or abdominal injuries and patients who have been ventilated with a bag and mask technique. The insertion of a gastric tube facilitates the abdominal examination of these patients and reduces the risks of aspiration.

An intra-abdominal bleed should be suspected if the ribs overlying the liver and spleen are fractured (numbers 5–11), the patient is haemodynamically unstable, or if there are seatbelt marks, tyre marks, or bruises over the abdominal surface. However, the detection of abdominal tenderness is unreliable if there is a sensory defect from neurological damage or drugs, or if there are fractures of the lower ribs or pelvis. In these cases, a diagnostic peritoneal lavage or ultrasound should be carried out to help rule out an intraperitoneal injury (see Chapter 11). Ideally the former should be performed by the general surgeon who will be responsible for any subsequent laparotomy.

Extremities

The limbs are examined by inspection, palpation, and then movement. All the long bones must also be rotated and, if the patient is conscious, he or she should be asked to move each limb actively.

Upon completion of the examination, the presence of any bruising, wounds, and deformities must be noted along with any crepitus, instability, neurovascular abnormalities, compartment syndrome, or soft tissue damage (Figure 1.17) (see

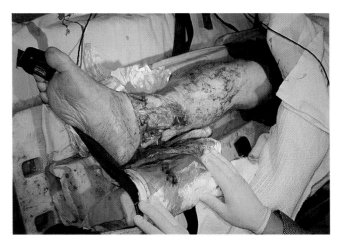

Figure 1.17 Open fracture of right tibia and fibula. There is extensive soft tissue loss and impaired perfusion of the foot.

Chapter 15). As time delays can result in tissue loss, gross limb deformities need to be corrected and the pulses and sensation rechecked before any radiographs are taken.

Any wounds associated with open fractures must be swabbed and covered with a non-adherent dressing. Different surgeons will need to examine the limb, so a Polaroid photograph of the wound before it is covered will reduce the number of times the dressings have to be removed. This is turn will lessen the chances of the wound becoming infected.

All limb fractures need splintage to reduce fracture movement and hence reduce pain, bleeding, formation of fat emboli, and secondary soft tissue swelling and damage. In the case of femoral shaft fractures, a traction splint should be used (see Chapter 14).

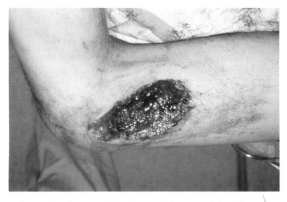

Figure 1.18 Gunshot wound to the medial aspect of the left knee. In addition to the skin loss there was significant damage to the popliteal artery and vein.

Soft tissue injuries

The whole of the patient's skin must be examined to determine the number and extent of soft tissue injuries. Each breach in the skin needs to be inspected to determine the site, depth, and the presence of any underlying structural damage that may require surgical repair during the definitive care phase (Figure 1.18). However, once the clinical state of the patient stabilises, superficial wounds can recleaned, irrigated, and dressed. A detailed description on the management of soft tissue injuries is given in Chapter 15.

Spinal column

A detailed neurological examination needs to be carried out at this stage to determine if there are any abnormalities in the peripheral nervous system. Motor and sensory defects, and in male patients the degree of priapism, can help indicate the level and extent of the spinal injury.

If the cord has been transected above the spinal origin of the sympathetic nervous system, hypotension results from peripheral vasodilatation. The degree of vasodilatation depends on how little sympathetic tone remains. A cervical transection of the cord removes all vasoconstrictor tone and thus leads to profound hypotension. However, this neurogenic shock is not associated with a tachycardia because the sympathetic innervation of the heart has been lost (see Chapter 10).

A detailed description of the diagnosis, treatment, and nursing care of this type of condition is described in Chapter 10.

Back

If a spinal injury is suspected, the patient should only be moved by a well-coordinated log-rolling technique or a vertical lift (Figure 1.19). Usually the former is used, and the patient

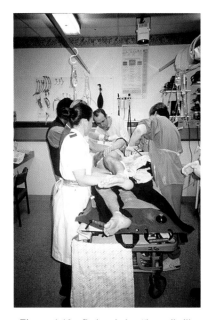

Figure 1.19 Patient being "log-rolled".

is turned away from the examiner who takes this opportunity to clear away all the debris from under the patient. The whole of the back is then assessed from occiput to heels; bruises and open wounds should be looked for. The back of the chest must be auscultated, the area between the buttocks inspected, and the vertebral column palpated for bogginess, malalignment, and deformities in contour. The examination finishes with palpation of the longitudinal spinal muscles for spasm and tenderness. The patient is then log-rolled back into the supine position.

The nursing team leader will also need to make an initial assessment of the skin using a pressure sore scoring system, for example the Waterlow system (Figure 1.20). In the elderly,

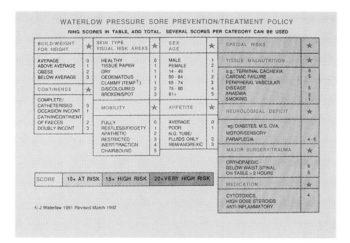

Figure 1.20 Waterlow Scoring System.

and other high-risk patients, meticulous attention to prevention of pressure sores must be paid from the outset. The patient may have spent a considerable time in one position before being rescued and, if surgery is required, may have to remain in the same position for several more hours. It is therefore important to remove the patient from the spinal board as soon as possible and to note the length of time in any one position. A designated team member should then move whatever can be moved every thirty minutes, by the use of hip lifts for example. This needs to be taken into consideration when the patient's definitive care plan is compiled.

Analgesia

Pain control is a fundamental aspect of the initial management of trauma patients. This is not only for humanitarian reasons but also because pain can reduce the tolerance of the patient to hypovolaemia [5,14]. However, analgesia can mask important clinical signs and symptoms. For example systemic analgesia can hide a fall in the level of consciousness from a rise in intracranial pressure. Furthermore in extremity injuries, systemic and regional analgesia can mask the symptoms of rising compartment pressure. It is therefore essential that the specialist teams involved in the patient's definitive care are informed so that early signs are not missed. It is also important to maintain careful monitoring of the patient's status once the analgesia has been administered.

Good communication, explanation, and gentle handling are important preliminaries to pain relief. Correct immobilisation of injured limbs can also be very effective. In addition, the team should be proficient in providing the other common types of analgesia such as Entonox, morphine, and regional analgesia [15].

Entonox

This gaseous mixture of 50% oxygen and 50% nitrous oxide, can be effective as a short-term analgesic agent, for example

during splinting, manipulation, and extraction. It is contraindicated when there is a pneumothorax or a fracture to the base of the skull.

Morphine

Morphine sulphate is a potent analgesic agent. It should be administered intravenously, in dilution with normal saline to produce a solution of 1 mg/ml. After a starting bolus (usually 5 mg for a 70 kg male), 1 mg increments can be given each minute until the patient's pain is relieved. The analgesic and respiratory depressant effect of the administered medication must be monitored continuously, particularly if it is suspected that any other drugs (including alcohol) have already been taken.

There is no place for oral or intramuscular analgesia in the trauma patient because both sites have poor perfusion. This leads to limited absorption of the drug initially and bolus absorption following resuscitation. As morphine may cause nausea and vomiting, an antiemetic such as metaclopramide should also be administered intravenously prior to the initial bolus.

Regional analgesia

This can be extremely effective if skilfully administered to the patient suffering limb trauma or specific areas of soft tissue injury. However, it must be borne in mind that regional analgesia can totally desensitise a limb and so mask the signs of rising compartment pressures. Consequently, this type of analgesia should only be administered with caution. Furthermore, the clinician must be very sensitive to any circulatory changes in the limb after the regional anaesthesia has been administered.

Radiography

All blunt trauma patients require cervical spine, chest, and pelvic radiographs in the resuscitation room. The lateral cervical spine x-ray is used to exclude 85% of the cervical abnormalities, but to do so it needs to show all seven cervical vertebrae as well as the C7–T1 junction (Figure 1.21). To facilitate this, one of the team members should pull the patient's

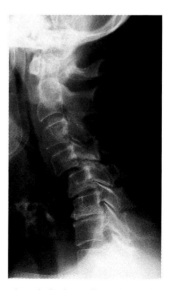

Figure 1.21 Lateral cervical spine radiograph showing all seven cervical vertebra as well as the base of the skull and the top of T1. There is a bifacet dislocation of C5 on C6.

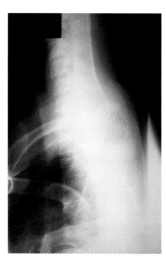

Figure 1.22 A normal swimmer's view of the cervical vertebra. Note there is no displacement of the lower cervical and upper thoracic vertebral bodies.

arms towards the feet as the radiograph is taken. A "swimmer's view" can be used if this fails to give an adequate view (Figure 1.22).

At the end of the secondary survey further radiographs will need to be taken to help identify all the skeletal and spinal abnormalities (see Chapters 10, 13 and 14). When these are carried out depends on the condition of the patient. If the patient is hypoxic or haemodynamically unstable, then these problems must be addressed first. Once the patient's condition stabilises, radiographs of particular sites of injury can be performed along with other specialised investigations. This may involve transporting the patient to specialised areas of the hospital for MRI, CT, or angiography. It is an important part of the team leaders' responsibilities to determine the priorities of these investigations. This should take into account the state of the patient, the investigations available in the hospital, and the advice from the different specialists involved in the patient's care.

Medical history

At the end of the secondary survey, the medical team leader must fully assess the patient's medical history because this can have a profound effect on what sort of definitive care is required. An AMPLE medical history is therefore needed (see box below). Part of this information will have already been acquired by the doctor from the ambulance personnel as well as from the relative's nurse.

AMPLE history
A Allergies
M Medicines (current)
P Past medical history
L Last meal (time of)
E Events leading to the incident

The most basic details necessary to evaluate a trauma patient are the time and exact mechanism of injury. The pre-injury health details should also be obtained because it can have a profound effect on the patient's outcome. In a recent survey of trauma patients attending the Emergency Department of Hope Hospital in Salford, 45% were found to have significant pre-existing medical conditions [16] (see Chapter 25). If it is not possible to obtain this information from the patient or relatives, inspection of previous hospital records or direct communication with the general practitioner will be helpful.

Assimilation of information

As the condition of the patient can change quickly, repeated examinations and constant monitoring of the vital signs are essential. The circulation nurse, responsible for recording the latter at 15 minute intervals, must be vigilant and bring any deterioration in the respiratory rate, pulse, blood pressure, conscious level, and urine output to the immediate attention of the team leaders.

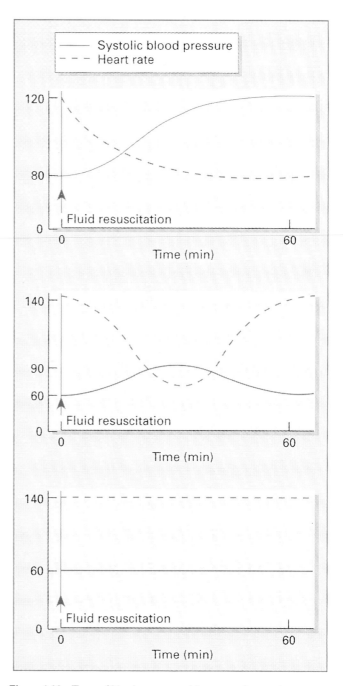

Figure 1.23 Types of blood pressure and heart rate changes that may occur following resuscitation.

By the end of the secondary survey, the answers to the following questions must be known:

● **Is the patient's respiratory function satisfactory?**
If it is not adequate then the cause must be sought and corrected as a priority (see Chapters 2 and 3).

● **Is the patient's circulatory status satisfactory?**
It is essential that the trauma team recognises shock early in its progress and intervenes aggressively. It is equally important to evaluate the patient's response to the resuscitative measures (Figure 1.23) (see chapter 5).

If there has been less than 20% of the blood volume lost, the vital signs usually return to normal after less than 2 litres of colloid (or 6 litres of crystalloid). If they then remain stable the patient is probably not actively bleeding. However, care and constant supervision is needed in these cases because these trauma victims may deteriorate later.

Transient responders are patients who are actively bleeding or recommence bleeding during the resuscitation. Therefore their vital signs initially improve but then decline. They have usually lost over 30% of their blood volume and require an infusion with typed blood. Control of the bleeding source invariably requires an operation.

In a shocked patient, the total lack of response to the infusion suggests that either the condition is not due to hypovolaemia, or the patient has lost over 40% of their blood volume and continues to bleed faster than the rate of the fluid infusion. The history, mechanism of injury, and the physical findings will help determine which is the most likely. The former needs invasive techniques in order that the pulmonary and central venous pressures can be monitored. In the case of major haemorrhage, an operation and a blood transfusion are urgently required. The source of the bleeding is usually in the chest, abdomen or pelvis.

● **What is the extent and priorities of the injuries?**
The ABC system is used to categorise injuries so that the most dangerous is treated first. For example, problems with the airway must be corrected before those of the circulation.

● **Have any injuries being overlooked?**
The mechanism of injury and the injury pattern must be considered to avoid overlooking sites of damage. It is important to remember that blunt trauma rarely "skips" areas. For example if an injury has been found in the thorax and femur, but not in the abdomen, then it may have been missed. The patient must be re-examined.

● **Are tetanus toxoid, human antitetanus immuno-globulin, or antibiotics required?**
This will depend on both local and national policies which should be known by the team leaders.

Documentation

The medical notes must be written up at the end of the resuscitation by the medical team leader. At the same time the charts, vital signs, fluid input and output information, drug administration, and preliminary nursing care documentation are all collated by the nursing team leader. A purpose-designed single trauma sheet can facilitate this process (Figure 1.24).

The relative's nurse can then brief the team leaders about the condition of any relatives or friends who are in the department on the patient's behalf. The medical team leader should accompany the nurse back to the relative's room, to talk to them. However, if this doctor has had to go urgently with the patient, another clinician, fully versed with the situation, should be sent instead.

If the patient is unconscious, clothing and belongings may provide essential information. Usually the rescue personnel will have sought the trauma victim's identity before arrival at hospital. However, whether the patient's name is known or not, some system of identification is required, not least so that drugs and blood can be administered safely. This becomes more important when there are several patients in the resuscitation room. If identity bracelets are impractical, then indelible markers can be used to write a number on the patient's skin.

Any possessions brought in with the patient must be handed over to the nursing staff by the rescue personnel. These must be kept safely, along with the patient's clothing and property. At the end of the secondary survey, or during it if there are hands to spare, all these articles must be searched. A check is needed for any medical alert card or disc, a suicide note and any medicine bottles or tablets.

Jewellery and, when appropriate, dentures, need to be removed from the patient and stored in a labelled valuables bag or envelope. This should be with the patient's permission if conscious. Rings and other constrictive jewellery must also be removed as the fingers may swell. If this is not possible, they should be cut off. At an appropriate moment, preferably by nurses outside the trauma team, the property is collected, checked, recorded, signed for, and locked away.

If a criminal case is suspected, all clothing, possessions, loose debris, bullets and shrapnel are required for forensic examination. These too must be collected, labelled, placed in waxed bags, and signed for prior to releasing them to the appropriate authorities according to established procedures.

Definitive care

Once the patient has been adequately assessed and resuscitated, definitive care can start. In many cases this will require either an operation(s) and/or intensive care management. It is therefore very important that the transition from the resuscitation room to these areas is done as smoothly as possible.

In deciding the order of treatment in this phase, the trauma team leader needs to take into account the:

● presence of any immediately life-threatening conditions;
● presence of any limb-threatening conditions;
● physiological state of the patient;
● resources of the hospital;
● likelihood of having to transfer from the hospital for further specialist care.

It is therefore essential that all the injuries are known. However, it may be that certain life- or limb-threatening conditions have to be treated before all the appropriate investigations can be carried out. For example, a large extradural haematoma will need to be drained before the patient's suspected Colles' fracture is confirmed radiologically.

As around 95% of UK trauma patients are victims of a blunt force, many have sustained multiple injuries [17]. A further consideration therefore is the logistics of carrying out several procedures and how well the patient can cope physiologically. It may be appropriate in certain cases of significant multiple injuries to carry out a staged operative procedure with the patient returning to the Intensive Care Unit between theatre sessions. This will enable the operations

BLOODS	RESULTS	BLOODS	RESULTS
☐ Hb		☐ WCC	
☐ Hct		☐ PLTS	
☐ Na		☐ BS	
☐ K		☐ Urea	
☐ BM			

	Time %O₂			
☐ ABG	pO²			
	pCO²			
	pH			
	BE			
☐ Other				

PRIMARY SURVEY

ASSESSMENT	RESUSCITATION

ASSESSMENT

☐ **AIRWAY**
- ☐ Normal   Gag Y/N
- ☐ Unconscious
- ☐ Facial fractures

CERVICAL SPINE
☐ Normal ☐ Suspect injury ☐ Firm collar ☐ In line traction

☐ **BREATHING**

RR ON ARRIVAL.................../min
- ☐ Trauma   (blunt/penetrating)
- ☐ Pneumothorax (open / closed / tension)
- ☐ Haemothorax
- ☐ Flail segment

☐ **CIRCULATION**

SYSTOLIC BP ON ARRIVAL ....mmHg
- ☐ Haemorrhage
  - ☐ External
  - ☐ Internal
    - ☐ Chest
    - ☐ Abdomen
    - ☐ Pelvis

☐ **DYSFUNCTION**

GCS ON ARRIVAL...................
- ☐ Alert
- ☐ Responds to verbal commands
- ☐ Responds to pain
- ☐ Unresponsive

  Pupils equal : Y / N

RESUSCITATION

- ☐ Spontaneous
  Mask/mask + airway _ _ _ %O²
- ☐ Ventilated   ☐ ETT - *size* _ _
- ☐ N-G tube

- ☐ Chest drain
  Left   Right
  Size _ _ _   *Size* _ _ _ _

IV (1)- *site* _ _ _ _   *Size* _ _ _ _
IV (2)- *site* _ _ _ _   *Size* _ _ _ _

Blood ordered   ☐ 0 Neg
Time _ _ hrs   ☐ Grouped
               ☐ X-match
               ☐ G + S
- ☐ Pressure dressings
- ☐ Arterial blood gases
- ☐ ECG monitor

- ☐ In line stabilisation of
  whole spine

X-RAYS   Findings
- ☐ C-spine
- ☐ CXR
- ☐ Pelvis
- ☐ SXR
- ☐ Long bones
- ☐ Spine
- ☐ C.T. scan

DRUGS	Dr. sig.	Sig. given
☐ Tet. tox. 0.5 ml	·	
☐ Humo. Tet. 250 units		
☐ Analgesics		
☐ Antibiotic		
☐ Anaesthetic drugs		

SECONDARY SURVEY
Tick pulses present

Summary of Injuries

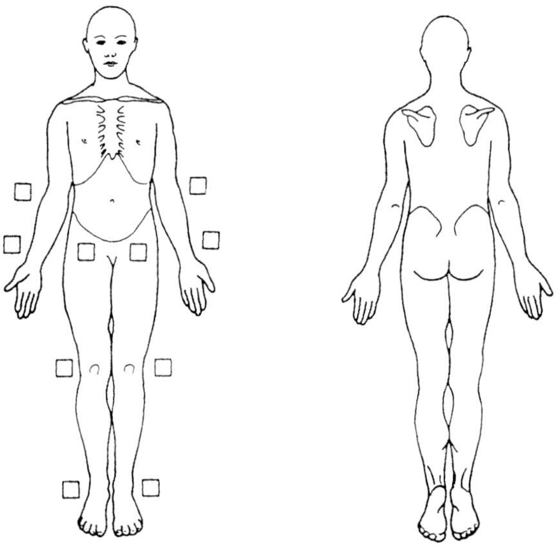

PERITONEAL LAVAGE
RBC _ _ _ _ /mm³   WBC _ _ _ /mm³
Bacteria _ _ _ Y/N   Food _ _ _ Y/N
Performed by _ _ _ _   Time _ _ _ _

USS abdo _ _ _ _ _ _ _ _ _

URINE (Cath / MSU / Other)
Blood _ _ _ _ _   Ketones _ _ _ _
Sugar _ _ _ _   Protein _ _ _ _

REFERRALS

	Grade	Time Called	Arrived
☐ Anaesthetist			
☐ Gen.surgeons			
☐ Orthopaedic			
☐ Neurosurg.			
☐ Thoracic			
☐ Plastic			
☐ Max. fac.			
☐ Other			

DISPOSAL TIME
Ward _ _ _ _ _ _ _ hrs
ITU _ _ _ _ _ _ _ hrs
Theatre _ _ _ _ _ _ hrs
CT scan _ _ _ _ _ _ hrs
Died _ _ _ _ _ _ _ hrs
Transfer _ _ _ _ _ _ hrs

Resuscitation led by :

Initially : _ _ _ _ _ _ _ _ _ _
Finally : _ _ _ _ _ _ _ _ _ _

Chart compiled by :

Name _ _ _ _   Signature _ _ _ _

Name _ _ _ _ _ **Age/D.O.B.** _ _ _ _ _
Address _ _ _ _ _ _ _ _ _ _
_ _ _ _ _ _ _ _ _ _
_ _ _ _ _ _ **A/E No:** _ _ _ _ _

Date _ _ _ _ **Time of arrival** _ _ _ _
Drugs _ _ _ _ **Allergies** _ _ _ _
PMH _ _ _ _ _ _ _ _ _ _
_ _ _ _ _ _ _ _ **Last ate** _ _ _ _

Figure 1.24 Trauma sheet.

INCIDENT DETAILS : Time
- Mechanism

- Pre-hospital care

Vital signs at scene :
BP [   ] Pulse [   ] RR [   ] GCS [   ]

NURSING DETAILS
Relatives   Name _ _ _ _ _ _ _ _ _ _ _ _ _ Phone no. _ _ _ _ _
             Address _ _ _ _ _ _ _ _ _ _ _ _ _ _ _ _ _ _ _
             _ _ _ _ _ _ _ _ _ _ _ _ _ _ _ _ _ _ Contacted Y/N
Other details

James
Driscoll
McCabe
1991

VITAL SIGNS   Hour
                                   Minute
Blood   180
pressure ↕   160
                                   140
                                   120
                                   100
                                   80
Pulse ●   60
                                   40
                                   20
                                   0
                        Respiratory rate
                        Temperature °C
             Arterial oxygen saturation (%)

Pupil
scale
(mm)

·1
●2
●3
●4
●5
●6
●7
●8

ACTIONS / EVENTS

	Hour
	Minute

PUPILS
+ Reacts
- No reaction
C Closed by swelling

	R	Size
		Reaction
	L	Size
		Reaction

	G.C.S.	
VERBAL	Orientated	5
	Confused	4
	Inappropriate words	3
	Incomprehensible sounds	2
	None	1
MOTOR	Obeys commands	6
	Localises pain	5
	Flexion to pain	4
	Decorticate movement	3
	Extension to pain	2
	None	1
EYE	Spontaneous	4
	To speech	3
	To pain	2
	None	1
	G.C.S. Total Score	

HAEMACCEL

I.V. Site 1				**I.V. Site 2**			
Time	Fluid	Vol.	Given	Time	Fluid	Vol.	Given

Total input IV site 1= [   ] ml   Total input IV site 2 = [   ] ml

TOTAL IV INPUT [=] [   ] ml

URINE OUTPUT		**OTHER LOSSES**	
Catheter / voided		Specify : _ _ _ _ _ _ _ _	
Time	Vol.	Time	Vol.

TOTAL URINE OUTPUT	**TOTAL OTHER LOSSES**
[=] [ ] ml	[=] [ ] ml

Department of Medical Illustration, S.H.A. H91071270

Figure 1.24 Trauma sheet (continued).

to be carried out when the patient is in the optimal physiological state.

Finally the team leader should consider if there is any advantage in carrying out certain treatments in patients who require transfer to another hospital for some of their injuries. For example, it would be essential that a haemodynamically unstable head-injured patient is not transferred to a Neurosurgical Centre until the source of bleeding is identified and treated.

Deciding on the optimum definitive care plan therefore requires accurate information on the patient's injuries and physiological state, clinical experience, and a good liaison with all the specialists involved in the patient's care.

Preparation for transfer of the patient

Communication

To facilitate a smooth transfer, it is important to ensure that the receiving facility and personnel have been contacted directly by the medical team leader. If an interhospital transfer is envisaged, the clinicians must also decide on the most suitable method of transportation and how the patient should be prepared for the journey. For example, it is difficult to subdue patients in the confined space of an aircraft. Therefore, if air transport is required, and the patient is confused or aggressive, the use of restraints (physical or pharmacological) should be considered prior to leaving.

Assessment

All aspects of the primary survey must be reassessed before the patient leaves and appropriate adjustments made. For example, the patient who tolerates an oropharyngeal airway should be intubated and ventilated so that the airway can be protected, and hypoxia and hypercarbia prevented. All cannulae, catheters, tubes, and drains must be secured.

Monitoring

Monitoring during the transfer period must be continued to ensure that ventilation and tissue perfusion are adequate. If a parameter needs to be monitored before transfer, it also needs to be monitored during transfer. Consequently a fully charged ECG monitor, automatic BP recorder, end-tidal CO_2 monitor, and pulse oximeter are essential.

Equipment and drugs

The trolley carrying the patient during transfer must also transport the suction system, oxygen supply, ventilator, portable blood pressure monitor, and defibrillator monitor. Airway adjuncts, needles, and drugs are usually carried separately by one of the medical team.

It is important to remember that portable ventilators use their gas supply as the power source. Therefore, an adequate amount of oxygen must be taken.

Transfer personnel

During transit, the patient needs to be accompanied by appropriately trained staff to enable them to monitor and intervene with any ventilatory or perfusion problems. If intubation equipment is involved, the most suitable personnel are the airway nurse and doctor.

Records

All the medical and nursing notes, radiographs, blood tests, identifying labels, and, if necessary, consent forms must be taken with the patient.

Relatives and friends

The nurse dealing with these people must inform them about the transfer. When the trauma victim is to be moved to another hospital, this nurse should also help the friends and relatives in their own transportation arrangements.

Final check

Before moving off, the team must ensure that the patient is appropriately covered and, for intra-hospital transfers, the lift, if needed, has been reserved.

Upon arrival

The transfer team must hand over to the doctor and nurse who will be in charge of the patient's definitive care. In this way important events during transfer, as well as a summary of the initial resuscitation, can be given to the personnel directly responsible for the patient. All documentation can be handed over at this stage and the transfer equipment retrieved.

Summary

In order to give the most efficient resuscitation, a group of doctors and nurses must be ready to meet the patient on arrival in the resuscitation room. These people must be coordinated by medical and nursing team leaders so that they are all aware of the tasks that they have to perform, and that these are carried out simultaneously.

The first priority is to detect and treat all the immediately life-threatening conditions. Following this, a detailed head-to-toe assessment can be completed. The team leaders can then list the patient's injuries and their priorities for both further investigations and definitive treatment.

References

1. Driscoll P, Monsell F, Duane L, Wardle T, Brown T. Optimal long bone fracture management. Part II – Initial resuscitation and assessment in the accident and emergency department. *Int J Orthopaed Trauma* 1995;**5**:110–17.
2. Driscoll P, Vincent C. Organising an efficient trauma team. *Injury* 1992;**23**:107–10.
3. Driscoll P, Vincent C. Variation in trauma resuscitation and its effect on patient outcome. *Injury* 1992;**23**:111–15.
4. Walker J, Driscoll P. Trauma team protection from infective contamination, in (Driscoll P, Gwinnutt C, Jimmerson C, Goodall O, eds) *Trauma resuscitation: the team approach*. London: Macmillan Press Ltd, 1993.
5. Rady M, Little R, Edwards D, Kirkman E, Faithfull S. The effect of nocicepetive stimulation on the changes in haemodynamics and oxygen transport induced by haemorrhage in anaesthetised pigs. *J Trauma* 1991;**31**:617–21.
6. Driscoll P. Changes in systolic blood pressure, heart rate, shock index, rate pressure product and tympanic temperature following

blood loss and tissue damage in humans. Leeds University, MD Thesis, 1994.

7. Little R, Kirkman E, Driscoll P, Hanson J, Mackway-Jones K. Preventable deaths after injury: why are the traditional "vital" signs poor indicators of blood loss. *J Accid Emerg Med* 1995;**12**:1–14.

8. Scalea T, Simon H, Duncan A *et al.* Geriatric blunt multiple trauma: Increased survival with early invasive monitoring. *J Trauma* 1990;**30**:129–34.

9. Burri C, Henkemeyer H, Passler H, Allogower M. Evaluation of acute blood loss by means of simple haemodynamic parameters. *Prog Surg* 1973;**11**:109–27.

10. Owens T, Watson W, Prough D, Kramer G. Limiting initial resuscitation of uncontrolled hemorrhage reduces internal bleeding and subsequent volume requirements. *J Trauma* 1995;**39**:200–9.

11. Bickell W, Wail M, Pepe P *et al.* A comparison of immediate versus delayed fluid resuscitation for hypotensive patients with penetrating torso injury. *N Eng J Med* 1994;**331**:1105–9.

12. Kaweski S, Sise M, Virgillo R. The effect of prehospital fluids on survival in trauma patients. *J Trauma* 1990;**30**:1215–18.

13. Krausz M, Bar-Ziv M, Rabinovich R *et al.* "Scoop and run" or stabilize hemorrhagic shock with normal saline or small-volume hypertonic saline? *J Trauma* 1992;**23**:6–10.

14. Kirkman E, Little R. Cardiovascular regulation during hypovolaemic shock: central integration, in (Secher N, Pawelczyk J, Ludbrook L eds) *The bradycardic phase in hypovolaemic shock.* London: Edward Arnold, 1994.

15. Driscoll P, Gwinnutt C, Nancarrow J. Analgesia in the emergency department. *Pain Rev* 1995;**2**:187–202.

16. Wardle T, Driscoll P, Oxbey C, Woodford M, Campbell F. Pre-existing medical conditions in trauma patients. *40th Ann Proc Ass Advanc Automotive Med* 1996;**40**:351–61.

17. Anderson I, Woodford M, Irving M. Preventability of death from penetrating injury in England and Wales. *Injury* 1989;**20**:69–71.

2 Management of the upper airway

Carl L. Gwinnutt
Consultant Anaesthetist, Hope Hospital, Salford

Anthony McCluskey
Consultant in Anaesthesia and Intensive Care, Stepping Hill Hospital, Stockport

OBJECTIVES

■ Understand the importance of continuing care of the airway.

■ Identify those patients who need tracheal intubation and how this may be facilitated.

■ Recognise the potential problems associated with the airway during transfer and in the operating theatre.

■ Understand the techniques of airway maintenance in patients on the Intensive Care Unit and the associated problems.

To manage victims of trauma successfully, one must treat the greatest threat to life first. Asphyxia from an obstructed airway will cause death faster than ventilatory insufficiency attributable to thoracic injuries. Both will cause death faster than exsanguination or an expanding intracranial haematoma. Therefore during initial resuscitation, it is the airway which commands first priority; the A of ABC.

On leaving the resuscitation room, the perception of the patient's needs often change. Patients are transferred around the hospital for investigations, to the operating theatre for surgery or direct to the ICU. Others may need transfer to another institution for definitive care. Some patients will by now be maintaining their own airway, while others will have been intubated for a variety of reasons. It is at this stage that the airway is often neglected, and yet should it become compromised, patients will suffer irreparable damage or death just as quickly as they would have done during their initial management.

At all times during the care of a patient leaving the resuscitation room, the airway retains its place of primary importance.

Assessment

Care of the non-intubated patient

Many trauma patients will leave the resuscitation room able to maintain their own airway. Although a secondary survey should have been performed to detect potential problems, occasionally this will not have been possible, for example because of the need for surgery. In such circumstances, airway deterioration may occur extremely insidiously and a quick assessment is mandatory before leaving the Resuscitation Room so that potential airway problems can be identified.

Examine the face and mouth

● Look at the facial hair and lips for any evidence of thermal injury.
● Inspect the tongue and mucous membranes for swelling or haematoma.
● Check for any continuing bleeding especially if the patient is supine.
● Identify the whereabouts of missing or broken teeth and the security of any loose ones.

Examine the neck

● Check the position of the trachea, particularly if a chest drain has been inserted.
● Note any bruises, swelling or wounds, and consider potential damage to underlying structures.
● Palpate the larynx for crepitus which indicates the possibility of a fracture.
● Watch during respiration for any tracheal tug or indrawing of the supraclavicular spaces.

Count the respiratory rate, during quiet breathing and speech

● Rates greater than 30 per minute may indicate increasing difficulty.
● Inspiratory stridor suggests supraglottic obstruction, expiratory stridor suggests bronchial obstruction.
● Note the quality of the patient's voice, the presence of hoarseness, and the number of words between breaths.
● Ask about dysphagia – it may be the only indication of swelling in the hypopharynx.

When this check has been satisfactorily completed and no evidence of airway compromise found, these patients should be transferred to their destination accompanied both by someone able to intervene and with the appropriate equipment. At a minimum this must consist of oro- and nasopharyngeal airways, a bag-valve-mask device, oxygen and suction. Monitoring of the patient will be dictated by their physical status, with perhaps the single most useful device being a pulse oximeter.

The decision to intubate

Under certain circumstances, it may be considered safer to intubate a patient before leaving the resuscitation room, even though an airway is being maintained and there appears to be no immediate threat to its patency or security. When the decision has been taken to intubate the patient, this is best performed by an experienced anaesthetist.

The commonest indications for this elective form of intubation are:

- Where there is a threat to the continuing patency of the airway, for example, following inhalation of hot or toxic gases that may cause the mucosa to swell, or as a result of compression from a haematoma developing in the neck.
- Where there is a threat to the security of the airway, for example, the head-injured patient with a reduced level of consciousness, who is tolerating an oral airway. This usually indicates the absence of the gag reflex predisposing to aspiration of any regurgitated gastric contents.
- Inadequate ventilation from exhaustion, as a result of the increased work of breathing caused by a flail chest, severe pulmonary contusion, or occasionally a coexisting medical problem, for example asthma.

The need for intubation in these circumstances will be amplified when:

- The patient faces a prolonged transfer to another centre for treatment.
- Access to the patient at any time is difficult, which prevents intervention in the case of deterioration, for example during helicopter transfer.
- Monitoring of the patient's condition is difficult, the classical example being during some modern radiological investigations.

The most common route for intubation in these situations is orotracheal, and it is usually accomplished with the assistance of drugs.

Management

Drugs

Drugs are administered to facilitate tracheal intubation and subsequently to ensure that the patient tolerates the presence of the tube and mechanical ventilation. This is achieved by rendering the patient unconscious and abolishing muscle activity using combinations of the following groups of drugs (Table 2.1):

- intravenous anaesthetic agents, sometimes referred to as hypnotics;
- opioid analgesics;
- muscle relaxants.

Table 2.1 Commonly used anaesthetic drugs

	Concentration	Bolus	Dose Infusion
Anaesthetic agents			
Etomidate	2 mg/ml	0.2–0.3 mg/kg	NOT USED
Thiopentone	25 mg/ml	2–7 mg/kg	NOT USED
Propofol	10 mg/ml	1.5–2.5 mg/kg	4–10 mg/kg/h
Midazolam	2 ml/ml	0.07–0.3 mg/kg	5–15 mg/h
Analgesics			
Morphine	Variable	0.1–0.15 mg/kg	5–15 mg/h
Fentanyl	50 µg/ml	1–3 µg/kg	1.5–5.0 µg/kg/h
Alfentanil	0.5 mg/ml	10 µg/kg	0.5–2 µg/kg/min
Alfentanil	5 mg/ml	NOT USED	
Muscle relaxants			
Suxamethonium	50 mg/ml	1.5 mg/kg	NOT USED
Atracurium	10 mg/ml	0.5–0.6 mg/kg	0.5 mg/kg/h

It is essential that hypovolaemia is corrected before the use of anaesthetic drugs. They all reduce myocardial contractility and cause vasodilatation in varying degrees leading to hypotension which is exacerbated by hypovolaemia.

Intravenous anaesthetic agents

Intravenous anaesthetic agents cause loss of consciousness in little more time than it takes to reach the brain from the site of injection. Generally, consciousness is regained a few minutes after administration unless further doses or an infusion is given. Of the drugs described, only propofol and midazolam are currently used in this way. The following is intended as a guide to the pharmacology of the drugs used. The dosages represent the range normally used; however, smaller doses will be required in the elderly and those in whom there is any degree of hypovolaemia.

Etomidate

This comes as a clear, 0.2% solution (20 mg in 10 ml). After 0.2–0.3 mg/kg (7.5–10 ml), consciousness is lost after 30–45 s and lasts for 4–8 min. Etomidate is considered by many to be the drug of choice in trauma patients as it is associated with the greatest degree of cardiovascular stability, thereby helping to maintain perfusion of vital organs. It also reduces cerebral oxygen requirements and cerebral blood flow, which helps control intracranial pressure. It does not cause histamine release and therefore allergic reactions are rare. It causes pain on injection, hiccoughs, and a high incidence of involuntary movement. It is not used repeatedly or by infusion as it causes suppression of the adrenocortical axis.

Thiopentone

This is a yellow powder which is dissolved in water to make a 2.5% solution (500 mg in 20 ml). The dose required is usually 2–7 mg/kg (6–20 ml) and consciousness is lost in 15–30 s lasting for 4–10 min. Extreme care has to be taken when thiopentone is used in trauma patients, the elderly, and frail, because of its marked depressant effect on the cardiovascular system and propensity to cause hypotension. In these circumstances, a dose as low as 0.5–1 mg/kg may be sufficient.

Apnoea lasting 20–30 s is common after administration. Thiopentone is generally regarded as the drug of choice for use in patients with isolated head injuries as it reduces intracranial pressure by the same mechanism as etomidate and it has marked anticonvulsant activity. Accumulation occurs with repeated doses which delays recovery.

Propofol

This is an emulsion (hence its white colour) of 1% (200 mg in 20 ml). The dose is 1.5–2.5 mg/kg (10–20 ml) and consciousness is lost in 30–40 s although the point at which this occurs is less clear than with the above agents. It lasts for 4–7 min after which there is rapid and full recovery. The main problem is that propofol can cause profound hypotension, particularly in the presence of any hypovolaemia, as a result of vasodilatation. It must therefore be used with extreme caution (if at all) in such patients. Apnoea is common, often for up to 60 s. It is occasionally painful on injection. The great advantage of propofol is that it is non-cumulative and can be used either by intermittent bolus doses or as a constant infusion to maintain unconsciousness *once resuscitation is complete*. Hence it is very popular for maintaining sedation in intubated patients over long periods on the ICU. The rate of infusion will vary depending upon the degree of sedation required but is usually in the range 4–10 mg/kg/h.

Midazolam

This is not a true intravenous anaesthetic agent, as it has a much slower onset. It is a water-soluble, short-acting benzodiazepine which comes as a 0.2% solution (10 mg in 5 ml). The dose required is usually 0.07–0.3 mg/kg. Consciousness is lost slowly over 40–60 s and lasts 10–15 min with a longer period of amnesia. Cardiovascular stability is relatively good. It is frequently used in intermittent doses (2–5 mg) to help maintain unconsciousness for short periods. Accumulation can occur if it is used by infusion over several days, leading to a delay in recovery when it is stopped.

Opioid analgesics

This is the term used to describe all drugs which have an analgesic effect mediated via the opioid receptors and includes both natural and synthetic compounds.

Morphine

The most versatile of all the opioids, morphine is most effective in the acute situation when it is administered intravenously. It is an effective analgesic against both visceral pain and the pain of trauma. In addition it has anxiolytic and sedative properties which make it useful in intubated patients. An initial dose of 0.1–0.15 mg/kg is titrated intravenously, and an effect is usually seen within 3–4 min, with further doses given as required. Over long periods it is more usual to use an infusion of 5–15 mg/h. Occasionally hypotension occurs as a result of vasodilatation secondary to histamine release. Nausea, vomiting, and delayed gastric emptying are side effects of all the opioids. Respiratory depression also occurs which, although it can be a problem in patients who are breathing spontaneously, is used to advantage in those being mechanically ventilated.

Fentanyl

This is a synthetic analgesic, 80–100 times as potent as morphine, but a single dose only lasts 20–40 min. It is similar in action to morphine, but more rapid in onset and with a greater degree of cardiovascular stability. It is administered as boluses of 1–3 µg/kg or as an infusion of 1.5–5 µg/mg/h for longer periods. Accumulation can occur in critically ill patients after prolonged infusions.

Alfentanil

This is a synthetic analgesic, related to fentanyl, but only one-fifth as potent. It has a very rapid onset of less than 1 min, and a bolus of 10 µg/kg lasts for 10–15 min. Marked respiratory depression can occur even with this small dose but it is cardiovascular stable. It is non-cumulative and therefore alfentanil is popular for use as an infusion at a rate of 0.5–2 µg/kg/min.

Muscle relaxants (neuromuscular blocking drugs)

These are administered to facilitate laryngoscopy and intubation by abolishing muscle tone and laryngeal reflexes. Once these drugs have been given, the patient will become apnoeic, thereby committing the anaesthetist to maintaining ventilation and intubation to protect against regurgitation and aspiration of gastric contents. Relaxants are divided into two groups based upon their pharmacological action.

Depolarizing relaxants: suxamethonium

This is the only drug used in this group. It comes in 2 ml ampoules (50 mg/ml). A bolus of 1.5 mg/kg is given intravenously which causes generalised twitching (fasciculation) followed by profound relaxation after 30–45 s, lasting for 3–5 min. Recovery occurs spontaneously as it is metabolised by plasma cholinesterase. Suxamethonium is the muscle relaxant of choice in an emergency as it has the most rapid onset of action. However, there are a number of potential problems associated with its use:

- Repeated doses cause vagal stimulation and severe bradycardia. Atropine must always be available and administered prior to a second dose.
- It may provoke a rise in the intraocular pressure resulting in the loss of vitreous in penetrating eye injuries.
- It is the commonest trigger of malignant hyperpyrexia. This is a rare disorder of muscle metabolism which causes a rapid rise in body temperature (> 2° C per hour).
- It may cause prolonged apnoea in patients who are plasma cholinesterase deficient.
- It may cause hyperkalaemia when administered after major crush injuries, burns > 24 h old, massive denervation injury, and pre-existing muscle dystrophies.
- It needs to be stored in the fridge to prevent breakdown.

Non-depolarizing relaxants: atracurium

A large number of drugs are available in this group but it is the authors' preference to use atracurium. It is available in 2.5 ml and 5 ml ampoules containing 10 mg/ml (25 mg and 50 mg respectively). In order to produce relaxation sufficient for intubation, 0.5–0.6 mg/kg needs to be given intravenously. This takes 90–120 s to be fully effective and subsequently lasts for 30–40 min. Smaller doses take progressively longer and last for a shorter period of time. Atracurium has no direct cardiovascular effects but occasionally cutaneous histamine release can cause mild hypotension. It is stored in the fridge as it undergoes very slow spontaneous degradation when exposed to room temperature for long periods. Its main use is for the maintenance of relaxation following the use of suxamethonium, or for use in those circumstances where suxamethonium is contraindicated. Atracurium is widely used as it does not have to be reconstituted and is non-cumulative. Intermittent doses of 0.1–0.2 mg/kg can be used to maintain relaxation but more commonly an infusion of approximately 0.5 mg/kg/h is used.

The rate of an infusion or the need for intermittent doses of a non-depolarising relaxant can be determined by monitoring the motor response following percutaneous stimulation of a peripheral nerve. This is most commonly achieved clinically by stimulating the ulnar nerve at the wrist with 55–60 mA with four stimuli at a frequency of 2 Hz and observing the response of the adductor pollicis muscle (the "train-of-four" response). The strength followed by the number of twitches declines with increasing intensity of neuromuscular block. The aim is usually to adjust the dose of relaxant to abolish all but one of the twitches to a train-of-four stimuli.

Reversal of neuromuscular block

At some point it may become necessary to reverse the effects of a non-depolarising muscle relaxant, either because the danger to the patency or safety of the airway has passed or an assessment of neurological function is necessary. Although the effects of these drugs do wear off spontaneously, they do so slowly over a prolonged period. Recovery can be accelerated by the administration of an anticholinesterase. This blocks the action of acetylcholinesterase, responsible for the breakdown of acetylcholine at cholinergic synapses. Increasing the concentration of acetylcholine restores normal neuromuscular function. In addition to an action at the neuromuscular junction, anticholinesterases function at parasympathetic nerve endings where they cause bradycardia, spasm of the bowel and bladder, and increase in bronchial secretions. Therefore, they must always be administered with a suitable dose of either atropine or glycopyrrolate.

The speed at which an anticholinesterase reverses the muscle relaxant will depend upon the intensity of the neuromuscular block when administered: the more intense the block, the slower the reversal. They will not reverse a very intense block, that is if it is given soon after a dose of muscle relaxant or when there is no response to a train-of-four stimuli.

Neostigmine is the commonest anticholinesterase used. A fixed dose of 2.5 mg i.v. is used in adults, and has a maximal effect in 5 min, lasting 20–30 min. It is administered with either 1.2 mg atropine or 0.5 mg glycopyrrolate.

Tracheal intubation

Strictly speaking, only a muscle relaxant need be administered to facilitate intubation, as this will abolish laryngeal reflexes, prevent any resistance by the patient, and allow the tube to be placed in the trachea! However, an anaesthetic agent is administered initially as intubation in a conscious, paralysed patient would not only be extremely unpleasant but potentially harmful as a result of local tissue trauma, reflex tachycardia, hypertension, and rise in intracranial pressure. The technique used is as follows.

Rapid sequence induction

Following trauma, gastric emptying is delayed and therefore all patients must be assumed to have a full stomach. If an intravenous anaesthetic and muscle relaxant are administered, there is a risk of regurgitation of the gastric contents coincident with loss of the protective laryngeal reflex; this places the patient in danger of pulmonary aspiration. Appropriate steps must therefore be taken to minimise these risks. In the following description it is assumed that an injury to the cervical spine has been excluded, the patient is on a tipping trolley, has intravenous access established, and is being monitored accordingly.

Where possible a naso- or orogastric tube is passed and used to remove any liquid contents from the stomach. All equipment needed for intubation is checked for availability and function, and the appropriate drugs drawn up into labelled syringes. Suction is switched on and placed at the patient's head. While this is happening, the patient breaths high flow oxygen via a well-fitting facemask for 2 min (pre-oxygenation). An assistant will be required to apply cricoid pressure and a check must be made to ensure that where and how to apply it is understood (see below).

The patient should be warned that they may first feel dizzy followed by a sensation of gentle pressure on the front of their neck and then they will "fall asleep". The chosen anaesthetic agent is then injected into a fast-running infusion, followed by the suxamethonium. As the patient loses consciousness (judged by loss of the eyelash reflex), cricoid pressure is applied. The oxygen mask is now held over the patient's face until the fasciculations cease, (usually 30–40 s) at which point relaxation is maximal. Laryngoscopy is now performed, the tracheal tube passed into the trachea, the cuff inflated, and the lungs ventilated, while the chest is auscultated in both axillae for breath sounds. If this is positive, cricoid pressure can be released and the tube secured. An alternative check for correct placement is measurement of the carbon dioxide concentration in expired gas; this should be greater than 2%.

Cricoid pressure (Sellick's manoeuvre)

The cricoid cartilage is the only complete ring of cartilage in the airway, and when pressure is applied to it anteriorly, it compresses the oesophagus against the body of the sixth cervical vertebra. This occludes the oesophageal lumen, preventing regurgitation, and reduces the amount of oxygen entering the stomach, should manual ventilation become necessary during the attempt to intubate. Pressure should be applied directly in the midline by an assistant, who uses the tips of the thumb and index finger. If pressure is applied incorrectly, the larynx can be displaced, making intubation more difficult. Cricoid pressure is effective in the presence of a gastric tube, but if the patient starts to vomit, it should be released to prevent the risk of oesophageal rupture from the high intraluminal pressure. Depending upon the circumstances the patient must be placed in a position to reduce the risk of aspiration, head down and lateral if possible, and the airway cleared of vomit with suction.

If the patient has a suspected or proven injury to the cervical spine, and orotracheal intubation is to be performed, it may be necessary to remove temporarily the immobilising device, for example the collar, to facilitate laryngoscopy and allow application of cricoid pressure. In such cases, manual immobilisation by a third person must be used to keep the head and neck in a neutral position. The person applying cricoid pressure may also place the other hand beneath the

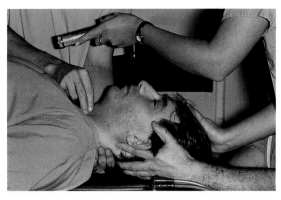

Figure 2.1 Rapid sequence induction. Note the application of cricoid pressure with counter pressure, while a further assistant immobilises the cervical spine.

cervical spine and apply gentle counterpressure (Figure 2.1). An alternative technique can be used to achieve intubation in these circumstances if there is any suggestion that intubation may be difficult (see below).

The use of intravenous anaesthetic drugs in not an appropriate technique in all patients, particularly where there is evidence of potential difficulty in maintaining the airway or performing intubation. This is often suggested by the presence of:

- any pre-existing conditions, for example a short immobile neck, receding mandible, limited mouth opening, protruding or unhealthy teeth, a large tongue;
- specific injuries, in particular to the cervical spine, limiting movement;
- evidence of airway obstruction, for example after severe facial trauma or burns to the airway;
- stridor at rest.

The administration of an intravenous anaesthetic and muscle relaxant, renders the patient apnoeic and totally dependent upon the physician to maintain and secure the airway and provide ventilation. Should this prove difficult or impossible, then the patient will become hypoxaemic, forcing the creation of cricothyroidotomy under less than ideal circumstances. Therefore, when any of the above conditions are present, there are two commonly used alternative techniques. Both require the skill of an experienced anaesthetist.

- Unconsciousness, muscle relaxation and abolition of reflexes is induced by an inhalational agent, frequently halothane in oxygen, with the use of the patient's own spontaneous ventilation. The inspired concentration is increased slowly while spontaneous ventilation is maintained. After several minutes of breathing 3–5% halothane, the patient can undergo laryngoscopy so that the airway can be assessed and intubation performed. If the larynx is visible, then either a tracheal tube is passed or a muscle relaxant administered, in the knowledge that intubation will be possible. The main disadvantages of this technique are that the inhalational agents cause dose-dependent myocardial depression and hypotension, and therefore they must only be used in patients who are fully resuscitated and stable. There may also be difficulty in some patients breathing an adequate concentration of anaesthetic to abolish laryngeal reflexes because of the respiratory depressant effect.
- The alternative is to keep the patient awake, anaesthetise the upper airway with local anaesthetic and perform direct laryngoscopy. This allows assessment of the upper airway and the larynx. If the larynx is visible, the patient can either

be rendered unconscious and a relaxant given, in the knowledge that intubation is possible, or the larynx can be anaesthetised and the tube inserted while the patient is awake. Alternatively, following anaesthesia of the airway, a fibreoptic bronchoscope can be passed and used as an introducer over which a tracheal tube can be passed into the larynx. This technique may have to be used if the larynx cannot be visualised directly. It also has the advantage of allowing visual confirmation that the tube is correctly positioned.

In the trauma patient, whenever there is difficulty anticipated with intubation, the physician must either have the skill and facilities for performing a cricothyroidotomy, or someone else who can perform the task must be immediately available.

The surgical airway

During the primary survey, as a result of all other attempts to secure the airway and achieve ventilation failing, it may have been necessary to create a surgical airway either by the insertion of a large-bore cannula or small tracheostomy tube through the cricothyroid membrane.

Needle cricothyroidotomy

This is only a temporary measure, allowing insufflation of oxygen through a 14 G (2 mm) cannula to prevent life-threatening hypoxaemia for 20–30 min. Therefore arrangements must be made urgently for the creation of a definitive airway before the patient leaves the resuscitation room, because of the time limitation and risk of the technique failing from the cannula becoming kinked or dislodged. Orotracheal intubation can be attempted by an experienced anaesthetist but if this fails, a cricothyroidotomy must be performed and a small diameter tracheostomy tube inserted (see below). At this stage, an emergency tracheostomy is not recommended because of the much greater incidence of complications and because it takes longer to perform than a cricothyroidotomy.

Surgical cricothyroidotomy

The insertion of a 4–6 mm tracheostomy tube through the cricothyroid membrane allows effective ventilation of the patient with either a self-inflating bag and valve or a mechanical ventilator. This technique allows oxygenation, elimination of carbon dioxide, and bronchial toilet to be carried out (with an appropriately sized catheter). Such an airway is satisfactory for up to 48 h, following which, if an airway is still necessary, it must be replaced.

The upper airway should first be inspected by direct laryngoscopy and the feasibility of tracheal intubation assessed. If this is not possible or undesirable, then arrangements should be made for a formal tracheostomy to be created by an ENT surgeon so that the trachea can be inspected for any potential damage caused during the establishment of the surgical airway.

Management of the airway during transfer

It has long been recognised that the transport of critically ill patients both around and between hospitals is hazardous and can cause a significant deterioration in their condition. Therefore it must be conducted in a careful and controlled manner by persons trained in the technique. The most vulnerable areas during any transfer are patients' airway and breathing, particularly if they have been intubated and are being mechanically ventilated.

Security of the tracheal tube

Unfortunately there is no guaranteed way of securing a tracheal tube. Whichever technique is used, the aim is to prevent the tube being accidentally removed or being inserted further than desired. The commonest method of securing the tube is to use a length of tape or bandage passed around the patient's neck and tied around the tube. The main problem with this method is that once the tape becomes wet with saliva or blood, the tube can slip through the tapes. Attempts to tighten the tapes around the patient's neck may simply apply pressure to the soft tissues and obstruct venous return from the head, causing an increase in the intracranial pressure. Furthermore the tape must not be tied to the 15 mm connector inserted into the end of the tube, as this can be pulled out and the tube is lost into the larynx or trachea.

An alternative is to use a length of adhesive tape ("Sleek"), wrapped around the tube and applied to the patient's face. Clearly this cannot be done if there is trauma or burns to the face, or if for some reason the tape will not adhere to the skin (Figure 2.2).

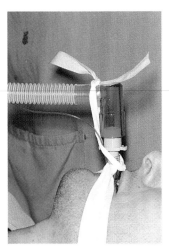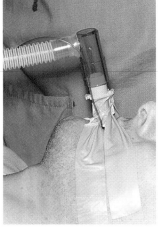

Figure 2.2 Methods of securing tracheal tubes. (a) Non-elastic tape, securely fastened to the tracheal and ventilator tubing, not the 15 mm connector. (b) Sleek applied around the tube and to the patient's face. A useful method in patients with head injuries.

Despite the best efforts, tracheal tubes "fall out". This is often due to the weight of the ventilator tubes attached to them or the use of excessively long ventilator tubing, which can cause it to be caught accidentally. Therefore, security of the tracheal tube can be improved by the use of appropriate lengths of lightweight ventilator tubing and ensuring it is adequately secured.

If a tracheostomy tube is in place, then this must be secured to prevent it becoming dislodged. This is best achieved by using cotton tapes which are tied with knots to the flanges on the tube, passed around the patient's neck and tied together, again with knots, not bows. In addition to this, some surgeons advocate suturing the flanges to the skin of the neck. Such measures are essential if the reason for the tracheostomy was failure to intubate the patient! Similar considerations apply to

the presence of a tracheostomy tube inserted through the cricothyroid membrane (Figure 2.3).

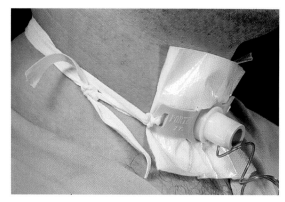
(a)

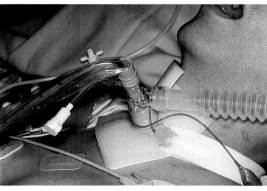
(b)

Figure 2.3 Methods of securing a tracheostomy tube. (a) Cotton tapes secured with knots. Compare with (b) on the ICU where Velcro fastenings are used.

Equipment

Because of the risk of accidental extubation of both an oro-tracheal tube or tracheostomy tube during transfer, the intubated patient must always be moved with equipment to allow reintubation (see box, page 31). This must be checked for completeness and function before departure. The most commonly ignored device is suction, which is already less than ideal, as portable units are generally inferior to the ones operated via the piped vacuum system.

In view of the absolute dependency of an intubated and ventilated patient on a whole variety of equipment, appropriate monitoring devices are required. Fortunately nowadays, most are available in battery-operated forms. However, they do not replace the need for careful clinical assessment of the patient. The extent of monitoring the airway and breathing in these patients will depend upon what is available, but pulse oximetry, end-tidal carbon dioxide, airway pressure, and a disconnect alarm should be regarded as a minimum (Figure 2.4). In some circumstances, constant infusions of drugs are used and therefore battery-operated syringe pumps which are fully charged will be required.

Drugs

The presence of a tracheal tube can be extremely distressing to a patient while being moved about and may cause hypertension and a tachycardia. In addition, coughing and breath-holding can impair ventilation. Consequently, a combination

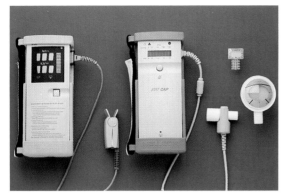
(a)

(b)

Figure 2.4 Equipment for transfer. (a) Pulse oximeter and infrared and chemical carbon dioxide analysers. (b) VentiPAC 5 portable ventilator with pressure gauge and disconnect alarm.

of an intravenous anaesthetic agent and opioid analgesic are given to overcome these problems.

Non-depolarising muscle relaxants are also used to facilitate ventilation, at the same time to reduce the risk of the patient extubating himself. However, it must be remembered that when these drugs are used, the patient is totally dependent on the ventilator and if failure goes unrecognised patients are rendered apnoeic and hypoxic. Hence the need for a disconnect alarm.

The temptation to just "draw up a couple of syringefuls" of the various drugs needed should be resisted, and ampoules of drugs must be taken, carried in crush-resistant containers, along with sterile needles and syringes. A "sharps" bin must be available for safe disposal of needles or ampoules.

Ventilation

Because of the additional work of breathing through a tracheal tube, most intubated patients will be mechanically ventilated. Modern transport ventilators are gas powered and use the cylinder oxygen as both the respiratory gas and the power source. Therefore the contents of small cylinders (for example, C & D) are used quickly, particularly when the patient is receiving 100% oxygen. Adequate spares must therefore be carried and checked for contents before departure. These ventilators have controls which allow tidal volume and respiratory rate to be determined approximately and can be used

to ventilate with either 100% oxygen or in an "airmix" mode, in which they deliver 45–60% oxygen. Once the patient has been attached to one of these ventilators, adequacy of ventilation must be checked preferably by arterial blood gas analysis or alternatively by measurement of oxygen saturation (with a pulse oximeter), end-tidal carbon dioxide, and expired tidal or minute volume.

Total reliance must never be placed on a mechanical ventilator. Although the devices themselves are increasingly reliable and robust, they still need a compressed gas supply to function and occasionally they can be damaged by careless use. Therefore a self-inflating bag valve must always accompany the patient to allow manual ventilation in the event of a ventilator failure.

All compressed gas is dry and consideration should be given to humidification. This is most easily achieved by using a heat and moisture exchanger (HME) placed between the tracheal tube and the ventilator tubing. As their name suggests, these devices function by collecting moisture from the expired gas and using it to humidify the inspiratory gases. This helps prevent drying of secretions which predisposes to their retention and subsequent chest infection.

The operating theatre

Patients often leave the resuscitation room and pass directly to the operating theatre, usually because of continuing haemorrhage. Despite the urgency of surgery, the importance of ensuring that the patient has a patent, secure airway must not be overlooked both in terms of maintaining oxygenation but also to allow a general anaesthetic to be administered. Once surgery commences further intervention in the airway may not be possible.

Theatre preparation

Before the arrival of the patient, the airway equipment must be checked. Apart from all of the routine equipment, this must include devices in case of difficulty with intubation, facilities for performing needle cricothyroidotomy and a surgical airway, and double lumen tubes if a thoracotomy may be required. The anaesthetic machine and ventilator should be checked in accordance with local policy. Finally the function of all the monitoring equipment is checked.

Patient's airway

A tracheal tube may have already been inserted during resuscitation. It is essential that it is checked for position by noting the length at the teeth or alveolar margin, listening for breath sounds, and measuring the end-tidal carbon dioxide. The integrity of the cuff is checked as is the volume of air and pressure within it. The diameter of the tube is noted and finally, if everything is satisfactory, it can be secured in place.

Occasionally it may be necessary to change the tracheal tube, usually because it is too short, the cuff is leaking, or one of a different type is required, for example a reinforced tube, because of the need to place the patient lateral or prone. Although this can be achieved by simply removing one tube, performing direct laryngoscopy, and reinserting another, often a single lumen tube is changed over an introducer. Following a period of preoxygenation, a 60 cm bougie is inserted through the existing tube, the tube removed leaving the bougie in place and then the new tube passed over the bougie into the trachea. This technique is particularly useful if there have been any difficulties with the initial intubation. At this stage a tracheal tube is not usually changed simply because of its small diameter at this stage, as the ventilator is doing the work of breathing.

If the patient is not already intubated, then an assessment similar to that described earlier is carried out, with indications noted where the procedure may be difficult. Typical signs may include trauma to the soft tissues of the face and neck, fractures of the midface, thermal injury to the upper airway, or the presence of actual or suspected cervical spine injury. In these circumstances one would consider:

- inhalational induction and direct laryngoscopy to assess the ease of intubation;
- awake intubation with topical anaesthesia;
- fibreoptic laryngoscopy and intubation;
- cricothyroidotomy or tracheostomy under inhalational or local anaesthesia.

Ventilation

When patients arrive with chest drains *in situ*, they must be checked to ensure that the drains are still functioning. Patients with multiple rib fractures require a chest drain inserted to prevent the development of a tension pneumothorax during mechanical ventilation because of the use of positive pressures. It is important to check that both lungs are being ventilated after the insertion of a tracheal tube, and the oxygen concentration of the inspired gases should be adjusted to maintain a saturation of > 95%. This may also require adjustment of the inspiratory to expiratory ratio (usually 1:2) and the use of PEEP (see later). The expired tidal volume must be measured as an index of ventilation, particularly if there is a persistent air leak from a bronchial tear. A double lumen may be required to isolate one lung and ensure ventilation in this situation if the leak is very large. If ventilation is difficult and the airway pressures are high, this may be due to:

- inadvertent endobronchial intubation. *Withdraw the tube and recheck; check chest x-ray.*
- Gastric dilatation splinting the diaphragm. *Pass a naso- or orogastric tube.*
- Pneumo/haemothorax. *Insert chest drain; check x-ray.*
- Diaphragmatic hernia.

The final check of adequacy of oxygenation and ventilation is the arterial blood gas analysis.

Intensive care unit (ICU)

Many trauma patients are often transferred to the ICU for further treatment, arriving either directly from the resuscitation room or more often via the operating theatre. They are frequently intubated on arrival and may remain so for periods of days or even weeks. This section will concentrate on the management of the trauma patient's airway which remains instrumented during care on the ICU. This will be considered under four headings:

- Indications for maintaining tracheal intubation.
- Different routes of tracheal intubation and tracheostomy, with their specific advantages and disadvantages.
- Sedation and analgesia.
- Hazards and complications of long-term tracheal intubation.

Indications for maintaining tracheal intubation

Irrespective of whether a patient is intubated immediately during resuscitation or at a later stage, the main indications for maintaining intubation on the ICU are:

- to maintain a patent upper airway;
- to secure the upper airway;
- to facilitate the delivery of high concentrations of oxygen;
- to allow mechanical intermittent positive pressure ventilation (IPPV).

Although any of these indications may occur in isolation, it is more usual for several or all of them to be present.

The presence of a tracheal or tracheostomy tube also provides access to the airway for the clearance of secretions in patients unable to cough because of their injuries or as a result of the administration of sedative, analgesic, or neuromuscular blocking drugs (see later).

Maintaining a patent airway

An impaired conscious level is the commonest reason for compromise of the patency of the patient's upper airway. In the initial phase, hypoxaemia and hypovolaemia alone or in combination will reduce conscious level, but by the time the patient reaches the ICU it is most likely to be due to the presence of either primary or secondary brain injury. The patency of the airway may also be jeopardised from swelling from both within the airway, for example secondary to thermal injury, or from without as a result of a haematoma in the neck owing to direct trauma. Although such problems may not have been present immediately, intubation may have been carried out expectantly, before distortion of the anatomy precluded it. Finally, the lack of a patent airway may be iatrogenic as a result of the use of sedative or muscle relaxant drugs to facilitate ventilation (see below).

Securing the upper airway

Protective upper airway reflexes will also be depressed as the conscious level falls, with the consequent risk of pulmonary aspiration of gastric contents and material from the upper airway itself (for example, blood or dislodged teeth). A cuffed tracheal or tracheostomy tube, when correctly positioned, will secure the airway, largely preventing gross pulmonary aspiration, although the protection afforded is not absolute and insidious aspiration of small volumes of contaminated material may still occur.

To facilitate the delivery of a high concentration of oxygen

Many trauma patients will require a high inspired concentrations of oxygen to overcome the hypoxaemia, consequent upon the ventilation/perfusion abnormalities from lung injury. This may arise directly as a result of trauma or secondary to metabolic lung injury, that is acute respiratory distress syndrome (ARDS) (see later). Concentrations approaching 100% are only attainable if the patient is intubated. Face masks with a high flow only deliver 45–50%. Even when a reservoir is attached this will only rise to around 70–80% depending upon the patient's respiratory pattern.

Common indications for mechanical ventilation in critically ill trauma patients

- Respiratory failure
  - aspiration pneumonia
  - inhalational injury
  - acute upper airway obstruction
  - high cervical spinal cord trauma
  - respiratory depression secondary to:
    - head injury
    - drugs
    - exhaustion
- Severe head injury
  - to allow hyperventilation which reduces Pa_{co_2}, cerebral blood volume and ICP
  - associated use of relaxants prevents surges of ICP from coughing and straining
- Chest injury
  - flail chest
  - pneumothorax, haemothorax
  - pulmonary contusion
- Multiple organ failure
  - optimises oxygen transport and reduces the work of breathing
- Severe left ventricular failure (secondary to myocardial contusion)
  - reduces preload and afterload and myocardial oxygen demand
- Following cardiopulmonary resuscitatiion
- Maintenance of organ function in patients diagnosed clinically as brain-stem dead pending harvesting

To allow mechanical intermittent positive pressure ventilation (IPPV)

This is by far the commonest reason for prolonged intubation of a trauma patient on the ICU. It may be because the patient's own ventilatory efforts are inadequate for their needs, ventilation is reduced by the administration of drugs, or ventilation is used as a therapeutic manoeuvre. Indications for mechanical ventilation of patients after major trauma are summarised in the box above.

Different routes used for tracheal intubation in the ICU

There are essentially three routes for intubating the trachea:

- orotracheal
- nasotracheal
- tracheostomy.

Orotracheal intubation is often the route of first choice as it is the simplest and most rapid to do. However, the nasal route has several potential advantages over the oral route in patients who require long-term tracheal intubation. A *nasotracheal tube* is usually better tolerated by patients and requires a lighter level of sedation. The fixation afforded by a nasotracheal tube is better than that of an orotracheal tube and oral hygiene is

easier and more effective with a nasotracheal tube. However, passage of a nasotracheal tube is technically more difficult and epistaxis is a frequent complication. Furthermore, the nasal route is contraindicated in the presence of possible basal skull fracture and clotting abnormalities. Theoretically, weaning from mechanical ventilation may be hampered owing to the increased work of breathing through the inevitably smaller nasotracheal tube; for example, the resistance to airflow of a size 7.0 (internal diameter 7 mm) tracheal tube is approximately three times that of a size 9.0 (internal diameter 9 mm). Against this, the reduced sedation requirements of a nasal tube may facilitate weaning and the increased work of breathing can be overcome by applying additional airway pressure support of 5–10 cm H_2O during inspiration. The advantages and disadvantages of both routes are summarized in Tables 2.2 and 2.3.

Table 2.2 Advantages and disadvantages of orotracheal intubation

Advantages	Disadvantages
Simple and quick method to perform	Intolerance by patient, may require deeper levels of sedation
Minimal risk of trauma	Difficult to maintain good oral hygiene Eating/drinking not possible Occlusion of the tube by kinking/biting Fixation less satisfactory

Table 2.3 Advantages and disadvantages of nasotracheal intubation

Advantages	Disadvantages
Usually well tolerated by patient	More difficult to insert
Fixation satisfactory	Epistaxis
Less likely to kink	Only possible to insert a smaller tube – increases work of spontaneous breathing, obstruction by secretions more likely
No possibility of bite occlusion	May cause sinusitis from blockage of nasal ostia
Oral hygiene improved	

Most tracheal tubes in use today are of the disposable, single-use plastic PVC or silastic variety. Plastic tubes are implant-tested and have a lower tendency to produce a tissue reaction; they mould themselves to the contours of the upper airway when warmed to body temperature; thus, they are more suited to longer term use. To seal the lower airway and lungs effectively from potential contaminants, the tracheal tube must have an inflatable cuff. There are two types of cuffs: the more modern low pressure–high volume and the older high pressure–low volume. The newer type is preferred as it exerts a lower pressure on the tracheal mucosa over a wider area when correctly inflated, thereby reducing the likelihood of ischaemic damage. Only sufficient air should be injected into the cuff to prevent leakage around it during the inspiratory phase of IPPV. The regular use of an aneroid manometer pressure gauge prevents the use of pressures greater than the capillary perfusion pressure of approximately 30 mmHg. An excessively high cuff pressure not only injures the tracheal mucosa but also prevents the cuff from acting as an emergency "blow-off" valve if the pressure within the breathing circuit becomes dangerously elevated.

It is important to select the size of tracheal tube appropriate to the patient and the route of intubation. Too small a size may require overinflation of the cuff to prevent air leakage, converting a low pressure cuff into a high pressure one. In addition, as already mentioned, smaller tubes have a higher airflow resistance. In contrast, too large a tracheal tube is more likely to cause pressure damage to the lips, nasal passages, and larynx. Furthermore, folds may be produced in a relatively underinflated cuff that allow channelling and aspiration of material from the pharynx (Figure 2.5).

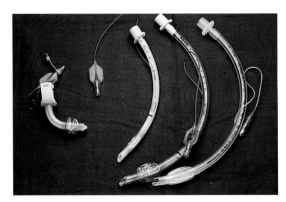

(a)

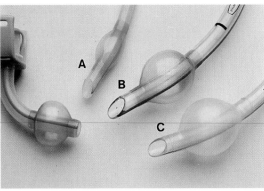

(b)

Figure 2.5 (a) Tracheal tubes and tracheostomy tube. (b) Detail shows high pressure–low volume cuff (A) and low pressure–high volume cuffs (B, C).

Tracheostomy is undertaken in certain defined circumstances that vary according to the institution, because of the higher associated morbidity and mortality when compared with tracheal intubation, principally caused by stomal haemorrhage and infection. Tracheostomy may be performed acutely to provide a definitive airway in those patients with upper airway obstruction where tracheal intubation is not possible. Examples of this would be patients who are being oxygenated via a needle cricothyroidotomy, especially children, or those with a fractured larynx. In both cases a surgical airway via the cricothyroid membrane is contraindicated. However, the most common use of tracheostomy is when the trachea must remain intubated for a prolonged period (for example, bulbar palsy secondary to acute cerebral injury) as the complications and risks associated with oral and nasal tubes increase and become unacceptable.

Opinions vary on the length of time before tracheostomy should be performed from approximately one to three weeks. Advocates of early tracheostomy quote a shorter duration of mechanical ventilation and ICU stay and a reduced incidence of pneumonia.

These benefits are probably a consequence of smaller sedation requirements and better toleration of enteral feeding.

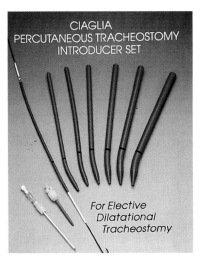

Figure 2.6 Equipment used for percutaneous dilatational tracheostomy.

However, it is known that the incidence of tracheal tube-induced laryngeal injury peaks before seven days and thus very early insertion of a tracheostomy would be required to avoid this. The decision to perform a tracheostomy must be individualised to the patient's specific circumstances and not governed by arbitrary time limits. Advantages and disadvantages of tracheostomy are summarized in Table 2.4.

Table 2.4 Advantages and disadvantages of tracheostomy

Advantages	Disadvantages
Very well tolerated by patient – facilitates weaning from ventilator	Relatively complex to perform – skilled, experienced operator essential
Fixation excellent	*Perioperative complications* Stomal haemorrhage
Good oral hygiene	Stomal infection
Accidental extubation more easily rectified	Malplacement in pretracheal tissues and oesophagus
	Later complications
Patient able to talk with "silver tube"	Deep erosion causing innominate artery haemorrhage, tracheo-oesophageal
Patient able to swallow, eat, and drink	fistula Sinus formation Tracheomalacia Tracheal stenosis

Until recently, the performance of a tracheostomy required the services of a surgeon and the transfer of a critically ill patient from the "safe environment" of the ICU to the operating theatre, often some distance away. However, it is becoming more common for intensivists themselves to perform tracheostomy on the ICU using one of two percutaneous techniques. The tracheostomy may be performed with a series of graded dilators railroaded along a Seldinger wire inserted into the trachea through a needle puncture (Figure 2.6). The tracheostomy tube is inserted once the track has dilated sufficiently to accommodate it. In the alternative approach, a special set of guidewire dilating forceps is used to produce the tracheostomy in a single action. Both percutaneous approaches are simpler and quicker than the classical approach, are safe when undertaken by experienced practitioners, and are associated with a lower incidence of complications.

Minitracheostomy tubes (for example, the *Portex Mini-Trach*) are small cuffless tubes with an internal diameter of 4 mm. They are inserted through an incision made into the cricothyroid membrane. Apart from their undoubted use in acute life-threatening upper airway obstruction, they have a relatively limited role on the ICU, particularly following the more widespread use of full-sized percutaneous tracheostomy. Their main use is in effecting adequate tracheobronchial toilet in patients with poor cough and sputum retention, but who do not require formal tracheal intubation or tracheostomy. These devices can be inserted under local anaesthesia using a combination of a small amount of local infiltration, bilateral superficial cervical plexus block along the anterior border of the sternomastoid muscles (see later), and an intravenous bolus of lignocaine, 1 mg/kg two minutes before the tube is inserted to reduce coughing.

Mechanical ventilation (IPPV)

During spontaneous ventilation, the descent of the diaphragm and expansion of the chest wall reduces the intrapulmonary pressure 1–2 cm H_2O below atmospheric pressure, and air flows into the lungs until the pressure in the alveoli is atmospheric. During mechanical ventilation, an intermittent positive pressure is applied to the ventilating gases so that they flow periodically into the lungs, hence *intermittent positive pressure ventilation* or IPPV. As in spontaneous ventilation, expiration occurs by passive recoil of the tissues of the lung and chest wall. Following major trauma there is often a fall in the compliance and increase in resistance of the lungs which impede gas delivery and distribution. In order to overcome this, ICU ventilators principally use complex electronics to control a flow of gas into the patient to ensure that the desired tidal volume is delivered.

Another problem that critically ill patients face is their tendency to develop areas of atelectasis. This is greatest when intra-alveolar pressures and volumes are at their lowest, that is end expiration when the lung volume equals the functional residual capacity (FRC). This leads to an increase in intrapulmonary shunting (blood flow to non-ventilated areas) and worsening hypoxaemia. Increasing the tidal volume alone is insufficient to rectify this problem; the need is to increase the FRC. This is achieved by maintaining a positive pressure in the lungs throughout the ventilatory cycle, that is applying a positive end-expiratory pressure or PEEP. This prevents the airway pressure falling to atmospheric and thereby reduces atelectasis. Unfortunately, although PEEP usually increases oxygenation, it may have an adverse effect on the cardiac output by reducing venous return. Clearly this will be magnified in the trauma patient who has not been adequately fluid resuscitated.

Many patients with severe injuries develop respiratory failure ($P_{O_2} < 60$ mmHg in ambient oxygen $\pm$ $P_{CO_2} \geq 50$ mm Hg). This may be due to direct thoracic trauma impairing the mechanics of ventilation or the subsequent pain associated with fractures of the thoracic cage. However, it more commonly follows the development of an acute metabolic lung injury – the acute respiratory distress syndrome (ARDS). After major trauma, circulating vasoactive and inflammatory mediators are released from damaged and ischaemic tissues (for example cytokines, complement, leukotrienes, and free radicals) causing an increase in the permeability of the pulmonary capillaries. Accumulation of extravascular lung water develops (non-cardiogenic pulmonary oedema) which can severely impede gas transfer across the alveoli.

The resulting hypoxia is unrelieved by high flow oxygen delivered by a face mask, and tracheal intubation and IPPV are required to improve oxygenation of the patient significantly by reliably delivering 100% O_2 to the lungs and allowing the

application of PEEP to increase the FRC of the lungs and reduce ventilation/perfusion mismatch. It may also have a role in limiting the accumulation of extravascular lung fluid.

Mechanical ventilation is therefore used after major trauma to help optimise oxygenation and is facilitated by the administration of potent narcotic analgesics and adequate sedation. In some circumstances, muscle relaxant drugs are used, most often in those patients with brain injuries.

Sedation and analgesia

Following major trauma, patients admitted to the ICU will require varying degrees of sedation and analgesia. These are not synonymous – a sedated patient may still be in pain while it is not necessary to be sedated to have good analgesia. Sedation and analgesia require different drugs and techniques and are necessary for different reasons.

Sedation is used to help patients tolerate the presence of a tracheal tube and mechanical ventilation. Furthermore, it will help patients who are confused and frightened by their surroundings, and reduce the risk of psychological trauma. When used appropriately, sedation should produce a calm, cooperative patient who is easier to nurse.

Analgesics are needed to provide pain relief from injuries sustained, postoperative pain, and any invasive procedures carried out on the ICU. In addition, intravenous opioids are frequently used for their anxiolytic and sedative properties; they are synergistic with sedatives thereby reducing the doses required. The respiratory depressant effect is also useful in patients undergoing mechanical ventilation.

As recently as 20 years ago, it was not uncommon for intubated, ventilated ICU patients to be heavily sedated, paralysed by the use of muscle relaxants and totally unaware of their surroundings. It is now recognised that such extremes are not only unnecessary but potentially harmful, being associated with immunosuppression, increased risk of infection, ileus, and renal and hepatic toxicity.

Nowadays, muscle relaxants are infrequently used, with sedation adjusted to produce a patient who is calm, awake, orientated, and tolerant of an artificial airway and ventilation. To assess this, various scoring systems have been described. The Ramsay Sedation Scale is widely used (Table 2.5). A

Table 2.5 Ramsay Sedation Score

Score	Conscious level
1	Restless and agitated
2	Cooperative, calm, orientated
3	Asleep, responds to verbal commands
4	Asleep, responds briskly to glabellar tap
5	Asleep, responds sluggishly to glabellar tap
6	No response

score of 2–4 would be satisfactory depending upon the time of day, clinical situation, and patient's needs.

The drugs used to achieve sedation and analgesia on the ICU are essentially the same as already described, with constant intravenous infusions of propofol, midazolam, and morphine being widely used. The use of muscle relaxants has been reduced by the rational use of sedation and improved design of ventilators. They are now used primarily in the initial stages of ventilation of patients with brain injury to ensure that the patient does not cough or "fight" the ventilator and that inflation pressures are kept low. This keeps the intrathoracic pressure low in order not to impede venous drainage of the brain, which in turn would raise the intracranial pressure. Furthermore, paralysis facilitates hyperventilation which may be used to reduce intracranial pressure in the acute phase.

Complications associated with long-term tracheal intubation

General considerations

The presence of an oro- or nasotracheal tube may be irritating to the patient and cause agitation, hypertension, cardiac dysrhythmias, and myocardial ischaemia. Accidental extubation by a confused patient may have disastrous results. It is often necessary for the patient to be adequately sedated if the tracheal tube is to be tolerated well. Sedation can cause further problems itself as some patients may not tolerate the cardiovascular depressant effects of sedative agents. The tube must be well secured, although tapes should not be too tight, particularly in patients with raised ICP, as jugular venous congestion may result. It is essential that the length of the tube measured at the lips or naris as appropriate is recorded so that migration of the tube in either direction is noticed immediately; modern tracheal tubes are marked at 2 cm intervals along their length. If the tube slips downwards, either endobronchial intubation or carinal stimulation may occur. The former will result in collapse of the contralateral lung and significant hypoxia; continuous pulse oximetry can be useful in alerting ICU staff. Carinal stimulation is usually intensely irritating to the patient and often causes severe agitation and cardiovascular upset.

As already outlined, one of the main reasons for intubation of patients on the ICU is mechanical ventilation. Despite its ability to improve oxygenation, it can have several adverse consequences. The raised mean intrathoracic pressure associated with IPPV reduces venous return to the heart, particularly in hypovolaemic patients; this causes a fall in cardiac output and arterial pressure. Pulmonary barotrauma may occur if inflation pressures are excessive, resulting in pneumothorax, pneumomediastinum, and surgical emphysema. IPPV is also associated with a reduction in the concentration of pulmonary surfactant. All these effects are magnified when PEEP is applied.

Nosocomial pneumonia

The development of nosocomial pneumonia is perhaps the most serious and frequent complication of prolonged tracheal intubation. Insertion of a tracheal tube bypasses the normal protective function of the glottis and the tube itself is a foreign body that acts as a nidus for micro-organisms to colonise. The normal clearance of secretions from the upper airway by ciliary action is impaired, owing partly to the presence of the tracheal tube. However, the immunosupressive effects of sedative and analgesic drugs, and of major trauma are also important. Stagnant secretions make an excellent culture medium.

The situation is often compounded owing to an overgrowth of bacteria from the stomach and upper gastrointestinal tract; unfortunately, even a correctly inflated tracheal cuff does not entirely prevent the passive aspiration of infected secretions (although aspiration is less likely with the high volume–low pressure variant). Normally, the production of gastric acid provides a sterile environment. However, as many critically ill patients are unable to tolerate enteral feeding, unopposed gastric acid may cause acute erosion or ulceration of the gastric mucosa. Thus patients on ICUs are often routinely prescribed prophylactic H_2-antagonists (cimetidine or ranitidine) or the proton pump inhibitor omeprazole. Studies have shown an increased incidence of nosocomial pneumonia in patients treated with H_2-antagonists. The most effective and physiological method of attaining a normal gastric acid environment which reduces the risk of both bacterial overgrowth and of acute ulceration of the gastric mucosa is to provide enteral nutrition, and it is current practice to attempt nasogastric feeding at an earlier stage than was previously the case. Where this is not possible, there is a move towards the use of mucosal protection agents (sucralfate) rather than gastric acid inhibitors which provide prophylaxis against gastric ulceration whilst maintaining the acid environment. The practice of selective decontamination of the gut using enteral, non-absorbed antibiotics (amphotericin B, tobramycin, polymyxin E) in combination with a systemic broad spectrum antibiotic appears to be waning.

Good nursing and medical care on the ICU will reduce the incidence of nosocomial pneumonia (see box). The use of sedative and analgesic drugs should be kept to the minimum required to produce a calm, cooperative, reasonably pain-free patient. The unnecessary use of heavy sedation further immunocompromises the patient. Where possible, opioids should be avoided by the appropriate use of regional and local anaesthetic techniques. Regular chest physiotherapy by the expert practitioner helps expectoration of secretions and prevention of atelectasis. The passage of suction catheters down the tracheal tube may itself introduce infection and cause airway trauma if it is not performed skilfully.

Prevention of nosocomial pneumonia

- Good basic standards – scrupulous washing of hands immediately before and after contact with the patient, wearing of gloves and aprons
- Regular, proficient chest physiotherapy
- Minimal level of sedation; avoidance/reduction in dosage of opioids by appropriate use of regional and local analgesia whenever possible
- Regular disinfection of ventilator tubing or use of disposable equipment
- Bacterial/viral filters between patient and ventilator
- Avoiding overuse of "prophylactic" broad-spectrum antibiotics; use of appropriate antibiotic therapy in conjunction with microbiological sensitivities obtained from sputum samples
- Optimising nutritional status of patient
- Enteral feeding whenever possible; H_2-antagonists associated with higher risk

Acute maxillary sinusitis

Nasal intubation may impede the normal drainage of the paranasal air sinuses with retention and stagnation of secretions leading to infection. The incidence of sinusitis appears to increase significantly after five days and head-injured patients are at particular risk as many of them have air/blood levels on CT scan. It is unfortunately difficult to diagnose as a high index of suspicion is required to make the necessary radiological diagnosis (plain skull x-ray or CT scan). Sinusitis should therefore always be considered in septicaemic patients with a nasotracheal tube *in situ* where the focus of infection is undetermined. Treatment requires removal of the nasotracheal tube, and nasogastric tube if present, and antibiotics.

Late complications

Complications which may occur after removal of the tracheal tube are listed in the box. Hoarseness is almost universal and self-limiting. However, true vocal cord paralysis may occur occasionally after a prolonged period of tracheal intubation from compression by the tracheal tube cuff. Temporary disorders of swallowing, with or without the added complication of laryngeal incompetence, are relatively common and it is therefore essential to ensure the adequacy of both before permitting the patient food and drink if aspiration is to be avoided.

Severe tracheal stenosis may occur in up to 10% of patients following prolonged (longer than 10 days) tracheal intubation, although the incidence has sharply declined since the widespread adoption of tracheal tubes with high volume–low pressure cuffs. Contributory factors include overinflation of the tracheal tube cuff, insertion of too large a tracheal tube (usually in children), repeated movement of the tube against the tracheal mucosa, and traumatic extubation. Tracheal stenosis is more common in patients following tracheostomy. However, while it is certainly true that narrowing will occur at the tracheostomy site as a direct consequence of the surgical procedure itself, there is evidence to show that the period of prolonged tracheal intubation preceding the performance of the tracheostomy is more important in determining the frequency and severity of tracheal stenosis.

Late complications of prolonged tracheal intubation

- Sore throat
- Hoarseness
- Dysphagia
- Laryngeal or subglottic oedema
- Laryngeal/tracheal ulceration
- Laryngeal web
- Polyp formation
- Recurrent laryngeal nerve palsy
- Laryngeal incompetence
- Vocal cord granuloma
- Tracheal stenosis
- Stricture of nasal passage
- Perforated nasal septum

Summary

On leaving the resuscitation room, the airway retains its place of primary importance. However maintained, constant vigilance is required to ensure early identification and correction of any problems. Where there is any concern about the patient's ability to maintain a patent airway, then tracheal intubation should be performed by those trained in the technique, but with the additional ability to create a surgical airway safely should this fail and compromise the patient. In those patients requiring long-term airway maintenance, tracheostomy is preferred, with percutaneous techniques becoming increasingly popular.

APPENDIX
PRACTICAL PROCEDURES

Tracheal intubation

Descriptions and pictures are not a substitute for acquiring the skill of intubation on anaesthetised patients under the direction of an anaesthetist. The following description assumes:

- all the necessary equipment for intubation is available and functioning (see box);
- the patient is being monitored appropriately and pre-oxygenated;
- there is **no injury** to the cervical spine.

Equipment required for orotracheal intubation

- Selection of cuffed tracheal tubes of different diameters (5.0–9.0 mm)
- Laryngoscopes – Macintosh, Magill, McCoy
- Magill forceps
- Syringe
- Lubricant
- Gum elastic bougie
- Stylet
- Tape/bandage to secure the tube
- Ventilator or bag-valve apparatus with reservoir
- SUCTION

Positioning

The optimal position of the patient's head for orotracheal intubation is with the neck flexed and the head extended at the altanto-occipital joint, often referred to as "sniffing the morning air". This is best facilitated by placing a small pillow under the head. The patient's mouth is then opened using the index finger and thumb of the operator's **right** hand, using a scissor action. The mouth is quickly examined and any debris removed using a rigid sucker (Yankeur type).

Laryngoscopy

The laryngoscope is always held in the operator's **left** hand; the blade is introduced into the mouth along the right side of the tongue, displacing it to the left side of the mouth. The tip is advanced until the right tonsillar fossa is identified, and then the blade is moved to the midline until the uvula is seen. The blade is advanced over the surface of the tongue until the epiglottis comes into view and then further until the tip lies in the gap between the base of the tongue and epiglottis – the vallecula. Force is then applied **in the direction to which the handle of the laryngoscope is pointing**, the effort coming from the operator's arm, not the wrist. The aim is to lift the tongue and epiglottis to expose the larynx. If successful this is seen as a triangular opening, apex anteriorly, with the whitish-coloured true cords laterally.

Intubation

With the tracheal tube held in the right hand, the tube is introduced into the right side of the patient's mouth, advanced and **seen to pass through the cords**. It should then be positioned such that the cuff lies just below the cords (some tracheal tubes have markings just above the cuff to help correct location). Holding the tube firmly in position, the laryngoscope is carefully removed, the cuff is the inflated, and ventilation commenced. Finally the position of the tube is checked with an appropriate method and, if the tube is in the trachea, it should be secured in place.

> The aim should be to complete intubation in approximately thirty seconds. If this cannot be achieved the patient must be preoxygenated before intubation is reattempted.

Nasotracheal intubation

An appropriately sized tube (usually 1.0 mm in diameter smaller, and 6 cm longer than an oral one) is well lubricated and introduced usually via the right nostril along the floor of the nose. In the supine patient it is therefore advanced vertically, with the bevel pointing medially to reduce the damage to the turbinates. As the tube reaches the nasopharynx, slight resistance may be encountered as the tube passes the protuberance of anterior tubercle of the first cervical vertebra. Once in the oropharynx, the tube can be visualised with a laryngoscopy as described above. The tube can now either be advanced into the larynx directly, or the tip can be picked up using a pair of Magill's forceps (designed so as not to impair the view of the larynx) and directed into the larynx. The procedure then continues as for oral intubation.

Difficult intubation

Occasionally intubation of the trachea is not straightforward, most often because the larynx cannot be seen at laryngoscopy. Although there are many anatomical variations which may cause this (see box), in the trauma patient it is most often secondary to an inability to position the head and neck in the optimal position because of a potential injury to the cervical spine (and the presence of a semirigid collar).

A variety of techniques can be used to help solve the problem of difficult intubation; the following are the most commonly used:

Common anatomical variants which may impede intubation
● Reduced neck movement
● Reduced mouth opening
● Receding lower jaw
● Short neck
● Prominent incisor teeth
● Narrow mouth
● High arched palate

● *Manipulation of the thyroid cartilage.* Often the larynx can be brought into view during laryngoscopy by downwards and upwards pressure. This should first be applied by the operator with the right hand (whilst laryngoscopy is performed with the left hand). Once the optimal view is obtained an assistant should be instructed to apply pressure at the same point and in the same direction. This manoeuvre must not be confused with cricoid pressure which is used to prevent regurgitation.

● *Use of a gum elastic bougie.* This device, which is 60 cm long with an anteriorly angled tip, can often be passed posterior to the epiglottis at laryngoscopy into the larynx, even when the latter structure cannot be directly seen. Often as it is advanced, correct placement is confirmed by being able to "feel" the tip run over the rings of cartilage in the trachea. Whilst the position of the laryngoscope is maintained, the tracheal tube is then passed over the bougie (railroaded). As the larynx is approached, the tube is rotated so that the bevel lies anteriorly to prevent it catching on one of the vocal cords. Once the tube is in place, the bougie is withdrawn, the cuff inflated, and the position of the tube checked with the use of an appropriate method.

● *Other types of laryngoscopes.* Sometimes a longer Macintosh blade is needed to reach the valecula or, alternatively, a straight blade (Magill) can be used to pass posterior to the epiglottis and lift it directly to reveal the larynx. A recent invention is the McCoy laryngoscope, the tip of which can be angled by a lever adjacent to the handle of the laryngoscope. This has the effect of increasing the "lift" at the base of the tongue, lifting the epiglottis more anteriorly to reveal the larynx.

● *Fibreoptic techniques.* Ultimately, if intubation cannot be achieved in any other way, it may be necessary to resort to the use of a fibreoptic intubating bronchoscope. This is introduced via either the mouth or nose and guided under direct vision into the trachea. A tracheal tube, previously mounted on the bronchoscope, can then be passed into the trachea, and the correct position confirmed. This technique can be used in awake patients in conjunction with local anaesthesia of the upper airway, or anaesthetised patients.

Surgical airway

This technique is used to provide a definitive airway, that is it allows oxygenation and elimination of carbon dioxide, when all other techniques have failed. While it is performed, high flow oxygen via a face mask or ventilation using a bag-valve-mask device must be continued.

Local anaesthesia

Where time allows, particularly in the conscious patient, consideration should be given to using local anaesthesia. Lignocaine 1% with adrenaline 1:100 000 is used; this has the added advantage of reducing bleeding. Two techniques can be used:

- Local infiltration of 1–2 ml over the cricothyroid membrane. Care must be taken not to inject too much or the local anatomy will be obscured.
- The nerves which supply the skin over the anterior surface of the neck can be anaesthetised by subcutaneous infiltration of local anaesthetic as they pass over the anterior border of the sternomastoid muscles (Figure 2.7). This technique has the advantage of not distorting the anatomy in the region of the cricothyroid membrane.

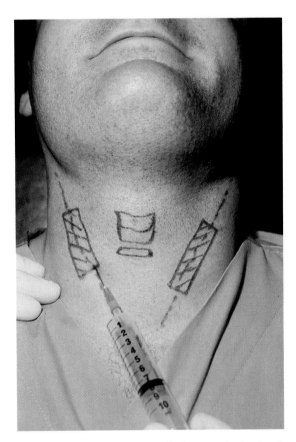

Figure 2.7 Infiltration of local anaesthetic along anterior border of sternomastoid muscles for surgical airway. Thyroid and cricoid cartilages are marked.

Surgical technique

The skin over the membrane is prepared and the larynx is immobilised by the operator with the index finger and the thumb of their non-dominant hand. A midline, 3–4 cm longitudinal incision is made, through the skin and subcutaneous tissues over the cricothyroid membrane. At this point, bleeding may be profuse, but time must not be wasted attempting to provide haemostasis. The operator should now insert a finger through the incision to reassess the position of the membrane and once confirmed, a transverse incision is made through it and a channel made with the use of the scalpel handle or a small self-retaining retractor. A 5.0–6.0 mm cuffed tracheostomy tube is then inserted; make sure that it passes into the trachea, not anterior to it into the pretracheal tissues. It is often easier to insert the tube initially from the side, rotating and advancing it to lie in the trachea.

Once in place, the obturator is removed, the cuff inflated, and the trachea suctioned to remove any inhaled blood and secretions. The tube can then be secured in place using the tapes provided. Bleeding usually stops spontaneously once any respiratory obstruction, hypoxaemia, and hypercarbia are relieved.

Further reading

American College of Surgeons Committee on Trauma. *Advanced trauma life support course for physicians.* Chicago: American College of Surgeons, 1993.

Atkinson R, Rushman G, Lee J. *A Synopsis of anaesthesia.* Bristol: John Wright, 1987.

Benumof JL. Management of the difficult adult airway. *Anesthesiology* 1991;**75**:1087.

Benumof JL, Scheller MS. The importance of transtracheal jet ventilation in the management of the difficult airway. *Anesthesiology* 1989;**71**:769.

Birmingham PK, Cheney FW, Ward RJ. Esophageal intubation: a review of detection techniques. *Anesthesia and Analgesia* 1986;**65**:886.

Bodenham AR. Editorial: Percutaneous dilational tracheostomy. *Anaesthesia* 1993;**48**:101.

Calvey TN, Williams NE. *Principles and practice of pharmacology for anaesthetists,* 2nd edn. London: Blackwell Scientific, 1991.

Cobley M, Vaughan RS. Recognition and management of difficult airway problems. *British Journal of Anaesthesia* 1992;**68**:90.

Driscoll PA, Gwinnutt CL, LeDuc Jimmerson C, Goodall O. *Trauma resuscitation: the team approach.* London: Macmillan, 1993.

Guidelines Committee of the American College of Critical Care Medicine; Society of Critical Care Medicine and American Association of Critical-care Nurses Transfer Guidelines Task Force. Special Article: Guidelines for the transfer of critically ill patients. *Critical Care Medicine* 1993;**21**:931.

King TA, Adams AP. Failed tracheal intubation. *British Journal of Anaesthesia* 1990;**65**:400.

Majernick JG, Bieniek R, Houston JB, Hughes HG. Cervical spine movement during orotracheal intubation. *Annals of Emergency Medicine* 1986;**15**:417.

Rotondo MF, McGonigal MD, Schwab W, Kauder DR, Hanson CW. Urgent paralysis and intubation of trauma patients: Is it safe? *Journal of Trauma* 1993;**34**:242.

3 Pulmonary trauma and chest injuries

Jonathon A. J. Hyde
Cardiothoracic Registrar, Queen Elizabeth Hospital, Birmingham

Ashok Shetty
Cardiothoracic Registrar, Queen Elizabeth Hospital, Birmingham

Roop Kishen
Consultant Intensivist, Hope Hospital, Salford

Timothy R. Graham
Cardiothoracic Consultant, Queen Elizabeth Hospital, Birmingham

---

OBJECTIVES

- To impart a knowledge of thoracic anatomy.
- To discuss the pathophysiology of chest trauma and mechanisms of injury.
- To describe how chest trauma is assessed clinically and with the help of imaging and endoscopic techniques.
- To discuss specific conditions associated with chest trauma.

In the United Kingdom, management of thoracic trauma has, until recently, been suboptimal, leading to unnecessary deaths and morbidity. This has resulted principally from a lack of formal guidelines. The introduction of the ATLS programme has revolutionised management of all forms of trauma; with thoracic trauma in particular, correct early management can significantly affect outcome, and the practice of ATLS guidelines regarding these injuries should continue to be encouraged [1]. However, care should be taken to treat each individual case on its own merit, since strict protocol-driven systems cannot predict all eventualities. The basic ATLS principles should attain stability in the early stages of presentation (that is, the primary survey), but the next problem is how subsequently to deal with the situation. There are a number of problems that arise in the "secondary survey" part of ATLS practice which involve the lungs and their ventilation, and if these are not addressed early, the outcome may be tragic. Pulmonary trauma has a variety of different, often misleading, clinical pictures.

Chest trauma is a factor in approximately 50% of fatal accidents, and in half of these, chest injury is the primary cause of death [2]. A report from Switzerland on the epidemiology of thoracic trauma in an industrialised society [3] demonstrated 12 thoracic injuries per day per million population, of which four required hospital admission. Their analysis of 1500 patients with thoracic injuries revealed chest wall injuries to be the commonest form of trauma sustained by these victims (Table 3.1). In the same report it was noted that chest trauma was usually associated with other injuries which accounted for the high mortality (Table 3.2).

Table 3.1 Proportion of injuries in chest trauma

Type of injury	Percentage affected
Chest wall	54
Flail chest	13
Pneumothorax	13
Haemothorax	20
Pulmonary injury	21
Miscellaneous	18

Table 3.2 Association of injuries in thoracic trauma

Organ system	Incidence (%)	Mortality (%)
Head and neck	42	26
Abdominal	32	31
Orthopaedic	46	24
Thoracic alone	29	11

Thoracic trauma can broadly be divided into penetrating and blunt injuries. Penetrating injuries are usually due to either stab wounds or missiles, depending on civilian or military practice, whereas blunt injuries can arise in a huge variety of situations. The most common of these in civilian life are deceleration (for example road traffic accidents), falls from a height, and direct impact. Patients who sustain catastrophic intrathoracic pulmonary injuries, such as laceration of a major airway, usually die at the site of the accident or are unsalvageable. Pneumothoraces, especially tension, should be easily recognised and treated expeditiously, or fatalities will

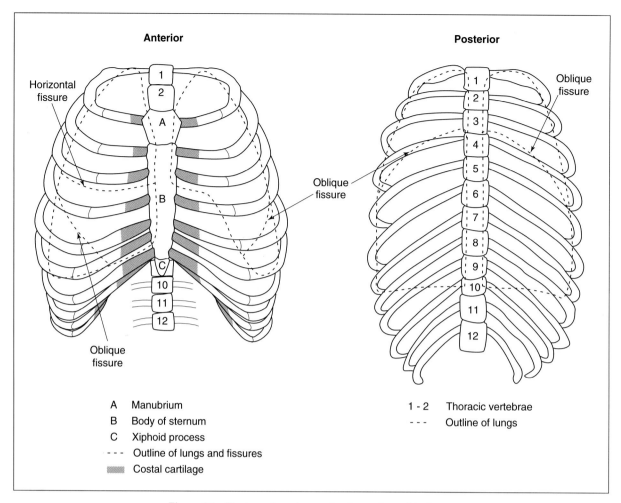

Anterior

Horizontal
fissure

1
2
A
B
C
10
11
12

Oblique
fissure

Posterior

Oblique
fissure

1
2
3
4
5
6
7
8
9
10
11
12

Oblique
fissure

A   Manubrium
B   Body of sternum
C   Xiphoid process
- - -   Outline of lungs and fissures
▨   Costal cartilage

1 - 2   Thoracic vertebrae
- - -   Outline of lungs

Figure 3.1 The bony thoracic cage showing outlines of the lungs.

result. Perhaps more difficult to manage is pulmonary contusion, which may develop insidiously over a period of days, and this is dealt with in detail later in this chapter.

Of all patients with thoracic trauma who manage to reach hospital alive, 85% can be successfully managed without any major surgical intervention [4]. The principles of management of patients who have sustained thoracic trauma include effective cardiopulmonary resuscitation and close monitoring, followed by early detection and correction of life-threatening injuries.

Applied anatomy

A thorough knowledge of the anatomy of all structures in and around the thorax is essential for personnel dealing with chest trauma. These structures are discussed separately:

Chest wall

The chest wall consists of the bony skeleton covered with its attached muscle and integument, and acts as a cage to protect the thoracic contents (Figure 3.1). The bony skeleton comprises 12 pairs of semicircular ribs attached to the sternum anteriorly through the costal cartilages. The exceptions to this are ribs 11 and 12 which are free anteriorly. The sternum consists of three parts: a short manubrium, a longer body, and a xiphoid process of variable length. It acts as a protective shield to the heart and great vessels. It gives attachment to the ribs and

clavicles in addition to the pectoral and abdominal muscles, and the muscles of the neck. The thoracic cage is covered by muscle, fascia, subcutaneous fat, and skin. The area inferior to the axilla is the thinnest part of the chest wall and is an appropriate site for insertion of chest drains (see page 46).

Diaphragm

The diaphragm consists of a central tendon and radially orientated muscle fibres which connect it to the chest wall. The diaphragm has three hiati (Figure 3.2). The *oesophageal* hiatus contains both vagal trunks and their branches in addition to the oesophagus. The *aortic* hiatus also contains the azygos vein and the thoracic duct. The *vena caval* hiatus is situated more cranially, and only contains the inferior vena cava. The diaphragm contributes significantly to respiration, a descent of 1 cm being equivalent to nearly 400 ml of tidal volume. During normal breathing, the diaphragm moves by about 1.5–2 cm and during deep breathing it can travel as much as 8–10 cm. During full expiration, the dome of the diaphragm may rise as high as the fifth intercostal space, which explains the incidence of diaphragmatic injuries in penetrating trauma, even when the entry wound is relatively high in the chest.

Tracheobronchial tree

The trachea extends from the cricoid cartilage, at the level of the sixth cervical vertebra, to the carina, at the level of the upper border of the fifth thoracic vertebra, where it bifurcates

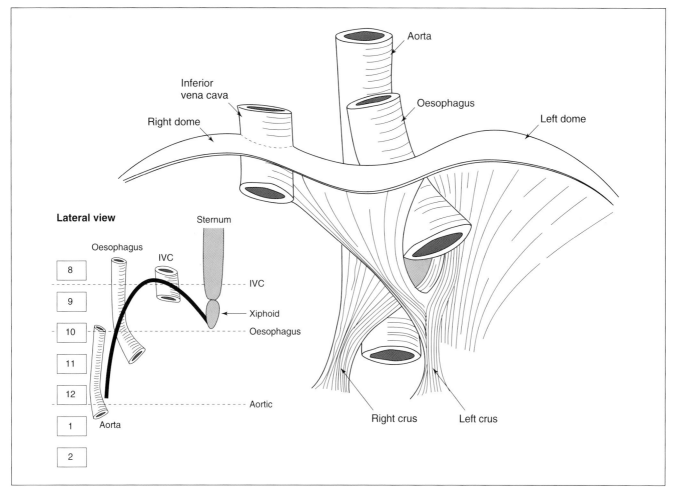

Figure 3.2 The openings of the diaphragm.

(Figure 3.3). The jugular veins are anterolateral to the trachea, whereas the common carotid arteries are posterolateral to it, with the vagus nerve lying in the groove between the artery and vein. The right main bronchus is shorter, straighter, and at a lesser angle to the trachea than the left. It lies just below the azygos–superior vena caval junction and behind the right pulmonary artery. The left main bronchus passes under the aortic arch abutting the pericardium and left atrium anteriorly.

Lungs and pleurae

The right lung contributes approximately 55% of the total lung mass and has oblique and transverse fissures which divide it into three lobes: upper, middle, and lower (Figure 3.4). The left lung is divided into upper and lower lobes by the oblique fissure. Both lungs are divided into bronchopulmonary segments corresponding to the bronchial branches, and are supplied by branches of the pulmonary arteries. The right and left pulmonary arteries pass superiorly in the hilum, anterior to the respective bronchus. There are superior and inferior pulmonary veins on each side, the right middle lobe being drained by the superior vein.

The pleural cavities are lined by two serous membranes into which the lung is invaginated. It is made up of connective tissue and lined with mesothelium, which secretes a small amount of serous fluid, lubricating the surface. The parietal pleura lines the inner wall of the thoracic cage. The visceral pleura is intimately applied to the surface of the lungs and is reflected onto the mediastinum at the hilum.

Pathophysiology

The main consequences of chest trauma are as a result of its effects on haemodynamic and respiratory function. Pulmonary pathophysiology and ventilation is dealt with here; haemodynamics are covered in Chapter 4. It must be understood, however, that there is some considerable overlap between the two systems, and changes in one may profoundly alter the function of the other.

Mechanics of ventilation

The respiratory system can be divided into two broad anatomical regions: the airways and the alveoli. This section will cover the mechanics of ventilation in delivery and removal of gases to and from the alveoli. The next section on gas exchange will cover the passage of gases across the alveolar membrane. The airways start branching at the trachea, with subsequent narrowing at each division until the terminal bronchioles, when the diameter remains constant at about 0.5–0.7 mm [5]. The lungs and chest wall are elastic in nature, and the functional residual capacity (FRC) is the volume at which the inward pull of the lungs balances the outward recoil of the chest wall. Any factors (such as injury or disease processes) that alter this fine balance will automatically have an effect on FRC.

Compliance is a measurement of "stiffness" and can be defined as change in volume divided by change in pressure.

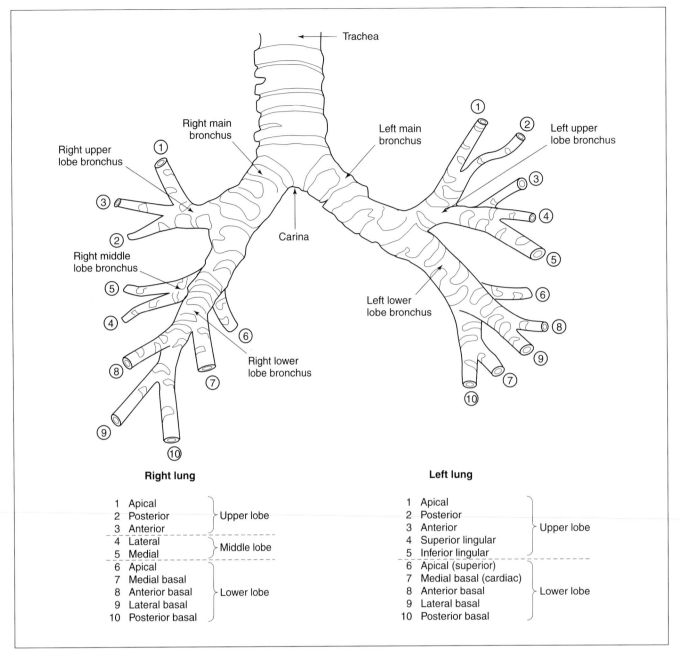

Figure 3.3 Tracheobronchial tree showing branches to bronchopulmonary segments.

Lung compliance decreases (that is, becomes stiffer) as volume increases, whereas the opposite is the case for chest wall compliance. This helps to maintain the critical balance, because conditions that lead to a loss of elastic tissue and decreased recoil cause increased compliance, and vice versa.

Total lung capacity (TLC) is the total amount of air within the lungs at maximal inspiration. The vital capacity (VC) is the volume obtained on full expiration from TLC. TLC is determined by a combination of inspiratory muscle strength, chest wall recoil, and lung recoil, and is equal to VC plus RV (residual volume).

The dead space is the volume of the airways that is ventilated but in which gas exchange does not occur, and can be divided into anatomical or physiological (which takes into account extra dead space created by processes such as ventilation/perfusion mismatch). Anatomical dead space in a healthy 70 kg man is approximately 150 ml.

For gas exchange to take place, it must be delivered to the alveoli, and this occurs by bulk flow down a pressure gradient. This gradient is dependent on airway resistance, and is the reason for their progressive decrease in diameter. Airflow in the larger airways is turbulent, but in the smaller ones laminar flow occurs; therefore, most resistance occurs in the large airways. This creates the necessary gradient, resulting in delivery of oxygen to the alveoli during inspiration, and removal of carbon dioxide during expiration. Any processes that disrupt this balance will affect adequacy of respiration.

Gas exchange

Gas exchange occurs at the alveolar level, and is dependent on a sufficient supply of oxygen. The Acinus is the basic unit of gas exchange, and comprises respiratory bronchioles, alveolar ducts, alveolar sacs, and alveoli [6]. The blood supply

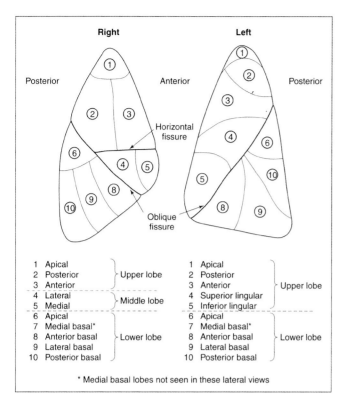

Right			Left		

1	Apical		1	Apical	
2	Posterior	Upper lobe	2	Posterior	
3	Anterior		3	Anterior	Upper lobe
4	Lateral		4	Superior lingular	
5	Medial	Middle lobe	5	Inferior lingular	
6	Apical		6	Apical	
7	Medial basal*		7	Medial basal*	
8	Anterior basal	Lower lobe	8	Anterior basal	Lower lobe
9	Lateral basal		9	Lateral basal	
10	Posterior basal		10	Posterior basal	

* Medial basal lobes not seen in these lateral views

Figure 3.4 Lateral (costal) views of the lungs showing the bronchopulmonary segments.

of the alveoli is specialised for the function of gas exchange, the pulmonary artery dividing in a similar way to the airways. An extensive capillary network is formed around the alveolus, with a gas–blood barrier of as little as 0.5 μm, which facilitates the process of respiration [7].

We have discussed the mechanisms by which gases reach the alveolus, and shall now deal with their passage to and from the blood stream. This takes place by simple diffusion. Diffusion depends on the concentration of the gases involved, the properties of the gas, the pressure gradient driving the process, and the area of the membrane across which it is to occur. Oxygen diffuses across the alveolocapillary membrane, the capillary plasma, and the red cell membrane, and then combines with haemoglobin. The reverse process occurs with carbon dioxide. The actual gas mixing in the alveolar spaces is a very rapid process, and the rate limiting step is not this, but the transfer of gases across the erythrocyte membrane. An important point to note here is that injuries or disease processes that affect diffusion have a marked effect on oxygen delivery. This is because carbon dioxide can diffuse across the erythrocyte membrane much more quickly than oxygen, and its removal, therefore, is less affected.

Control of ventilation

Respiration is a dynamic process which provides the cells with oxygen, removes carbon dioxide, and maintains acid-base balance. It is controlled within the central nervous system (CNS), and relies on a number of peripheral and central sensory detectors. The autonomic function is located in the brain stem, and voluntary control in the cerebral hemispheres [8]. The sensory detectors consist of chemoreceptors (aortic and carotid bodies), and mechanoreceptors (lungs and chest wall). The sensors provide the CNS with information about the respiratory and acid-base status of the body, and this in

turn acts on the effectors of respiratory function to create appropriate ventilation.

There are three separate respiratory centres in the CNS, called the pneumotaxic centre, the apneustic centre, and the medullary centre. The medullary centre consists of two areas of nuclei, one for inspiration and one for expiration. They can independently drive the respiratory muscles, but if destroyed result in cessation of autonomic breathing. Stimulation of the pneumotaxic centre inhibits inspiration and causes expiration to commence. The apneustic centre can end the inspiratory phase by negative inputs from the sensory detectors.

Information about the respiratory status of the body is largely dependent upon two factors: oxygen and carbon dioxide. The partial pressures of both of these need to be kept within very narrow physiological ranges and, if the values stray from these ranges, the sensors are triggered for an autoregulatory response. The oxygen sensors are mainly peripheral, almost exclusively in the carotid bodies. The carbon dioxide sensors are mainly in the CNS, but up to 30% may contribute from the periphery.

Defects in respiratory function

Hypoxia

Hypoxia is the commonest pathophysiological manifestation of any moderate to severe chest injury (see box). Since it is the dominant feature of chest injury, early interventions are designed to ensure that an adequate amount of oxygen is delivered to all portions of the lung capable of normal ventilation and perfusion. Hence, oxygen administration must be commenced immediately in all patients, using a mask and bag reservoir capable of delivering an Fi_{O_2} in excess of 0.85. Of course, in some circumstances, the patient will require immediate intubation and ventilation, to ensure the necessary oxygen requirement reaches vital tissues. Compromised respiratory function may arise from any of the following mechanisms (Table 3.3).

Causes of hypoxia in chest trauma

- Diminished blood volume
- Ventilatory failure
- Contusion of lung tissue leading to ventilation/perfusion mismatch
- Changes in the pressure relationships within the pleural space
- Displacement of mediastinal structures
- Collapse of the lung (pneumothorax)

A traumatic pneumothorax usually occurs secondary to pulmonary parenchymal, or tracheobronchial injury, and is rarely due to oesophageal injury. When an associated chest wall injury creates a direct communication between the inner thoracic cavity and the external environment, an *open pneumothorax* (sucking chest wound) results. This continuity between the thoracic cavity and atmospheric air leads to preferential influx of air through the chest wall defect, rather than through the tracheobronchial tree during inspiration, and similarly, its escape during expiration. The reason for this is that air will follow the path of least resistance, this being the larger diameter chest-wall defect. The implications are a progressive air-filling of the ipsilateral thoracic cavity during inspiration, with a consequent shift of mediastinal structures to the unaffected

Table 3.3 Mechanisms of impaired respiratory function

Feature	Mechanism
Airway obstruction	• Maxillofacial injury with oedematous soft tissue, or bleeding into the pharynx • Obtunded patient with the tongue falling back into the pharynx • Direct laryngeal injury with oedema and haemorrhage • Tracheal or bronchial obstruction due to direct injury, aspiration of blood, gastric contents or foreign bodies
Hypoventilation	• Pain from damaged tissues; skeletal and neuronal injuries can lead to shallow breathing with a relative increase in the dead space • Flail chest results in decreased efficiency of ventilation to a variable extent from paradoxical movement of the flail segment; however, most of the respiratory abnormalities associated with a flail segment are secondary to the associated contusion • Tracheobronchial injury leading to loss of effective ventilatory volume
Loss of lung volume	• Reduced cough secondary to pain and soft tissue injury, leading to retention of secretions and atelectasis • Diaphragmatic rupture, leading to herniation of abdominal contents into the thorax; this acts as a space-occupying structure in the thoracic cavity and may result in collapse of a lobe or even the whole lung • Tension pneumothorax • Haemothorax or pneumothorax

side. During expiration, the air efflux partially reverses this situation, as the affected lung receives air from the unaffected one.

A traumatic *tension pneumothorax* is produced secondary to laceration of the lung or airway, with escape of air into the pleural space. The difference from a simple pneumothorax is that in a tension pneumothorax, the airflow is unidirectional into the pleura on inspiration, but cannot escape during expiration due to the presence or formation of an effective flap valve. This causes a progressive accumulation of air in the pleura, with collapse of the ipsilateral lung, producing hypoxia, and shift of the mediastinum to the opposite side. In advanced cases hypoxia-induced myocardial failure can lead to low cardiac output states. It was originally believed that the associated mediastinal shift could restrict the venous return by kinking the vena cavae, leading to a low cardiac output state. However, studies performed more recently have shown this not to be so [9]. Other groups have suggested that unilateral tension pneumothorax does not directly lower cardiac output [10].

In most cases of traumatic tension pneumothorax, there will be a variable amount of surgical emphysema from dissection of air into tissue planes of least resistance. This will be more obvious if the aetiology is a tracheobronchial injury, when there is associated mediastinal emphysema. Though surgical emphysema can produce a grossly abnormal physical appearance, it rarely produces any clinically significant or pathophysiological changes.

Haemothorax following chest wall injury is often secondary to bleeding from intercostal vessels and less often from the internal mammary vessels. A significant, or life-threatening haemothorax is usually due to major lung parenchymal laceration, injury to the pulmonary hilum, or from aortic disruption or direct cardiac lacerations. Haemothorax following pulmonary parenchymal injury is often associated with a pneumothorax of variable degree, which contributes to the development of early hypoxia. The haemothorax, if large, will also occupy space in the thoracic cavity normally occupied by lung, and the subsequent collapse will worsen the hypoxia.

Impairment of gas exchange

Patients with a pulmonary injury can have major impairment of gas exchange owing to diffuse interstitial and alveolar haemorrhage, as seen following pulmonary contusion. Pulmonary contusion is one of the main factors responsible for the increased morbidity and mortality associated with chest trauma. Based on both experimental and clinical results, pulmonary contusion has been described as a progressive condition, with initial haemorrhage and oedema, followed by interstitial fluid accumulation and decreased alveolar membrane diffusion. These changes produce relative hypoxaemia, increased pulmonary vascular resistance, decreased pulmonary vascular flow, and reduced compliance. Richardson and associates have documented a decreased bacterial clearance in dogs who have sustained pulmonary contusion, suggesting that contused lungs are also more susceptible to bacterial infection [11].

Shunt

In patients with impaired respiratory function from pulmonary injury, the associated mediastinal shift secondary to haemothorax and/or pneumothorax, results in compression of the non-injured lung, further compromising ventilation. This ventilation–perfusion mismatch can lead to an intrapulmonary shunt of more than 30%, contributing significantly to the hypoxaemia, especially in the early stages. Later, this hypoxia-induced pulmonary vasoconstriction will divert the blood away from the non-ventilated alveoli leading to a reduction of the intrapulmonary shunt to below 5%.

Mechanism of injury

Blunt trauma

Blunt trauma can be caused by direct impact, shear forces, rotary forces, and deceleration. The severity of direct impact depends on the strength of force, duration of impact, and the size and site of the contact area on the patient. Hence, fractures of four or more ribs represent a serious and often life-threatening injury, even in the absence of other obvious damage. Shear forces can produce serious degloving injuries, as is often seen when the patient is run over by a motor vehicle. Deceleration injuries are usually associated with high-speed motor vehicle accidents or falls from a height. The use of seatbelts has contributed significantly to the reduction of incidence of chest injuries in vehicular accidents, particularly in frontal impacts, with one study demonstrating the differences in rib fractures between restrained and unrestrained drivers [12]. Fractures of the clavicle are usually of little significance except when the fractured end injures the subclavian vessels. They can also rarely be associated with injuries to the brachial plexus. Sternal injuries commonly occur following vehicular accidents. If seatbelts are used without shoulder restraints, there are frequently both sternal and vertebral injuries as the body is thrown sharply forward on sudden deceleration. Sternal injuries are commonly associated with costochondral dislocations of multiple ribs and the appearance of flail segments.

Penetrating trauma

Stab wounds confined to the chest wall are usually relatively benign, unless an intercostal or internal mammary artery has been injured. In these instances, there is often a significant and continuing haemorrhage leading to hypovolaema, and in most cases, a haemothorax. Gunshot wounds, particularly from high velocity weapons, can cause devastating injuries to the chest wall with significant tissue loss, most pronounced at the exit wound site.

Blast injuries

Blast injury of the lung (see Chapter 22) is caused by transmission of pressure waves through the tracheobronchial tree from an adjacent explosion. The severity of the injury depends upon the magnitude of the explosion and the proximity of the patient to the blast. The pulmonary damage usually consists of ruptured alveoli and capillaries with interstitial and intra-alveolar haemorrhage. It is a diffuse lesion which can, if severe, produce bronchovenous fistulae leading to large air emboli and sudden death. The commonest early symptom is a cough owing to excessive bronchial fluid; this may lead to progressive respiratory failure, so must be regarded with a high index of suspicion.

Clinical assessment

Early assessment and simultaneous resuscitation of the patient with respect to the organs injured, and potential consequences, are the most important part of trauma management. In all patients, an initial systematic assessment should be carried out including history regarding the time of the injury, mechanism of injury, and the subsequent course of events. This can be obtained either from the patient or from bystanders, relatives, police, or paramedical personnel. Personal health history, if available, is very valuable information as it can give some insight into the individual's response to shock and injury. In particular, history regarding previous cardiac, respiratory, and vascular status is of paramount importance. Assessment should also include information about the condition of the patient at the scene of the accident. It is important to establish immediately the presence or absence of all vital signs. In patients with chest trauma, this involves identifying the nature and extent of the damage, the organs involved and the effect on cardiac and respiratory function. In addition, one must assess the effect of the injury to extrathoracic organs on cardiorespiratory function. This includes common examples such as the effects of head injury on breathing, of maxillofacial trauma on airway patency, and of hypovolaemia from bleeding from any site. As in all cases of trauma, a standardised plan of action such as that recommended by the Advanced Trauma

Life Support (ATLS) programme should be followed. The recommendations divide management into the following categories, although it is important to note that the primary survey and resuscitation are simultaneous events:

1. primary survey
2. resuscitation
3. secondary survey
4. definitive care.

Primary survey

Essentially, this follows the standardised 'ABC' (airway, breathing, circulation) rules for resuscitation, which is fully described in Chapter 1.

The *breathing* pattern should then be carefully observed by exposing the chest completely. A complete examination should include observation, palpation, and auscultation. After noting any obvious external injuries, the quality of respiration and presence of any paradoxical chest wall motion, suggesting a flail segment, must be looked for carefully. Slow and shallow respiration may be due to central nervous system injury or sedation (including the effects of alcohol, although this must not be assumed). Tachypnoea of more than 24 breaths per minute in patients with a thoracic injury suggests respiratory dysfunction from pulmonary compromise or injury. Both lungs must be auscultated fully to identify adequate air entry in all zones.

The *circulation* is assessed by quickly but thoroughly evaluating the pulse (for rate, quality, and rhythm), blood pressure, pulse pressure, and peripheral tissue perfusion (skin colour, temperature, and capillary return). Cyanosis should be noted but no real information can be inferred by its presence, since it is haemoglobin-dependent. Heart sounds are auscultated and the presence of any murmur is noted. The neck veins should be examined, since engorgement may indicate cardiac tamponade or a tension pneumothorax but, even in these conditions, they may be empty if the patient is profoundly hypovolaemic.

The main purpose of this primary survey is to identify any immediately life-threatening injuries which must be treated as simply and quickly as possible (Table 3.4).

Secondary survey

Once the patient's condition has been stabilised and all immediate threats to life have been appropriately treated, a secondary survey must be performed, which involves further, detailed physical examination. This allows assessment of the extent of any injury to thoracic organs and allows evaluation of the effects of other injuries on cardiorespiratory function. It is important to realise that the secondary survey must not commence until there is no longer any immediate threat to life. It is at this stage that particular attention must be given to the identification of *potentially* life-threatening injuries (Table 3.5). This is the stage at which to perform a detailed physical examination. It is during this survey that the following essential investigations should be performed: a chest radiograph (erect if possible), an ECG, and arterial blood gases. Dependent upon the results, further definitive measures can be undertaken to optimise respiratory and cardiac function. If the patient's clinical status is at any stage seen to be deteriorating, it is important to return to the primary survey and resuscitation, in case a new threat to life has arisen, or has been missed. Further monitoring is also necessary to evaluate cardiac and pulmonary function more accurately. In appropriate cases,

Table 3.4 Immediate threats to life in thoracic trauma

Injury	Mechanism	Treatment
Tension pneumothorax	• One-way valve filling the thoracic cavity with air • Compression/displacement of mediastinum and opposite lung	• Clinical diagnosis • Needle decompression converts to simple pneumothorax • Chest drain
Open pneumothorax (sucking chest wound)	• Continuity between atmosphere and thoracic cavity • Air follows path of least resistance on inspiration • Effective ventilation impaired	• Occlusive dressing taped only on three sides creates a flutter valve • Chest drain
Massive haemothorax	• Accumulation of >1500 ml blood in thoracic cavity • Either hypovolaemic effects or mechanical compression causing tamponade	• Restore intravascular volume • Decompression with large-bore chest drain
Flail chest	• Isolated bony segment of chest cage, usually from multiple rib fractures, results in paradoxical chest wall motion • Pain may contribute to hypoxia	• Ventilation & humidified oxygen • Re-expand lung • Cautious fluid resuscitation • Analgesia
Cardiac tamponade	• Mechanical compression from blood in the pericardial sac	• Emergency pericardiocentesis • Fluid resuscitation • Emergency anterior thoracotomy (Chapter 4)

this includes central venous cannulation, urinary catheter placement, and strict fluid-balance recording, particularly in patients who have been hypovolaemic, where careful restoration of organ perfusion is crucial. Sometimes, Swan–Ganz catheterisation is required in order to monitor pulmonary artery pressures, and to derive cardiac output and vascular resistance indices. These patients and others who show abnormal features on chest radiography may require more specialised diagnostic tests and investigations, including echocardiography, CT scan, MRI scan, angiography, and endoscopy, dependent upon local availability. Further management and its timing will depend upon the information obtained from these investigations, the haemodynamic and respiratory status of the patient, and the extent of any associated injuries.

We shall now turn in more detail to the history and examination.

Regional assessment

Chest wall

When a patient has sustained a chest wall injury, a history of pain on deep breathing, coughing, or change of position are all highly suggestive of a rib fracture. On examination, the fractured area may be tender and elicit crepitus. Associated surgical emphysema may make this finding difficult to establish. A flail chest will often be obvious to the examining physician by its paradoxical movement during respiration, but can equally be very difficult to diagnose. When a part of the flail segment gets impacted under the adjacent rib cage, the movement may not be noticed but the bony irregularity will be obvious. This is called "stove-in-chest", and is a serious complication of rib fractures. A flail chest is produced when two or more consecutive ribs and/or the sternum are fractured or dislocated at more than one site, resulting in an isolated segment of chest cage. This discontinuity means that the segment moves paradoxically to the rest of the chest wall during the two phases of respiration. It is seen in 10–20% of all patients with chest trauma and carries a mortality of up

to 50% in elderly patients [3]. Flail segments may be located anteriorly, laterally, or posteriorly and may be of any size (Figure 3.5). Posterior flail segments are rare because of the thick muscular protection provided by the back muscles. The respiratory insufficiency following a large flail chest is predominantly caused by the associated pulmonary contusion (Figure 3.6). The impact required to produce such a flail segment must be substantial, and is transmitted to the underlying lungs. The earlier understanding that the paradoxical movement of a flail segment causes respiratory insufficiency owing to pendulous movement of gases from one lung to another across the carina, has been disproved by pneumotachographic studies [13].

Fractures of the sternum can also manifest with severe pain, aggravated by deep breathing and coughing. Clinically, there may be an area of tenderness. Bony irregularity can be appreciated on palpation along the length of the sternum. When this is secondary to a steering-wheel injury, a characteristic semicircular area of bruising on the anterior chest wall is frequently noticed.

In patients with a fractured clavicle, pain and bony crepitus can be elicited on even small movements of the shoulder. In addition, discontinuity along the clavicle and fullness of the supra- and infraclavicular fossae may be noticed. Scapular fractures can be difficult to diagnose as they are the least symptomatic and not readily accessible owing to the thick padding of surrounding muscles. However, they are extremely important because it takes a huge amount of force to fracture the scapula, and are frequently associated with significant damage to other, apparently unharmed organs.

Certain injuries of the bony thorax are specifically associated with injury to underlying structures and should alert the physician to the possibility of their presence (Table 3.6)

Tracheobronchial tree

Tracheobronchial injuries usually manifest themselves with rapidly progressive surgical emphysema and shortness of breath owing to the associated pneumothorax and reduction

Table 3.5 Potential threats to life in thoracic trauma

Injury	Concerns	Specific management
Pulmonary contusion	• Progressive respiratory failure	• Oxygenation • Ventilation if severe
Myocardial contusion	• Arrhythmias • Myocardial infarction • RV dysfunction	• Cardiac monitoring • Serial enzyme measurement
Aortic disruption	• Contained haematoma • Persistent bleeding and hypotension • Rupture and sudden death	• Fluid resuscitation • Consider angiography • Consider TOE, MRI and CT scan
Diaphragmatic rupture	• Abdominal visceral herniation • Mechanical compression of thoracic organs • Often late diagnosis	• NGT insertion and CXR • Upper GIT contrast studies
Tracheobronchial rupture	*Trachea:* • Airway obstruction • Pneumomediastinum *Bronchus:* • Usually fatal	• Airway maintenance • Oxygenation • Chest drain(s) • Bronchoscopy
Oesophageal rupture	• Mediastinitis • Empyema following delayed rupture into pleura	• Oesophagoscopy • Contrast studies

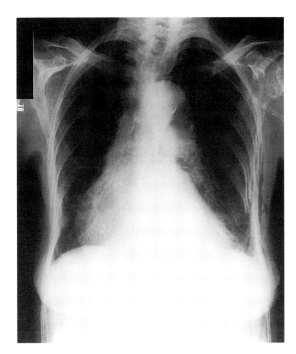

Figure 3.5 Plain chest radiograph showing a left-sided flail segment spanning four ribs.

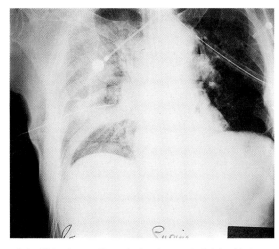

Figure 3.6 Plain chest radiograph showing marked right-sided pulmonary contusion.

in tidal volume. When the distal bronchus is totally obliterated, the subsequent collapsed lobe or lung causes worsening shortness of breath. Mediastinal emphysema can be diagnosed on auscultation by a crunching noise synchronous with the heart beat (Hamman's sign), but associated surgical emphysema or sternal fracture can mask this finding, as, more commonly, can a noisy environment. These injuries are often very serious, and require immediate confirmation and surgical treatment.

Table 3.6 Incidence of thoracic injuries with associated fractures

Fracture site	Underlying injury	Incidence (%)
First rib	Heart and great vessels	15
Scapula	Brachial plexus	13
	Great vessels	13
	Pulmonary contusion	54
Sternum	Cardiac contusion	80
	Great vessels	5–12

Imaging and investigations

Chest radiograph

This is the most important basic investigation and is mandatory for any patient with a chest injury. If the patient is haemodynamically stable, a posteroanterior (PA) view with the patient in an erect posture, is best followed by a lateral view if the situation allows. In other patients, in which the situation does not allow such delay, it should be performed at the bedside. It has been reported that only 50% of rib fractures may be evident on initial chest radiographs. Fractures of the first three ribs suggests significant kinetic energy release and should raise suspicion of aortic injury. Fractures of the lower four ribs should make one look carefully for intra-abdominal injuries, particularly the liver, spleen, and kidney. In addition, the radiograph may show evidence of fractures of the clavicle, sternum, and scapula, and may suggest the presence of flail chest.

A pneumothorax may be missed on a chest radiograph, particularly when there is significant surgical emphysema. Hence, whenever a pneumothorax is suspected, a chest radiograph in full expiration is ideally requested. This reduces the amount of air in the lung and therefore provides better contrast between the air in the pleura and the lung. A pneumothorax is identified on a radiograph by a rim of complete translucency, without any lung markings present on the lateral aspect (Figure 3.7). When the pneumothorax is large, the lung may collapse

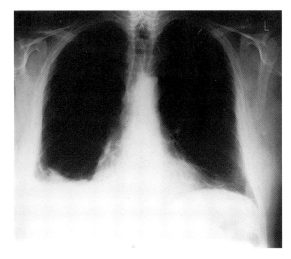

Figure 3.8 Erect chest radiograph showing blunting of the right costophrenic angle, suggestive of a haemothorax.

identified by increased density of the hemithorax, to the point of a "white-out", if massive (Figure 3.9). Further accumulation of blood will obliterate the diaphragmatic contour and, with a haemopneumothorax, a gas–fluid level may even be seen.

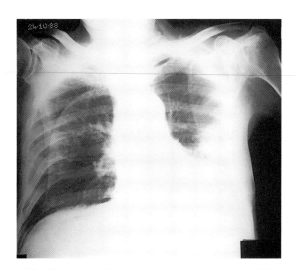

Figure 3.7 Plain chest radiograph showing an approximately 50% right-sided pneumothorax.

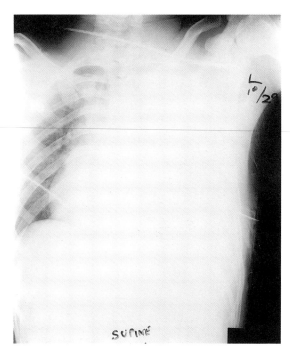

Figure 3.9 Supine chest radiograph showing a massive left-sided haemothorax.

towards the hilum with a shift of mediastinal structures towards the opposite side. It has been estimated that when the rim seen is 1 cm on the radiograph, the pneumothorax is about 10% of total lung volume. When the volume of the lung appears to occupy only half of the pleural space, it is referred to, by convention, as a 50% pneumothorax. It should be noted, however, that because of the contour of the chest, a 10% pneumothorax on radiograph may be closer to 50% loss of lung volume, and a 50% pneumothorax may be closer to 80 or 90% loss of lung volume. Therefore, treatment should be on a clinical basis, and the radiograph should simply act as a guide, or as confirmation.

In an erect chest radiograph, a haemothorax can be diagnosed by obliteration of the costophrenic angle, requiring at least 300–400 ml of blood in the pleural space (in the erect position) (Figure 3.8). In a supine patient, a haemothorax is

Pulmonary parenchymal injury can present with variable features on a chest radiograph. Pulmonary lacerations will manifest with the presence of a pneumothorax initially, and further features develop insidiously with the relevant injury. In addition there may be a well-defined opacity in the lung substance with convexity at the upper edge, which is indicative of intrapulmonary haemorrhage. Pulmonary contusion may appear in various ways, ranging from an infiltrate in the involved segment of the lung from diffuse haemorrhage into the lung tissue, to a complete "white-out" of the hemithorax. Serial chest radiographs are very important, as this condition can develop insidiously, and may eventually require ventilation of the patient. An infiltrate appearing in subsequent, serial chest films may also suggest aspiration pneumonia, and the

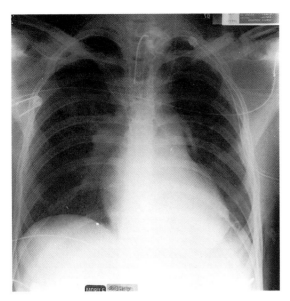

Figure 3.10 Plain chest radiograph demonstrating pneumomediastinum (clearly shown along the left border of the heart).

history is, once again, an important factor in distinguishing the two. A pulmonary haematoma is also often difficult to differentiate from pulmonary contusion because there will be a degree of extravasation of blood into the lung substance surrounding a haematoma. The contusion resolves first, leaving a sharply defined density, the haematoma, which then resolves slowly over several weeks. A pneumatocoele can easily be identified by a chest radiograph as a cyst-like cavity, and fluid or blood can collect in the space, which is then seen as a gas–fluid level.

In cases of blast injury, chest radiographs usually demonstrate diffuse infiltrates in both lung fields. There is often an associated pneumothorax or pneumomediastinum. In patients with traumatic asphyxia there will be infiltrates bilaterally owing to diffuse interstitial haemorrhage. These patients also frequently have radiographic evidence of pulmonary oedema.

Lung torsion is rare, but can present on serial chest radiographs as an area of increasing density. One report stated that the commonest finding was atelectasis secondary to bronchial obstruction, and pulmonary contusion with associated venous engorgement [14].

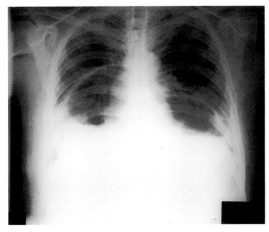

Figure 3.11 Plain chest radiograph showing bilateral diaphragmatic rupture.

Injuries of the trachea and bronchi can be suspected when any of the first four to five ribs are fractured and there is simultaneous radiographic evidence of mediastinal, pericardial, or subcutaneous air (Figure 3.10). It should be noted that 25% of patients with a tracheobronchial injury are reported to have a normal chest radiograph initially.

The plain chest radiograph has a low specificity for diagnosing penetrating diaphragmatic injuries. Following a penetrating injury, it is diagnostic in only 5% of cases. It can be helpful in the cases of blunt injury where a large defect has allowed herniation of abdominal contents which can clearly be seen in the thorax (Figure 3.11). The chest radiograph is found to be normal in about a third of cases with diaphragmatic injuries, and non-specific in nearly two-thirds of cases. Radiographic suspicions of diaphragmatic injury include haemothorax, elevated hemidiaphragm, blunted costophrenic angle, and a clear outline of a hollow viscus in the thorax, or an abnormally located nasogastric tube in the chest.

Computed axial tomography (CT)

This is becoming increasingly popular in the assessment of patients with major trauma for two main reasons: there is considerable expertise now available in the acute situation, and the information obtained may be very specific. The limitations of this procedure include higher expense and variable delay involved in arranging the procedure, as well as the unavoidable fact that the patient must be removed from direct resuscitative support. Hence, this procedure cannot be indicated in haemodynamically unstable patients, however potentially valuable the results. A screening body scan (wide spacing of slices) performed when a patient is undergoing an abdominal or cranial CT scan, can provide additional information regarding occult pneumothoraces, mediastinal haematomata and the presence of pericardial fluid. A minimal haemothorax may be recognised in the apex as a pleural cap. The detection of such a haemothorax is an indication for further monitoring of the pleural space for associated injuries, for example a ruptured diaphragm or an aortic disruption.

In patients with a tracheobronchial injury, a CT scan can identify small peribronchial or peritracheal accumulations of air that would suggest the possibility of rupture. It can readily diagnose a tracheal tear in patients with indwelling endotracheal tubes if the balloon is seen to herniate. Its usefulness in parenchymal lung injury is limited and, in most cases, will not add much new information to that provided by the chest radiograph. However, an area of consolidation can be assessed to demonstrate potential lack of viability of lung tissue, presence of air-filled cysts, and localised areas of parenchymal damage. This information may be helpful with management and monitoring.

In the presence of gross diaphragmatic rupture, the plain chest radiograph can readily detect abnormalities, but the presence of a major chest wall injury, a haemothorax, or a pneumothorax may obscure the diagnosis. CT scanning is useful in clarifying such pathology since it can demonstrate even small visceral hernias, which may otherwise not clinically declare themselves immediately.

Magnetic resonance imaging (MRI)

MRI is the most recent modality of investigation to prove useful in the assessment of thoracic structures. Its spatial resolution is equal to that of CT scanning, and an additional advantage is that solid structures can be differentiated from blood vessels without the use of intravenous contrast materials.

Its unique advantage is its capability for imaging in a variety of different planes, from only a single scan. Its use in identifying cardiac abnormalities is currently being evaluated, especially by synchronising the image with ECG monitoring. MRI has also been used in selected cases to some degree of success, to identify diaphragmatic defects. Though the quality of the image is far superior to other conventional techniques, the disadvantages include an extended period of patient isolation, and incompatibility with ventilators and intensive monitoring or resuscitation. The above factors severely limit its use for thoracic trauma, where the patient's condition is often unstable.

Endoscopy

Endoscopy can provide valuable information in patients with oesophageal or tracheobronchial injuries. It can, in fact, be the only diagnostic tool for confirmation of a suspected serious and life-threatening injury. The two main forms used in cases of thoracic trauma are bronchoscopy and oesophagoscopy.

Indications for bronchoscopy in patients who have sustained chest trauma are:

● haemoptysis;
● subcutaneous emphysema without pneumothorax;
● unresolving or massive airleak through chest drains;
● persistent pneumothorax or pneumomediastinum.

Specific conditions

Pneumothorax

Simple pneumothorax

Patients who have sustained a pneumothorax present with varying degrees of shortness of breath and sharp chest pain, particularly on inspiration. Cyanosis may be noticed in extreme cases, particularly in the instance of an undiagnosed tension pneumothorax, where the patient is *in extremis*. There are several clues to a suspected diagnosis of pneumothorax, not least of which is the history. On examination, the ipsilateral chest wall may show external evidence of blunt or penetrating trauma. Expansion of the chest will be limited and the trachea may be deviated away from the affected side if the pneumothorax is significant. On auscultation, air entry will be diminished or absent, and a hyper-resonant percussion note will be present. These signs and symptoms will be more pronounced in patients with a tension pneumothorax, who will soon start to show signs of profound haemodynamic deterioration, such as hypotension, tachycardia, and ultimately cardiac arrest. Similarly, a haemothorax will produce shortness of breath and all the previously mentioned signs of respiratory distress, as well as signs of hypovolaemia if the blood accumulates rapidly in the pleural space. It is very common for traumatic lung damage to result in both blood and air in the pleural space. This condition is a haemopneumothorax. Patients may also complain of a pleuritic type of chest pain owing to irritation of the parietal pleura by blood. Clinical examination will reveal reduced or absent breath sounds, with reduced chest expansion and a dull percussion note over areas with an accumulation of blood or clot. In addition, there may be evidence of mediastinal shift to the opposite side, if the haemothorax is large.

The aim of chest tube drainage is to relieve the symptoms and to encourage the lung to expand as quickly as possible, which will help in sealing minor or moderate air leaks by adherence to the chest wall. In many cases, surgery under general anaesthesia will subsequently be required for a range of procedures including debridement and stabilisation of the chest wall. Removal of the chest tube is best performed when there has been no air leak for at least 24 hours, even when coughing is present, and the lung is shown to be fully expanded on a chest radiograph. For removal, the patient is asked to perform the Valsalva manoeuvre after a full inspiration, and the tube is promptly pulled out (after the anchoring stitch is divided), with the skin edges approximated between the thumb and index finger. The mattress stitch, or purse-string, is now tied and the wound covered with a small dressing. A chest radiograph should be repeated in order to look for any air that may have entered the pleural cavity during removal, and for the possibility of recurrence of the pneumothorax.

Subcutaneous emphysema is usually associated with a traumatic pneumothorax and will usually resolve over a period of 7–10 days following satisfactory chest drainage (Figure 3.12). Occasionally, a part of the injured lung can get trapped in the chest wall, and acts as a one-way valve that decompresses into the subcutaneous tissue, producing massive and un-resolving subcutaneous emphysema. If the site of injury can be isolated, this can be treated by an incision over the area needing relief, then should be followed by the insertion of an intercostal drainage tube. When gross subcutaneous emphysema is from a mediastinal source, as can happen with major airway injuries, a suprasternal incision should be made to open the pretracheal space. This can dramatically decompress such a situation. Rarely, thoracotomy will be necessary to control a pneumothorax in the acute situation, especially when it is caused by a major airway injury. Indications for a thoracotomy for the treatment of a pneumothorax are:

● massive airleak with difficulty in maintaining adequate volume;
● failure of the lung to expand;
● persistent air leak for more than two weeks.

Tension pneumothorax

This is identified by:

● respiratory distress;
● tachycardia;

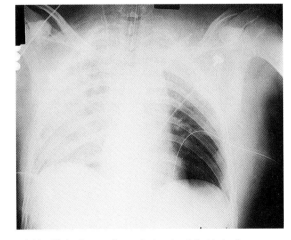

Figure 3.12 Plain chest radiograph showing left-sided subcutaneous (surgical) emphysema.

- tracheal deviation to the contralateral side;
- unilateral absence of breath sounds on the affected side;
- distended neck veins;
- cyanosis (in extreme cases).

In addition, a hypertympanic percussion note can be elicited over the chest wall on the affected side, although this is often difficult in practice in a noisy emergency room. A tension pneumothorax is a clinical diagnosis, not a radiological one, and requires immediate decompression by insertion of a large-bore needle or cannula into the second intercostal space in the midclavicular line anteriorly. A rush of air confirms the diagnosis and will usually save the patient's life. At this stage, the clinical picture should change, since the tension pneumothorax has been converted to a simple one. Following establishment of intravenous access, a routine intercostal drainage tube can then be formally inserted to relieve the pneumothorax thus formed.

Open pneumothorax (sucking chest wound)

This is readily diagnosed in a patient who shows signs of respiratory distress in the presence of a large chest wall defect and it is usually clinically obvious. The mechanism and pathophysiology have been described earlier.

In patients with an open pneumothorax and compromised respiratory function, the wound should immediately be covered with a gauze dressing, taped only on three sides, creating a one-way flutter valve to prevent the development of a tension pneumothorax. An intercostal chest tube must be inserted immediately into a relatively clean site, usually away from the wound, to allow re-inflation of the lung, following which the wound can be cleaned and redressed with a totally occlusive dressing. After completion of this procedure, a chest radiograph is repeated to verify the tube position and to check for any residual pockets of air or fluid, which should be addressed if present. Formal surgical closure can be undertaken when the patient's condition is stable.

Haemothorax

Any haemothorax diagnosed on an erect chest radiograph should be treated by intercostal tube drainage, as the amount of blood required to produce such a radiographic finding will be at least 500 ml. A chest tube will also allow monitoring of the amount of blood loss and, as long as a large calibre (32F or larger) tube is used, will prevent the development of a clotted haemothorax with its associated sequelae such as fibrothorax and/or empyema. The chest tube should be inserted through the fifth interspace in the anterior axillary line. Failure of blood to drain completely would suggest either a clotted haemothorax, or a subpleural accumulation of blood, and this will require a formal thoracotomy if significant, because large amounts will not resolve completely. Thoracotomy is also indicated for haemothorax in the presence of:

- hypovolaemic shock with >1000 ml of drainage immediately after insertion of the chest tube;
- total blood loss >1500 ml, even when not associated with other signs;
- continued blood loss of >200 ml/h for 4 hours.

The presence of a continued bleed of approximately 100 ml/h after the initial drainage may suggest a clotting abnormality, possibly from large volume blood transfusions or even disseminated intravascular coagulation (DIC). If suspected, this should be investigated immediately and rectified

accordingly with platelets and/or coagulation factors. Chest drains may be considered for removal if the drainage is less than 100 ml in a 12-hour period, there is no air leak, and the chest radiograph is clear.

A *massive haemothorax* is defined as the loss of 1500 ml or more of blood into the chest cavity, or the loss of 200 ml/h of blood for four consecutive hours. The presenting signs are hypovolaemic shock associated with absence of breath sounds and dull percussion note on the affected side of the chest. The neck veins may either be collapsed from hypovolaemia, or distended from mechanical effects of the volume load in the hemithorax. The initial management comprises simultaneous restoration of the intravascular volume deficit, and decompression of the chest cavity. Fluids should be administered rapidly (dependent on premorbid medical conditions, of course) through more than one large-calibre venous access lines. The choice of fluids used is debatable, but both crystalloid and colloid infusions will suffice until type-specific or cross-matched blood is available. A large-bore chest drain (32F or larger) should be used to prevent the possibility of clot blocking the tube. Drainage should be carefully monitored, as sudden "dumping" of a large volume via the drain may relieve a paradoxically beneficial, tamponading effect on the bleeding source, and cause profound hypotension. If there is continuing blood loss through the drain, of the quantity mentioned above, exploratory thoracotomy is indicated. This should be performed by an experienced general surgeon, or ideally a cardiothoracic surgeon if one is available.

Chest wall injuries

Flail chest

Flail chest is recognised by paradoxical movement of the chest wall. It is due to an isolated portion of the chest wall losing bony continuity with the rest of the thoracic cage. The flail segment, if large, causes severe disruption to normal chest wall function. In these patients, acute respiratory distress is usually due to the associated lung contusion which frequently accompanies such an injury. The result of the paradoxical movement and an underlying lung contusion can be a severe hypoxia, which may be further exacerbated by blood loss from rib fractures. Diagnosis is often not immediately apparent, particularly if there is splinting of the chest wall. It can sometimes be suspected by elicitation of fracture crepitus and uncoordinated respiratory movements, and confirmed on a chest radiograph (which in itself may be unreliable). If there is an associated pneumothorax, it is drained immediately. The basis of treatment is to combine full expansion of the lung with good oxygenation.

However, progressive hypoxia in spite of oxygen supplementation, often requires intubation and support with mechanical ventilation. Exhaustion, hypoxia, and associated injuries may also be indications for ventilatory support. Adequate analgesia is essential in these patients to allow self-ventilation and the ability to cope with as much active physiotherapy as possible. Fluid balance is a particularly difficult task in patients with lung contusion, because the injured lung is particularly susceptible to fluid overload and also the undercorrection of hypovolaemia. Patients who have sustained a flail chest are initially managed with adequate analgesia and early mobilisation. The use of sandbags or external traction to reduce paradoxical movement should be discouraged as it will restrict chest expansion and limit mobility. Use of "internal splinting" by means of positive pressure ventilation to stabilise the flail segment is the treatment of choice for these injuries.

Mechanical ventilation is often required when there is significant associated pulmonary contusion leading to respiratory failure, which can develop insidiously at any time after the injury.

Rib injuries

A "simple" rib fracture, without injury to the lungs or other intrathoracic structures, is common following many trivial injuries, especially in elderly persons suffering from osteoporosis. Simple rib fractures require adequate analgesia for satisfactory management. Pain relief is very important, especially in elderly patients, to ensure a normal respiratory pattern, otherwise shallow breathing with ineffective coughing will lead to atelectasis, infection, and ultimately respiratory failure, if not recognised. Strapping of the chest wall was originally believed to provide pain relief by immobilising the fractured ends of the ribs, but since it will not allow movements to occur in a normal plane, this practice has been abandoned [15]. In addition, it can promote atelectasis by restricting the expansion of the lung. Non-opiate analgesics, either oral or parenteral, should be used in these patients. Opiates can adversely affect ventilation and the clearance of secretions by their actions on central respiratory pathways in the brain. If the pain relief is not satisfactory, intercostal nerve blockade is sometimes considered. Intercostal block is performed with 0.25–0.5% bupivacaine, and is infiltrated beneath the inferior borders of all the fractured ribs, plus one rib above and one below, to prevent pain from the overlap of innervated fields. It should be administered posteriorly at the level of the angle of the ribs. If the patient has sustained costochondral separation and/or sternal fractures, the local anaesthetic should be instilled parasternally beneath the anterior aspect of the ribs: 1–2 ml of the anaesthetic agent injected into each space is sufficient.

Patients who are admitted to the hospital with a chest wall injury as part of their injury complex, and have pain as a primary problem, are optimally managed with epidural analgesia. In a randomised trial, treatment with epidural (compared to intravenous fentanyl) improved maximum inspiratory pressure and vital capacity, with an increased Pa_{O_2} and a reduced Pa_{CO_2}. Contraindications for this procedure include open wounds in the midline posteriorly and bleeding or coagulation disorders. Fractures of the sternum are similarly managed by the optimisation of pain relief, but when the fragments are unstable or grossly uneven, operative reduction and wiring are necessary to facilitate normal breathing patterns.

Operative stabilisation of rib fractures can be undertaken when a thoracotomy is required for other lesions, and/or the patient is having a general anaesthetic for another procedure. Fractures can be stabilised using Kirschner wires, wire sutures, staples, and steel plates. In the experience of one group [15], this procedure was performed in 12 patients without parenchymal injury or brain injury, and it was found that these patients spent an average of eight days less on the ventilator than patients who did not have operative stabilisation. In general, however, practice is moving away from stabilisation.

Prognoses of chest wall injuries are variable. In one report [16], it was found that a poor prognosis in cases of trauma to the chest wall was determined by the severity of the injury, other associated injuries, blood transfusion, presence of bilateral flail chest, and an age >50 years. In another report [17], long-term disability, including chest tightness, chest wall pain, dyspnoea, abnormal spirometry, and poor return to gainful employment, were seen in >50% of patients with significant flail chest who had required ventilation. Operative stabilisation of the chest wall may be performed in an attempt to minimise these long-term sequelae in appropriate cases.

Diaphragmatic injuries

Blunt injury of the diaphragm results from a forceful blow to the abdomen or thorax that produces a sudden increase in pressure differential and a burst type of injury. These tears are radial and often lead to herniation of abdominal contents into the chest, adversely affecting respiration. Automobile accidents are the commonest cause of such lesions, side impact collisions being three times more likely to produce diaphragmatic ruptures than frontal collisions. Frontal impact with a severe thoracic blow results in a downward burst type of injury. All these injuries select the weakest points in the diaphragm, which are the embryological points of attachment, especially in the costosternal or paravertebral regions.

Blunt rupture of the diaphragm is uncommon and the reported incidence is from 0.08 to 3% [18]. The left hemidiaphragm is more prone to disruption from blunt trauma than the right, probably owing to the dispersion of force by the dome of the liver on the right [19]. In 1968, rupture of the right diaphragm was reviewed [20] and it was noticed that autopsy studies of trauma victims who died in the field demonstrated an equal frequency of right- and left-sided diaphragmatic rupture. As the right-sided injuries were usually more severe, with injury to other organs (probably the liver), many of these victims did not survive long enough to reach hospital for diagnosis and treatment. The precise mechanism of blunt diaphragmatic injury is not well understood, although a pleuroperitoneal pressure differential appears to be required to produce the typical damage. The proposed factors which make the diaphragm vulnerable to such a bursting type of injury may be the fact that the diaphragm has a lower compliance when loaded with a non-uniform pressure gradient, and the central tendon is inextensible. Kearney and colleagues identified a significant correlation between the direction of impact, the intravehicular position of the victim at time of impact and the side of the diaphragm ruptured [21].

Penetrating diaphragmatic injuries are often missed as they are usually far less symptomatic on presentation. It has been reported that 19% of thoracoabdominal stab wounds will penetrate the diaphragm. Again, the left diaphragm is more often involved than the right, but this is probably because most assailants are right-handed and attack face to face. The important thing to note about penetrating injuries of the diaphragm is that a small tear may enlarge slowly, even over many years, resulting in abdominal visceral herniation into the chest at a much later date. Most penetrating injuries of the diaphragm are initially asymptomatic. The most suggestive sign of diaphragmatic injury is the proximity of the entry wound on the surface. Two groups [20,22] defined specific anatomical zones with graded probabilities of diaphragmatic injury. The main areas of concern are below the fourth intercostal space anteriorly, below the sixth space laterally, and below the eighth space posteriorly. The symptoms can range from shoulder or ear pain, pleuritic chest pain, tachycardia, dyspnoea, an acute abdomen, or drainage of bile, enteric contents, or urine from the chest tube. Demetriades et al. [22], in their study on penetrating injuries of the diaphragm, however, claimed that there is no real correlation between the site of entry and the presence of diaphragmatic injury.

Blunt injuries and larger tears to the diaphragm are usually associated with injury to other organs, and the principal symptoms relate to the organs involved. In addition, herniation of the intra-abdominal contents into the thorax is often seen in patients with blunt disruption, clinical manifestations of which are shortness of breath from bowel occupying the thoracic cavity and compressing lung, and occasionally acute abdomen from strangulation of bowel loops through the tear.

Diagnostic peritoneal lavage (DPL) is often used as a safe diagnostic tool in patients with diaphragmatic injury. However, the lavage is often negative when there is a combination of abdominal organ and diaphragmatic injury, in fact more so than when there is abdominal injury alone. This could be due to the fact that an associated diaphragmatic injury directs the flow of blood towards the chest with its negative intrathoracic pressure, leaving the abdomen relatively dry. It is considered, therefore, that a poor quantity return of lavage fluid may be taken as a positive sign of diaphragmatic injury. One study [23] found a 29% false negative peritoneal lavage rate in blunt diaphragmatic injuries (with the use of $100\,000$ red cells/cm^3 as a positive lavage) and a 100% false negative rate in those cases where the diaphragm was injured in isolation.

Other tests for diagnosing diaphragmatic injuries include contrast gastrointestinal studies, contrast and pneumo-peritoneography, and radiolabelled peritoneography. Contrast gastrointestinal studies are sensitive, only if herniation of a hollow viscus into the thorax has already occurred. This will give a false negative result with any peritoneography studies, as the herniated viscus will block the defect. When other methods have failed to identify the damage, intra-abdominal instillation of technetium sulphur colloid may be a helpful diagnostic technique.

Diaphragmatic injuries, however trivial, should always be surgically repaired, otherwise there is the permanent possibility of incarceration or strangulation of a bowel loop. Even more likely is the progressive widening of the defect, with movement of bowel into and occupying space that should contain lung. This may develop unnoticed over years, until symptoms (usually respiratory) present. If a diaphragmatic injury is identified during diagnostic studies before laparotomy, the best approach is the vertical midline incision. This allows excellent exposure of the injured hemidiaphragm and the contralateral diaphragm, and allows for diagnosis and repair of any other intra-abdominal damage. If there is an associated chest injury requiring thoracotomy, a thoracoabdominal incision is most suited; it allows optimum access to both cavities, and enables the diaphragmatic repair to take place from whichever side is most appropriate.

Tracheobronchial tree

Injuries to the tracheobronchial tree are usually only seen in major chest trauma. The cervical trachea is usually involved, and the mechanism of injury is most commonly penetrating. Severity of penetrating trauma depends upon the agent involved, its trajectory and, most importantly, its velocity (see Chapter 22). Blunt trauma can, however, also result in tracheobronchial injury (see box). Most patients with a major airway injury will die at scene as a result of asphyxia, aspiration of blood, or intrapulmonary haemorrhage. However, when the transection, even if complete, becomes sealed off by soft tissues, survival is possible. Even in these instances, it must be remembered that patients can succumb to late effects such as infection, granuloma formation, and stenosis. Airway injuries usually produce significant surgical emphysema secondary to pneumomediastinum or pneumothorax. They may also produce pneumopericardium or haemothorax.

Treatment of tracheobronchial injuries depends upon the site of trauma. Injuries to the cervical trachea can be approached through a cervical collar incision or an oblique incision over the medial border of the sternocleidomastoid muscle. Injuries to the left side of the distal trachea or the left main bronchus need a left thoracotomy for satisfactory and safe access. Most other tracheal injuries are easily approached through a right thoracotomy. Occasionally a partial or complete

---

Non-penetrating causes of tracheobronchial trauma

- A direct blow to the hyperextended neck.
- Sudden forceful compression of the chest in the anteroposterior direction, resulting in a simultaneous increase in its lateral diameter. The lungs, being in contact with the parietal pleura, are dragged laterally resulting in traction forces on the carina, causing a laceration or transection of the trachea or a mainstem bronchus. These injuries nearly always occur within 2 cm of the carina.
- A sudden increase in intratracheal pressure against a closed glottis results in linear rupture of the tracheobronchial tree because the greatest wall tension is generated in the airways with the largest diameter (Laplace's law).
- Acceleration or deceleration injury produces a shearing force on the tracheobronchial tree between the relatively stationary areas of the cricoid cartilage and the carina.

---

median sternotomy may have to be undertaken, especially when injuries to other mediastinal structures are suspected. Tracheal lacerations are usually sutured by a direct single layer repair (after the edges have been trimmed and cleaned with 3/0 or 4/0 vicryl or PDS. Rarely, resection of a segment of trachea may be necessary owing to extensive devitalisation. Up to 6 cm of trachea may be excised and joined by end-to-end anastomosis after mobilisation, without compromising the blood supply. This may require cervical dissection, mediastinal and hilar dissection, division of the inferior pulmonary ligament, and occasionally incision into the pericardium. It is important to have senior anaesthetic input for treatment of these injuries, as the administration of general anaesthesia may be technically exacting.

Pulmonary injuries

The incidence of pulmonary injuries following all forms of chest trauma can vary between 50 and 68% [24–26]. There are several specific types of parenchymal lesions seen resulting from chest injury, and a number of conditions causing impaired gas exchange without affecting the parenchyma itself.

Pulmonary contusion

Pulmonary contusion is defined as haemorrhage in the lung parenchyma owing to direct damage from external trauma. The haemorrhage is often localised and adjacent to the site of rib fractures, but not always, and care must be taken to assess the clinical situation and radiographs for evidence of this condition. Pulmonary contusion secondary to blunt trauma is often associated with a pneumothorax and/or haemothorax.

Prognosis with pulmonary contusion is very variable. When the contusion is limited to small areas of lung, resolution of the infiltrates usually occurs within a week or two, but extensive injuries will compromise pulmonary function significantly and will require ventilatory support. Fluid resuscitation in pulmonary contusion is a paradox and presents management difficulties, since the damaged lung is very prone to fluid overload [27]. We would advocate extreme caution in these injuries, in spite of published work to the contrary [28]. Though initial experiments have shown the benefits of steroids in pulmonary contusion, it is not suported by subsequent results [29]. Other studies have shown that bacterial clearance in contused lungs is further suppressed by steroids, and that large doses of steroids may aggravate pulmonary failure after hypovolaemic shock. The recommended management of pulmonary contusion, therefore, will be aggressive treatment of any associated injuries and cautious crystalloid and blood administration to restore normal tissue perfusion, with selective application of mechanical ventilation based on the presence of associated injuries and poor gas exchange. Ventilatory support may be indicated in many instances (see box).

In the Vietnam war, Fischer and associates [30], concluded that pulmonary resection in patients with severe contusion lessened morbidity and improved survival. This remains to be confirmed in civilian practice.

Blast injuries, with their diffuse pulmonary parenchymal damage can lead to respiratory failure requiring mechanical ventilation, probably with positive end expiratory pressure (PEEP) to maintain satisfactory oxygenation. In extreme cases, extracorporeal gas exchange mechanisms such as extracorporeal membrane oxygenation (ECMO) and $ECCO_2R$, may be considered, although results under these circumstances are poor, and it is generally a salvage procedure which requires cardiothoracic surgical and anaesthetic input.

Indications for ventilation in pulmonary contusion

- Clinical respiratory insufficiency (tachypnoea >30 min, increased work of breathing and fatigue)
- Laboratory evidence of ventilatory insufficiency or hypoxaemia (Pa_{O_2} <60 mmHg or $F_{I_{O_2}}$ >0.45)
- Multiple organ injuries including head injury and/or circulatory shock

---

Aspiration

The term "aspiration pneumonia" can cover a variety of different clinical syndromes, but for the purposes of this chapter we shall deal only with the aspiration of gastric contents or pharyngeal matter associated with trauma. The airway is normally protected from foreign matter by an interaction of anatomical and physiological mechanisms, but if these are disrupted, aspiration may ensue. The most common cause for disruption of these mechanisms is depressed consciousness, such as after a severe head injury. There are a number of predisposing factors that may heighten an individual's risk to aspiration in the event of a head injury, and these should not be overlooked [31]. They include advanced age, laryngeal pathology, gastro-oesophageal reflux disease, gastrointestinal ileus, and bowel obstruction. Of course, factors that contribute to a decreased level of consciousness must also be considered. These include alcohol and narcotic ingestion, and exposure to toxic fumes.

The important steps in the development of aspiration pneumonia are the introduction of foreign (usually gastric) contents into the airways, and the subsequent development of pulmonary infection (pneumonitis). The pneumonitis may be infective, from the inhalation of microbial flora, or chemical from aspiration of gastric acid. There is generally a contribution from both aetiologies, but the role of hydrochloric acid in the development of the subsequent aspiration syndromes must be emphasised. The lower the pH, the worse and more immediate the effects, and animal models have shown that a pH of 1.5 is associated with immediate damage to the respiratory epithelium [32]. Such damage is always associated with secondary infection from dysfunction of normal defence mechanisms. The quantity is also important, small volume aspirations being associated with an insidious onset of asthmatic symptoms after 24 to 48 hours. Large volume aspirates are much more serious, and usually result in a systemic cardiorespiratory response. The acid damages the alveolar capillary barrier, increasing permeability, or "leakiness".

This disease process has been extensively studied, both in animal models and in clinical observations, and the outcome usually falls into one of four groups [33,34] (see box).

Management can present many problems, but is essentially supportive. Bronchoscopy and lavage is helpful, and in the majority of situations, intubation and ventilation is necessary. Fluid resuscitation can present a particular problem, since large volumes are often required, particularly if there are concurrent injuries. This needs to be weighed up against the fact that the lungs are now "leaky" and susceptible to pulmonary oedema much more readily. Early antibiotic therapy is not usually required, since the gastric acid lowers the pH to the point of "sterility", indeed the results of trials have not demonstrated any benefit from their use [35]. If, after a few days, purulent sputum is produced, along with the appearance of a pyrexia, superimposed infective pneumonia must be suspected, and appropriate antibiotic therapy commenced.

Potential outcomes of aspiration

1. Rapid death from refractory respiratory failure within days.
2. Progressive improvement to recovery within days.
3. Initial stabilisation followed by secondary bacterial pneumonia.
4. Prolonged ARDS with multiple organ dysfunction syndrome.

Acute respiratory distress syndrome (ARDS)

Acute respiratory distress syndrome (ARDS) has been defined as an acute arterial hypoxaemia [36]. It presents as a progressively worsening respiratory failure, usually resulting from gastric aspiration, or capillary leak from shock or severe sepsis [37]. It should always be considered as a potential problem in the multiple trauma victim, particularly those who have had a significant chest injury, or who are mechanically ventilated. It should also be noted that it is a condition that can present insidiously at any time after the accident, and it is not uncommon for a previously apparently well patient to rapidly develop respiratory distress. The commonest presentation usually has sepsis as its aetiology, and presents with worsening hypoxia associated with patchy radiographic changes 24 to 72 hours after the injury or event. Several clinical stages have been identified, from the early appearances of pulmonary oedema to the later stages of respiratory failure [38].

ARDS is a condition with an extremely high morbidity and mortality and must be recognised at the earliest possible stage. Patients who develop ARDS have a very high risk of developing multiple organ failure, which contributes to the high rate of mortality. Although extracorporeal membrane oxygenation (ECMO) has been suggested and well tried as a method of managing these patients, no studies have yet demonstrated it to have an advantage over conventional ventilatory support [39]. Management is largely supportive and, although much research has gone into finding an intervention that will interrupt the pathophysiological sequence leading to its development, there is still no solution.

Pulmonary laceration

This is defined as a tear in the pulmonary parenchyma and is the predominant feature following penetrating injury. Blunt injury can also result in laceration when great force is involved, leading to penetration of the lung by fractured rib ends or bursting tears from a severe crush injury.

Most pulmonary parenchymal injuries produce a pneumothorax and/or a haemothorax, which should be managed by the insertion of an intercostal drainage tube, as mentioned. In cases of penetrating trauma, about 5% of patients with a pulmonary laceration will require formal operative treatment for persistent bleeding, clotted haemothorax, persistent air leak, or failure of the lung to expand. In addition, significant haemoptysis suggests deep lung laceration involving airways, and is an indication for surgery. About 50% of patients requiring a thoracotomy following pulmonary laceration can be managed by simply suturing the laceration, with or without plication. Other cases require formal pulmonary resection, particularly when associated with haemoptysis and major vascular or bronchial injury. In some instances, for example when there is heavy bleeding and tissue damage, a lobectomy or pneumonectomy is the easiest option, and may be life-saving.

Embolism

Air embolism with hypotension and arrhythmia or cardiac arrest also suggests a severe injury and requires operative intervention. When air embolism is suspected, the hilum should immediately be occluded with a vascular clamp or tourniquet after the inferior pulmonary ligament has been divided. Under these circumstances, some surgeons have advocated the use of a hilar snare, which can give better haemostasis without injury to delicate hilar structures. Following this, the systemic arterial pressure should be raised with the use of pressor agents such as dopamine or adrenaline, to facilitate the flushing out of any air that may have entered the coronary arteries. Temporary use of systemic anticoagulation with heparin may be useful, as clotting has been shown to aggravate the vascular obstructive problems associated with coronary air embolism. Depending on the damage to hilar structures, lobectomy or even pneumonectomy may be required in extensive lacerations, as mentioned above.

Haematoma and pneumatocoele

A pulmonary haematoma is a collection of blood in a space within the lung tissue. It is usually associated with contusion of variable extent surrounding it, and frequently with pulmonary laceration. As with any haematoma, it is particularly prone to infection.

A pneumatocoele is a cyst-like cavity that is filled with air, and usually results from a small bronchial injury associated with disruption of the lung parenchyma. It increases in size on positive pressure ventilation (PPV). It can frequently produce haemoptysis and, if it becomes infected, will produce an abscess.

Pulmonary haematomata can be managed "conservatively", except when associated with severe haemoptysis, when they may require segmentectomy or lobectomy. Pneumatocoeles can similarly be managed by conservative means. In both of these conditions, persisting haemoptysis may necessitate pulmonary resection.

Asphyxia

Traumatic asphyxia is produced by severe or sudden compression of the chest against a closed glottis, resulting in a sudden pressure rise in the venous system of the upper body. This will lead to massive engorgement of these veins with extravasation of blood into the surrounding tissues. Simultaneously, diffuse interstitial haemorrhage occurs within the substance of the lungs, compromising oxygenation, and leading to respiratory distress.

Torsion

Lung torsion is a very rare form of pulmonary injury with only three trauma-linked cases reported in the literature. It has been postulated that sudden compression of the chest wall may displace the lower lobe (blood-filled) in an upward direction, tearing the inferior pulmonary ligament. The upper lobe, which is lighter, gets sucked into the vacuum space created in the lower hemithorax, thus resulting in the injury.

Summary

Although 25% of all trauma deaths in the UK directly result from a chest injury, the majority of cases can be adequately treated by nothing more complex than chest needle or drain insertion. It is crucial that no further harm is done to the patients who make it thus far. As we have discussed, there is a wide variety of conditions that can affect the pulmonary apparatus, each arising from a range of aetiologies. Hypoxia remains the common denominator in the majority of these, and has several contributing factors. Every effort must be made to prevent the development of hypoxia, and if it does occur, to remedy the situation immediately. Chest injuries are often concurrent with damage to other body systems, that frequently present with a more dramatic external manifestation. In such situations it is essential to stick to the "ABC" system and not get side-tracked, since problems with "Airway" and "Breathing" will kill the patient most rapidly. Adoption of a rationalised, standard approach will allow events to become stabilised, and progression to definitive care.

References

1. American College of Surgeons, Committee on Trauma. Thoracic trauma, in *Advanced Trauma Life Support Program for Physicians: Instructor Manual*. Chicago: ACS, 1993.
2. Lo Cicero J, Mattox KL. Epidemiology of chest trauma. *Surg Clin N Amer* 1989;**69**:15.
3. Besson A, Segesser F, in *Colour atlas of chest trauma and associated injuries*, vol. 1 (Oradell, ed.). New York: NJ Medical Economics, 1983.
4. Irving M, in *ABC of major trauma* (Skinner D, Driscoll P, Earlam R, eds). London: BMJ Publications, 1991.
5. Bastacky J, Hayes TL, Schmidt BV. Lung structure as revealed by microdissection. *Am Rev Respir Dis* 1983;**128**(S7).

6. Fraser RG, Pare JAP, Pare PD. *Diagnosis of diseases of the chest.* (3rd edn). Philadelphia: WB Saunders, 1988.

7. Weibel ER. *Morphometry of the human lung.* Berlin: Springer-Verlag, 1963.

8. Muscedere J, Zamel N, Slutsky AS. Physiology, in (Griffith Pearson F, ed.) *Thoracic surgery*, vol. 1. New York: Churchill Livingstone, 1995.

9. Rutherford RB, Hurt Jr HH, Brickman RD. The pathophysiology of progressive tension pneumothorax. *J Trauma* 1968;**8**:212.

10. Gustman P, Yenger L, Warner A. Immediate cardiovascular effects of tension pneumothorax. *Am Rev Resp Dis* 1983;**127**:171.

11. Richardson JD, Woods D, Johanson WG. Lung bacterial clearance following pulmonary contusion. *Surgery* 1979;**86**:730.

12. Newman RJ, Jones IS. A prospective study of 413 car occupants with chest injury. *J Trauma* 1984;**24**:129.

13. Trinkle JK, Richardson JD. Management of flail chest without mechanical ventilation. *Ann Thoracic Surg* 1975;**19**:355.

14. Stratmeirer EH, Barry JW. Torsion of the lung following thoracic trauma. *Radiology* 1954;**62**:726.

15. Sheikh AA, Culbertson CB. Emergency department thoracotomy in children: rationale for selective application. *J Trauma* 1993;**34**:323.

16. Shorr RN, Rodriguez A, Inchek MC. Blunt chest trauma in the elderly. *J Trauma* 1989;**29**:234.

17. Wilson SE, Murray C, Antonenko DR. Non-penetrating thoracic injuries. *Surg Clin N Amer* 1977;**57**:17.

18. Boulanger BR, Mirvis SE, Rodriguez A. Magnetic resonance imaging in traumatic diaphragmatic rupture: case reports. *J Trauma* 1992;**32**:89.

19. Carter BN, Giuseffi J, Felson B. Traumatic diaphragmatic hernia. *Am J Radiol* 1951;**65**:56.

20. Epstein LI, Lempke RE. Rupture of the right hemidiaphragm due to blunt trauma. *J Trauma* 1968;**8**:19.

21. Kearney PA, Rouhana SW, Burney RE. Blunt rupture of the diaphragm: mechanism, diagnosis, and treatment. *Ann Emerg Med* 1988;**18**:828.

22. Demetriades D, Kakoyiannis S, Parekh D. Penetrating injuries of the diaphragm. *Br J Surg* 1988;**75**:824.

23. Freeman T, Fisher RP. Inadequacy of peritoneal lavage in diagnosing acute diaphragmatic rupture. *J Trauma* 1976;**16**:538.

24. Moghissi K. Laceration of the lung following blunt trauma. *Thorax* 1971;**26**:223.

25. McNamara JJ, Messersmith JK, Dunn RA. Thoracic injuries in combat casualties in Vietnam. *Ann Thorac Surg* 1970;**10**:389.

26. Graham JM, Mattox KL, Beal AC. Penetrating trauma of the lung. *J Trauma* 1979;**19**:665.

27. Hyde JAJ, Rooney SJ, Graham TR. Fluid management in thoracic trauma. *Hospital Update* 1996;**22**:448–52.

28. Bongard FS, Lewis FR. Crystalloid resuscitation of patients with pulmonary contusion. *Am J Surg* 1984;**148**:145.

29. Franz JL, Richardson JD, Grover FL. Effect of methylprednisolone sodium succinate on experimental pulmonary contusion. *J Thorac Cardiovasc Surg* 1974;**68**:842.

30. Fischer RP, Geiger JP, Guernsey JM. Pulmonary resection for severe pulmonary contusion secondary to high velocity missile wounds. *J Trauma* 1974;**14**:293.

31. Hodder RV, Cameron R, Todd TRJ. Infections, in (Griffith Pearson F, ed.) *Thoracic trauma*. New York: Churchil Livingstone, 1995.

32. Wynne JW, Ramphal R, Hood CI. Tracheal mucosal damage after aspiration: a scanning electron microscope study. *Am Rev Respir Dis* 1981;**124**:728.

33. Bynum LJ, Pierce AK. Pulmonary aspiration of gastric contents. *Am Rev Respir Dis* 1976;**114**:1129.

34. De Paso WJ. Aspiration pneumonia. *Clin Chest Med* 1991;**12**:269.

35. Murray HW. Antimicrobial therapy in pulmonary aspiration. *Am J Med* 1979;**66**:188.

36. Ashbaugh DG, Bigelow DB, Petty TL, Levine BE. Acute respiratory distress in adults. *Lancet* 1967;**2**:319–23.

37. Lennartz H. Extracorporeal venovenous long-term bypass for lung assist (ELA) in adults, in (Lewis CT, Graham TR, eds.) *Mechanical circulatory support*. London: Edward Arnold, 1995.

38. Moore F. Clinical pathologic review of ARDS, in (Moore FD, Lyons JH, eds.) *Post-traumatic pulmonary insufficiency*. Philadelphia: WB Saunders, 1969.

39. Zapal WW. Extracorporeal membrane oxygenation in severe acute respiratory failure: a randomised prospective study. *J Am Med Ass* 1979;**242**:2193.

4 Mediastinal trauma

Jonathon A. J. Hyde
Cardiothoracic Registrar, Queen Elizabeth Hospital, Birmingham

Ashok Shetty
Cardiothoracic Registrar, Queen Elizabeth Hospital, Birmingham

Timothy R. Graham
Cardiothoracic Consultant, Queen Elizabeth Hospital, Birmingham

---

OBJECTIVES

- To describe applied mediastinal anatomy.
- To discuss pathophysiology and mechanism of injury to the mediastinum.
- To describe imaging techniques and other investigations available for mediastinal injury.
- To discuss the specific conditions associated with mediastinal injury.

Trauma to the chest is associated with a very high morbidity and mortality, and must be taken seriously and with a high index of suspicion, even when external features are absent.

The incidence of thoracic trauma and deaths associated with it has been mentioned previously. As with pulmonary injuries, the aetiology of mediastinal injuries can be divided into blunt and penetrating. Both of these can be caused by a wide variety of factors, and may vary substantially in severity and presentation. The heart itself is always surrounded with a certain amount of mystique, which is understandable, but should not mean that it is avoided or ignored. All medical practitioners exposed to trauma should be able to manage and stabilise a patient with a cardiac or great vessel injury until experienced, specialised help arrives. This does not require any great skill or expertise, and can usually be attained by simple measures alone, the failure to perform which may have tragic consequences

Applied anatomy

As with pulmonary trauma, anatomical knowledge and understanding of the structural relationships is vital. The mediastinum is the area extending from the sternum anteriorly to the spine posteriorly, and contains all the thoracic viscera except the lungs. It is divided into distinct zones for anatomical purposes (Figure 4.1). These are:

- *superior mediastinum* (above the upper level of the pericardium)
- the lower portion beneath this layer, divided into the:

- *anterior mediastinum*
- *middle mediastinum* (containing the pericardial sac and its contents)
- *posterior mediastinum.*

The important components are discussed separately.

Heart and pericardium

The heart lies in the middle mediastinum, extending from the level of the third costal cartilage to the xiphisternal junction (Figure 4.2). The majority of the anterior surface of the heart is represented by the right atrium and its auricular appendage

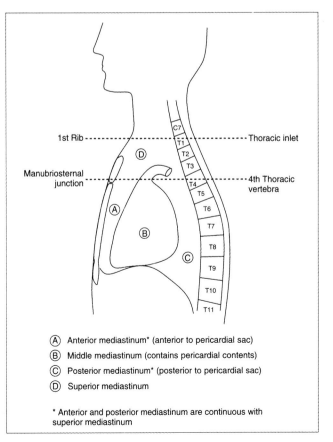

(A) Anterior mediastinum* (anterior to pericardial sac)
(B) Middle mediastinum (contains pericardial contents)
(C) Posterior mediastinum* (posterior to pericardial sac)
(D) Superior mediastinum

* Anterior and posterior mediastinum are continuous with superior mediastinum

Figure 4.1 Divisions of the mediastinum.

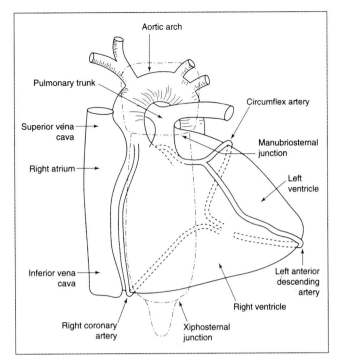

Figure 4.2 The heart from anteriorly with the sternum super-imposed.

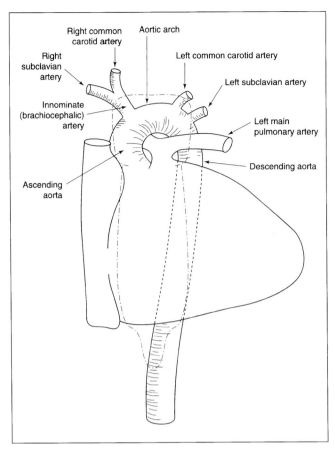

Figure 4.3 The thoracic aorta with its relationship to the heart, sternum and great vessels.

superiorly, and the right ventricle inferiorly. The aorta emerges from the cranial aspect and crosses to the left as the arch. The pulmonary artery extends cranially and bifurcates in the concavity of the aortic arch. The left pulmonary artery is attached to the concavity of the arch of the aorta, just distal to the origin of the left subclavian artery. This attachment is the ligamentum arteriosum, the obliterated remnant of the fetal ductus arteriosus. The pericardium invests the heart, is attached to the diaphragm inferiorly and extends along the right and left pulmonary arteries.

Aorta and great vessels

The thoracic aorta is divided into three parts: the ascending aorta, the arch, and the descending aorta (Figure 4.3). The ascending aorta is intrapericardial for most of its length. The aortic arch begins at the level of the origin of the innominate artery and ends at the origin of the left subclavian artery. The descending aorta then continues to the diaphragm, which it traverses at the level of the 12th thoracic vertebra. The innominate artery passes from the proximal aortic arch and runs superolaterally to the right, posterior to the innominate vein. It branches behind the right sternoclavicular joint into the right common carotid and right subclavian arteries. The left common carotid artery and the left subclavian artery are the other great vessels.

Oesophagus

The oesophagus is approximately 25 cm long, extending from the pharynx to the stomach, and is the narrowest part of the alimentary tract (Figure 4.4). It starts at the level of the 6th

cervical vertebra in the midline, and finishes at the level of the 11th thoracic vertebra, about 2.5 cm to the left of midline. The cervical and thoracic oesophagus are surrounded by loose areolar tissue in a single plane, which facilitates the rapid spread of infection throughout its length, should it rupture.

Thoracic duct

The thoracic duct arises from the cisterna chyli, which overlies the 1st and 2nd lumbar vertebrae, and lies posteriorly and to the right of the aorta (Figure 4.5). It ascends through the hiatus between the aorta and the azygos vein, anterior to the right intercostal branches of the aorta. Here it overlies the right sides of the vertebral bodies, and injury to this part of the duct may result in right-sided chylothorax. It drains into the venous system at the junction of the left subclavian and internal jugular veins.

Pathophysiology

As mentioned in the previous chapter, the main consequences of chest trauma are as a result of its effects on haemodynamic and respiratory function. We shall now deal with the patho-physiology of the alterations in haemodynamics and their sequelae.

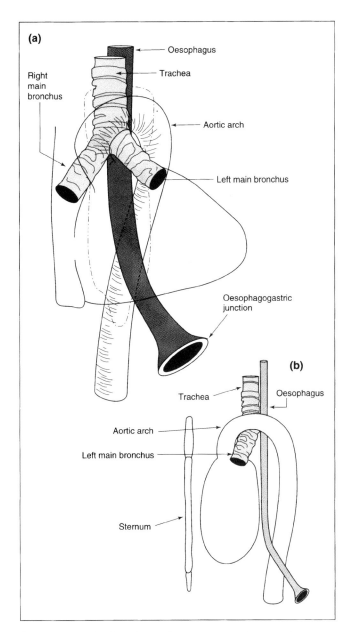

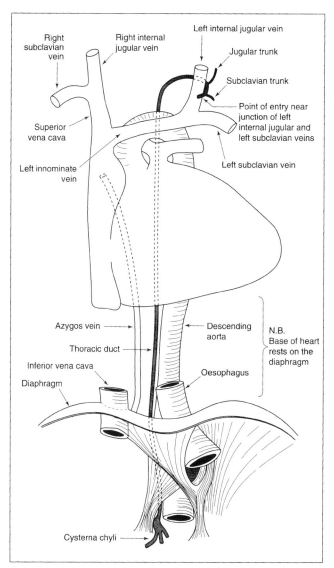

Figure 4.5 Schematic representation of the thoracic duct.

Figure 4.4 (a) The thoracic oesophagus and its relationships. (b) Schematic lateral representation of (a). The heart lies anteriorly to all depicted viscera.

Hypovolaemia

Profound hypovolaemia as a result of exsanguination in chest trauma, is most often seen with aortic transection, great vessel rupture, pulmonary hilar injury, or cardiac laceration not producing tamponade. This will lead to a low cardiac output state which adversely affects the other consequences of chest injury such as hypoxaemia, cardiac tamponade, congestive cardiac failure, and myocardial ischaemia and infarction.

Cardiac tamponade

When a pericardial tear is large and not sealed off by clot, the associated bleeding from a cardiac laceration can lead to huge exsanguination and haemothorax. If the haemorrhage is contained by the pericardium, however, cardiac tamponade will rapidly result from the accumulation of blood and clot in the rigid pericardial cavity. The intrapericardial pressure (which is equal to the intrapleural pressure) is normally several millimetres lower than right and left ventricular end diastolic

pressures (LVEDP), which helps in the diastolic filling of the heart. The accumulation of blood and clot in this confined space will increase the intrapericardial pressure, thus reducing the pressure gradient between the intracavity and intrapericardial pressures. This will produce significant restriction to cardiac filling, producing the phenomenon of cardiac tamponade. Initially, the decrease in stroke volume (due to reduced diastolic filling) is compensated for by increased adrenergic tone which produces a tachycardia, increased contractility, and increased systemic vascular resistance. This maintains the critical perfusion pressure at the cost of a falling cardiac output. With continuing increase in intrapericardial pressure (that is, no relief of the tamponade), the compensatory mechanisms will eventually fail, causing hypotension. The resulting fall in coronary perfusion causes selective hypoperfusion of the subendocardium, further compromising the stroke volume and producing a worsening low cardiac output state. The whole cycle self-perpetuates resulting in cardiac arrest if not urgently relieved.

Myocardial dysfunction

There are a number of situations that can arise in which the ability of the heart to function as an efficient pump is compromised. These conditions may originate from a variety

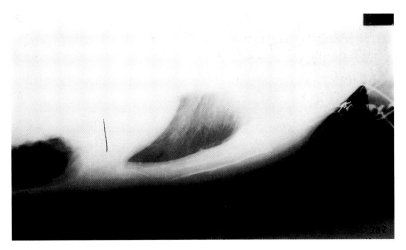

Figure 4.6 Lateral radiograph demonstrating complete manubriosternal dislocation.

of different causes, but uniformly lead to a decrease in cardiac output, with its resulting sequelae.

Myocardial contusion

Myocardial contusion following blunt injury can lead to decreased cardiac contractility and decreased compliance of the ventricle, resulting in a low cardiac output state from myocardial failure. Pathologically, these lesions may range from localised areas of haematoma on the epicardial surface, to widespread disruption of myocardial fibres. Extravasation of red blood cells and tissue fluid results in a reduction in the local microcirculation. Associated coronary artery injury or injury to smaller vessels within the contused area can lead to tissue necrosis and infarction, as collateral formation is usually very poor in acute cases.

Myocardial ischaemia and infarction

Patients who have sustained multiorgan trauma, have their myocardial function further compromised by reduced coronary perfusion from hypovolaemia and hypoxaemia, ultimately leading to congestive cardiac failure. Infarcted areas in either the free wall of the ventricle or in the septum can rupture leading to haemopericardium and cardiac tamponade, or ventricular septal defect. Approximately 20% of patients with myocardial contusion suffer from arrhythmias. These arrhythmias vary widely, and include supraventricular tachycardia, atrial fibrillation, ventricular ectopics, and sinus tachycardia. It is also possible to develop conduction defects ranging from bundle branch block to complete heart block. Myocardial infarction following coronary artery damage and/or occlusion can produce cardiogenic shock or myocardial failure. Arrhythmias can also compromise cardiac function secondary to increased irritability of the myocardium which follows ischaemia or infarction.

Valvular injury and intracardiac shunts

Traumatic injury to valves may result in acute volume overloading of the ventricle. This can lead to congestive cardiac failure, if the regurgitation produced is significant. Similar pathophysiology is associated with congestive cardiac failure caused by intracardiac shunts. Acute insufficiency of the tricuspid valve, however, often goes unnoticed in the presence of more obvious associated injuries. Hence, these lesions are most commonly diagnosed months to years after the trauma, when patients may develop non-specific symptoms of dyspnoea, fatigue, and a previously unnoticed systolic murmur.

Mechanism of injury

Cardiac injury can be equally severe in blunt or penetrating trauma. Both forms of trauma are associated with a very high mortality. It has been reported that 89.2% of 102 patients with a mixture of blunt and penetrating cardiac injuries were dead on arrival at hospital [1]. It is vitally important to recognise cardiac injuries early, since appropriate early treatment can be life-saving.

Blunt cardiac trauma

Blunt trauma to the heart can be secondary to direct force, compression, deceleration, and blast, or burst may occur from increased intravascular pressure associated with sudden compression of the abdominal contents. Automobile accidents are the commonest cause of blunt injuries, and commonly produce compression of the heart between the sternum and vertebrae from direct impact against the steering wheel during rapid deceleration. Myocardial contusion is therefore, frequently noticed in association with sternal fractures (Figure 4.6), and has been reported to be as high as 30% [2]. The junction of the manubrium and body is the commonest site of a sternal fracture, although it can also occur transversely through the body of the sternum.

Penetrating cardiac trauma

Penetrating injuries are the commonest form of cardiac injury and are associated with an extremely high mortality. Among 532 cases of penetrating injury reported in South Africa recently, 76.5% of the patients were dead before arrival at hospital. Amongst penetrating cardiac injuries, gunshot wounds are associated with a fourfold higher mortality than stab wounds (see box).

Cardiac injuries can be divided into various types (Table 4.1).

Assessment and management

As with pulmonary trauma, early assessment and simultaneous resuscitation of the patient with respect to the organs injured, and potential consequences, are the most important part of trauma management. The same systematic evaluation should be performed on all trauma patients, and subsequent treatment

---

Reasons for high mortality with gunshot wounds

- A high velocity bullet is particularly destructive since it displaces on its axis in flight setting up immense shock waves and resultant cavitation, as well as a transient negative intrathoracic pressure which aspirates foreign materials into the track
- Higher incidence of multiple and complex wounds of the heart
- Higher incidence of associated injuries to the great vessels, pulmonary hila and solid abdominal viscera
- A more severe physiological condition of patients on arrival in hospital, with higher incidence of exsanguination and profound hypovolaemia

---

Table 4.1 Types of cardiac injury

Structure	Injury
Myocardial injuries	Contusion Infarction Arrhythmias Rupture Septal perforation Intracardiac shunts
Coronary artery injuries	Perivascular haematoma and vessel occlusion Intimal laceration and flap formation Thrombosis Division
Valvular injuries	Rupture of cusps Rupture of papillary muscles or chordae tendinae
Pericardial injuries	Haemopericardium and tamponade Pericardial rupture and cardiac herniation

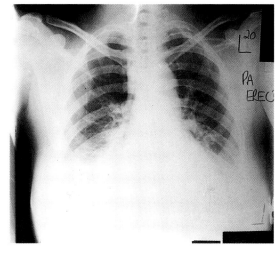

Figure 4.7 Plain chest radiograph showing suggesting traumatic disruption of the aorta. Note typical features: widened mediastinum, right paratracheal stripe, bilateral pleural caps, small right haemothorax.

tailored appropriately. This should follow the ATLS guidelines, commencing with "primary survey and simultaneous resuscitation", as alluded to earlier. Descriptions of the accident from witnesses can also provide very useful information. In all injuries the principal concerns are impaired respiratory and haemodynamic function, however, the likelihood of these being present are considerably higher with a chest injury.

Imaging

Chest radiograph

This is a very important basic investigation and is mandatory for any patient with a chest injury. If the patient is haemodynamically stable, a posteroanterior (PA) view with the patient in an erect posture, is ideal, but in practice these views are often performed on the supine patient in the A&E department.

In cardiac injuries, the chest radiograph can show cardiomegaly in patients with myocardial failure. In cardiac tamponade, the urgency of the clinical situation should not usually allow time for radiography, but rarely the classical "water bottle sign" may be seen, which is due to a widened cardiac shadow in a normal mediastinum.

The chest radiograph is a particularly valuable investigation in patients with a suspected aortic disruption, as it may show widening of the mediastinum, amongst other features (Figure 4.7). The specifity of this test is rather low, however, as only 25–35% of patients with radiographic widening of the mediastinum will prove to have actual transection of the thoracic aorta or disruption of the great vessels. There are several other radiographic features of aortic disruption although none is pathognomonic (see box). Aortic ruptures

from blunt injury are frequently associated with multiple rib fractures, flail chest, pneumothorax, haemothorax, and pulmonary contusions.

Fractures of the first two ribs (which are strong, short and relatively well protected) are associated with aortic injury in 5–15% of cases. An aortic injury must be suspected in patients with a haemothorax (particularly left-sided) who do not show any evidence of rib fractures or pulmonary injury. Confirmation of the nature and site of suspected injury of the aorta must be sought as a priority with further investigations (see page 62).

Radiographic features of aortic disruption

- Widened mediastinum
- Apical haematoma (pleural cap), especially on the left
- Fractured first or second ribs
- Shift of trachea to the right
- Compression and downward displacement of the left main bronchus to > 40% of normal
- Elevation of the right main bronchus
- Blunting or obliteration of the aortic knuckle
- Left haemothorax with no obvious other cause
- Obliteration of the aortic "window" on lateral views
- Deviation of the nasogastric tube in the oesophagus to the right.

Similarly, patients who sustain injury to the great vessels can show radiographic evidence of a haemothorax, or fracture of the clavicle and the first or second ribs. Deviation of the trachea or oesophagus away from the side of injury may also be a helpful sign. These injuries also need urgent confirmation by further investigations.

Blood in the pleural cavity (that is, a haemothorax) can be identified on an erect chest radiograph by obliteration of the costophrenic angle (Figure 4.8). This appearance on an

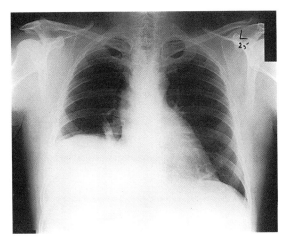

Figure 4.8 Erect chest radiograph showing right-sided haemothorax.

erect film requires at least 300–400 ml of blood in an adult. In a supine patient, a haemothorax can be identified by increased density or "whitening" of the hemithorax, representing the spread of blood throughout the posterior part of the chest (Figure 4.9).

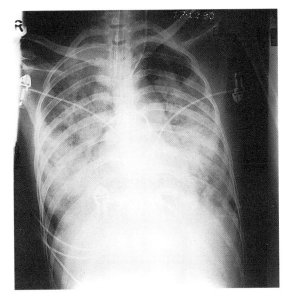

Figure 4.9 Supine chest radiograph showing bilateral haemothoraces (more pronounced on the right).

A chest radiograph is not very informative in oesophageal injury, especially when there is associated damage to the lungs and airways. If such an injury is suspected a soluble contrast study is usually required for diagnosis. Injury to the thoracic duct can be shown as a rapidly accumulating pleural effusion (chylothorax) and is associated with a high incidence of spinal injuries (Figure 4.10).

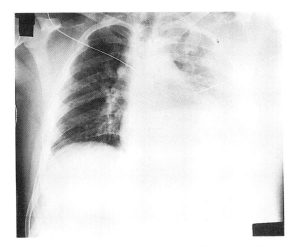

Figure 4.10 Plain chest radiograph showing fluid in the left thoracic cavity. This is a chylothorax, but could easily be confused with a haemothorax.

Computed axial tomography (CT)

The limitations of CT scanning for trauma has previously been mentioned in Chapter 3. The delay, expense, and isolation need to be weighed against the need for the specific information that would be obtained. Hence this procedure cannot be indicated in haemodynamically unstable patients, however potentially valuable the results.

In myocardial injuries, information obtained by a CT scan compares favourably with echocardiography in its ability to detect pericardial fluid. On CT scan, pericardial fluid usually occupies the superior pericardial recess and rarely extends inferiorly to surround the base of the heart. If it does, it strongly suggests cardiac injury, and attention may be directed towards identification and appropriate treatment.

Arguably, the main value of CT scanning in chest trauma, is in its ability to identify aortic and great vessel injury, as it can distinguish a widened mediastinum caused by haemorrhage from that caused by other aetiologies (Figure 4.11).

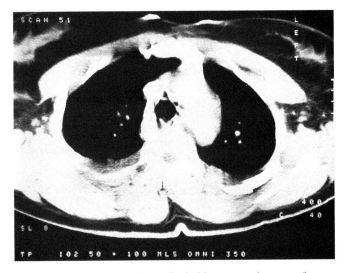

Figure 4.11 CT scan showing mediastinal haematoma in a case of traumatic disruption of the thoracic aorta.

It can also detect occult mediastinal haemorrhage in the presence of a normal chest radiograph. Congenital abnormalities and anatomical variations, which can produce non-specific abnormalities on chest radiographs, can also be detected easily. CT detection of any mediastinal haemorrhage may indicate the need for an aortogram, although the aortic contour may appear to be sharply preserved, because the adventitia is the last layer to rupture. In the majority of cases, particularly trauma, such a finding would indicate immediate surgical exploration and repair. False positive radiographic results in the suspected diagnosis of aortic tears can result from artefacts, and CT scanning is therefore useful, as it negates the need for angiography when there is no evidence of mediastinal haemorrhage, and supports the need for angiography or surgery when this is present.

In patients with a suspected injury to the thoracic duct, CT scanning with opacification of the duct by oral ingestion of ethiodised oil and a 50% fat emulsion has been used with some success. Other methods used to identify thoracic duct injury include nuclear lymphangiography with ingested ^{123}I-heptadecanoic acid, which offers a lower resolution evaluation of anatomic variations and the level of duct disruption. A subcutaneous injection of [99]T-sulphur colloid in the interdigital space of the feet can also give similar information.

There are several documented comparisons of chest radiography and CT in the literature, the overall consensus being that CT scans of the chest should not be performed as a routine procedure in patients who have sustained thoracic trauma, but only when clinically indicated [3–5].

Magnetic resonance imaging (MRI)

MRI has been mentioned in Chapter 3, and has become increasingly useful for assessment of cardiac abnormalities. Its use in the trauma situation is probably limited, however, for similar reasons to CT scanning.

Endoscopy

Endoscopy is a useful adjunct to all the routine investigations, and can usefully be employed in several instances of trauma. It is particularly valuable if it can be performed at the bedside with a portable unit.

Oesophagoscopy is usually only used when a contrast swallow is negative in patients with clinical suspicion of an oesophageal injury. *Thoracoscopy* and *laparoscopy* are very sensitive and specific methods of identifying diaphragmatic or solid organ injuries. Their main drawbacks include the requirement of general anaesthesia, and in the case of laparoscopy, concern about the safety of positive pressure pneumoperitoneum in a trauma patient with a possible diaphragmatic injury. Insufflation of the peritoneum in the absence of an intact diaphragm can produce a tension pneumothorax, or even carbon dioxide embolism if there are major hepatic or venous injuries (seen in 35–45% of patients with diaphragmatic injuries). The consequences of either of these events are catastrophic, and therefore the procedure can only be indicated if there is absolute certainty about the integrity of the diaphragm.

Suspected oesophageal or tracheobronchial ruptures are potentially life-threatening injuries, that need urgent confirmation. Contrast radiography and endoscopy are the only ways of achieving this, and endoscopy lends itself far better to the unstable, multiply injured patient in whom transfer would be hazardous.

Electrocardiogram (ECG)

The ECG has a very non-specific value in the assessment of patients with chest trauma. It can, however, be very useful in patients with minimal external injuries who have sustained significant blunt myocardial damage, as it is the best diagnostic test to predict severity and clinical impact of myocardial contusion. The development of new Q waves or heart block are the most reliable signs of significant cardiac injury, and serial ECGs are important for monitoring and assessing the progress of any cardiac injury. The incidence of ECG evidence of cardiac injury after blunt trauma has been estimated to be between 17 and 38%. The presence of a new arrhythmia usually indicates myocardial damage, which is seen in as many as 20% of patients following blunt chest trauma. The commonest arrhythmias seen, are supraventricular tachycardia, atrial fibrillation, ventricular ectopic beats, and ventricular fibrillation. Conduction defects, in the form of bundle branch block or complete heart block usually indicate sinus node or right coronary artery injury.

Cardiac enzyme analysis

The *creatinine kinase* (CK) isoenzyme is neither specific nor sensitive for cardiac injury as it is frequently raised in patients with blunt trauma from skeletal muscle injury. The *myocardial band* (MB) fraction, which used to be considered specific for cardiac tissue, can also be elevated in injury to many other tissues, including skeletal muscle, urinary bladder, liver, stomach, pancreas, prostate, uterus, colon, small bowel, and lung. It is also raised in cases of renal failure. More recent work has shown *troponin* to be considerably more specific to myocardial injury. Troponin T has been evaluated in terms of myocardial injury following infarction, but Troponin I is thought to be more specific for myocardial contusion.

Echocardiography

Echocardiography is arguably the most useful screening test for suspected cardiac injuries. *Transthoracic echocardiography* (TTE) can provide information about both wall and septal motion, valvular and chordal integrity, presence of a pericardial effusion, mural thrombi, and the ejection fraction. In addition, the use of Doppler with colour flow mapping gives accurate information regarding the haemodynamic effects of valvular injury and it can detect an intracardiac shunt with more accuracy.

Availability of *transoesophageal echocardiography* (TOE) has increased the diagnostic accuracy of echocardiography, particularly in patients with a poor transthoracic window caused by extensive surgical and mediastinal emphysema. TOE can give more accurate information about valvular lesions, septal defects, intracardiac shunts, and the possibility of concomitant injury to the great vessels. TOE is of particular use in patients with suspected aortic injury. It can be performed rapidly and safely at the patient's bedside, eliminating the delay and risk involved with transfer to another department, and its value in the hands of an experienced operator has been well validated [6]. The conclusions are that the main benefits of TOE are:

- portability
- ease of performance
- freedom from radiation
- improved speed of diagnosis
- lack of need for contrast
- improved accuracy.

On the negative side, its drawbacks include:

- availability of the instrument
- willingness and experience of the operator to perform the procedure under emergency circumstances

- need for a cardiologist, radiologist or experienced surgeon to interpret the results.

Echocardiography is a valuable adjunct to the diagnostic tools available in the management of thoracic trauma. As more personnel develop the necessary skills required for its use and interpretation, it is increasingly being used at an early stage.

Angiography

Angiography is still regarded as the "gold standard" in the evaluation of all vascular injuries. An abnormal chest radiograph with a widened mediastinum in a patient who has sustained chest trauma is often considered an indication for angiography, to rule out aortic disruption, regardless of the high false positive rate (Figure 4.12). Vascular injury may

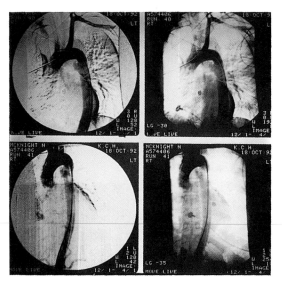

Figure 4.12 Aortic angiogram demonstrating a leak suggestive of traumatic disruption of the thoracic aorta.

present as vessel laceration or division in penetrating trauma, and avulsion, intimal flap formation, or obstruction from blunt trauma. Angiography may demonstrate such injuries manifest by frank extravasation, false aneurysm formation, arteriovenous fistula, spasm, dissection, partial or complete thrombosis, and distal embolism. Occasionally the changes may only include a small intimal flap or irregularity, but it is, nonetheless, important information. Rarely, but particularly following blast injuries, an aortogram may appear normal in spite of significant injury to the vessel, as this type of injury can damage the external layers without affecting the intima. In patients who sustain a ruptured thoracic aorta, the possibility of producing complications by the transfemoral approach must be considered.

Valvular leaks and intracardiac shunts can be identified by aortography or ventriculography. Similarly, pulmonary artery injury can be delineated by a pulmonary angiogram, with the use of the femoral vein for access.

Nuclear medicine

Radioisotope scans, particularly technetium pyrophosphate for detection of myocardial injury, is found to have very poor sensitivity and thus is not used routinely.

Specific conditions

Cardiac injuries

Cardiac injuries manifest primarily with haemodynamic abnormalities, varying with the severity of the damage and structures involved. Certain signs are non-specific, and present with many of the previously mentioned injuries, not only involving the heart. These include tachycardia, hypotension, and tachypnoea. Others are more specific to particular injuries. These include hypovolaemia from haemorrhage into the pleural cavity, or the signs of tamponade, if there has been a bleed into the pericardium. Hypovolaemia presents with tachycardia, pallor, air-hunger, and hypotension with collapsed neck veins. Patients with cardiac tamponade will also develop a tachycardia. In established cases of tamponade, there may be hypotension, muffled heart sounds, and distended neck veins, the classical combination of *Beck's triad*. It may be difficult to appreciate these signs in patients with multi-organ injury and surgical emphysema from a pneumothorax. *Pulsus paradoxus*, a drop in systolic blood pressure during inspiration in excess of the accepted 10 mmHg, is actually an exaggeration of the normal physiological response rather than a true paradox. *Kussmaul's sign* (a rise in venous pressure with inspiration when breathing spontaneously) is a true paradoxical venous pressure abnormality associated with tamponade. Evidence of blunt or penetrating trauma may be seen in the chest wall. In penetrating trauma, the wound of entry may be anywhere in the chest or abdomen dependent upon the length of the weapon and velocity of the missile. With blunt injuries, fractures of the sternum or the anterior ribs may be noticed. Patients with cardiac injury can also present with myocardial contusion, myocardial infarction, myocardial laceration, intracardiac shunts or, valvular damage. These will be commonly manifested by signs of congestive heart failure, such as acute shortness of breath with pulmonary oedema, raised JVP, tachycardia and, in many cases, hypotension. In addition, 20% of patients with myocardial contusion will develop various forms of supraventricular arrhythmias.

Treatment of cardiac injuries depends on the type of injury and the chambers involved. In pericardial lacerations, which can be seen following blunt injury, herniation or torsion of the heart can lead to severe haemodynamic embarrassment; this requires operative reduction and repair of the tear. In patients with an associated pneumothorax, occasionally a tension pericardium can develop. This may be treated by the placement of a catheter in the pericardial cavity in addition to routine drainage of the pneumothorax.

Myocardial contusion

Myocardial contusion has been reported to occur in as many as 30% of patients with severe blunt chest trauma, but ECG changes including ischaemia and arrhythmias can be seen in more. Frank infarction is not uncommon after severe contusions. Coexistent sternal or rib fractures are frequently seen in these cases.

Treatment of myocardial contusion is basically supportive with bed rest, oxygen supplementation, and careful monitoring of haemodynamics. This should include serial ECG and cardiac enzyme measurement, and cardiac monitoring until resolution, as a fatal arrhythmia can occur at any time. In patients with deteriorating clinical parameters, right and left heart filling pressures and cardiac output should be measured and optimised by pharmacological means. This necessitates insertion of a Swan–Ganz pulmonary artery catheter. Close monitoring of electrolytes, and anti-arrhythmic agents and pacemakers have reduced the incidence of death from arrhythmias. In refractory cases of low cardiac output, not responding to inotropic support, mechanical support in the form of an intra-aortic balloon pump (IABP) or ventricular assist device (VAD) may need to be considered.

Myocardial ischaemia (infarction)

Coronary artery lacerations mainly occur with penetrating cardiac trauma and are often fatal owing to sudden ischaemia-induced myocardial infarction. This ischaemia can often be complicated by hypovolaemia and cardiac tamponade if a significant bleed occurs. Occasionally, blunt injury may lead to coronary artery injury, the left anterior descending (LAD) artery being the commonest vessel affected, either directly or by torsion of the heart. Complete occlusion of this vessel is usually fatal, but in most cases the injury is limited to intimal damage and flap formation, or stenosis from intramural haemorrhage and perivascular contusion.

Myocardial infarction secondary to coronary artery injury is usually managed conservatively, as the extensive nature of associated organ injuries usually contraindicates the use of heparin or thrombolysing agents. However, isolated coronary artery injuries, when associated with injuries to other chambers requiring operative intervention, can be manged by coronary artery bypass grafting.

Myocardial laceration

Myocardial lacerations and ruptures usually result from penetrating injuries. The right ventricle, lying anteriorly, is most commonly involved, followed by the left ventricle, right atrium, and left atrium, in descending order of frequency. Prehospital mortality from penetrating cardiac trauma is extremely high, with a worse outcome if the left ventricle is involved or if cardiac tamponade occurs. Isolated myocardial rupture can result from blunt trauma and has a 65% immediate mortality. The atria are less commonly involved in blunt trauma, because the blood gets forcefully, but easily, displaced into the more compliant systemic or pulmonary venous bed.

Myocardial laceration almost always requires emergency surgery to relieve the tamponade or to control the haemorrhage. As the availability of expertise (instruments, equipment, lighting, and personnel) is limited in the emergency room, the surgery should be performed in the operating theatre whenever the patient's haemodynamic status allows. When it is necessary to perform this procedure in the emergency room, immediate relief of the tamponade and control of the source of bleeding with finger pressure should suffice to allow stabilisation of haemodynamics for urgent transfer to theatre. If facilities for surgery are not readily available, intermittent pericardiocentesis (by the placement of a catheter in the pericardial space and aspiration of blood when necessary to improve the haemodynamic condition) may be performed until provision is made for formal thoracotomy.

Intracardiac shunts and valvular disruption

Intracardiac shunts are rare, but are usually seen following a penetrating cardiac injury. They most frequently take the form of aorto-right ventricular shunts, coronary artery-intracavity shunts or aortopulmonary artery shunts. Rarely, ventricular septal defects can be produced by direct penetrating injuries. Blunt cardiac injuries may produce an intracardiac shunt, owing to disruption of the ventricular septum, by forceful compression against a closed valve during diastole. The free wall is more often ruptured in such injuries as a higher force is required to disrupt the septum. A ventricular septal defect can occur as a delayed event after blunt cardiac injury, if severe contusion of the septum is followed by cell death and necrosis. The atrial septum can also be ruptured by a similar mechanism, but this is extremely rare.

Amongst valvular injuries, the aortic valve is most commonly affected in cases of penetrating trauma. Blunt trauma can cause rapid displacement of blood during diastole with a torsional effect on the aortic root, lacerating aortic or mitral leaflets, papillary muscles, or chordae tendinae. In the aortic valve, the left coronary or the non-coronary cusps are more often involved than the right coronary cusp. Similarly, the tricuspid valve can be affected, leading to gross incompetence, but is a rare lesion with less than 100 cases reported in the literature.

If a patient is suffering from an intracardiac shunt, and marked haemodynamic decline occurs, immediate surgery under cardiopulmonary bypass is strongly recommended. Rarely, a small ventricular septal defect will close spontaneously, so echocardiographic monitoring is important. Similarly, valve injuries causing significant valvular regurgitation and cardiac failure need immediate repair or prosthetic replacement of the valve. In the absence of congestive cardiac failure, supportive treatment is advocated until other associated injuries are rectified.

Foreign bodies

Foreign bodies, usually bullets and similar missiles, can be lodged in the myocardium and may be a source of endocarditis. Migration into systemic or pulmonary circulation is rare, but if it does occur, a potentially fatal embolus results.

Foreign bodies in the chambers of the heart, usually following gunshot injuries, do not warrant emergency surgery, when they are situated in the right side of the heart, but may be removed electively when the patient is well. In the left-sided chambers, they should be removed as soon as possible to prevent embolisation, particularly cerebral. This will require cardiopulmonary bypass, and the early involvement of cardiothoracic surgeons is essential in all such cases.

Pericardium

Isolated pericardial injury is rare. The associated cardiac damage is usually extensive and determines the course of the injury. The pericardium can rupture over the diaphragmatic or the pleural surfaces following blunt trauma and the heart can then herniate through the rent and cause torsion of the great vessels, with a resulting low cardiac output state.

In all of the above immediate threats to life, several large venous access sites, either peripheral or central, must be obtained, even if this involves a venous cutdown. Blood is drawn for cross-matching, typing, and all routine and any other indicated laboratory tests. Fluid resuscitation is continued in patients with hypovolaemic shock, but it should be remembered that overloading may cause a catastrophic deterioration in certain conditions. These are cardiac tamponade and pulmonary contusion, as mentioned above, and traumatic disruption of the aorta, discussed later. Oxygen therapy is always essential, to ensure that maximal oxygenation of tissues takes place.

Cardiac tamponade

Cardiac tamponade is usually caused by a penetrating injury and results from blood filling the fibrous pericardial sac, thus creating a mechanical embarrassment to the heart. The pericardium is fixed and only a small amount of blood will interfere with cardiac filling, therefore removal of as little as 20 ml of this by pericardiocentesis may dramatically improve cardiac function, and therefore the clinical condition. Frequently, however, the blood in the pericardium will have clotted by the time of attempted aspiration, giving a false negative "dry tap". The most common signs of tamponade include hypotension, muffled heart sounds, and an elevated jugular venous pulse (distended neck veins), which may be absent if the patient is hypovolaemic. Immediate management includes cautious resuscitation with volume replacement (fluid overloading may exacerbate the compression), but if this leads to deterioration in the clinical condition and there is a strong suspicion of tamponade, pericardiocentesis *must* be performed. It should be stressed again that cardiac tamponade is a clinical, and *not* a radiological diagnosis, and if suspected, an urgent call-out should be made to a cardiothoracic surgeon or, if not available, an experienced general surgeon. Pericardiocentesis is usually performed via the subxiphoid route, and if positive, should be followed by an emergency operation in theatre as soon as possible, to evacuate the blood and clot, and to control and repair the source of bleeding.

Emergency thoracotomy

A matter of some considerable contention in the acute situation, is the indication for "emergency room thoracotomy" (ERT) or "scene thoracotomy", if it occurs out of the hospital. ERT is an aggressive attempt to save a trauma victim who is in immediate danger of dying. The decision to perform this procedure involves scientific, ethical, social, and economic issues. The prognostic factors, survival levels, and cost-benefits must be considered before recommending such a procedure. Current indications for ERT are controversial, and it has been claimed that it is a hopeless procedure which should not be performed under any circumstances. More recently it has been suggested that the only correct indications are after a penetrating injury where there have been established vital signs present on arrival at the scene, and where there is no alternative, because of rapid clinical deterioration. Essentially, the urgent relief of tamponade is the basic life-saving step in ERT, and can buy time to enable transfer to theatre. Prognosis of ERT depends upon the mechanism of injury, the clinical condition of the patient when first seen, extent and effectiveness of prehospital resuscitation, transportation time, and procedural factors. There are several studies and reports in the literature, which look at survival rates and prognostic factors of this procedure [7–10]. Survival is acknowledged to be considerably better for patients sustaining penetrating trauma compared to those sustaining blunt trauma. The large study by Boyd *et al.* confirms our earlier recommendation that all patients with no established vital signs at scene, and patients with blunt injury without vital signs on arrival at the emergency room, should not be offered ERT [7,11].

The reasons for the extremely poor outcome in blunt trauma patients are a combination of several factors. A substantial number of these patients die of brain injury, from either direct brain insult or prolonged hypoxia prior to and during resuscitation. Blunt trauma is also associated with a very high incidence of multiple injuries, making the surgical treatment lengthier and more complicated. Disseminated intravascular coagulation is present in a substantial number (up to 70%) of these patients; this could partly be due to the associated hypovolaemia, and partly the extensive soft tissue injury.

Patients with penetrating cardiac injuries, who decompensate on, or just before, arrival, benefit most from ERT, although this number is small because the prehospital mortality of such injuries is nearly 85% [12,13].

Complications suffered by survivors of ERT are rare and mostly iatrogenic. It should be noted that the personnel performing the procedure are frequently not trained surgeons, a factor that will increase the incidence of complications. These include:

- laceration of the lung whilst the pleura is opened;
- phrenic nerve injury;
- injury to the myocardium or coronary arteries when the pericardium is opened;
- laceration of the myocardium during myocardial compression.

In conclusion, the authors would strongly discourage the use of ERT after blunt chest trauma, since most studies have shown a uniformly dismal outlook [10]. If the procedure is to be usefully performed, it should ideally be undertaken by a well trained and coordinated trauma team and planned simultaneously with all other resuscitative measures. It is particularly important to have a cardiothoracic surgeon present or contacted as soon as possible. Scene thoracotomies should almost always be avoided and in viable cases of thoracic trauma, the "swoop and scoop" policy should be adopted to give the best chance of a successful outcome.

Aortic and great vessel injuries

Aortic injuries commonly manifest with shock and signs of a haemothorax or cardiac tamponade, depending upon the site of injury. Indeed, the majority of patients who have sustained a traumatic aortic injury die at the scene. Changes associated with aortic injury depend upon the site of rupture. Patients with a disruption of the intrapericardial section of the ascending aorta will usually develop cardiac tamponade. Extrapericardial ascending aortic rupture produces a mediastinal haematoma followed by a haemothorax, usually on the right side. Small penetrating injuries often close spontaneously secondary to associated hypotension, when the adventitial fragments tend to swell and fold into the area of injury. Subsequently, with restoration of blood pressure, the site can either rebleed immediately or after some delay. Resuscitation protocol therefore presents a dilemma, and immediate recognition and treatment is essential. If undiagnosed, a false aneurysm may result and gradually enlarge, producing symptoms owing to either pressure effects on the adjacent structures or sudden death from rupture.

Injury to the aortic arch may not be obvious initially if the adventitial layer remains intact, when the damage is contained in the form of a mediastinal haematoma. Consequently, tamponade is rare in these patients, and apart from a transient period of hypotension responding well to fluid therapy, clinical signs are notoriously absent. It is therefore crucial to have a high index of suspicion in patients with a typical history of a deceleration-type accident, or a fall. This will lead to a series of urgent radiological investigations (page 57).

Patients with small penetrating injuries, who survive the initial period, may develop a pseudoaneurysm which can manifest with sudden hypvolaemia and death if there is an early or late rupture into the pleural cavity or pericardium. All such injuries present a dilemma in resuscitation: if there is a contained haematoma, which is purely restrained by the adventitial layer, overzealous fluid replacement will cause a rise in pressure sufficient to cause rupture, but under-replacement will cause hypotension and its sequelae. A fine balance needs to be reached, and prompt diagnosis and treatment is essential. Patients with damage to the aorta may also present with a continuous murmur if the aneurysm erodes into the pulmonary artery or the vena cava. Occasionally these patients can present with a catastrophic haemoptysis or haematemesis resulting from erosion into an airway or the oesophagus respectively.

Diagnosis of aortic injury requires immediate suspicion. In penetrating injuries to the left hemithorax, anterior chest or neck, one should always suspect aortic injury. Similarly, aortic rupture should be suspected in patients with refractory hypovolaemia without external thoracic trauma or evidence of other vascular injuries. Symptoms associated with aortic rupture include severe retrosternal or interscapular pain from an expanding mediastinal haematoma. Other symptoms may be hoarseness of the voice from compression of the recurrent laryngeal nerve, dysphagia from compression of the oesophagus, and paraplegia or paraparesis from compression of intercostal branches supplying the anterior spinal artery. These patients can also present with ischaemia, and even infarction, of various intra-abdominal organs or extremities owing to the occlusion of respective main branches of the aorta.

Clinically, patients with an aortic injury may have fractures of the sternum, ribs, or vertebrae. They can also have haematomata at the base of the neck, tracheal deviation, upper arm hypertension relative to hypotension in the legs, bruits in the chest and neck vessels, a haemothorax, or even stridor. The upper body hypertension, which is seen in nearly 50% of patients with acute aortic transection, may be due to:

- a combination of partial or complete occlusion of aortic flow caused by the divided intima;
- intrusion of haematomata onto the aortic lumen causing extrinsic compression;
- stimulation of arch baroreceptors;
- activation of the renin–angiotensin pathway from renal hypoperfusion.

If an aortic injury is confirmed, formal surgical repair at the earliest opportunity is indicated.

Patients with injuries to the large intrathoracic vessels will usually succumb to a massive haemorrhage and die instantly. When the injury is partial, however, with the adventitia remaining intact, they can present with haematomata in the supra- or infraclavicular regions causing an absent or low volume pulse on the affected side. When there is an associated injury to the trachea or oesophagus, patients can present with haemoptysis or haematemesis respectively. Such patients are also vulnerable to brachial plexus injury, vagus, or recurrent laryngeal nerve damage, and can present with motor and/or sensory loss in the extremities, hoarseness of voice, and dysphonia. Venous injuries can produce haematomata with oedema of the neck and arm, and even development of superior vena cava syndrome (SVCS).

Penetrating injuries of the aorta are often fatal. Blunt injuries are usually due to deceleration in road traffic accidents or falls from heights. The most common mechanism of injury is horizontal deceleration, which produces traumatic disruption of the aorta. This occurs in the region of the ligamentum arteriosum, just distal to the origin of the left subclavian artery, in over 85% of cases, as the aorta is relatively firmly fixed at this point. Only adventitial continuity prevents sudden death from massive exsanguination in these patients. The haematoma produced is contained in a small area; therefore cardiac tamponade is rare and apart from a moderate transient hypotension which responds well to fluids, symptoms and signs are notoriously absent. In a minority of patients, the rupture occurs in the ascending aorta or, rarely, in the descending aorta near the diaphragm.

Vertical deceleration can produce damage to the vessels of the aortic arch (in addition to the ascending aorta), secondary to acute lengthening stress of the great vessels at their origin.

Compression injury of the chest wall with displacement of the heart downwards and to the left, may produce ascending aortic ruptures. Similarly, upward displacement of the heart and mediastinal structures from a cranially directed impact to the lower chest or upper epigastrium may rupture the descending aorta.

Traumatic aortic ruptures are usually fatal, and timely diagnosis is the key to survival. Mortality risk increases with time in patients with an undiagnosed aortic rupture. Ascending aortic ruptures have a near 100% mortality and only 10–20% of patients with injuries to the proximal descending aorta survive long enough to reach hospital [14]. False aneurysm formation in surgically untreated survivors or where the condition has not been recognised, will be symptomatic within three years of the event in 50% of patients, with delayed rupture occurring up to 30 years later.

The great vessels from the arch of the aorta can similarly be injured by both blunt and penetrating trauma. Penetrating trauma to the intrathoracic vessels is usually fatal, unless small, and in these cases false aneurysm is invariably formed. Mechanisms of blunt trauma responsible for injury to the intrathoracic components of the great vessels include direct compression, shear forces, and deceleration forces. Direct compression of the anterior chest can injure the innominate and left common carotid arteries by forcing them against the vertebral column. Blunt injury to the subclavian arteries is usually associated with fractures of the clavicle or first rib and must always be suspected when such a fracture is diagnosed. These injuries are slightly more common at present because of shoulder harness seatbelts. The subclavian artery, like the superior mesenteric artery, is more deficient in collagen in its media compared with other vessels; this makes it more vulnerable to avulsion and compression type injuries.

Injuries to the great veins are more common than currently reported, particularly subclavian and axillary vein injuries. Penetrating trauma is responsible for 83% of such injuries, with 17% due to blunt trauma.

Patients who have sustained an aortic injury have a 90% survival rate following surgical intervention, if they are haemodynamically stable at the time of operation. Hence, surgery is to be recommended to all patients with such injuries, except those with very severe associated injuries, or elderly patients with serious pre-existing medical conditions. Resuscitation in these patients must be undertaken with particular caution, maintaining controlled hypotension sufficient to keep organ perfusion at an acceptable level. This may involve control of relative hypertension with alpha-blockers, as well as extreme caution with fluid replacement, because too high a pressure may cause rupture of the single adventitial layer or dislodge a clot, leading to sudden massive exsanguination.

Oesophageal injuries

Oesophageal injuries are uncommon because of its protected position in the posterior mediastinum. In a series of 600 penetrating chest wounds reported by Oparah and Mandal [15], there were only three oesophageal perforations. The cervical oesophagus is more vulnerable to injury than the thoracic section, and associated damage to the trachea and great vessels is common in such instances. Blunt oesophageal injury is also uncommon; indeed, Beal *et al.* [16] have reported an incidence of 0.001% oesophageal injuries in all blunt trauma admissions amongst 96 reports since 1900. Automobile accidents were the commonest cause and the cervical oesophagus was involved in 70% of the cases in which it occurred.

Isolated oesophageal injuries are rare. They usually occur as a result of a penetrating wound to the chest, but a spontaneous burst or rupture following a crush injury is not uncommon. Symptoms suggesting an oesophageal injury are pain on deglutition and pyrexia from spillage of oesophageal contents into the mediastinum, and subsequent infection (mediastinitis). Patients will often complain of intense back pain secondary to this mediastinitis. Oesophageal injuries can produce surgical emphysema, pneumothorax, or signs of peritonitis depending upon the site of rupture. If the oesophageal contents leak into the pleural cavity, an empyema may ensue, with well-recognised signs and symptoms. All cases of traumatic oesophageal tears with pleural contamination should initially be treated with a large-bore chest drain, and subsequently repaired surgically. This should be performed via a cervical, thoracic and/or abdominal incision according to the site and mechanism of injury.

If the oesophagus is found to have an injury, management should follow certain basic principles (see box). Approaches to the injured oesophagus depend upon the level at which the damage has occurred. Cervical oesophageal injuries can be approached by an incision along the anterior border of sternocleidomastoid muscle. If the neck vessels and the sternocleidomastoid muscle are retracted laterally, and the larynx with trachea medially, the pharynx and cervical oesophagus can be clearly exposed. A tear should be closed transversely after the edges have been trimmed and confirmation that they are viable. Synthetic absorbable sutures (vicryl, Dexon or PDS) are preferred for closure. The wound should always be closed over a drain, because of the high probability of contamination of the area.

Patients who have sustained high velocity oesophageal injuries with extensive tissue loss, should have oesphageal exclusion in the form of cervical oesophagostomy and gastrostomy, combined with drainage of the mediastinal contents by tube thoracostomy. Continuity can be re-established when the infection has been controlled, using stomach, colon, or a loop of jejunum. In such patients, some groups have recommended oesophageal exclusion and diversion in continuity by the use of umbilical tape or a silastic band tied around the distal oesophagus and beneath the vagal fibres. A cervical oesophagostomy allows complete diversion. After resolution of the acute process, the distal band can be removed and oesophageal continuity restored.

Thoracic duct injuries

Injury to the thoracic duct is usually due to blunt trauma. It most commonly occurs following either a fall from a height, direct compression or hyperflexion and hyperextension spinal injuries. Its principal manifestation is a chylous effusion which can present itself at the time of injury or as a delayed event, with increasing shortness of breath, hypovolaemia, or ascites. If disruption or avulsion occurs, a chylothorax will result that may insidiously compromise respiratory function. This classically presents as a milky fluid discharged through the chest drain. This should be sent for analysis: the presence of chylomicrons will act as confirmation.

Blunt abdominal trauma can cause ductal rupture, commonly in the region of the 9th or 10th thoracic vertebra, leading to chylous ascites. Susceptibility to injury is much greater when the duct is full after a fatty meal. Penetrating injury to the duct is often associated with injury to adjacent structures (see page 56) and can often be fatal.

It is usually possible to treat these injuries conservatively, with the use of a chest drain, dietary supplementation, and assistance, and precautions taken to avoid infection, such as antibiotics. Serial chest radiographs are routinely used to monitor progress.

Management of patients with a thoracic duct injury is principally by insertion of a large-bore chest drain (at least 32F) connected to suction to prevent tubal obstruction from viscous chyle. This will ensure complete expansion of the lung to encourage pleural adhesion. Obliteration of pleuromediastinal space is encouraged and the closure of the chylous fistula is facilitated. The flow of chyle should be reduced by substitution of dietary fat with medium-chain triglycerides; these are absorbed directly into the portal venous system. In patients with persistent leakage, total parenteral nutrition must be considered. There is no consensus of opinion regarding how long conservative management should be continued. In general, it is advisable that operative treatment is recommended for the indications shown in the box.

When operative intervention is necessary, a low thoracic duct ligation at the level of the diaphragm, is the procedure of choice regardless of the site of leak. When the location of the fistula can be identified, the duct should be ligated above, as well as below, the fistula. Both animal experiments and clinical experience have shown that, owing to the tendency of the lymphatics to develop collaterals, ligation of the thoracic duct does not produce any permanent abnormalities [17].

Double cream or olive oil administered through a nasogastric tube, four hours before the operation, will cause marked increase in the flow of chyle, thus facilitating identification of the site of leakage. If the duct cannot be located, all the tissue between the aorta and azygos vein should be mass ligated at the level of the oesophageal hiatus; this will control the leak in >90% of patients. Induced pleurodesis, irrespective of the

---

Management principles in oesophageal injury
• Operative repair within 12 hours of injury
• Prevention of further contamination by fasting or oesophageal exclusion
• Broad spectrum antibiotics
• Nutritional support
• Prompt drainage of secondary leaks

Indications for surgery after traumatic thoracic duct injury
• Chyle drainage >1500 ml/day for 5 days in an adult
• Drainage >100 ml/year of child/day for 5 days in a child
• Drainage >200 ml/day after 14 days
• Development of metabolic complications
• When intrathoracic exploration is required for injury to other structures

method used, has not been very successful. A pleuroperitoneal shunt has been successfully used in refractory cases, although there are conflicting reports in the literature regarding their use [18]. Some believe that pleuroperitoneal shunting should be used as an intermediate stage between failed non-operative management and operative ligation, with a thoracotomy avoided if possible.

Summary

Although the mediastinum contains the "clockwork" of the body, many patients survive to reach hospital after severe chest trauma. It is this self-selected group of patients who need urgent, appropriate treatment, with recognition of both immediate and potential threats to life. Many of these patients will go on to require definitive specialised procedures, but they can nearly all be kept alive and stabilised by the emergency department personnel until this can occur. A standardised approach to management of the trauma patient, such as the ATLS, will ensure that mediastinal injuries are picked up early, and requires no specialist skills or knowledge of an area that is still mysterious to many practitioners.

References

1. Kulshrestha P, Iyer KS, Sampath KA. Cardiac injuries – a clinical and autopsy profile. *J Trauma* 1990;**30**:203.
2. Kissane RW. Traumatic heart disease. *Circulation* 1952;**6**:421.
3. McGonigal MD, Schwab CW, Kauder DR. Supplemental emergent chest computed tomography in the management of blunt torso trauma. *J Trauma* 1990;**30**:1431.
4. McLean TR, Olinger GN, Thorsen MK. Computed tomography in the evaluation of the aorta in patients sustaining blunt thoracic trauma. *Surgery* 1989;**106**:596.
5. Poole VG, Morgan DB, Cransten PE. Computed tomography in the management of blunt thoracic trauma. *J Trauma* 1993;**35**:296.
6. Kearney PA, Smith DW, Johnson SB. Use of transoesophageal echocardiography in the evaluation of traumatic aortic injury. *J Trauma* 1993;**34**:696.
7. Boyd M, Vanek VW, Bourguet CC. Emergency room resuscitative thoracotomy: when is it indicated? *J Trauma* 1992;**33**:714–21.
8. Harnar TJ, Oreskovich MR, Copass MK. Role of emergency thoracotomy in the resuscitation of moribund trauma victims. *Am J Surg* 1981;**142**:96.
9. Vig D, Simon E, Smith RF. Resuscitation thoracotomy for patients with traumatic injury. *Surgery* 1983;**94**:554.
10. Jahangiri M, Hyde JAJ, Griffin SJ, Lewis CT, Magee PG, Wood AJ. Emergency thoracotomy for thoracic trauma in the accident and emergency department: indications and outcome. *Ann Roy Coll Surg Eng* 1996;**78**:221–4.
11. Trunkey DD. Chest wall injuries, in (Blaisdell FW, Trunkey DD, eds) *Cervicothoracic trauma II*. New York: Thieme, 1994.
12. Steichen FM, Dargan EL, Efron G. A graded approach to the management of penetrating wounds to the heart. *Arch Surg* 1971;**103**:574.
13. Mattox KL, Beal AC, Jordan GL. Cardiorrhaphy in the emergency centre. *Cardiovasc Surg* 1974;**68**:886.
14. Berkoff HA, Hurley EJ. Aortic injury, in (Blaisdell FW, Trunkey DD, eds) *Cervicothoracic trauma*. New York; Thieme, 1994.
15. Oparah SS, Mandal AK. Operative management of penetrating wounds of the chest in civilian practice. *J Thorac Cardiovasc Surg* 1979;**77**:162.
16. Beal SL, Pattmeyer AW, Spisso JM. Esophageal perforation following external blunt trauma. *J Trauma* 1988;**28**:1425.
17. Valenzuela GJ, Hewitt CW, Kramer GL. Effects of sustained lymph drainage on cardiovascular lymph in sheep. *Am J Physiol* 1989;**256**:867.
18. Millison JW, Kroni L, Rheuban KS. Chylothorax: an assessment of current surgical management. *J Thorac Cardiovasc Surg* 1985;**89**:221.

5 Shock

Carl L. Gwinnutt
Consultant Anaesthetist, Hope Hospital, Salford

Peter Nightingale
Consultant in Anaesthesia and Intensive Care, Withington Hospital, Manchester

OBJECTIVES

■ To understand the physiological mechanisms that ensure adequate tissue oxygenation.

■ To understand the physiological changes which occur in the shocked patient.

■ To recognise and be able to treat the patient who remains in a state of shock after initial resuscitation.

The term shock should be reserved to define the state of *inadequate oxygen delivery to the tissues*. In the resuscitation room, the presence of shock is determined with the use of clinical parameters of the primary survey, and initial treatment is symptomatic. Oxygen and intravenous fluids are given, the aim being to restore rapidly the ability of the circulatory system to deliver oxygen to the vital organs before irreparable damage occurs. Patients cannot remain permanently in a state of shock, they will either recover or die. It has been said that shock is "a momentary pause on the way to death", a pause which allows the trauma team an opportunity to intervene.

Unfortunately, in some patients, the initial resuscitation manoeuvres fail to restore adequate tissue oxygenation, that is, they remain in shock. In order to ensure their survival, the cause of shock must be identified so that treatment can be directed more specifically. In order to achieve this, an understanding of the mechanisms responsible for maintaining oxygen delivery to the tissues in the normal situation is required.

Oxygen delivery and utilisation

Blood flow to the tissues

This is dependent upon:

- blood flow to the tissues;
- oxygen carriage by the blood;
- tissue oxygen consumption.

This is determined by the adequacy of the heart as a pump, and by the distribution of blood flow between the organs as a result of neurohumoral factors and local regulation of flow.

The heart's functions as a pump is measured as the volume of blood each ventricle ejects per minute. This is called the *cardiac output* (CO) and is the product of the volume of blood ejected per beat – *stroke volume* (SV) and the heart rate (beats/minute) – and is expressed in litres per minute. The output of the two ventricles must be the same over a short period of time otherwise the entire circulating volume would end up in either the systemic or pulmonary circulation!

$$\text{Cardiac output} = \text{stroke volume} \times \text{heart rate}$$
$$\text{Normal adult value} = 4.0\text{--}6.0\,\text{l/min}$$

In order to compare patients of different sizes, cardiac output is indexed to body surface area (BSA) and is called the *cardiac index* (CI), which is the cardiac output per square metre of body surface area, and expressed in l/min/m²:

$$\text{Cardiac index} = \frac{\text{cardiac output}}{\text{body surface area}}$$
$$\text{Normal adult value} = 2.8\text{--}4.2\,\text{l/min/m}^2$$

The cardiac output is affected by a variety of factors, of which the most important are:

- heart rate
- preload
- myocardial contractility
- afterload.

Heart rate

An increase in the heart rate will increase cardiac output. However, as the rate increases, it is the diastolic phase of the cardiac cycle which is predominantly shortened. As this is the period during which ventricular filling occurs, once the rate rises above about 160 beats/min in the young adult, the reduced diastolic time reduces ventricular filling, leading to a progressively smaller stroke volume.

The critical heart rate at which this fall in output occurs is also dependent on the age of the patient and condition of the heart; for example, rates over 120 beats/min may cause inadequate filling in the elderly.

An increase in heart rate is termed a *positive chronotropic effect*, and is mediated either directly by the sympathetic nervous system, or indirectly by the release of catecholamines from the adrenal medulla. The converse, a decrease in heart rate, is called a *negative chronotropic effect*, and is usually the result of vagal activity on the sinoatrial node and atrioventricular node.

Alternatively it may be secondary to drug administration, for example beta blockers.

> An increase in the heart rate will only lead to an increase in the cardiac output if it is kept below a critical level

Preload

Starling's Law of the Heart states that "the energy of contraction is proportional to the initial length of the cardiac muscle fibre". The initial length of a cardiac muscle fibre is termed the "preload" and relates to the distension of the ventricles at the end of diastole. This is determined by return of venous blood to the heart, which in turn is affected by the circulating blood volume, gravity, sympathetic stimulation, intrathoracic, and intra-abdominal pressures.

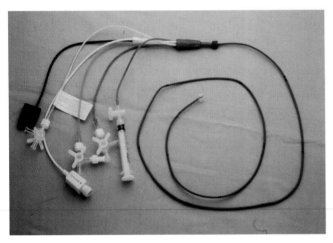

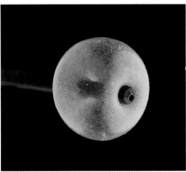

Figure 5.1 Pulmonary artery flotation catheter (PAFC). (Insert shows detail of tip with balloon inflated). Channels on catheter: pink, balloon inflation; blue, proximal opening (CVP); yellow, distal opening (PAP); white, thermistor (cardiac output); black, fibreoptic (Sv_{O_2}); clear, infusion port.

The greater the preload, the greater the energy of contraction, and hence stroke volume. However, this is only true up to a point because of the molecular structure of the contractile elements of muscle. Beyond this point, further cardiac distension results in a smaller contraction.

Measurement of preload

Clinically, it not possible to measure cardiac muscle fibre length to determine the degree of stretching produced by blood in the ventricle at the end of diastole. Nevertheless, with standard invasive haemodynamic monitoring, it is possible to estimate circulating blood and cardiac volumes. Measurement of the pressure in the superior vena cava or right atrium, that is the central venous pressure (CVP), has long been used as an index of circulating volume. However, it reflects the interaction between right ventricular function and rate of venous return and so bears little direct relationship to blood volume except at extremes. Current haemodynamic monitoring is based upon measurement of pressures in the pulmonary artery with the use of a specialised multilumen catheter called a pulmonary artery flotation catheter (PAFC) (Figure 5.1). This is often referred to as a "Swan–Ganz" catheter after its inventors. At its distal end there is an inflatable balloon and a temperature thermistor. There is also one lumen which opens at the tip beyond the balloon.

The catheter is inserted via the internal jugular or subclavian vein into the right side of the heart, and positioned in the pulmonary artery by using the blood flow out of the right ventricle. At the same time the pressure trace is monitored via the distal lumen to confirm correct placement (Figure 5.2). Once in a branch of the pulmonary artery, the balloon is inflated, isolating the distal lumen from the right side of the heart (Figure 5.3).

At this point, the pulmonary artery trace disappears to be replaced by the pulmonary artery occlusion pressure trace (PAOP), or wedge pressure, which is normally 9–12 mmHg. The PAOP is an indirect measure of the back pressure from the left atrium and is considered to be proportional to the *left ventricular end-diastolic pressure* (LVEDP) which in turn is related to the *left ventricular end-diastolic volume* (LVEDV).

As with CVP monitoring, there are reservations against using pulmonary artery occlusion pressure (PAOP) to assess intravascular volume status, although here the relationship is slightly stronger (Figure 5.4).

Ideally LVEDV should be measured. However, it is easier to estimate LVEDP, as described above, which is assumed to reflect preload. Nevertheless, the relationship between the two is neither simple or linear, and is affected by a variety of often rapidly changing factors during resuscitation (Figure 5.5).

As LVEDP increases, so does ventricular performance, but if a critical value is exceeded the ventricle begins to fail (Figure 5.6).

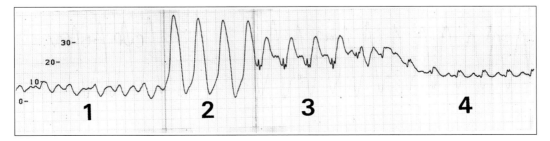

Figure 5.2 Pressure tracing obtained during insertion of PAFC. Section 1, right atrium; section 2, right ventricle; section 3, pulmonary artery; section 4, "wedged".

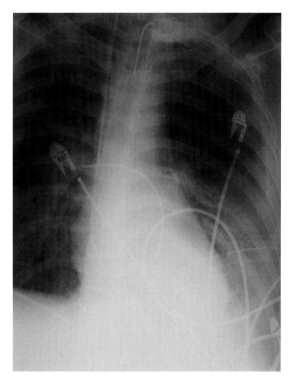

Figure 5.3 Chest x-ray showing typical position of PAFC in a main branch of the right pulmonary artery.

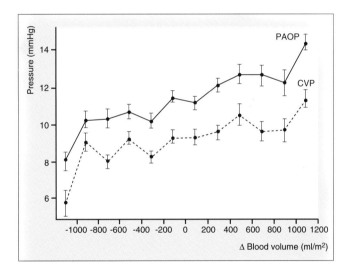

Figure 5.4 Changes in the pulmonary artery occlusion pressure PAOP) and central venous pressure (CVP) with changes in blood volume.

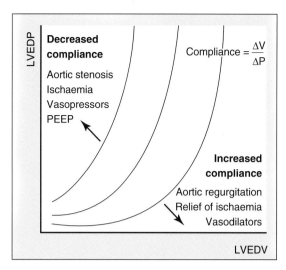

Figure 5.5 Variations in compliance of the left ventricle and relationship between left ventricular end-diastolic volume (LVEDV) and pressure (LVEDP).

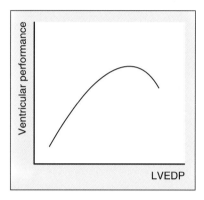

Figure 5.6 Relationship between LVEDP and ventricular performance. (This is often referred to as a "Starling curve".)

Clearly, inference of ventricular and circulating blood volumes from pressures is limited. It has recently become possible to measure *right ventricular end-diastolic volume* (RVEDV) at the bedside with the use of a modified pulmonary artery catheter. This variable is usually indexed to body surface area (RVEDVI, ml/m^2), and has been shown to provide better information about cardiac filling, and to correlate better with cardiac index, than PAOP. In one study CI increased in two-thirds of patients with a low RVEDVI (<90 ml/m^2) as a result of fluid administration, irrespective of the PAOP which ranged from <12–>18 mmHg.

In addition to measuring the pressures in the pulmonary artery, these catheters can be used to measure the cardiac output with a thermal dilution technique. This allows other haemodynamic variables to be calculated, including stroke volume, systemic, and pulmonary vascular resistance. A further modification is the addition of fibreoptic channels which allow continuous measurement of mixed venous oxygen saturation (see pages 72–73).

The blood volume

The normal circulating blood volume in an adult is approximately 70 ml/kg (lean body mass). It is regulated by a complex interaction of neural and humoral mechanisms. Activation of the renin–angiotensin–aldosterone system results in sodium retention and an increase in circulating volume along with stimulation of areas in the hypothalamus responsible for thirst, thus increasing fluid intake. In addition, stretch receptors in the atria influence the release of antidiuretic hormone (ADH) thus reducing water excretion, whilst under conditions of increased intravascular volume atrial myocytes secrete atrial natriuretic peptide, the actions of which generally oppose those of ADH and angiotensin.

At any one time, depending on the diameter of the vessels, 50% or more of the circulating volume may be in the venous system. This is under the influence of sympathetic activity, mediated by both humoral and nervous stimulation, and other local factors, particularly products of metabolism. A change of vessel diameter from maximum to minimum can effectively "increase" the venous return by approximately 1000 ml.

Myocardial contractility

This relates to the force and rate at which myocardial fibres contract for a given initial length, and it has a major influence on stroke volume and hence cardiac output. Substances which affect contractility are termed *inotropes* and can be either positive or negative in their actions. Again, contractility cannot be measured but only inferred indirectly as a result of the effect on stroke volume and cardiac output.

Positive inotropes produce a greater contraction at a given end-diastolic volume (or more accurately muscle fibre length), which is equivalent of shifting the curve in Figure 5.6 upwards and to the left. The sympathetic nervous system, the natural catecholamines, and beta-agonist drugs such as dobutamine have positive inotropic activity. Anything which reduces contractility is termed a *negative inotrope*, examples including myocardial damage, hypoxia, acidosis, anti-arrhythmic drugs, and anaesthetic agents. The effect of inotropic activity is summarised in Figure 5.7.

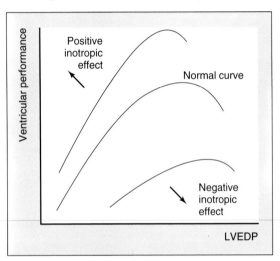

Figure 5.7 The effect of positive and negative inotropes on ventricular performance.

Afterload

As the ventricular muscle contracts, the pressures within the left and right ventricles increase until they exceed those in the aorta and pulmonary artery respectively; the aortic and pulmonary valves open and blood is ejected. Any impedance to flow generates an end-systolic wall stress, often called the afterload. It is not possible to measure this in clinical practice, but an estimate of peripheral loading conditions on the ventricle is obtained by calculating the *systemic vascular resistance* (SVR). This is calculated as the pressure difference between arterial and venous systems divided by the cardiac output (compare this with Ohm's Law, R = V/I).

$$\text{Systemic vascular resistance} = \frac{(MAP - CVP) \times 80}{\text{cardiac output}}$$

$$\text{Normal value} = 770\text{--}1500 \ \text{dyn/s/cm}^5$$

(The factor of 80 is used to convert values in mmHg into SI units.)

> Reducing afterload for a given preload will allow the ventricular muscle to shorten more quickly and extensively, increasing stroke volume and cardiac output

Empirically, it would seem that a reduction in the SVR or afterload would be beneficial. However, if there were a total loss of vascular tone, the capacity of the circulation would become such that the total blood volume would be insufficient to fill it, and flow through organs would be dependent upon their intrinsic resistance. Some organs would receive more than normal amounts of oxygenated blood (for example, skin) at the expense of others which would receive less (for example, brain). To prevent this, vascular tone is constantly regulated by sympathetic innervation and local mechanisms to ensure that blood goes to those organs which are least tolerant to hypoxia (see page 72).

Oxygen carriage by the blood

This is dependent on oxygen reaching the alveoli (Chapter 3) and its uptake into blood flowing through the pulmonary capillaries. This and the cardiac output (see above) determine oxygen delivery to the tissues.

Oxygen uptake into the blood

Insufficient oxygen dissolves in simple solution in plasma to meet tissue requirements. Blood contains haemoglobin at a concentration of approximately 15 g per 100 ml which facilitates oxygen uptake. Each molecule of haemoglobin can carry four molecules of oxygen, and when this occurs the haemoglobin is said to be 100% saturated. The net result of this is that each gram of haemoglobin can carry 1.34 ml of oxygen and each 100 ml of blood, which contains 15 g haemoglobin, carries:

$$15 \times 1.34 = 20.1 \ \text{ml of oxygen}$$

This is termed the *haemoglobin oxygen capacity* and is approximately 60 times greater than if oxygen was simply dissolved in plasma.

The relationship between percentage saturation of haemoglobin and partial pressure of oxygen (P_{O_2}) is a sigmoid curve (Figure 5.8), the *oxyhaemoglobin dissociation curve* (ODC), although it clearly relates to the association also!

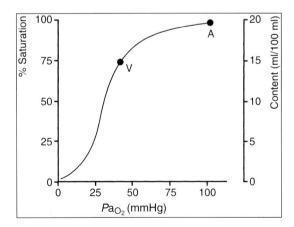

Figure 5.8 The oxyhaemoglobin dissociation curve (ODC). The normal values for arterial (A) and venous (V) blood are indicated.

The rapid uptake of oxygen from the alveoli occurs on the steep part of the ODC where small changes in P_{O_2} cause large changes in haemoglobin saturation. By the time a P_{O_2} of 100 mmHg (13.3 kPa) is reached, haemoglobin is 97.5% saturated (the normal healthy state). Beyond this the curve flattens out and little further increase in saturation occurs despite exposure to a high P_{O_2}. At a P_{O_2} of 250 mmHg (33 kPa), haemoglobin is effectively fully saturated. In addition to the steepness of this pressure gradient, release of oxygen from the haemoglobin is facilitated by an alkaline environment (low H^+), low partial pressure of carbon dioxide (P_{CO_2}), low concentrations of 2,3-diphosphoglycerate (2,3-DPG) in the red blood cells, a low temperature, and carbon monoxide, all of which shift the ODC to the left. (The opposite of these factors reduces the affinity – see below).

Although the vast majority of oxygen carried in the blood is in combination with haemoglobin, a small amount dissolves in the plasma. The volume dissolved is directly proportional to the P_{O_2} and is approximately 0.003 ml/100 ml blood per mmHg.

Therefore the total volume of oxygen carried in the blood is the sum of that combined with haemoglobin plus that dissolved in the plasma. This is called the *oxygen content.*

The oxygen content of the arterial blood will depend on the:

- haemoglobin concentration;
- oxygen carrying capacity of the haemoglobin;
- saturation of haemoglobin with oxygen;
- amount dissolved in the plasma.

This can be expressed as:

$$O_2 \text{ content per 100 ml blood} = (Hb \times 1.34 \times \text{saturation}) + (0.003 \times P_{O_2})$$

At a P_{O_2} of 100 mmHg:

$$
\begin{aligned}
O_2 \text{ content per 100 ml} \\
\text{arterial blood } (CaO_2) &= (15 \times 1.34 \times 97.5\%) \\
&\quad + (0.003 \times 100) \\
&= 19.5 + 0.3 \\
&= 19.8 \text{ ml}
\end{aligned}
$$

Although increasing the haemoglobin concentration increases oxygen content, the advantage of this may be offset by an increase in blood viscosity which may impede blood flow. The normal haemoglobin concentration is usually just above the point at which oxygen transportation is optimal. A slight fall in haemoglobin concentration, and hence viscosity, may improve flow and actually increase oxygen transportation.

In comparison, venous blood has a partial pressure of oxygen (Pv_{O_2}) of 40 mmHg (5.3 kPa) and is still 75% saturated:

$$
\begin{aligned}
O_2 \text{ content per 100 ml} \\
\text{venous blood } (Cv_{O_2}) &= (15 \times 1.34 \times 75\%) + (0.003 \times 40) \\
&= 15.07 + 0.12 \\
&= 15.2 \text{ ml}
\end{aligned}
$$

Transport of oxygen to the tissues

Having considered the cardiac output and oxygen content of the blood individually, we can now consider them together to determine the total volume of oxygen delivered to the tissues:

$$
\begin{aligned}
\text{Oxygen delivery } (D_{O_2}) &= \text{cardiac output} \\
&\quad \times \text{arterial oxygen content} \\
&= 5000 \text{ ml/min} \times 19.8 \text{ ml/100 ml} \\
&\sim 1000 \text{ ml/min}
\end{aligned}
$$

This variable is also referred to as the *oxygen flux.*

To eliminate the effect of patient size, oxygen delivery (D_{O_2}) is normally indexed to body surface area by substituting cardiac index for cardiac output:

$$
\begin{aligned}
D_{O_2}(\text{ml/min/m}^2) &= \text{cardiac index } (\text{l/min/m}^2) \\
&\quad \times \text{arterial oxygen} \\
&\quad\quad \text{content } (\text{ml/100 ml}) \\
&\quad \times 10^{\dagger}
\end{aligned}
$$

Normal value = 500–700 ml/min/m^2.

($^{\dagger} \times 10$ converts O_2 content per 100 ml to per litre.)

The most important feature of this equation is that oxygen delivery is the result of *multiplying* the cardiac output by the oxygen content. Therefore, if either, or more importantly both of these parameters fall, there will be a significant reduction in oxygen delivery.

Tissue oxygen consumption

When arterial blood arrives at the tissue level, it enters an environment where the P_{O_2} is much lower. Capillary P_{O_2} is approximately 20 mmHg (2.7 kPa) and cellular P_{O_2} 2–3 mmHg (0.4 kPa). Diffusion of oxygen occurs down this partial pressure gradient despite the affinity of haemoglobin for oxygen. In addition to the steepness of this pressure gradient, release of oxygen from the haemoglobin is facilitated by local conditions: the increased P_{CO_2}, the slightly more acidotic environment, and any increase in temperature, shifts the ODC to the right by, thus decreasing the affinity of haemoglobin for oxygen.

Under normal circumstances, not all the oxygen is removed from the haemoglobin. At rest, the whole body *oxygen consumption* (V_{O_2}) is about 140 ml/min/m^2 (250 ml/min) and the normal value of D_{O_2} is about 560 ml/min/m^2 (1000 ml/min) assuming a normal cardiac index of 2.8 l/min/m^2 and haemoglobin of 15 g/dl. Therefore tissues are taking up only 25% of the oxygen delivered to them. This is known as the *oxygen extraction ratio* (OER). As a result of only 25% of the oxygen being extracted, mixed venous blood is still 75% saturated despite the partial pressure of oxygen in venous blood (Pv_{O_2}) having fallen to 40 mmHg (5.3 kPa). This means that there is still a good deal more oxygen that can be extracted from the circulating blood. This is summarised in Figure 5.9.

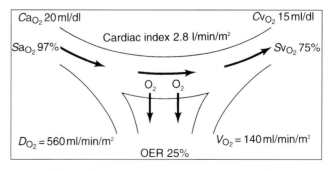

Figure 5.9 Summary of oxygen delivery and uptake.

If oxygen demand does not change, consumption of oxygen can be maintained over a wide range of oxygen deliveries. This relationship is usually depicted diagrammatically with

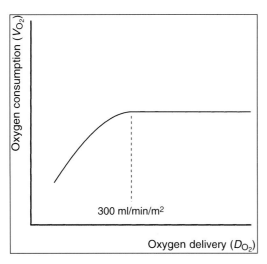

Figure 5.10 Relationship between oxygen delivery (D_{O_2}) and consumption (V_{O_2}). Note the critical value for delivery below which consumption falls.

D_{O_2} on the 'x' axis and V_{O_2} on the 'y' axis (Figure 5.10). Under normal circumstances, increased oxygen demand is met by increasing delivery, primarily by increasing cardiac output. However, should oxygen delivery fall, for example, because of anaemia, reduced cardiac output or hypoxia, then oxygen consumption can also be maintained by increasing oxygen extraction. Below a delivery of about 300 ml/min/m² oxygen extraction is maximal and oxygen consumption will fall as it is now directly dependent on the rate of delivery to the tissues.

Because calculation of both D_{O_2} and V_{O_2} involves the variables CI and Hb, this can give rise to a false relationship when they are plotted against one another. If V_{O_2} cannot be directly measured by indirect calorimetry, it may be better to plot OER on the 'x' axis and cardiac index on the 'y' axis since they do not share common variables, therefore reducing the possibility of a mathematically induced relationship.

Tissue and cellular effects of shock

Whatever the cause of shock, if it remains inadequately treated, or worse, unrecognised, tissue oxygenation becomes increasingly compromised and anaerobic metabolism occurs. This results in the formation of lactic acid which eventually leads to intracellular and systemic acidosis. In the later stages, microcirculatory changes lead to stagnation of blood flow and a further impairment of tissue perfusion. In addition, the hydrostatic pressure within the capillaries increases because blood can still perfuse the capillaries but cannot escape, and as a consequence further intravascular fluid is lost through the capillary wall into the interstitial space thereby compounding the problem. Eventually the damage leads to the development of multiple organ dysfunction syndrome (MODS), one of the commonest causes of late death after trauma.

Compensatory mechanisms

Fortunately, during shock, the body compensates in an attempt to satisfy tissue oxygen demand by:

- increasing the cardiac output;
- increasing oxygen extraction;
- increasing the oxygen content of the blood.

Increasing the cardiac output

In an attempt to increase the cardiac output, a variety of mechanisms come into play which help maintain or increase intravascular volume. Hypovolaemia is detected by volume receptors situated within the heart, and baroreceptors in the carotid sinus and aortic arch. These trigger an increase in sympathetic activity originating from the vasomotor centre in the medulla. The potential fall in cardiac output is limited as a result of the positive inotropic and chronotropic effects, and venous return is increased as a result of venoconstriction. Furthermore, as a result of the increased sympathetic activity, blood pressure is maintained, with a gradual increase in the diastolic component. A redistribution of blood occurs from the skin, gastrointestinal tract, and muscles, to the brain, heart, and kidneys, which are often referred to as the vital organs. This gives rise to the classical clinical picture of the shocked patient:

- sweaty, from increased sympathetic stimulation;
- pale and cool peripherally, from diminished skin blood flow;
- reduced gastrointestinal motility (ileus) from reduced blood flow;
- a rapid thready pulse from vasoconstriction decreasing the pulse pressure.

Stimulation of the adrenal medulla leads to an increased release of systemic catecholamines, enhancing the effects of direct sympathetic discharge on the heart and the precapillary sphincters of non-essential organs to help maintain perfusion of the vital organs. This selective perfusion also leads to a lowering of the hydrostatic pressure in capillaries serving non-essential organs, thereby encouraging the redistribution of fluid from the interstitial space to the intravascular space to help maintain the intravascular volume.

At the same time, a reduction in renal blood flow is detected by the juxtaglomerular apparatus in the kidney, which releases renin. Within a few minutes, this leads to the formation of angiotensin II, which in turn increases the secretion of aldosterone. Together with antidiuretic hormone (ADH) released from the pituitary, these hormones increase the reabsorption of sodium and water by the kidney, reducing urine volume and maintaining circulating blood volume. Renin, angiotensin II, and ADH also produce generalised vasoconstriction, which increases venous return, and are also partly responsible for mediating the symptom of thirst in the conscious patient.

Insulin and glucagon are also released to assist the supply and use of glucose by the cells. In addition the body attempts to enhance the circulating volume by releasing osmotically active substances from the liver. These increase plasma osmotic pressure, and so cause interstitial fluid to be drawn into the intravascular space.

Increasing oxygen extraction

Under normal circumstances, for example during exercise, an increased oxygen demand is met by increasing oxygen delivery. Similarly, during shock, the main compensatory mechanisms which take place within the circulatory system aim at maintaining blood flow via the mechanisms described above. If these mechanisms are inadequate and delivery falls, as often happens when shock is inadequately treated, there is increased extraction of oxygen from the blood and hence a fall in regional venous saturation. This is very difficult to assess clinically, but an average value can be obtained by measuring the *mixed venous oxyhaemoglobin saturation* (Sv_{O_2}). This can be done either by removing specimens of blood via a catheter within the pulmonary artery or more commonly using a modified PAFC. This has two fibreoptic channels to allow continuous measurement; one channel transmits near infrared light which is reflected by passing red cells, a second channel conducts the reflected light to a photodetector that determines the oxygen saturation of the haemoglobin. This is a global value and is affected by the venous blood from all organs as it returns to the heart. Under normal circumstances it is approximately 75%. Acute falls to below 70% indicate that global delivery of oxygen is becoming inadequate.

Increasing oxygen content of the blood

Although shock is associated with an increased rate and depth of respiration, this has little effect on oxygen uptake from the lungs into the blood. Haemoglobin in blood passing ventilated alveoli is already 97.5% saturated and the slight rise in alveolar P_{O_2} which occurs as a result of the hypocarbia produced by hyperventilation can only increase this by 1%.

Autoregulation

Certain organs are able to regulate their own blood supply despite variations in perfusion pressure, This is termed *autoregulation* and is most evident in the brain and kidneys. The exact mechanism remains unclear, but it is probably a combination of intrinsic activity of smooth muscle in the arteriolar walls responding to changes in pressure, and the vasodilator effects of metabolites accumulating as a result of reduced perfusion. Clearly, this can only happen over a limited range as there is a maximum to both the extent of vasoconstriction limiting flow and vasodilatation increasing it. Finally, an increase in temperature causes vasodilatation ensuring that metabolically active tissues receive an increased flow of blood to deliver adequate supplies of oxygen and substrate.

Types of shock

Following multiple trauma, the following types of shock occur, either alone or in varying combinations:

- Hypovolaemic
  - haemorrhage
  - crush injury
  - burns
- Cardiogenic/obstructive
  - myocardial infarction
  - myocardial contusion
  - cardiac tamponade
  - tension pneumothorax
  - pulmonary embolus
- Septic
  - perforated bowel
  - infected wounds
  - aspiration
  - gut translocation
- Neurogenic
  - high spinal cord lesion.

Rarer causes of shock include air embolism and anaphylaxis.

The cardiorespiratory response to major trauma is complex. Oxygen demand is high (unless there is concurrent hypothermia), and increases in oxygen extraction are seen. If global oxygen delivery is inadequate, as is often the case, Sv_{O_2} will fall. However, reductions in regional blood flow are difficult to quantify and severe occult tissue hypoxia can occur with few apparent indications. Mixed venous oxygen saturation may only fall slightly as the venous effluents from other organs may maintain a relatively normal value.

Once the initial resuscitation in the Emergency Room and definitive surgery in the Operating Theatre have finished, the patient will often require transfer to the Intensive Care Unit (ICU) for further management. The rest of this chapter will address the role of the ICU in identifying and treating the various causes of shock.

ICU admission

The principles of care for patients on the ICU is no different to medical care in general. All patients will need to have a full history taken, a thorough examination, and then laboratory or other investigations. The main difference is the degree of monitoring performed. Many patients arrive on the ICU with varying degrees of vascular access, catheters, drains, and an endotracheal tube in place. These must be initially checked for position, function, and security before progressing.

The history

Commonly this is unavailable from the patient and other sources of information must be used. A comprehensive hand-over must be obtained from the doctors and nurses who have cared for the patient so far, in particular details of the mechanism of injury (see below). Further information may become available from sources such as the family, GP, and old hospital notes, particularly with respect to any pre-existing medical problems.

The following should be established and recorded:

- identity of patient;
- mechanism of injury;
- time since injury;
- initial conscious level and vital signs;
- any delays in resuscitation;
- type and volume of fluid therapy so far;
- how much blood is still available;
- nature and adequacy of surgery;
- what investigations have been performed and any results.

The physical examination

In addition to establishing the patient's current physical condition, the ICU is often the setting for performing the secondary survey – a head to toe examination (see Chapter 1). Bear in mind the mechanism of injury in order not to miss any potentially life-threatening injuries or other minor injuries.

Establishing monitoring

Initially this will usually consist of ECG and non-invasive blood pressure measurement. In addition, the following are frequently used and established as indicated:

- Respiratory function
  - pulse oximetry
  - arterial and mixed venous blood gases
  - end-tidal CO_2
  - tidal and minute volumes
  - airway pressures

- Cardiovascular function
  - intra-arterial pressure
  - central venous pressure (CVP)
  - pulmonary artery pressures (PAOP)
  - cardiac output
  - mixed venous oxygen saturation (Sv_{O_2})
- Renal function
  - hourly urine output
  - urine sodium and osmolality
- Neurological function
  - conscious level (Glasgow Coma Scale score)
  - pupils – size and briskness of reaction to light
  - processed EEG
  - intracranial pressure
- Metabolic indices (by indirect calorimetry)
  - oxygen consumption (V_{O_2})
  - carbon dioxide production (V_{CO_2})
  - energy expenditure.

The best monitoring of the patient is frequent clinical examination.

Large blood vessels should be used initially for invasive monitoring, both for ease and speed of access (for example, the femoral artery and vein). This is particularly true in the hypotensive or cold patient. If a subclavian line is inserted for central venous access, the side already having a chest drain *in situ* is preferable, if other injuries and considerations permit.

Inserting monitoring lines is not a therapeutic procedure – it must not take precedence over treatment.

Consideration should be given to changing vascular lines inserted in non-sterile conditions but it is important to ensure that replacements are functional before others are removed.

Additional investigations

Further investigations will depend on clinical circumstances and may include:

- Haematology — FBC, platelets, clotting studies, cross-match
- Blood chemistry — Arterial and central or mixed venous blood gases, electrolytes, urea, creatinine, sugar, lactate, osmolality, cardiac enzymes, amylase, myoglobin, alcohol, albumin, amylase
- Microbiology — Blood and urine cultures, peritoneal contents, wound swabs, sputum
- Urine — Blood, myoglobin
- X-rays — Repeat chest x-ray ± lateral view, lateral thoracolumbar spine if trunk injury, swimmer's view of C-spine, odontoid peg, facial views (and skull if no CT), others as indicated by injuries
- Angiograms — Thoracic aorta, abdominopelvic vessels, limb vessels
- CT scans — Head and neck, facial bones, chest/abdomen and pelvis
- Ultrasound — Abdomen and pelvis if injury to trunk
- Echocardiography
- 12-lead ECG
- Peritoneal lavage

- Compartmental pressures
- Intra-abdominal pressure.

When these stages have been completed, it is now possible to address further management.

Diagnosis and management of shock

The probability of survival after admission to the ICU will depend upon:

- severity and type of injury;
- appropriate care at the scene;
- resuscitation after admission;
- adequacy and appropriateness of initial surgery;
- pre-existing serious disease;
- age (as an indirect reflection of cardiac reserve);
- incidence of complications and quality of care on the ICU.

Late deaths on the ICU following multiple trauma are associated with a systemic inflammatory response syndrome (SIRS), either with or without documented infection (sepsis). This leads to the multiple organ dysfunction syndrome (MODS) in which the acute respiratory distress syndrome (ARDS) plays a major role. Precipitation and continuation of these events is strongly linked with failure to relieve tissue hypoxia adequately, particularly during the initial resuscitative phase. Pulmonary embolism remains the other important late cause of death. Optimum care on the ICU will therefore be aimed at quickly stopping any further deterioration by reversing tissue hypoxia, with the goal of reducing the incidence of MODS.

The first consideration, as always, is to *ensure a secure airway and adequate oxygenation*. Hypoxia and hypoventilation are common following multiple trauma. Tracheal intubation should be performed early rather than waiting for any deterioration. The reasons for intubation are many and include trauma or burns to the upper airway, head injury, flail chest, pulmonary contusion, and protection of the airway. Patients can aspirate even if not in coma (defined as a Glasgow Coma Scale score < 8). This is especially true in those who are hypotensive.

Remember to keep the neck immobilised with in-line stabilisation during intubation unless cervical injury has been ruled out.

ARDS is a common complication after major trauma and the incidence may be reduced by early intubation and mechanical ventilation. Goris has devised an ARDS prevention scale (Table 5.1), a total score of 10 or more points indicating that prophylactic intubation should be performed.

A high inspired oxygen fraction should be used initially, to ensure at least 95% oxyhaemoglobin saturation, and later tailored according to measurement of Pa_{O_2}. Tracheostomy should be performed as a planned procedure, either during initial surgery when the airway has been compromised and intubation is likely to be prolonged, or some days later when the patient is more stable. Percutaneous tracheostomy is becoming increasingly popular and can be performed on the ICU.

Maximum effort is directed at optimising cardiac output, haemoglobin level, and arterial blood pressure to ensure *adequate tissue perfusion*. This will involve ensuring adequate access to the circulation, control of haemorrhage, restoration

Table 5.1 ARDS prevention scale of Goris

1	2	3	4	5	6	10
# Foot # Ankle # Wrist # Rib # Mandible	# Forearm # Le Fort II	# Humerus # Tibia # Vertebra # Le Fort III Ruptured spleen > 4 units blood	Ruptured liver Initial SBP <80 GCS 8–14	# Femur # Pelvis $Pa_{O_2} < 60$	Perforated bowel	Aspiration Flail chest GCS < 8

Abbreviations: #, fracture; GCS, Glasgow Coma Scale score; SBP, systolic blood pressure. Score calculated from sum of points for all injuries sustained. Total score >10 suggests prophylactic intubation.

of the circulating volume, and the use of complex pharmacological support including inotropes and vasodilators.

Hypovolaemic shock

This is the commonest cause of shock after trauma and is usually secondary to haemorrhage. The degree of hypovolaemia will be exacerbated if there are extensive soft tissue injuries. Up to 25% of the volume of tissue swelling following trauma is accounted for by leakage of plasma into the interstitial space around an injury, so called "third space loss". The effect of loss of volume from the circulation from either cause is to reduce venous return to the heart which in turn reduces preload, cardiac output and oxygen delivery to the tissues.

The severity of the *initial* fluid deficit, and the success of resuscitative efforts, can be gauged initially by clinical assessment of the patient. Four categories of shock have been described using this approach (Table 5.2).

However, these are only a crude estimate of volume status, are dependent on compensatory mechanisms, and may lead to inadequate administration of fluids during resuscitation. This is not uncommon in those patients who are unable to mount the normal compensatory mechanisms such as the elderly, those with pre-existing cardiovascular disease or taking medications such as beta blockers or calcium antagonists, or those with pacemakers. Furthermore, not all young patients show the classic hypotension/tachycardia response to hypovolaemia. Pregnant patients may respond atypically because of their increased circulating blood volume, while young athletic individuals normally become hypotensive only following significant haemorrhage. Occasionally, after haemorrhage alone, a hypovolaemic patient may present with a bradycardia – a well described, but often not appreciated physiological response. However, if there is coexisting tissue damage then this phenomenon is either blocked or greatly reduced.

Estimating the true amount of blood lost is problematical since external losses prior to admission are notoriously difficult to quantify, and there is a tendency to overestimate. Haemorrhage may also be concealed when it occurs with:

- haemothorax
- abdominal bleeding
- multiple closed long bone fractures
- retroperitoneal bleeding
- pelvic fractures.

The clinician has to rely upon both the clinical state of the patient and subsequently the results of invasive monitoring to assist in estimating the volume of blood lost. The priorities are to maintain adequate venous access, restore circulating blood volume, and stop further haemorrhage so as to maintain oxygen transport to the tissues.

Adequate venous access

A minimum of two short, wide-bore cannulae are required to allow the rapid administration of blood and other fluids. If limb veins are used, sites proximal to the injuries should be chosen so that administered fluids are not lost from damaged veins and fractured bones. Use of a Seldinger technique will facilitate the insertion of large-bore cannulae, particularly if the central veins are used.

Restore circulating blood volume

Initial therapy aims to restore blood volume rapidly by liberal fluid administration. Debate over the choice of fluid for resuscitation has raged for years and will not be repeated here.

Table 5.2 Categories of hypovolaemic shock

Grade	1	2	3	4
Blood loss (litres)	<0.75	0.75–1.5	1.5–2.0	>2.0
Blood loss (% BV)	<15%	15–30%	30–40%	>40%
Heart rate	<100	>100	>120	140 or low
Systolic BP	normal	normal	decreased	decreased + +
Diastolic BP	normal	raised	decreased	decreased + +
Pulse pressure	normal	decreased	decreased	decreased
Capillary refill	normal	delayed	delayed	delayed
Skin	normal	pale	pale	pale/cold
Respiratory rate	14–20	20–30	30–40	>35 or low
Urine output (ml/hr)	>30	20–30	5–15	negligible
Mental state	normal	anxious	anxious/confused	confused/drowsy
Fluid replacement	colloid	colloid	blood	blood

Any available fluid will be effective if the quantity used is adapted to its diffusion space; that is, normally three to five times more crystalloid has to be given than colloid. A consensus view is emerging that, when significant replacement is required (greater than 3 litres), the fluid should consist of crystalloid and colloid with the latter becoming more dominant as replacement volumes increase. In Europe, artificial colloids, especially gelatins, dextrans, and starch solutions are often used much earlier than in other parts of the world. By the time the multiple trauma patient reaches the ICU, it is probable that the fluids being given will be predominantly blood and relatively short-acting colloids. Gelatins are popular because of the absence of any effect on blood coagulation and their osmotic diuretic effect. In burn patients albumin is widely used. Glucose solutions should be avoided because of their large volume of distribution, potential for causing hyponatraemia, and worsening cerebral oedema and reperfusion injury. Platelets and clotting factors should be given to replace deficits if a coagulopathy is present as determined by laboratory investigations.

Stop further haemorrhage

This may involve any of the following, alone or more often in combination:

- appropriate surgery, especially abdominal and thoracic;
- external fixation of fractures, especially those involving the pelvis;
- arterial embolisation;
- balloon tamponade of large veins;
- blood components, eg platelets, clotting factors.

Hypothermia

Hypothermia is common after multiple trauma, and is due to a variety of causes (see box below). It is often associated with a coagulopathy or worsening acidosis; therefore all fluids administered should be warmed. As core temperature increases vasodilatation occurs revealing the need for further fluid administration.

Causes of hypothermia in major trauma

- Alcohol: blunts vasoconstrictor response
- Immobility: reduces heat production
- Intemperate climate: heat lost before admission
- Head injury: impairs thermoregulation
- Prolonged exposure: loss during resuscitation and surgery
- Anaesthetic drugs: impair thermoregulation, stop shivering

Myoglobinuria

This is commonly seen after multiple trauma and even if it is not grossly apparent initially, blood or urine should be sent for myoglobin estimation. If present it will be necessary to maintain a high flow of alkaline urine to prevent precipitation of myoglobin in the renal tubules. Sodium bicarbonate is given to maintain urine pH > 6.5, and acetazolamide (250 mg b.d.) may also be given to avoid an excessive increase in blood pH. A urine output as high as 300 ml/h has been recommended and involves the use of mannitol and perhaps a loop diuretic.

In the absence of pre-existing cardiac disease or cardiac injury, patients are generally tolerant of liberal fluid therapy. Where this is not the case, the margin for error is much narrower. Nevertheless more damage is likely to be caused in the long term from inadequate fluid therapy than from overtransfusion. The persistent use of clinical variables such as heart rate, systemic blood pressure, central venous pressure, and urine output results in many patients remaining inadequately fluid resuscitated by the time of ICU admission. Attempts to improve cardiovascular function should always therefore initially be made by further fluid administration. The more widespread adoption of relatively non-invasive modes of monitoring cardiac function, for example oesophageal Doppler probes, is recommended.

Many of the patients admitted to the ICU have undergone prolonged initial resuscitation, which often involves major surgical procedures. Others have failed to improve, or have deteriorated after an initial response (see box below). Whatever the reason for admission, resuscitation now becomes more complex and invasive assessment of the patient's cardiovascular status is frequently necessary to assess the haemodynamic state. This allows a more accurate diagnosis, with rational therapy guided by more precise monitoring.

Common reasons for poor response or deterioration after initial resuscitation

- Underestimation of initial blood loss or concealed bleeding
- Failure to recognise co-existing cardiogenic or obstructive shock
- Air or fat embolism
- Irretrievable head injury
- Unrecognised neurogenic shock
- Resuscitation fluids not entering the circulation

Assessing regional perfusion remains difficult, gastric tonometry being the only widely accepted method, used as a guide to splanchnic perfusion. Globally, the balance between oxygen delivery and consumption can be obtained by measurement of mixed venous oxygen saturation, values persistently below 60% indicating inadequate global perfusion. Although a less accurate substitute, central venous oxygen saturation may be used whenever a central line is inserted. An increase in the central venous to arterial P_{CO_2} gradient may also be indicative of an inadequate cardiac output and is easily obtained (normal ≤ 6 mmHg).

Oxygen content is ensured by an adequate level of haemoglobin which is > 95% saturated. During resuscitation and stabilisation a high inspired oxygen is usually employed (often 100%) to maintain a high Pa_{O_2} to maximise oxygen diffusion gradients and haemoglobin saturation. It is difficult to define an ideal haemoglobin level because tissues have a different optimum haematocrit for maximum oxygen delivery. A haemoglobin level of 10–12 g/dl is generally acceptable; higher or lower values may be chosen depending on oxygenation status and cardiac output.

Cardiac output is manipulated by fluid therapy, positive inotropes, and very occasionally vasodilators. Dobutamine remains the commonest inotrope and an infusion of 2–15 µg/kg/min is usually required. Numerous other drugs are available with a variety of therapeutic profiles, the majority act as vasodilators, and it is essential that there is an adequate circulating blood volume before they are given. Failure to ensure this may result in severe tachycardia and catastrophic falls in blood pressure. Dopamine usually causes vaso-constriction and may have unpredictable effects on cardiac output and blood pressure. It does not reduce the incidence of acute renal failure in the critically ill patient and increasingly it is being shown to have adverse effects on regional blood flow, endocrine, and immune function, and there is doubt about its routine use for prolonged periods.

Mean arterial pressure (MAP) may be low, normal, or high after blood volume has been optimised. A high or normal MAP does not necessarily indicate adequate resuscitation has been achieved because there may be marked vasoconstriction with a low cardiac output. This may be seen with hypothermia and high levels of circulating catecholamines, both of which commonly occur after multiple trauma. Treatment consists of sedation, analgesia, and rewarming with further fluid re-placement as vasodilatation occurs. A low blood pressure is more common and may be related to an inadequate cardiac output, a vasodilated state or both. Vasodilatation following resuscitation from shock of any aetiology may be related to reperfusion injury and a systemic inflammatory state. Treat-ment consists of fluids and vasoconstrictors (see page 78).

Constant re-evaluation of the patient's cardiovascular and respiratory functions is required. If these do not stabilise after replacement of the estimated losses then other problems or injuries, which may have been missed, should be searched for.

Cardiogenic shock

Both incidental myocardial infarction and cardiac contusions can lead to cardiogenic shock if 40% of the ventricular myocardium has been affected. The diagnosis should be sus-pected if there is poor response to fluid therapy and the ECG shows ST segment changes. Tests for myocardial damage such as creatinine kinase estimations are not helpful, but echocardiography will pick up regional wall motion ab-normalities and any valvular dysfunction.

Treatment requires invasive monitoring to measure cardiac output and filling pressures. Use of a right ventricular ejection catheter enables right ventricular volumes to be calculated and may be helpful because these patients often benefit from judicious controlled fluid therapy. Combined drug therapy is frequently needed, typically dobutamine plus a pulmonary vasodilator such as glyceryl trinitrate (2–10 mg/h). However, it is not uncommon to need a vasopressor such as noradrenaline (0.2–1.0 mg/h) to help maintain blood pressure and ensure adequate coronary perfusion.

Obstructive shock

This occurs as a result of mechanical obstruction to either venous return to the heart or to the outflow of blood, usually from the right ventricle.

Impairment of venous return

The rate at which blood returns to the heart is dependent on the pressure gradient between the peripheral veins and the right atrium. Any condition which reduces this gradient by raising right atrial pressure will lead to a fall in venous return to the heart and reduce ventricular filling and cardiac output. Any degree of hypovolaemia will worsen these haemodynamic effects. Note that if the CVP is being monitored, it may not necessarily be high if the patient is also severely hypovolaemic.

Common causes include tension pneumothorax, cardiac tam-ponade, or high levels of mean airway (intrathoracic) or abdominal pressure.

Pneumothorax is not an uncommon occurrence following trauma, both *de novo* and following blockage of chest drains with fibrin and blood clot. It may also be a sequela to the insertion of catheters into the central veins. In the supine patient x-ray changes are often subtle. The mechanically ventilated patient is at an increased risk of the pneumothorax tensioning. The diagnosis of a tension pneumothorax should be made if there is hyper-resonance and diminished breath sounds, but the first sign may be a fall in blood pressure or cardiac output. The ventilator pressure (if in volume-controlled mode) will be elevated, but in pressure-controlled mode the tidal volume will fall. Tracheal deviation away from the pneumothorax may be seen, but is usually a late sign. Tension pneumothorax is an emergency and treatment should proceed without x-ray confirmation.

Definitive treatment consists of a large chest drain (at least 26FG) in the midaxillary line in the fifth interspace. If the situation is urgent a large-bore cannula (at least 16G) should be placed in the second interspace, anteriorly, in the mid-clavicular line (see Chapter 3).

Cardiac tamponade impedes ventricular filling. It is more common in penetrating injuries when a high index of suspicion is warranted (see Chapter 3). The classical presentation is of hypotension with tachycardia unresponsive to fluid therapy and there may be arterial pulsus paradoxus. Strikingly, how-ever, the neck veins are engorged with venous pulsus paradoxus (Kussmaul's sign). If a CVP line is *in situ* a rapid *x* axis descent may be seen due to atrial relaxation but a slow *y* axis descent as ventricular filling is retarded. Urgent echocardiography will confirm the clinical diagnosis.

Treatment is by pericardial aspiration, usually by the subxiphisternal route, under ECG, echocardiographic, or radiological guidance. A Seldinger technique can also be used to leave a cannula in the pericardial space for repeat aspiration. However, surgery will usually be required for definitive treat-ment.

A *high mean airway pressure*, which may be needed in post-traumatic ARDS to ensure adequate oxygenation, may also reduce venous return. Treatment is by reducing the PEEP level as much as can be tolerated, with volume loading and inotropes to improve cardiac output.

Continued retroperitoneal or intra-abdominal bleeding, or distended oedematous bowel, may lead to a marked *increase in intra-abdominal pressure*. This may interfere with renal perfusion, compress the inferior vena cava and lead to a fall in venous return to the heart. A transduced gastric or bladder pressure >15 mmHg is associated with a decrease in renal function and pressures >25 mmHg require urgent decompression. The abdomen must be opened and packed to stop the bleeding. The abdomen should be left open until the patient is more stable.

Obstruction to cardiac ejection

In the acute phase after trauma, this is most likely to be due to fat emboli secondary to fractures or amniotic fluid embolus from the pregnant uterus. Air embolism may occur following "blast injury" (see Chapter 22), if the veins in the neck are lacerated or a large volume of air enters the circulation via a cannula. A major pulmonary embolus, secondary to venous thrombosis, obstructing right ventricular ejection is an un-common cause of shock immediately after trauma. A diagnosis of a major obstruction to the right ventricle outflow should be considered if there is:

- ECG evidence of acute right heart strain (right BBB, $S_1Q_3T_3$ pattern);
- elevated right ventricular pressures;
- acutely elevated CVP with tricuspid regurgitation (large v wave);
- fall in cardiac output/end-tidal CO_2.

Treatment of fat embolism is supportive with emphasis on maintenance of adequate oxygenation. If it recurs, urgent consideration should be given to the fixation of any fractures. Rapid identification should be made of the source of air emboli and the patient ventilated with 100% oxygen to encourage absorption. Treatment of pulmonary embolism secondary to thrombus is better with thrombolysis rather than heparin alone. The risks of bleeding have to be weighed against the dismal prognosis of such a large pulmonary embolus. After fluid resuscitation, noradrenaline should be used to maintain aortic diastolic pressure and hence improve coronary artery perfusion pressure. If the facilities are available thoracotomy and embolectomy may be considered.

Septic shock

Shock following trauma is associated with a high incidence of positive blood cultures, particularly gram-negative organisms, probably gut-related. Other sources of infection include dirty wounds, peritoneal soiling, and pulmonary aspiration.

In septic shock there is a failure of peripheral circulatory tone. Following fluid resuscitation the cardiac output is usually high, but not high enough to compensate for the low SVR since MAP remains low and there are signs of organ hypoperfusion. Ventricular dysfunction is present despite the high cardiac output because there is reversible depression of the ejection fraction. Although oxygen demand is high, there appears to be a failure of peripheral oxygen utilisation, perhaps related to a maldistribution of blood supply, and the Sv_{O_2} is high. In addition, there is systemic capillary leakage allowing protein, sodium, and water to move from the interstitial to the intracellular space, worsening hypovolaemia.

Treatment consists of plasma volume expansion, normally with colloid solutions (the use of albumin has not been shown to influence outcome), blood transfusion to compensate for the dilutional anaemia so produced, and vasopressors.

> Vasopressors are not a substitute for adequate fluid therapy, but septic shock, by definition, does not respond to fluids alone.

In septic shock, the vasodilated patient (SVR <800 dyn/s/cm^5) whose cardiac index is deemed inadequate (<3.5 l/min/m^2) should receive noradrenaline because it also has a moderate inotropic effect. Adrenaline (0.2–10 mg/h) is another possible choice. If the cardiac index is high (>5 l/min/m^2), phenylephrine (2–10 mg/h) can be used as a pure vasopressor. The effects and dose response curves of all vasoactive drugs used in the ICU can be unpredictable so the lowest dose should be used initially and titrated to effect; large doses may, however, be necessary. Titration is usually to a blood pressure which produces adequate organ function whilst maintaining an acceptable cardiac index (usually ≥ 4.5 l/min/m^2) and hence oxygen delivery. In the septic, hyperdynamic, fluid-resuscitated patient, vasopressors have been shown to improve renal function. An MAP of 80 mmHg is usually satisfactory but higher

levels may be necessary in the patient with peripheral vascular disease or hypertension.

Neurogenic shock

The vasomotor centre controls vascular tone, with impulses transmitted to the peripheral vasculature via the sympathetic nerves. These nerves leave the spinal cord segmentally from T1 to L2. Transection of the spinal cord above T1 results in loss of vascular tone with vasodilatation of both the capacitance and resistance vessels. This causes pooling of blood which reduces venous return and lowers cardiac output. Consequently there is marked hypotension (blood pressure = cardiac output × peripheral resistance). In isolated spinal cord injury, the systolic blood pressure is usually around 90 mmHg, which is sufficient to maintain perfusion of the cord and prevent further hypoxic damage. However, coexisting injuries may cause hypovolaemia and exacerbate the fall in blood pressure, thereby placing the cord at risk. A lesion above T1 will also result in loss of the cardioaccelerator fibres which originate from T1 to T5. This leaves vagal tone unopposed and causes a bradycardia of around 50 beats per minute. Furthermore, a lesion at this level will interrupt the outflow to the adrenal gland, thereby reducing the reflex secretion of catecholamines and eliminate the systemic vasoconstrictor and cardiostimulatory response to hypovolaemia.

The resultant overall picture of neurogenic shock which follows a spinal cord injury above T1 is one of hypotension, bradycardia, and low central venous pressure with warm, dry peripheries secondary to vasodilatation and loss of sweating. Gradually the patient becomes hypothermic.

The initial management consists of ensuring adequate venous access and the administration of intravenous fluids, crystalloids, colloids, or blood depending upon the presence or absence of other injuries. If a bradycardia is severe and symptomatic, glycopyrrolate 0.2 mg, repeated as necessary, or atropine up to 1 mg can be given intravenously. Atropine is more likely to cause drying and thickening of secretions which may exacerbate respiratory dysfunction, cause an ileus and, if multiple doses are given, can have adverse effects on the central nervous system. Consideration should be given to the early establishment of intra-arterial monitoring of blood pressure, as non-invasive methods are unreliable at low pressures, and repeated arterial samples will be required to assess pulmonary function. Excessive volumes of intravenous fluids must not be administered if the blood pressure does not respond, because of the risk of precipitating pulmonary oedema. Such patients will require the use of vasopressors and inotropes and, in order to guide therapy appropriately, a pulmonary artery flotation catheter should be inserted. Monitoring with central venous pressure has been found unreliable in these circumstances.

The systemic vascular resistance will be low (<700 dyn/s/cm^5), consistent with loss of vascular tone. Fluids should be administered to maintain a pulmonary artery occlusion pressure of approximately 12 mmHg and, if the blood pressure remains low, then an infusion of an alpha adrenergic agonist such as noradrenaline can be used. Dopamine (2–5 µg/kg/min) may also be used to maintain the blood pressure at pre-injury levels, and improve tissue perfusion. Both agents have positive inotropic actions.

A significant number of patients will develop pulmonary oedema during the first week post-injury, despite careful control of fluid therapy. This is thought to be due to damage to the pulmonary endothelium which occurs following a brief but massive sympathetic discharge at the time of injury, causing extreme hypertension. The risk of pulmonary oedema is increased by excessive administration of fluids, particularly crystalloids, hypoxia, or a concurrent myocardial injury.

It must be remembered that patients with this type of injury are extremely intolerant of being tilted and great care must be exercised when they are moved. This is particularly true if they have to be transported around the hospital for investigations or treatment.

Summary

Following multiple trauma, survival from shock depends upon administering oxygen, restoring the circulating blood volume, and identifying and treating those conditions which reduce venous return or impair cardiac function. This approach can reduce the incidence of multiple organ dysfunction syndrome and death, but must be instigated as soon as possible. It may require sophisticated equipment for diagnosis, rational therapy, and monitoring the response to treatment, which at all times is aimed at ensuring adequate tissue perfusion with oxygenated blood.

Further reading

Abou-Khalil B, Scalea TM, Trooskin SZ, Henry SM, Hitchcock R. Hemodynamic responses to shock in young trauma patients: Need for invasive monitoring. *Crit Care Med* 1994;**22**:633–9.

American College of Surgeons Committee on Trauma. *Advanced trauma life support course for physicians: course manual.* Chicago: American College of Surgeons, 1993.

Baek S-M, Makabali GG, Bryan-Brown CW, Kusek JM, Shoemaker WC. Plasma expansion in surgical patients with high central venous pressure (CVP); the relationship of blood volume to hematocrit, CVP, pulmonary wedge pressure, and cardiorespiratory changes. *Surgery* 1975;**78**:304–15.

Bauman MH, Sahn SA. Tension pneumothorax: Diagnostic and therapeutic pitfalls. *Crit Care Med* 1993;**21**:177–8.

Beards SC, Watt T, Edwards JD, Nightingale P, Faragher EB. Comparison of the hemodynamic and oxygen transport responses to modified fluid gelatin and hetastarch in critically ill patients: A prospective, randomized trial. *Crit Care Med* 1994;**22**:600–5.

Diebel L, Wilson RF, Heins J, Larky H, Warsow K, Wilson S. End-diastolic volume versus pulmonary artery wedge pressure in evaluating cardiac preload in trauma patients. *J Trauma* 1994;**37**: 950–5.

Driscoll PA, Gwinnutt CL, LeDuc Jimmerson C, Goodall O. *Trauma resuscitation: the team approach.* London: Macmillan, 1993.

Goris RJA. The injury severity score. *World J Surg* 1983;**7**:12–18.

Hanique G, Dugernier T, Laterre PF *et al.* Significance of pathologic oxygen supply dependency in critically ill patients: comparison between measured and calculated methods. *Intens Care Med* 1994;**20**: 12–18.

Hutton P, Clutton-Brock T. The benefits and pitfalls of pulse oximetry. *BMJ* 1993;**307**:457–8.

Jansen JRC. The thermodilution method for the clinical assessment of cardiac output. *Intens Care Med* 1995;**21**:691–7.

Johnson KD, Cadambi A, Seibert GB. Incidence of Adult Respiratory Distress Syndrome in patients with multiple musculoskeletal injuries: effect of early operative stabilization of fractures. *J Trauma* 1985;**25**: 375–84.

Lang RM, Borow KM, Neumann A, Janzen D. Systemic vascular resistance: an unreliable index of left ventricular afterload. *Circulation* 1986;**74**:1114–23.

Little RA, Kirkman E, Driscoll P, Hanson J, Mackway-Jones K. Preventable deaths after injury: why are the traditional 'vital' signs poor indicators of blood loss. *J Accident Emerg Med* 1995;**12**:1–14.

Martin C, Papazain L, Perrin G *et al.* Norepinephrine or dopamine for the treatment of hyperdynamic septic shock? *Chest* 1993;**103**: 1826–31.

Moulton C, Pennycook AG. Relationship between Glasgow coma score and cough reflex. *Lancet* 1994;**343**:1261–2.

Mythen MG, Webb AR. The role of gut mucosal hypoperfusion in the pathogenesis of post-operative organ dysfunction. *Intens Care Med* 1994;**20**:203–9.

Ruokonen E, Takala J, Kari A, Saxen H, Mertsola J, Hansen EJ. Regional blood flow and oxygen transport in septic shock. *Crit Care Med* 1993;**21**:1296–303.

Shippy CR, Appel PL, Shoemaker WC. Reliability of clinical monitoring to assess blood volume in critically ill patients. *Crit Care Med* 1984;**12**:107–12.

Shoemaker WC, Appel PL, Kram HB *et al.* Prospective trial of supranormal values of survivors as therapeutic goals in high risk surgical patients. *Chest* 1988;**44**:1176–86.

Steltzer H, Hiesmayr M, Mayer N, Krafft P, Hammerle AF. The relationship between oxygen delivery and uptake in the critically ill: is there a critical or optimal therapeutic value? *Anaesthesia* 1994;**49**: 229–36.

Sugrue M. Intra-abdominal pressure. *Clin Intens Care* 1995;**6**:76–9.

Williams JF, Seneff MG, Friedman BC *et al.* Use of femoral venous catheters in critically ill adults: Prospective study. *Crit Care Med* 1991; **19**:550–3.

Wo CCJ, Shoemaker WC, Appel PL, Bishop MH, Kram HB, Hardin E. Unreliability of blood pressure and heart rate to evaluate cardiac output in emergency resuscitation and critical illness. *Crit Care Med* 1993;**21**:218–23.

6 Head injury

Douglas Gentleman
Honorary Consultant Neurosurgeon, Ninewells Hospital, Dundee, and Consultant, Centre for Brain Injury Rehabilitation, Royal Victoria Hospital, Dundee

Rona Patey
Consultant Anaesthetist, Aberdeen Royal Infirmary

OBJECTIVES

- To review the main scientific principles which underpin clinical practice in the management of severe head injury.

- To recognise that the initial order of clinical priorities in managing a seriously head-injured patient is the same as for any other seriously injured patient.

- To appreciate the critical importance of cerebral oxygenation and perfusion after head injury, and the need to maintain these at all stages of management.

- To understand the types of intracranial complication that can follow head injury, and how these are diagnosed and treated.

- To recognise which patients need a neurosurgical consultation with a view to transfer to the neurosurgical unit, and how to conduct that transfer safely.

A million people attend hospital each year in the UK after a head injury, 100 000 are admitted, and 10 000 are transferred to a neurosurgical unit. Behind these bald statistics lie two clinical problems:

- how to identify as early as possible the patient at risk of complications;
- how to prevent that patient's primary brain injury being compounded by a secondary insult that might threaten life or the quality of survival.

Brain damage and the challenge to clinicians

As we learn more about the pathological changes after trauma to the brain, so the conventional distinction between primary and secondary brain damage becomes increasingly blurred.

The events at the moment of injury that cause primary brain damage also trigger a cascade of biochemical and electrochemical damage which continues over subsequent hours and days – a process we may soon be able to modify with neuroprotective drugs [1]. However, it is still useful to think in terms of a "window of opportunity" in which clinicians can act to limit the total amount of brain injury.

Primary damage – the initial injury

Mechanical "deceleration" forces acting on the brain at the moment of injury transfer energy to the brain and cause primary brain damage. This ranges from temporary loss of function of individual neurones to gross anatomical disruption of neural pathways, and the clinical picture ranges from mild concussion to instant death. The cerebral microcirculation is also damaged. The conscious level varies with the amount of primary brain damage, and focal neurological signs can reflect damage to particularly susceptible areas of the brain.

Secondary damage – the continuing insult

The chemical environment of the damaged surviving neurones is altered by ion fluxes across cell membranes, the accumulation of metabolites such as lactate, and the generation or release of harmful substances like free radicals and excitotoxic neurotransmitters. This causes more neuronal damage and disequilibrium of the neuronal environment.

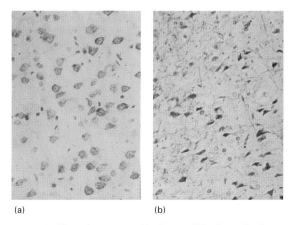

(a) (b)

Figure 6.1 (a) Normal neurones with plump cell bodies and pale cytoplasm. (b) Dead neurones after hypoxia and ischaemia, with pyknotic cell bodies and dark cytoplasm.

This continuing damage is made worse by any interruption of the oxygen supply to the injured brain. The well-established causes of secondary brain damage (see box) all do their harm by starving the injured neurones of oxygen during the critical hours or days that follow injury, so that they become more likely to die than to recover [2,3] (Figure 6.1). Either the blood contains too little oxygen, or cerebral blood flow is inadequate to meet neuronal needs.

Normally autoregulation by the cerebral vessels keeps blood flow constant over a wide range of systemic arterial pressure. A serious head injury impairs or abolishes autoregulation, and blood flow then simply varies with cerebral perfusion pressure – the difference between mean systemic blood pressure and intracranial pressure (ICP). The blood supply to injured neurones then becomes vulnerable to low blood pressure or high ICP, making it vital to maintain an adequate blood pressure and to control ICP after serious head injury.

Causes of secondary brain damage

- Intracranial haematoma (especially if surgery is delayed)
- Diffuse brain damage from:
  - hypoxaemia (for example, a blocked airway)
  - hypercarbia (for example, hypoventilation)
  - shock (for example, blood loss from injuries)
  - post-traumatic meningitis
  - epileptic seizures
  - neurochemical damage

The clinicians who treat a seriously head-injured patient must break the chain of continuing damage, to give surviving neurones the best chance to recover. The priorities are to give oxygen, to ensure an adequate circulation, and to reduce raised ICP. Managing a seriously head-injured patient is the work of many hands, and these principles apply whether the patient is in the resuscitation room, the ambulance, the CT scanner, the operating theatre, or the intensive care unit [4].

In the resuscitation room

Decisions and actions taken in the resuscitation room profoundly influence the outcome from serious head injury.

Initial assessment and resuscitation must follow the principles of Advanced Trauma Life Support (ATLS) [5], which are now accepted worldwide (see Chapter 1). The aim is to identify and correct life-threatening complications of injury in the order that they threaten life (see box below). It is more important to ensure that the injured brain is being perfused with enough oxygenated blood by identifying and correcting an obstructed airway, inadequate ventilation, and hypovolaemia than to carry out a detailed neurological assessment, however obvious the head injury.

Priorities in resuscitation

A Airway (with cervical spine control)
B Breathing
C Circulation (with haemorrhage control)
D Disability (neurological assessment)
E Exposure of the whole body and environmental considerations

---

Airway, breathing, and circulation

Airway and cervical spine control

The top priority is always to secure and maintain a clear airway and provide a good oxygen supply, whilst protecting the cervical spine. High flow oxygen (12–15 1/min) should be given to every trauma patient, with the use of a tight-fitting face mask (often called a "trauma mask") which has an oxygen reservoir bag. Exactly what airway care is needed depends on the injury and the patient's response, and may escalate from basic airway manoeuvres to provision of a definitive airway with mechanical ventilation (see Chapter 2).

The cervical spine must be protected during all airway manoeuvres, especially after high energy collisions or falls, with blunt trauma above the clavicle, and in an unconscious patient. The neck is held immobile in line with the body, either by an assistant or by securing it with a rigid cervical collar, sandbags, and tape; many patients are now brought to hospital secured in this manner on a long spine board (see Figure 1.5). Aligned immobilisation of the spine is maintained when the patient is turned for examination and treatment. A lateral cervical spine film should be taken early on, but a normal film does not exclude the possibility of spinal injury.

Breathing

Ventilation is assessed clinically to identify problems which need immediate treatment to save life (see Chapter 2). Arterial blood gases should be measured. Pulse oximetry is useful for giving an ongoing assessment of patient oxygenation, but can mislead if peripheral perfusion is poor, the probe is dirty or incorrectly applied, or in the very restless patient. It also gives no information about P_{CO_2}.

It is never too early to call for anaesthetic help with a seriously head-injured patient, as threats to airway patency or ventilation must be corrected as soon as possible to minimise secondary brain damage. Establishment of a definitive airway (most commonly by orotracheal intubation) usually involves a controlled rapid sequence intravenous induction (to minimise the threat of aspiration if there is regurgitation), with care taken to protect the cervical spine. Indications for intubation (immediately or before transfer to a neurosurgical unit) are shown in the box below. The decision to intubate a head-injured patient is also a decision to ventilate, and will usually involve drugs for sedation, analgesia, and muscle relaxation.

Circulation

Delay in recognising and treating exsanguinating haemorrhage from the trunk or extremities continues to cause some head-injured patients to die. This can easily be missed unless examination is systematic and thorough. Failure to control blood loss leads to hypovolaemic shock, cerebral hypoperfusion, and ischaemic secondary brain damage.

Pulse rate and pressure, respiratory rate, capillary refill time, and urinary output are much more useful than simply measuring blood pressure when the circulation is assessed in a trauma victim (see Chapter 5). Frequent assessment is necessary during resuscitation. Direct measurement of arterial and central venous pressure helps to monitor resuscitation, especially if cardiovascular instability is marked or in the patient with significant pre-existing disease.

| Indications for intubation and ventilation after head injury |

- Immediate
  - coma (not obeying, not speaking, not eye opening): GCS <8
  - loss of the protective laryngeal reflexes
  - ventilatory insufficiency (as judged by arterial blood gases):
    - hypoxaemia: $Pa_{O_2} < 9\,kPa$ on air, *or* $Pa_{O_2} < 13\,kPa$ with supplementary oxygen
    - hypercarbia: $Pa_{CO_2} > 6\,kPa$
  - spontaneous hyperventilation causing $Pa_{CO_2} < 3.5\,kPa$
  - respiratory arrhythmia
- *Before transfer*
  - deteriorating conscious level, even if not in coma
  - bilaterally fractured mandible
  - copious bleeding into mouth (for example, from skull base fracture)
  - seizures
  - if the patient is to be transferred by air

The patient should be catheterised and urine output regularly monitored. A gastric tube (orogastric rather than nasogastric if skull base injury cannot be excluded) minimises the risks of gastric dilatation and regurgitation, reduces the ventilation pressure, and improves the circulatory response to fluid therapy. Beware the very cold patient, for example one who has been lying out all night or has been injured in a mountain accident. These trauma victims may not respond to resuscitation until warmed up.

Fluid resuscitation begins with a rapid bolus of warmed electrolyte solution, and blood is transfused if it is estimated that over 15% of the blood volume has been lost. All sources of blood loss need to be identified, in order to estimate the circulatory deficit and guide surgical priorities. In an unconscious patient, a high index of suspicion is needed for chest, abdominal, and pelvic injuries [6]. Shock which responds transiently or not at all to initial fluid resuscitation usually implies that major haemorrhage has not been controlled. The patient may need to go to theatre for this, and full neurological assessment must wait until this has been achieved.

Neurological assessment in the resuscitation room

As emphasised above, this is done only after the airway, breathing, and circulation have been assessed and secured, and any necessary life-saving interventions carried out.

A fall in conscious level gives the earliest warning of worsening cerebral function, whether from an intracranial expanding lesion or extracranial problems like hypoxaemia, hypercarbia, or hypovolaemia. The Glasgow Coma Scale (see box below) is used throughout the world and measures three distinct aspects of conscious level: the eye opening response, the best motor response, and the best verbal response. Each aspect is stratified and described in unambiguous terms. It can also be assigned numerical values and summated to yield a Glasgow Coma Scale score which ranges from 3 to 15.

Conscious level must be measured early and often, and recorded on a neurological observation chart. Measurements at 10–15 min intervals rapidly establish a trend, that is valuable both for monitoring and for communication with others. It is vital to react promptly to observed changes, especially to deterioration.

It is essential that focal neurological signs are detected and acted upon quickly, as they reflect critical brain compression and can be followed by rapid deterioration. A dilating pupil can mean an expanding intracranial haematoma on the same side of the brain. Unilateral limb weakness can mean a haematoma on the opposite side of the brain. A conscious

| Glasgow Coma Scale |

- Eye opening response
  - spontaneous
  - to speech
  - to pain
  - no response
- Best motor response (in the upper limbs)
  - obeys commands
  - localises to painful stimuli
  - withdraws from painful stimuli
  - spastic flexion
  - extension
  - no response
- Best verbal response
  - orientated
  - confused
  - inappropriate words
  - incomprehensible sounds
  - no response

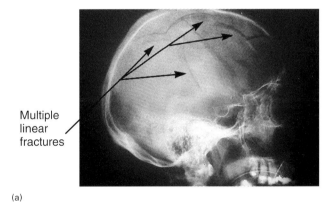

(a)

(b)

Figure 6.2 (a) Extensive linear fractures. (b) Linear fractures extending into the skull base.

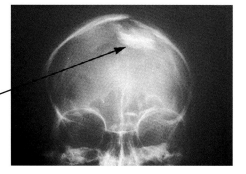

"Double density" caused by bone fragment projected through skull

(a)

Depressed fracture

(b)

Figure 6.3 (a) Depressed skull fracture: "double density" projection. (b) Depressed skull fracture: tangential view.

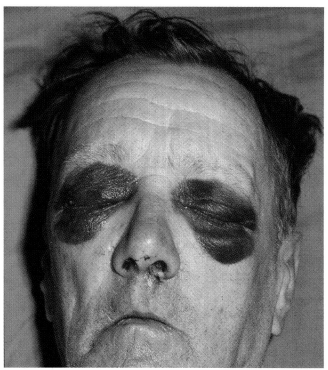

(a)

(b)

Figure 6.4 (a) Skull base fracture: periorbital haematomas. Eyes closed by swelling and bruising ("panda" or "racoon eyes"). (b) Skull base fracture: mastoid haematoma (Battle's sign).

patient can exhibit difficulty with the understanding or expression of speech (dysphasia). Other focal neurological signs are rarely useful soon after a serious head injury.

Conscious level and the pattern of limb movements cannot be measured in a patient who has been pharmacologically paralysed for endotracheal intubation and ventilation. However, this is always an acceptable price to pay to achieve cardiorespiratory stability in a seriously injured patient, especially before transfer to a CT scanner or a neurosurgical unit. It then becomes especially important to make repeated assessments of pupil size and reaction.

Further assessment in the resuscitation room

Scalp wounds

The more damage is visible on the outside of the head, the more there may be on the inside. It is important to ask about the mechanism of injury, to help decide whether the skull may have been fractured or penetrated.

External bleeding from scalp lacerations (see Figure 1.12) is controlled by pressure. Such bleeding is only rarely profuse enough to cause hypovolaemic shock, so that in a shocked patient it is vital to look elsewhere for the cause. Occasionally an area of scalp is avulsed, which a plastic surgeon may be able to re-implant.

The wound should be cleaned in the resuscitation room – removing dirt, hair, and any loose foreign bodies – assessed and, if necessary, carefully explored with a gloved finger, and closed with sutures or Steristrips. If neurological deterioration demands rapid transfer to the neurosurgical unit, the wound is simply covered and compressed to control haemorrhage and prevent further contamination.

Skull films

Skull fractures can be of the vault or base, linear or depressed, and simple or compound. Figures 6.2–6.4 show some examples. Only 5% of head-injured attenders at A & E departments prove to have a fracture, but this greatly increases the risk of intracranial complications [7]: haematoma (linear fracture) or infection (depressed or basal fracture). At the very least, a patient found to have a skull fracture must be admitted to hospital for a period of observation, and not sent home from the A & E Department.

Indications for skull films are shown in the box below.

Indications for skull films (if a CT scan is not to be done)

- History of high velocity injury (road accident, fall from height)
- History of assault with a weapon
- Unconsciousness at any time since injury
- Any alteration of consciousness at hospital
- Focal neurological signs
- Skull penetration (CSF leak, obvious skull depression, stab/shot)
- Marked bruising or laceration of the scalp

Skull films are redundant when a decision can be taken on clinical grounds that the patient needs a CT scan or referral to the neurosurgeons (see section below on referral). However, they are especially useful when the patient's neurological condition does not suggest the need for a CT scan, creating a danger that the seriousness of the head injury is underestimated and the patient sent home with potentially disastrous consequences.

Skull films can easily locate metallic foreign bodies without the artefact seen on a CT scan (Figure 6.5a), but a scan is superior for locating bone fragments or non-metallic foreign bodies (Figure 6.5b). The mechanism of injury and the condition of the patient should influence the choice of investigation when a foreign body is suspected.

Increasingly a scan is now done before referral to the neurosurgical unit, as more general hospitals acquire scanners. The scan can then aid decisions on the need and timing of transfer, and an image transfer system to the neurosurgical unit can be valuable. The range and significance of CT scan findings is discussed later.

Deterioration in the resuscitation room

The commonest reasons for deterioration are disturbances of the airway, ventilation or circulation, or a fit. The ABC priorities need to be reviewed: checks should be made that the airway is clear, breathing is adequate, enough oxygen and fluids are being given, and that haemorrhage has been controlled.

A fit can cause dramatic deterioration, and is managed by protecting the airway and waiting for the fit to stop; only if it

is prolonged (> 2 min) or repeated should anticonvulsants be given. Intravenous diazepam (5–15 mg) aborts a seizure (at the risk of respiratory depression), and phenytoin (5–10 mg/kg) by slow intravenous injection (with continuous ECG monitoring) prevents more fits.

If none of these complications is found or if focal neurological signs develop, brain compression from a haematoma or swelling is likely. The patient should be intubated and ventilated to control Pa_{O_2} and Pa_{CO_2}, given mannitol (0.25–1.0 g/kg) to lower ICP, and urgently transferred to the neurosurgical unit.

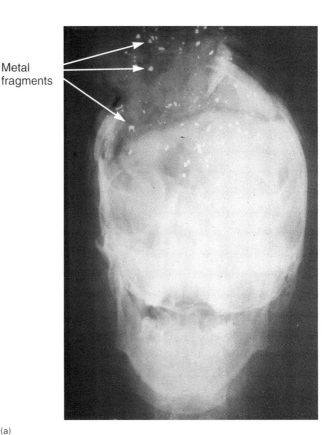

(a)

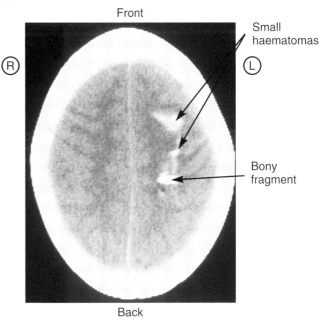

(b)

Figure 6.5 (a) Plain skull film: metallic foreign bodies. Severe blast injury to head; multiple metal fragments in brain with much of top of skull missing. (b) CT brain scan: bone fragments from penetrating brain injury.

Burrhole exploration of a presumed extradural haematoma in a general hospital seldom saves life. More often the haematoma proves to be intradural or the burrholes are misplaced, and time is wasted that would be better spent getting the patient to the neurosurgeon.

Referral to the neurosurgeon

After resuscitation, the critical decision is whether the patient should be referred to the neurosurgeon for advice and possible transfer. There should never be any hesitation about seeking neurosurgical advice about the management of a head-injured patient.

Delayed referral from general hospitals has been known for some time to cause avoidable death and disability after serious head injury [8]. Guidelines for use in the UK (see box below) were published in the early 1980s [9] and have been refined and extended since [10]. These identify patients at risk of developing complications, especially intracranial haematoma, and encourage early referral and transfer for investigation and treatment before clinical deterioration takes place.

Criteria for referral to the neurosurgeon

- *Immediate* (after initial assessment and resuscitation)
  - any altered level of consciousness, if there is a skull fracture
  - persisting coma, even without a skull fracture
  - unexplained deterioration of conscious level
  - development of focal neurological signs
  - any abnormality on a CT scan
- *Urgent* (within 6–8 h of admission)
  - persisting confusion, even without a skull fracture
  - compound depressed skull fracture (or other penetrating injury)
  - suspected CSF leak from nose or ear

Safe transfer to the neurosurgical unit

At any time after a serious head injury, a blocked airway, inadequate breathing, or seizures can rapidly cause cerebral hypoxia or hypercarbia, and continued blood loss from undiagnosed or undertreated injuries can cause shock. These complications must be pre-empted or corrected to prevent secondary brain damage.

Transfer to the neurosurgical unit exposes a seriously head-injured patient to great danger, as respiratory, cardiovascular, or neurological complications can develop and pose a real threat [11]. This threat is as real during a short transfer as during a long one. Even moving the patient a short distance in a hospital to the CT scanner or ICU must be taken seriously and done with care. To minimise the risk, the patient must be stabilised before transfer, and be sent with staff and equipment able to detect and manage any crisis en route [12,13]. Making the patient stable enough to transfer safely (see box below) is the endpoint of initial assessment and resuscitation.

What is needed to achieve stability before transfer

- Airway: clear, protected
- Breathing: adequate ventilation
- Circulation: adequate perfusion, blood loss stopped

This section will deal with what is needed to maintain stability and safety during the journey itself, and is summarised in the box below.

The escort

A suitably experienced doctor and a trained nurse (or paramedic) must accompany every seriously head-injured patient during transfer, even over short distances. An intubated and ventilated patient requires an escort with anaesthetic training and skills.

What is needed for a safe journey

- Trained escort
- Functioning monitors with an adequate power supply
- Drugs and adequate oxygen
- Intubation equipment
- Intravenous lines
- Ambulance
- Trolley

The escorts must familiarise themselves with the patient before the journey starts: the extent and severity of injuries, the management to date, and the patient's response. Clearly it helps if they have been involved in the resuscitation room. They must have the training and skills needed to deal with problems en route, including airway compromise, respiratory arrest, repeated epileptic fits, rising ICP with incipient coning, and falling blood pressure. They must be familiar with the equipment available during the journey.

Monitoring equipment

In the relatively cramped, dark, and noisy environment of a moving ambulance, clinical monitoring must be supplemented electronically and recording continued. For a patient with an altered conscious level, the minimum monitoring is pulse oximetry, continuous invasive blood pressure measurement, ECG, and end-tidal CO_2 monitoring. All equipment used during transfer must be serviced regularly to ensure it works when needed.

The patient needs high flow oxygen throughout the journey. The ambulance must carry two full oxygen cylinders, whose size depends on the length of the journey; for example, a cylinder containing 680 litres of oxygen will last just over an hour at a flow rate of 10 l/min. Before and after transfer, arterial blood gases are measured; during transfer the trend in oxygen saturation is monitored by pulse oximetry. Transcutaneous cerebral oximeters using near infrared spectroscopy to measure cerebral oxygenation are not yet of proven benefit.

In a ventilated patient, a capnometer continuously measuring end-tidal P_{CO_2} indicates whether the ventilation set is achieving the ideal Pa_{CO_2} (4.0–4.5 kPa). A higher Pa_{CO_2} will raise ICP by vascular engorgement, while a lower P_{CO_2} may induce patchy cerebral ischaemia by vasoconstriction. Correlation of end-tidal P_{CO_2} with arterial P_{CO_2} may be confirmed with arterial blood. The ventilator itself should have a pressure dial to indicate inflation pressure and a blow-off valve to avoid barotrauma to the respiratory tree.

A seriously injured patient has a labile cardiovascular system. This requires the same monitoring during transfer as before it (blood pressure, pulse rate, urine output, central venous pressure) to assess whether fluid resuscitation is adequate. Intra-arterial lines with an appropriate monitor allow continuous accurate measurement of blood pressure. There must be reliable intravenous access throughout the journey to infuse fluids, blood, or drugs. All lines must be secured and clearly labelled to prevent avulsion or confusion.

Occasionally an ICP monitor is inserted before transfer. Monitoring ICP on its own is of less value than combining blood pressure and ICP data electronically to give a continuous measurement of the cerebral perfusion pressure (CPP).

Drugs, tubes, and lines

It is important to anticipate any emergencies which may occur on route, to carry the necessary drugs and equipment, and to ensure that the escorting doctor and nurse are familiar with these and the problems which may arise from their use.

The ambulance must carry the full range of drugs needed to deal with emergencies (see box below) especially those needed for ventilation or cardiac resuscitation. A protracted seizure can be aborted with intravenous diazepam (5–15 mg), but this can depress respiration. Phenytoin (5–10 mg/kg) by slow intravenous injection prevents repeated seizures, but cardiac monitoring is needed because of toxicity. If clinical signs suggest rising ICP, an infusion of the osmotic diuretic mannitol (0.25–1.0 g/kg) lowers ICP for 20–60 min, gaining some more time for the transfer.

Drugs the ambulance must carry

- Drugs needed to institute and maintain ventilation
  - depolarising and non-depolarising muscle relaxants
  - short-acting analgesics
  - intravenous sedatives
- Drugs needed for cardiac resuscitation
- Anticonvulsants
- Mannitol

Any head-injured patient can deteriorate during transfer and need intubation or rapid fluid infusion. Tubes and lines inserted before the journey can fall out or obstruct. The ambulance must therefore carry a full range of endotracheal tubes, two working laryngoscopes, a full range of cannulae (including wide bore), and crystalloid solution (such as Hartmann's solution). In a ventilated patient a self-inflating bag (such as an Ambu bag) allows ventilation to be continued if the oxygen supply or the ventilator fails. Blood cross-matched before the journey should travel in the ambulance, not in a separate taxi.

Method of transport

The patient should be moved the minimum number of times between trolleys or beds in order to minimise discomfort or further injury, with care taken not to kink, obstruct, or pull out tubes and lines. These manoeuvres must never be hurried, and enough people must be recruited to move the patient and all attached monitors and equipment safely. It is helpful to have a fully equipped trolley for the transfer of seriously ill or injured patients to specialist centres. Ideally its equipment should run off the ambulance's power supply but, if not, the monitoring equipment must have adequate battery time.

The circulation is labile after a serious head injury, and the physical disturbance caused by movement into and out of the ambulance and the journey itself can cause fluctuations in blood pressure and cerebral perfusion pressure. The patient should be placed head first and 10–15° head-up in the ambulance, to minimise the effect of changes of speed and direction during the journey. The ambulance crew should be asked to provide a smooth ride at constant speed, even if the patient's neurological state is causing concern (see Chapter 24).

Despite improvements in design, ambulances can still be cramped, noisy, dark, and cold, and the escorts must be able to adjust to this, positioning themselves and their equipment sensibly and working with the maximum economy of movement. If a life-saving procedure like endotracheal intubation has to be carried out on route, it is more sensible to stop the ambulance briefly than to attempt heroics under poor conditions that expose the patient to the risks of failure or delay in carrying out the procedure.

Occasionally head-injured patients are transferred by helicopter or aeroplane. Problems of space, noise, and cold are even more obvious (see Chapter 24). Hypoxaemia must be anticipated, as the atmospheric pressure of oxygen falls with increasing altitude (even in a pressurised aircraft). Precautionary intubation and ventilation should be given careful consideration before departure if a patient is to be transferred by air.

At the neurosurgical unit

The handover

Good communication is vital when the patient is handed over at the neurosurgical unit, and if this is neglected there can be needless problems. The escorting doctor and nurse must be able to tell the neurosurgical staff what has been done so far: the injuries identified, treatment given for these, the patient's response, assessments of conscious level and focal neurological signs, and all drugs and intravenous fluids given. Medical and nursing records, observation charts, drug prescription sheets, blood results, x-ray films, and scans should be taken to the neurosurgical unit and left there.

Clinical re-assessment

The neurosurgical doctors and nurses must reassess the patient on arrival to establish their own baseline observations, using the same order of priorities as in the resuscitation room. Even with optimum care during transfer serious problems – airway compromise, pneumothorax, hypovolaemic shock – can develop insidiously. The patient must not be taken to the scanner until this assessment has been made. If a problem is identified it must be dealt with before the patient is moved from the neurosurgical reception area.

The neurological examination need only be brief. Conscious level and limb responses are assessed (unless sedative or paralysing drugs have been given for intubation and ventilation), and the pupils are checked for size, symmetry, and reaction to light. All responses are recorded on an observation chart.

Diagnosing intracranial complications: CT and MR scans

The purpose of transferring seriously head-injured patients to the neurosurgical unit is to diagnose and treat intracranial complications like haematoma and brain swelling. Except in infants, the skull is a rigid box of bone; consequently a small rise in intracranial volume can be accommodated by squeezing CSF and venous blood out of the head, but further rises rapidly raise ICP (Figure 6.6), threaten cerebral perfusion and

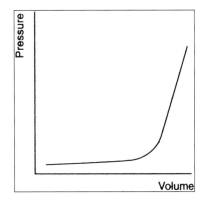

Figure 6.6 Intracranial pressure–volume relationship.

oxygenation, and compress and distort the brain (Figure 6.7). Speed in diagnosis and treatment is therefore vital to limit secondary brain damage.

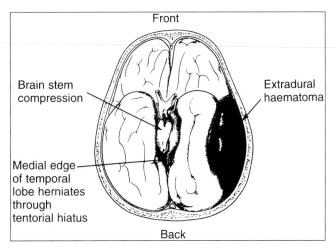

Figure 6.7 Brain compression and distortion from a large extradural haematoma.

Most patients undergo a CT scan of the brain. This technology revolutionised head-injury management (and neurosurgery generally) when introduced into clinical practice in the 1970s, and the speed and quality of images have greatly improved since then. Modern CT scanners can show a wide range of post-traumatic intracranial pathology [14] (see box overleaf). Some of these are illustrated below (see Figures 6.8–6.13).

A scan is done soon after arrival at the neurosurgical unit (unless already done at the referring hospital). Findings determine whether the patient goes straight to theatre, to the intensive care unit, to the ward, or back to the referring hospital. While the scan is being done, life support must be maintained and the patient carefully monitored to detect and correct any complications quickly.

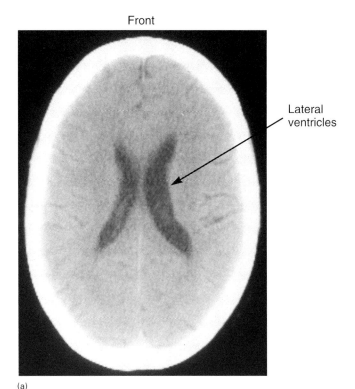

(a)

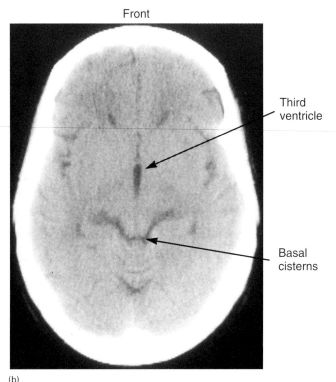

(b)

Figure 6.8 CT brain scan: normal axial sections. (a) Axial section at the level of the lateral ventricles. (b) Axial section at the level of the IIIrd ventricle and basal cistern.

Magnetic resonance imaging (MRI) outperforms CT in showing lesions of the skull base, posterior fossa, and spine, and the detailed anatomy in and around cerebral lesions. However, the role of MRI in acute head-injury management has so far been limited by availability, patient safety, and imaging time, although advancing technology may change this. Certainly MRI is much the more sensitive for showing lesions of primary brain damage and early diffuse brain swelling (15) (Figure 6.14).

Types of intracranial pathology seen on CT or MR scan

- Haematoma
  - extradural
  - intradural:
    - subdural
    - intracerebral
    - mixed (burst lobe)
- Brain swelling
  - generalised:
    - loss of cortical sulci and fissures
    - effacement of third ventricle
    - effacement of basal cisterns
  - focal:
    - shift of brain and ventricles
- Evidence of primary brain damage

Front

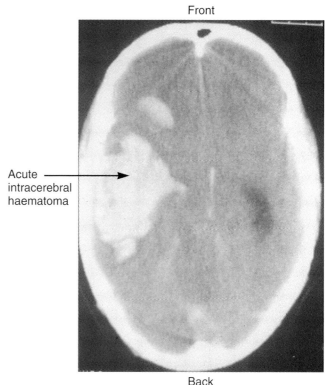

Acute intracerebral haematoma

Back

Figure 6.11 CT brain scan: large acute intracerebral haematoma.

Front

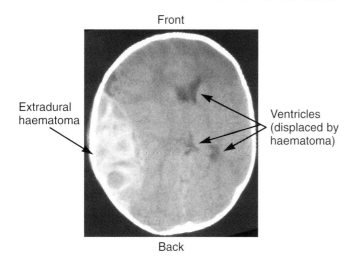

Extradural haematoma

Ventricles (displaced by haematoma)

Back

Figure 6.9 CT brain scan: acute extradural haematoma.

Front

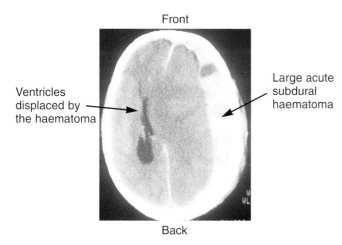

Ventricles displaced by the haematoma

Large acute subdural haematoma

Back

Figure 6.10 CT brain scan: acute subdural haematoma.

Front

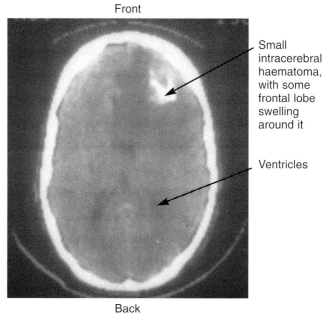

Small intracerebral haematoma, with some frontal lobe swelling around it

Ventricles

Back

Figure 6.12 CT brain scan: small acute intracerebral haematoma with some brain swelling.

Few patients with compound depressed skull fractures and basal fractures who are neurologically well are scanned, as their management is unlikely to be altered.

Managing intracranial complications

Interpreting a CT brain scan after head injury requires knowledge of the normal appearances and how the injury can alter these. Figure 6.8 shows typical axial sections from a normal CT brain scan: the cerebral hemispheres and the ventricular system are symmetrical; there is no distortion of any normal structure; the sulci and basal cisterns are clearly seen (excluding raised ICP), and there is no lesion such as an area of blood or damaged brain.

Haematomas

Acute haematomas produce high radiodensity areas on CT scan, and often distort and displace the adjacent brain and midline structures like the ventricles. They are either extradural (Figure 6.9) or intradural; the latter can be subdural (Figure 6.10), intracerebral (Figure 6.11), or mixed ("burst lobe"). Intracerebral haematomas and burst lobes usually affect the frontal or temporal lobes.

To operate or not?

Management depends on the clinical progress and on the location, size, and mass effect of the haematoma. All but the very smallest extradural haematomas are evacuated surgically, as are intradural haematomas large enough to compress and distort surrounding brain and to raise ICP. A poor or deteriorating neurological condition indicates the need for immediate surgery, and speed is then of the essence.

A small intradural haematoma not significantly distorting or compressing the adjacent brain is left alone, especially in a neurologically stable patient (Figure 6.12). If there is doubt as to what to do, the ICP can be monitored for several days by a catheter or solid state transducer implanted through a burrhole. A high or rising ICP (> 20 mmHg) suggests that the patient is likely to deteriorate if the haematoma is not evacuated [16]. At any stage neurological deterioration or failure to improve can indicate the urgent need for operation.

Surgical technique

A haematoma consists of clotted blood, which cannot be removed through a half-inch-wide burrhole, but only through a larger window cut in the overlying skull. A craniotomy or trephine is cut with a drill or bone saw, and the bone flap is replaced at the end of the operation. Less often, bone is simply nibbled away piecemeal around a burrhole to form a craniectomy.

An extradural haematoma is found immediately beneath the skull, and often arises from a tear of the middle meningeal artery in the middle cranial fossa. In order to reach an intradural haematoma, the dura is opened and reflected in flaps. This may expose a subdural haematoma arising from a cortical draining vein, torn as it traverses the subdural space to the superior sagittal sinus. Under the subdural clot the surface of the brain itself may be intact, or may be severely disrupted to form a mixture of blood and pulped brain tissue (burst lobe). A purely intracerebral haematoma is reached by making a corticotomy down to the clot.

Whatever the location of the haematoma, it is removed by gentle suction and irrigation, bleeding point(s) are secured by diathermy or metal clips, and diffuse ooze from the raw brain surface is controlled by tamponade with cotton wool balls. Non-viable brain tissue is removed, but less severe damage to the brain parenchyma is dressed with a monolayer of a haemostatic material like Surgicel. The dura is carefully closed with sutures to prevent CSF leaks and the intracranial spread of infection. The bone flap is replaced wherever possible, but sometimes diffuse brain swelling prevents this.

Complications

The main complications after surgical evacuation of an intracranial haematoma in the first 24–48 h are diffuse brain swelling and the re-collection of a haematoma. Both complications raise ICP and reduce the benefits of surgery. They are detected by clinical observation and/or ICP monitoring,

and can be confirmed by a further scan. A postoperative haematoma (either at the site of the previous clot or under the bone flap) may need a second operation. Damaged lobe(s) of the brain can swell during or after the operation, and this is managed as for diffuse brain swelling (see below).

The outcome depends more on the preoperative condition of the patient than on the site of the haematoma. The greater

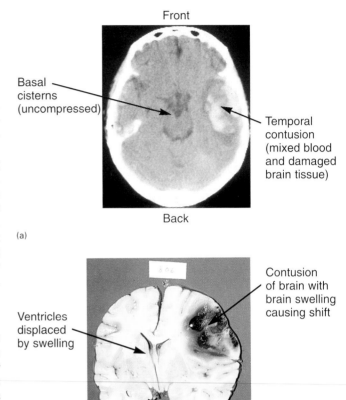

(a)

(b)

Figure 6.13 (a) CT brain scan: left temporal cerebral contusion. (b) Autopsy specimen: right frontal contusion with brain shift.

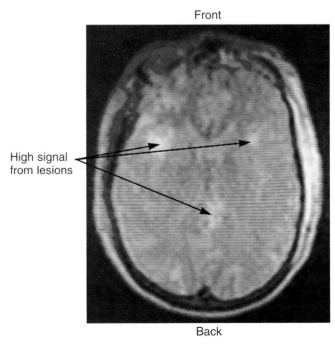

Figure 6.14 MR brain scan: scattered lesions of primary brain damage.

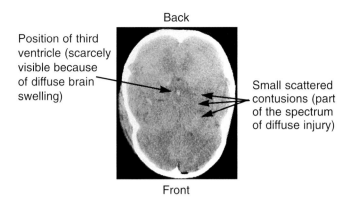

Figure 6.15(a) Diffuse brain injury: effacement of the third ventricle by swelling.

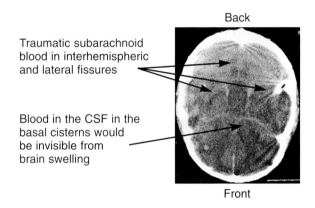

Figure 6.15(b) Diffuse brain injury: effacement of the basal cisterns by swelling and traumatic subarachnoid haemorrhage.

the depth and duration of altered consciousness and focal signs, the poorer the outcome. Increasing age also has an adverse effect.

Brain swelling and raised ICP

The scan may show no haematoma, but swelling of all or part of the brain. Generalised brain swelling follows either widespread brain damage from the initial trauma, or else a systemic insult (hypoxia, hypercarbia, or shock). Focal swelling reflects local contusion of the brain, especially the frontal or temporal lobes (Figure 6.13). As with a haematoma, focal swelling distorts and shifts the brain away from itself – best seen with midline structures like the ventricles.

Brain swelling causes areas of low or mixed radiodensity within the brain. These changes are often ill-defined on a CT scan until a few days after injury. An MR scan often shows more detail early on, because its signal intensity is highly sensitive to the local changes in the brain water content which will lead to swelling (Figure 6.14).

It is possible to deduce from a CT or MR scan that ICP is high. The cortical sulci, basal cisterns, and third ventricle are progressively effaced as ICP rises and CSF is forced out of the head in attempted compensation (Figure 6.15). When ICP becomes very high and CPP (mean blood pressure minus ICP) falls below critical levels the cerebral substance often has a "ground-glass" appearance on CT scan; this has a poor prognosis.

Management

Surgical treatment is unlikely to control raised ICP when there is generalised brain swelling, but can have a role with focal swelling from contusion. Swollen and contused tissue can be excised, especially from less eloquent brain areas like a frontal lobe.

The treatment of brain swelling and high ICP requires intensive and often complex monitoring and intervention, and therefore the facilities of an intensive care area [17,18]. ICP can be measured easily and reliably by an implanted catheter or solid state transducer, but on its own this information is of limited value. CPP is a more useful index of the patient's progress and response to treatment. Jugular venous oxygen monitoring is technically demanding but useful for assessing cerebral metabolic rate and the adequacy of oxygen supply. The value of direct cerebral oximetry by near infrared spectroscopy in head-injured patients remains to be proved.

The mainstay of intensive therapy is pharmacological. Mechanical ventilation (and often hyperventilation) with muscle relaxant and sedative drugs is used to maintain Pa_{O_2} and Pa_{CO_2} at optimal levels. Cerebral metabolic rate can be lowered by barbiturates or the anaesthetic agent propofol. Cerebral perfusion can be promoted with the use of inotropic and vasoactive drugs to raise mean arterial pressure, and mannitol or other diuretics to reduce brain water content. Fluid balance, haemoglobin concentration, blood sugar level, nutrition, and temperature are also carefully controlled to maintain a stable internal environment and provide the neurones with the most favourable conditions for recovery.

Primary brain damage

Severe primary brain damage causes characteristic CT scan appearances (see box below). These lesions are not directly treatable, and their importance is as markers of widespread microscopic damage to the neural tracts and cerebral microcirculation. Most of this damage is not visible on a CT scan, although MR can show it more clearly (Figure 6.14). Indeed the CT scan may show almost no abnormality even when the patient has clearly suffered a very severe head injury.

Management of severe primary brain damage is supportive in the intensive care unit, as described above for brain swelling. The prognosis is related to the quantum of damage (as reflected by the depth and duration of coma) and to whether or not secondary complications supervene.

CT signs of severe primary brain damage

- Small haematomas (often multiple and scattered)
  - deep hemisphere white matter
  - basal ganglia
  - corpus callosum
  - upper brain stem
- Traumatic subarachnoid or ventricular haemorrhage
- Generalised brain swelling

Penetrating wounds of the brain

A penetrating brain wound is one which breaches the skull and the meninges, giving pathogenic bacteria a portal of entry into the brain. Missile wounds from gunshot or shrapnel are common in war zones, and the brain can also be stabbed. Most penetrating brain injuries in the UK are of two types:

fractures of the skull base, and compound depressed fractures of the skull vault.

Many of these patients are neurologically well, as brain damage tends to be focal and conscious level is little impaired. These injuries can easily be overlooked or underestimated, and to avoid this it is crucial to ask about the mechanism of injury and to assess any overlying wound and skull films with care.

Skull base fracture

This is usually diagnosed clinically, not on films, by examining for periorbital haematoma (Figure 6.4a), mastoid haematoma (Battle's sign) (Figure 6.4b), haemotympanum, or the leakage of CSF (often blood-stained) from the nose or ear. These signs may not become obvious until a few days after injury as bruising and discoloration develop and as the soft tissue swelling which plugs the fracture site resolves. A skull film may show a linear vault fracture which extends into the base (Figure 6.2b) or even intracranial air (Figure 6.16).

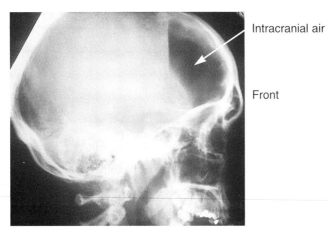

Intracranial air

Front

Figure 6.16 Plain skull film: intracranial gas (indicating skull base fracture).

Occasionally a severely head-injured patient exsanguinates through the nose and mouth because a skull base fracture has damaged the carotid or jugular vessels, and severe skull base fractures are found at autopsy in many fatal cases.

The force needed to fracture the skull base is likely also to damage the mucosa lining adjacent cavities (pharynx, sinuses, nose, and ears), allowing endogenous organisms (especially *Pneumococcus* spp.) to migrate through the breach in the skull and dura to cause meningitis or a brain abscess. Antibiotic prophylaxis can be given for one to seven days to prevent this, although some neurosurgeons now doubt that this is necessary. Benzylpenicillin is the drug of choice; erythromycin is a useful alternative for patients allergic to penicillin, and cephalosporins and sulphonamides are also effective. Persistent CSF leaks from the nose or ear are repaired surgically a week or two after injury, when local swelling has subsided.

Depressed vault fracture

Conscious level is normal in most patients with a depressed vault fracture but because of underlying brain contusion there may be focal signs, for example hemiparesis. The history is of a direct blow to the head, often involving assault with a weapon. The wound which almost always overlies the fracture needs careful assessment for evidence of bony depression or the presence of brain tissue or CSF. Skull films should include

a view tangential to the fracture to show the depressed bone fragment (Figure 6.3b).

The complications of depressed fractures are infection and epilepsy. The overlying wound should be explored within 24 hours of injury to remove dirt and hair, debride devitalised tissue, and elevate the bone fragments (unless they are only minimally depressed). Judgement about the need for elevation is needed if the fracture overlies a major venous sinus. Non-compound depressed fractures are elevated only if the cosmetic

Front

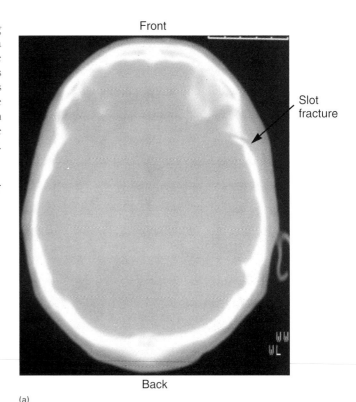

Slot fracture

Back

(a)

Front

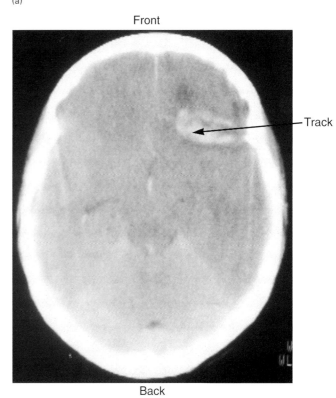

Track

Back

(b)

Figure 6.17

Top

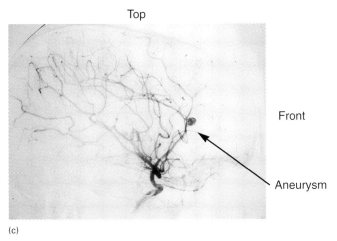

Front

Aneurysm

(c)

Top

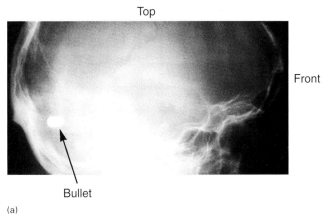

Front

Bullet

(a)

Front

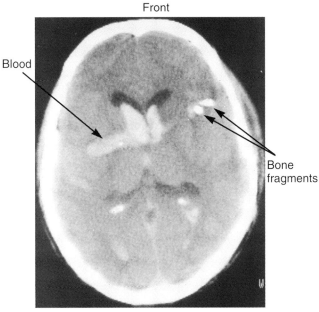

Blood

Bone
fragments

(b)

Figure 6.17 Stab wound of brain. (a) CT brain scan: "slot" fracture (scan set on bone windows). No detail of brain is seen. (b) CT brain scan: haematoma along track of weapon. Same patient as (a). (c) Cerebral angiogram: traumatic false aneurysm from stab wound. Same patient as (a). (Courtesy of Mr Michael du Trevou.)

deformity would be unacceptable, as on the forehead. Broad-spectrum antibiotics are given for a few days. If neglected, 10–20% of these injuries are complicated by meningitis, brain abscess, or empyema. Surgical treatment does not reduce the risk of epilepsy, which is increasingly likely with post-traumatic amnesia over 24 hours, focal neurological signs, a dural tear, or a fit in the first week after injury. Many neurosurgeons advise long-term prophylactic anticonvulsants for patients with depressed fractures who have multiple risk factors.

Other penetrating brain injuries

Stab wounds of the head can be missed at first, and an accurate history is crucial. Plain films often fail to show the slot-shaped fracture at the point where the skull has been penetrated, but a CT scan with window settings for bone may show it (Figure 6.17a), while the track of the blade is seen with window settings for brain (Figure 6.17b). Treatment may involve antibiotics, wound exploration and debridement, or intracranial surgery to control haemorrhage or to excise a traumatic aneurysm from one of the cerebral vessels (Figure 6.17c).

The damage caused by bullets and other missiles varies with the type of weapon and its distance from the victim, as energy transfer (and thus brain damage) is proportional to the square of the projectile's velocity as it enters the brain (see Chapter 22). Neurological impairment therefore varies enormously. Plain films show metallic projectiles (Figure 6.18a), while a CT scan shows their tracks, swelling, contusion, or haematomas (Figure 6.18b). Survival is often brief with high velocity injuries, but if the patient is thought to be viable when seen at hospital the entry and exit wounds can be explored to remove bone fragments and devitalised tissue and to control haemorrhage. It is often fruitless to seek the missile fragments themselves. In order to minimise brain swelling, these patients are all ventilated postoperatively in the ICU, and broad-spectrum antibiotics are given because of the risk of intracranial infection.

The future

It is likely that novel "neuroprotective" drugs will soon become available for clinical use [1]. Some will block neuronal cell

Figure 6.18 Missile wound of brain. (a) Plain skull film: intracranial bullet. (b) CT brain scan: haematoma and bone fragments along the track of the missile.

surface receptors for excitotoxic neurotransmitters, for example the NMDA antagonists which prevent the harmful effects of glutamate. Others will scavenge toxic ions and molecules like free radicals. These drugs may transform the management of the diffusely injured brain in the ICU, which remains limited and unsatisfactory, and offer new hope for modifying continuing damage after serious head injury.

However, neuroprotective drugs will not reduce the need to protect the injured brain at all times from the harmful effects of hypoxaemia, hypercarbia, shock, high ICP, and other causes of secondary brain damage. A successful outcome for seriously head injured patients will continue to depend heavily on doing the right things in the first 24 hours after injury [4,19].

Summary

The care of a seriously head-injured patient in the first 24 hours after injury involves many people. It is important that they base their clinical practice on a good understanding of how the brain is affected by injury.

Outcome is strongly influenced by the quality of early management ensuring:

- the perfusion of the brain with adequate amounts of well-oxygenated blood;
- control of raised ICP;
- prompt recognition and referral of patients needing neurosurgical assessment;
- safe transfer to the neurosurgical unit.

The contribution of the neurosurgical team is to diagnose and treat intracranial complications like haematoma or penetrating injury, with CT scanning as the mainstay of diagnosis. Treatment in the first 24 hours after injury may involve both intracranial surgery and intensive therapy.

Teamwork, good communication, and a well-organised service are all important in head injury management. Above all, sound clinical principles must be applied at all times.

References

1. Faden AI, Salzman S. Pharmacological strategies in CNS trauma. *Trends Pharmacol Sci* 1992;**13**:29–35.
2. Jenkins LW, Moszynski K, Lyeth BG *et al.* Increased vulnerability of the mildly traumatised rat brain to cerebral ischemia: the use of controlled secondary ischemia as a research tool to identify common or different mechanisms contributing to mechanical and ischemic brain injury. *Brain Res* 1989;**477**:211–24.
3. Ishige N, Pitts LH, Hashimoto T, Mishimura MC, Bartkowski HM. Effect of hypoxia on traumatic brain injury in rats. *Neurosurgery* 1987;**20**:848–58.
4. Gentleman D. Preventing secondary brain damage after head injury: a multidisciplinary challenge. *Injury* 1990;**21**:305–8.
5. American College of Surgeons Committee on Trauma. *ATLS Course Manual.* Chicago: American College of Surgeons, 1997, Chapter 6.
6. McLaren CAN, Robertson C, Little K. Missed orthopaedic injuries in the resuscitation room. *J Roy Coll Surg (Edin)* 1983;**28**:399–401.
7. Mendelow AD, Teasdale G, Jennett B *et al.* Risks of intracranial haematomas in head-injured adults. *BMJ* 1983;**287**:1173–6.
8. Rose J, Valtonen S, Jennett B. Avoidable factors contributing to death after head injury. *BMJ* 1977;**ii**:615–18.
9. Briggs M, Clarke P, Crockard A *et al.* Guidelines for initial management after head injury in adults: suggestions from a group of neurosurgeons. *BMJ* 1984;**288**:983–5.
10. Teasdale GM, Murray G, Anderson E *et al.* Risks of acute traumatic intracranial haematoma in adults and children: implications for managing head injuries. *BMJ* 1990;**300**:363–7.
11. Gentleman D. Causes and effects of systemic complications among severely head injured patients transferred to a neurosurgical unit. *Int Surg* 1992;**77**:297–302.
12. Gentleman D, Dearden M, Midgley S, Maclean D. Guidelines for resuscitation and transfer of patients with serious head injury. *BMJ* 1993;**307**:547–52.
13. Munro HM, Laycock JRD. Inter-hospital transfer: standards for ventilated neurosurgical emergencies. *Br J Intensive Care* 1993;**3**:210–14.
14. Marshall LF, Marshall SB, Klauber MR, Van Verkum Clark M. A new classification of head injury based on computed tomography. *J Neurosurg* 1991;**75**:S14–S20.
15. Jenkins A, Teasdale G, Hadley MDM, Macpherson P, Rowan JO. Brain lesions detected by magnetic resonance imaging in mild and severe head injuries. *Lancet* 1986;**ii**:445–6.
16. Galbraith S, Teasdale GM. Predicting the need for operation in the patient with an occult traumatic intracranial haematoma. *J Neurosurg* 1981;**55**:75–81.
17. Chan KH, Dearden NM, Miller JD, Andrews PJ, Midgley S. Multimodality monitoring as a guide to treatment of intracranial hypertension after severe brain injury. *Neurosurgery* 1993;**32**:547–52.
18. Jones PA, Andrews PJ, Midgley S *et al.* Measuring the burden of secondary insults in head injured patients during intensive care. *J Neurosurg Anesthesiol* 1994;**6**:4–14.
19. Langfitt TW, Gennarelli TA. Can the outcome from head injury be improved? *J Neurosurg* 1982;**56**:19–25.

7 Maxillofacial trauma

Iain Hutchison

Consultant Oral and Maxillofacial Surgeon, St Bartholomew's Hospital and The Royal London Hospitals

---

OBJECTIVES

- To understand the applied anatomy of the face in relation to facial trauma.

- To be able to institute appropriate emergency management and preliminary investigation for facial injuries.

- To be able to examine the face and diagnose facial injuries.

- To know the definitive investigations required for specific facial injuries.

- To understand the correct management of specific facial injuries.

- To be able to manage dental trauma and facial lacerations.

Facial injuries occur frequently. They may involve soft tissues alone, bone alone, or both in combination. The mouth and nose constitute the upper part of the airway and digestive tract and are therefore important in speech, breathing, mastication, and swallowing. Furthermore, facial appearance is very important in our society and affects how we are perceived by others and how we feel about ourselves. Therefore, failure to return a patient's face to its pretrauma form, or the development of unsightly scars, usually results in patient dissatisfaction and psychological and social disturbance.

Although life-threatening problems require urgent management and chest, abdominal, and neurological injuries take precedence, the maxillofacial surgeons should be involved in the management of all patients with facial injuries from the outset. This allows the maxillofacial treatment to be planned in conjunction with any other necessary treatment. Furthermore, the maxillofacial team are often able to assist in controlling bleeding and ensuring the airway in difficult cases. If the facial surgeons are not involved in A & E, communication problems frequently ensue when the seriously injured patient is admitted. It is often assumed by the admitting team that the maxillofacial surgeons have been informed about the patient, and several days lapse before the facial surgeons are then asked to see the patient for the first time. This delay results in less than optimal treatment for the facial injuries. The patient is left with residual facial deformities which, when the patient has fully recovered from life-threatening chest, neurological, or abdominal injuries, leave permanent physical and psychological scars and disabilities.

Anatomy

The facial bones protect the eye and upper aerodigestive tract, and are adjacent to the skull, brain, ear, and cervical spine. The bones of the middle third of the face, the nose, maxillae, ethmoids, and zygoma, are relatively weak in the anteroposterior plane. They articulate with the base of the skull. This articulation is weak so that strong blows to the anterior part of the face may cause separation of the facial bones from the base of the skull. Following this, the facial bones slide downwards and backwards to obstruct the airway. The tongue is attached to the posterior aspect of the mandible. Therefore, comminuted mandibular fractures may result in loss of this attachment with consequent posterior displacement of the tongue and obstruction of the airway. Finally, teeth, bone fragments, dentures, blood, and vomit may all be inhaled following facial trauma, with blockage of the airway (Table 7.1).

Table 7.1 Airway obstruction and its treatment

Cause	Treatment
Maxillary fractures	Disimpact
Midline mandibular fractures	Tongue suture
Inhaled objects: teeth; dentures; bone; blood; vomit	Examine, bronchoscopy, clear

The chin point, nose, and cheek bone (zygomatic) prominence are all prominent parts of the face. They sustain more trauma and are more frequently fractured.

The blood supply of the face is excellent. Therefore, no bone or soft tissue should be discarded until a maxillofacial surgeon has been consulted.

The teeth are firmly attached to the lower and upper jaw (mandible and maxilla respectively). Displacement of these jaws following fractures will therefore result in a malocclusion which is uncomfortable for the patient and obvious to the observing clinician. The occlusion also serves as a marker for the correct alignment of the jaws.

The sensory supply to the face is from the trigeminal nerve which runs through the bones of the face. Therefore, fractures of these facial bones commonly result in anaesthesia in the classical distribution of the trigeminal nerve branches:

- with mandibular fractures the ipsilateral chin is often numb;
- with maxillary and zygomatic fractures the ipsilateral cheek, nose, and upper lip are affected.

The facial nerve is rarely involved with bony trauma. However, lacerations in the parotid region sometimes result in damage to the facial nerve with consequent weakness of the muscles of facial expression on the affected side. They can also cause salivary fistulae and sialoceles.

Aetiology

Road traffic accidents (RTAs) used to account for the majority of facial injuries in the UK. However, this proportion has fallen with the introduction of better road systems, seatbelt and alcohol legislation, as well as attention to improving the safety of motor vehicles, for example airbags. Assault now accounts for a larger proportion of facial injuries. Domestic violence, where women and children are assaulted by their partners and parents respectively, is a particularly insidious form of assault because it recurs with increasing severity. Therefore, where domestic violence is suspected, social agencies should be called so that the problem is recognised and managed [1,2]. Accidents can happen in the home, at work, and whilst playing sports. Also, certain groups of patients, such as epileptics and alcoholics, are at risk of recurrent facial injury. Road traffic accidents (RTAs) and violent assault are frequently associated with excessive alcohol consumption [3].

Aetiology of facial trauma

- Road traffic accidents (RTAs)
- Assault
  - domestic
  - social/recreational
  - work
  - sport
- Accident
  - domestic
  - sport
  - industrial
- Risk groups
  - alcoholics
  - epileptics

Emergency management

As with injuries at other sites, the first priority in facial injuries is to ensure that the airway is maintained, the patient is breathing, and that there is no state of circulatory collapse. There is also an increased risk of cervical spine injuries when severe facial injuries have occurred. The usual precautions should therefore be taken (cervical collar and no movement) until a cervical spine injury has been excluded.

Several specific problems can occur in facial injuries which compromise the airway (Table 7.1). The mouth and nose constitute the upper airway and these may be obstructed by blood or vomit. The mouth should be cleared of all debris with the use of a good light and powerful suction. Alternatively, the index finger of one hand is passed down the inside of the cheek to the back of the mouth and the finger hooked towards the midline to bring forward the debris that sits over the tongue in the centre of the mouth. If the anterior attachment of the tongue is lost in midline mandibular fractures, and it

drops back obstructing the oropharynx, a 2/0 black silk suture is passed through a large portion of the tongue's dorsal surface and brought out of the mouth and taped to the side of the

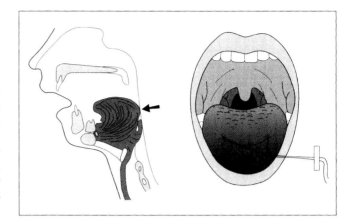

Figure 7.1 If the tongue has dropped back obstructing the airway after disruption of the mandibular midline, a 2/0 silk suture is passed through the tongue dorsum and taped to the side of the face to hold the tongue forwards.

face (Figure 7.1). If maxillary fractures at the Le Fort I, II and III levels result in backward displacement of the upper jaw obstructing the pharynx, a finger is passed through the mouth behind the soft palate pulling the fractured maxilla

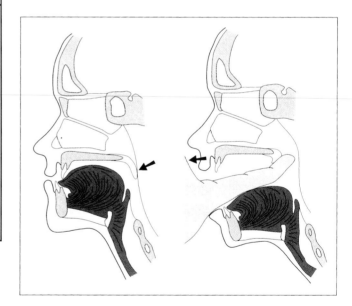

Figure 7.2 If the maxilla has been impacted down and back, causing upper airway obstruction, it should be disimpacted forwards with the left index finger behind the soft palate and the right index finger and thumb around the upper premaxilla or incisor teeth.

forwards into its correct position (Figure 7.2). If this is not possible, then gentle pulling on the anterior part of the maxilla in the region of the incisor and canine teeth may succeed in pulling the maxilla forwards. Failing this, the insertion of a nasopharyngeal airway can create a competent nasal airway. This tube must be kept patent by regular suction.

Wherever possible, the patient should be nursed sitting up or on one side to ensure a patent airway. One dose of intravenous steroids, such as 8 mg of dexamethasone, can be used to reduce oedema in the upper airway. If it is suspected that foreign bodies have passed into the tracheobronchial tree, a chest radiograph should be arranged and bronchoscopy used to remove the foreign material.

If the patient is not breathing spontaneously or if there is anxiety about maintaining an airway, endotracheal intubation is, paradoxically, often easy with good light and suction because the jaw fractures often enable easier access to the larynx. However, beware if the patient is conscious and maintaining an airway, and a decision is made to perform endotracheal intubation. The use of anaesthetic and paralysing agents can cause catastrophic loss of the functioning airway, which would be now difficult to visualise and intubate. When oral or nasal endotracheal intubation is not possible, cricothyroid puncture may be attempted but this is usually difficult because of neck swelling; in this case a tracheostomy may be necessary.

Bleeding

It is unusual for facial injuries to result in life-threatening haemorrhage. Soft tissue injuries are frequently associated with profuse initial haemorrhage which stops after a few minutes following direct pressure. However, small puncture wounds are sometimes associated with jagged tears in underlying arteries or veins and will continue to bleed unabated. This bleeding may not appear dramatic but simply present as a chronic persistent trickle of blood through the puncture wound. The severity of blood loss is often overlooked and requires specific management including intravenous fluid replacement. The wound must be opened widely so that the underlying vessel involved can be ligated. Where extensive soft tissue lacerations have occurred with obvious bleeding vessels, these may be temporarily ligated or clipped with an artery clip. In neck lacerations, where there is a suspicion of carotid artery or jugular vein damage, ultrasound Doppler or angiography must be arranged urgently followed by direct vessel repair of the carotid artery or ligation of the veins under general anaesthetic.

It is even rarer for closed facial bone injuries to cause major haemorrhage, but there are exceptions to this. In maxillary fractures, there may be significant blood loss from the nose. This is due to damage to the maxillary and anterior ethmoidal arteries. Once again, this does not present as pulsatile bleeding, but as a constant steady trickle of blood from the anterior airways. This is managed with anterior and posterior nasal packs [4]. Foley catheters with 10–20 ml balloons are passed down both nostrils, the balloons inflated with water or normal saline when they are in the nasopharynx, and the catheters pulled forwards under tension, blocking the choana (back of the nose) with the balloons. The catheters are then tied together, and BIPP or tulle gras packs are forced into the nose to arrest the bleeding. Alternatively, epistats with their double inflatable balloons achieve the same effect and are easier to use.

The patient may have profuse bleeding from the mouth from soft tissue lacerations and underlying fractures. This is best managed by suturing of the lacerations. Alternative methods for achieving haemostasis include under-running of retracted bleeding vessels with sutures and plugging intrabony blood vessels with oxidised cellulose. Occasionally, the patient may also have lost sufficient blood to have developed a consumptive coagulopathy, in which case blood products such as fresh frozen plasma and platelets must be administered, in conjunction with the local measures outlined above, to arrest the haemorrhage. Very rarely, the oral and nasal bleeding may be due to extensive skull base fractures with bleeding from the clivus through the posterior pharyngeal wall. These patients are usually moribund and arresting the haemorrhage with posterior nasal packs simply causes a rise in intracranial pressure.

When the patient is bleeding significantly from the face, or there are other major injuries, two large cannulae must be inserted into central or peripheral veins to ensure adequate venous access. Blood is taken for urgent cross-match, and plasma expanders are used to ensure adequent tissue perfusion whilst blood is awaited (see Chapter 5).

Examination of the face and investigations

A thorough history should be obtained including the cause of the trauma, whether there has been a loss of consciousness and whether domestic violence was involved. Adequate notes must be taken and, if possible, photographs should be obtained in view of possible later litigation.

Patients may complain of eye problems such as blindness, double vision or restriction of eye movement. There may be pain or anaesthesia in various facial parts. Teeth may not meet correctly and patients may be unable to open their mouth.

The examination follows a systematic pattern starting at the top of the head and extending down to the supraclavicular region and progressing from the front of the face to the back of the head. Lacerations, potential foreign bodies, swelling or depressions, bruising, deformity, or leakage of blood or other fluids from the ear, nose, or mouth should be sought first. This is followed by palpation for sites of tenderness, abnormal mobility, underlying crepitus or surgical emphysema, and alterations in sensation over the facial skin. Significant measurements should be taken, such as the distance between the two medial canthi (intercanthal distance).

Inspection

The forehead is examined first followed by the eyes.

For the *eyes*, particular attention is devoted to:

- visual acuity
- pupillary size and response to light and accommodation
- conjunctival lacerations
- periorbital swelling
- subconjunctival ecchymosis
- eye movements
- double vision
- exophthalmos/enophthalmos
- palpebral fissure shape and angulation
- intercanthal distance
- epiphora.

Distinguishing features of nasoethmoidal fractures (Figure 7.8)
• The intercanthal distance is increased – in the adult the distance is > 36 mm in this fracture
• The ridge created by the medial canthal ligament is lost
• The eyelids are displaced laterally and have a mongoloid slant
• The palpebral fissure itself becomes almond-shaped
• The patient may have epiphora from nasolacrimal damage
• The nasal apertures often point forward with a markedly obtuse nasolabial angle (Figure 7.8b)
• There may be a CSF leak [5]

Subconjunctival ecchymoses are recorded including their lateral extent; for example, zygomatic fractures are often associated with lateral subconjunctival ecchymosis with no posterior margin. The shape of the palpebral fissure should be assessed and the attachment of the medial canthal ligament. The patient may have epiphora (leakage of tears) if there has been trauma to the medial canthal region with damage to the nasolacrimal apparatus.

The *ears* are examined for:

● cerebrospinal fluid (CSF) leak
● auricular haematoma
● bleeding: anterior wall – mandibular condylar fracture, posterior wall – middle cranial fossa fracture.

If there is blood leaking from the external auditory meatus (EAM), the meatus itself should be examined. Tears on the anterior wall of the EAM are indicative of mandibular condylar neck fractures whilst tears on the posterior wall suggest a base of skull fracture. Haematoma over the mastoid process (Battle's sign) is found in fractures of the petrous temporal bone. If there is blood medial to the tympanic membrane, this also indicates a middle cranial fossa fracture.

The *nose* is examined for:

● swelling
● deformity
● bilateral black eyes
● epistaxis (sometimes unilateral)
● airway patency
● septal haematoma
● CSF leak.

The CSF usually separates from the blood to produce a tramline effect along the upper lip with two streaks of blood running outside the central clear CSF. The patency of the nasal airway needs to be tested.

The *cheekbone* is examined for alteration in shape, either depression or swelling. The face can normally be sub-divided into equal thirds horizontally: the distance between the hairline and glabella is equal to the distance from the glabella to the junction of the upper lip and the nose (nasion) which is in turn equal to nasion to chin point.

The middle third of the face may be lengthened with respect to the other two-thirds when maxillary fractures have occurred.

The function of all the branches of the seventh cranial nerve (*facial nerve*) to the forehead, eyelids, cheeks, lips, and chin should be assessed by asking the conscious patient to wrinkle his brow and nose, shut his eyes tight, smile, and whistle.

The outline of the lower *jaw* should be assessed, although fractured mandibles usually present as swellings at the affected site rather than altered contour. Patients may be unable to open their mouth fully. This should be recorded. The mouth is then examined for haematomas, lacerations, loose bodies, fractures of the teeth, and malocclusion.

Finally, the *neck* is examined for lacerations, swelling and respiratory difficulty which can manifest with use of the accessory respiratory muscles (sternomastoid) (see Chapter 2).

Palpation

The forehead, cheek, nose, upper lip, and lower lip are checked for alteration in sensation. The forehead is then assessed gently for abnormalities of contour and bony steps. Crepitus may be detected overlying a fractured anterior wall of the frontal sinus when surgical emphysema occurs. Palpate the superior orbital rims bilaterally, continuing around the lateral orbital rim and feeling particularly at the frontozygomatic suture for tenderness and separation. Palpate the zygomatic arches for depression. This examination continues forward onto the zygomatic prominence and along the inferior orbital rim. Look for steps and tenderness at the zygomaticomaxillary suture (Figure 7.3). The medial canthal ligaments are felt at their attachment to the lateral nasal wall. They should be palpable as a ridge. The frontonasal suture and nasal bones are palpated for mobility, steps, and tenderness. The patency of the nasal airways can then be assessed individually.

The temporomandibular joints are palpated on the face and intra-aurally for tenderness and crepitus. The palpation continues along the posterior border of the mandibular ramus and its inferior border to the midline. Gentle bimanual palpation is performed across potential mandibular fracture sites, fingers placed on the teeth adjacent to the fracture site and thumbs under the mandibular border, when gentle distraction may be performed. Individual teeth should be tested for fractures and mobility.

Mobility of the maxilla is tested with the left hand over the nose or zygomaticomaxillary suture to feel for movement, whilst the right hand holds the anterior maxillary teeth or gums, and attempts to mobilise the maxilla. If there is a fracture of the middle third of the face at the Le Fort I level, the nose will remain still whilst the maxillary alveolus with its teeth moves forwards; with fractures at the Le Fort II level there will be mobility of the nose, upper teeth, and upper jaw relative to the frontal bone and zygoma, which can be palpated at the frontonasal and zygomaticomaxillary sutures. Fractures at the Le Fort III level will produce movement at the fronto-zygomatic suture when attempts are made to mobilise the upper jaw by using the fingers of the right hand on the upper teeth. All lacerations should be measured and important distances such as the medial canthal ligament distance to the midline of the nose or the intercanthal distance should also be recorded. The neck is palpated for surgical emphysema and the position of the trachea is palpated. It should obviously lie in the midline.

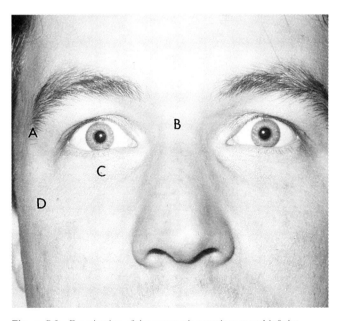

Figure 7.3 Examination of the zygomatic prominence and inferior orbital rim. Point A overlies the frontozygomatic suture; point B overlies the frontonasal suture; point C overlies the zygomaticomaxillary sutures on the inferior orbital rim, and point D overlies the cheek bone prominence.

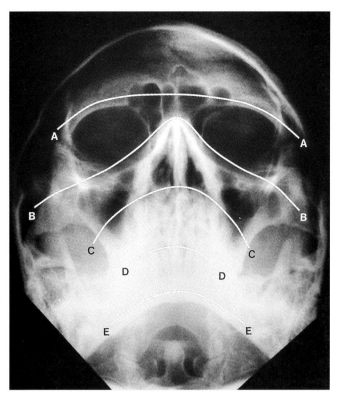

Figure 7.4 The straight occipitomental radiograph (OM) should be examined along five lines: line A shows the frontozygomatic and frontonasal sutures, the superior orbital rim, and the frontal sinus; line B shows the zygomatic arches and prominences and the inferior orbital rims; line C shows the coronoid process of the mandible, the lateral antral walls (zygomatic buttress) and the nasal septum; line D shows the teeth; line E shows the lower border of the mandible.

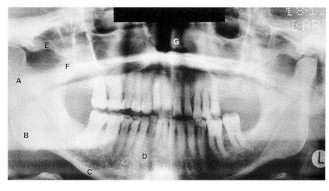

Figure 7.5 The orthopantomogram should be scrutinised at seven points for fractures: A: condylar neck; B: angle; C: mandibular horizontal body; D: parasymphyseal region; E: zygomatic arch; F: coronoid process; G: nasal septum.

The orthopantomogram (OPG) (Figure 7.5) and lateral oblique (LO) (Figure 7.6) views will show the mandible. A straight posteroanterior (PA) view of the head and face will show the skull and lower border of the mandible (Figure 7.7). Intraoral radiographs, such as the occlusal and periapical views, are appropriate for dentoalveolar injuries. A reverse Towne's view is useful for viewing the mandibular condylar necks.

Where possible, the views are taken with the x-ray beam passing posteroanteriorly. This will reduce the radiation dose to the eye and improve the clarity of the facial bones on the radiograph. Unfortunately, with a seriously ill patient, the radiographs are often taken with the patient supine when the x-ray beam passes anteroposteriorly. If poor views are

Investigation

Radiology

Views are taken of:

- Midface
  - occipitomental (OM) 0–45°
  - occipitofrontal (OF) 25°
  - brow-up lateral
- Lower jaw
  - OPG
  - PA jaws
  - lateral oblique
  - Towne's
- Dentoalveolar
  - intraoral.

Radiology is the mainstay of facial investigations. Soft tissue views are indicated when it is suspected that there are foreign bodies within the tissues. If there is a possibility of inhalation of foreign bodies or teeth, chest radiographs should be arranged. Cervical spine views are indicated in severe trauma to the face and when there is a possibility of spinal injury.

The standard view for the bones of the midface is the occipitomental view (OM) (Figure 7.4). This is taken with various angulations of the x-ray tube from 0° (horizontal) to 45° OM. Where there is a possibility of a Le Fort II or III fracture, then a "brow-up" lateral radiograph should be obtained to look for fluid levels in the sphenoid sinus. This is indicative of a skull base fracture.

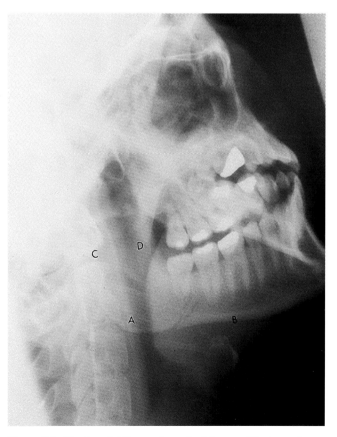

Figure 7.6 The lateral oblique radiograph of the mandible shows: A: mandibular angle; B: mandibular body; C: mandibular condylar neck; D: coronoid process. In this case, there is fracture through the third molar socket.

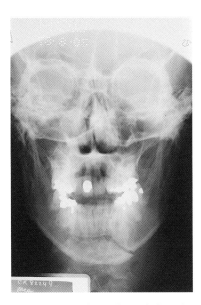

Figure 7.7 The posteroanterior jaw radiograph shows lateral displacement of fracture lines in the mandible as shown by this fracture through the left parasymphyseal region.

obtained with this technique, it is not worthwhile repeating the views until the patient has been seen by a maxillofacial surgeon.

CT scans

CT scanning is helpful in the management of severe maxillofacial trauma. Therefore, if patients are undergoing CT scan for neurological trauma, it is often appropriate to continue the investigation with fine 2 mm cuts through the facial bones so that coronal reconstructions of these scans can be performed. In most circumstances, the coronal view provides the best information for facial trauma followed by the sagittal and axial views. Examples where CT scanning is most helpful is in nasoethmoid and orbital wall trauma.

Ultrasound

Ultrasound may be indicated where fluid collections are suspected such as in post-traumatic sialoceles. These present as swellings, usually over the parotid gland after lacerations involving the gland have been closed by simple suture. They usually develop two to three days after the trauma. If a salivary gland injury is suspected at the time of presentation, a sialogram or instillation of methylene blue into the duct will demonstrate the site of the leak and aid in repair.

In certain circumstances full blood count, and urea and electrolytes should be measured. Group and cross match for blood transfusion will be necessary in the severely injured patient. If there is a suspected leak of CSF from the nose or ear, this fluid may be tested for glucose. Unfortunately, blood concentrations of glucose are higher than CSF concentrations so that if it is mixed with blood the test becomes invalid. It may be collected for research investigations such as Tau protein, but this test is not widely available.

Specific injuries

Nasal pyramid

Trauma to the nose is exceedingly common. The patient may sustain fractures to the nasal bones themselves or dislocation of the nasal septum or a combination of both. It is usually caused by a direct blow to the nose.

Presentation

The patient presents with nasal swelling and deformity and blockage of the nasal passages. Palpation over the nasal bones reveals tenderness and a step deformity. The patient will also often have discomfort over the anterior nasal spine. The anterior nares should be examined for septal haematoma, which manifests as a soft blue swelling over the septum.

Radiology

Lateral views of the nasal bones frequently show a fracture line. When patients have previously sustained a fractured nose there may be confusion as these fractures rarely heal by ossification so that the old fractures lines will still be present on radiographs.

Management in A & E

This usually involves simple measures to arrest nasal haemorrhage. Septal haematomas should be drained with a small incision, and a nasal pack inserted to compress the mucosa onto the underlying cartilage. If the patient has no nasal swelling it is reasonable to arrange an urgent maxillofacial or ent opinion so that the patient may have the fractured nasal bones reduced immediately. Otherwise, the patient should attend a maxillofacial trauma or ent clinic the next day when arrangements can be made to reduce the fractures within one week to ten days. Simple analgesics are used to relieve pain.

Ultimate management by maxillofacial surgery

The septum must be correctly reduced prior to manipulation of the nasal bones. External splints usually suffice, but occasionally with severe nasal bone comminution internal supports with angle irons may be necessary. If treatment of the fractured nose is delayed beyond three weeks, it is usually not possible to reduce the fracture with simple measures. The patient will probably have to undergo a septorhinoplasty as an elective measure to correct the cosmetic and functional disability.

Nasoethmoidal fractures

Signs of nasoethmoidal fractures include:

- flat deformed swollen nose
- epistaxis
- widened intercanthal distance
- loss of medial canthal ridge
- flattened naso-orbital valley
- almond-shaped eyes
- mongoloid slant to eyes
- nostrils pointing forward
- epiphora.

This is a relatively rare injury. Unfortunately, it is often misdiagnosed as a simple nasal fracture. As a result it is undertreated leaving severe permanent deformity. In fact, this injury results from severe anterior trauma to the nasal bones when they are pushed back through the ethmoid bones with

resultant lateral displacement of the lamina papyracea of the ethmoid bones.

Presentation

The patient has swelling over the nasal bridge and epistaxis as in simple nasal fractures. The critical distinguishing features are listed in the box.

Management in A & E

The patient has usually sustained a severe injury and an urgent maxillofacial opinion should be sought so that the patient can undergo treatment within the first couple of days after injury. If there is no neurological, airway, or circulatory damage, then opiates may be used to relieve pain.

Radiology

The occipitofrontal radiograph taken at 25° shows disruption of the lamina papyracea of the ethmoid bones (Figure 7.9).

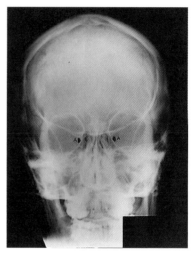

Figure 7.9 Point A marks the lamina papyracea of the ethmoid bones which fracture in nasoethmoid injuries.

Ultimate management

This fracture must be managed by open techniques. The fracture of the nasoethmoid region can be approached by incisions directly over the fractures or by a bicoronal flap. The essence of the technique is to lift the nasal bones out from the disrupted ethmoid sinuses. The medial canthal ligaments are often still attached to fragments of nasal bone. The nasal bones are fixed in their correct position using a combination of wires, microplates, or intranasal angle irons holding the nasal bones forward. If the medial canthal ligaments are detached, they are fixed with transnasal wires, passed to the opposite medial canthal region and tied over a microplate at this site. With old nasoethmoid injuries, the position of the medial canthal ligaments must be overcorrected with transnasal wires passed markedly posterior and superior to the opposite medial canthal ligament.

Zygomatic fractures

Presentation

Signs of *zygomatic fractures* include:

● swollen black eyes (periorbital haematoma)
● double vision

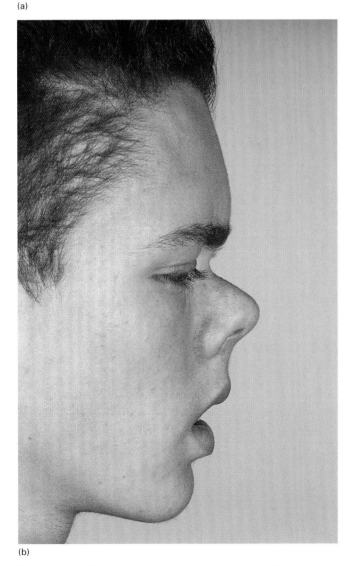

Figure 7.8 (a) This patient has a unilateral left nasoethmoidal fracture. He has flattening of the left naso-orbital valley, loss of the medial canthal ridge, widening of his left nose to medial canthal distance, and an almond shape to his left eyelids. (b) This patient with a bilateral nasoethmoid fracture demonstrates the classic severe flattening of the nasal bridge with an obtuse nasolabial angle and forward pointing nostrils.

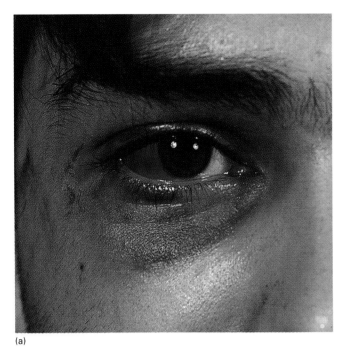

(a)

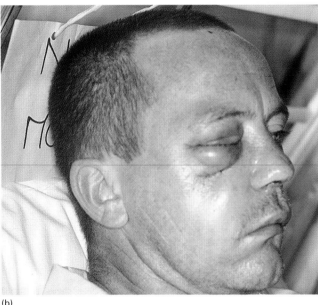

(b)

Figure 7.10 (a) This patient with a fractured right zygoma demonstrates the lateral subconjunctival ecchymosis caused by disruption of the lateral orbital wall formed by the zygoma. (b) This patient with a fractured right zygoma has flattening of his cheekbone prominence, right unilateral epistaxis (bleeding into the ipsilateral maxillary sinus following fracture of its walls which are formed by the zygoma), periorbital haematoma, and numbness of his right cheek.

- flattened zygomatic prominence
- tenderness and separation at zygomatic sutures
- ipsilateral epistaxis
- lateral subconjunctival ecchymosis (Figure 7.10a)
- infraorbital nerve (cheek) paraesthesia
- limitation of jaw opening.

The patient presents with pain and swelling over the affected zygoma, lateral subconjunctival ecchymosis where the posterior extent is not visible, ipsilateral infraorbital paraesthesia with numbness of the affected cheek, nose, upper lip, and upper gingivae and teeth. There may be unilateral epistaxis on the affected side, limitation in jaw opening because of compression of the depressed zygoma on to the temporalis

muscle tendon, double vision, and limitation of ipsilateral eye movement. The cheekbone prominence is often flat (Figure 7.10b). If there is severe disruption of the zygoma with marked displacement, the patient may have enophthalmos, dropping of the globe of the eye and pupillary level, with an anti-mongoloid slant of the eyelids on the affected side.

There may be tenderness and palpable bony separation and steps over one or all of the zygomatic sutures with other bones: that is, the fronto-zygomatic suture, zygomatico maxillary suture, the zygomatic buttress intraorally and the zygomatic arch.

Radiology

Plain occipitomental (OM) radiographs at 0° and 40° should be taken as these will demonstrate separation at the affected sutures. The straight OM (0°) shows the inferior orbital and lateral orbital rims (Figure 7.11), whilst the 40° more tilted x-ray beam gives a better view of the zygomatic arch. There is

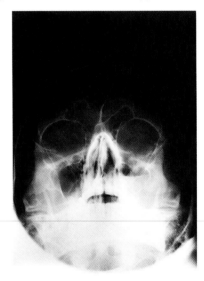

Figure 7.11 Straight occipitomental view showing separation at the left frontozygomatic suture, deformity of the left inferior orbital margin with separation at the zygomaticomaxillary suture and an opaque blood-filled left maxillary sinus, all typical of a fractured left zygoma.

usually blood in the affected maxillary sinus from a fracture in the sinus wall. This manifests as a fluid level on the radiograph. There may also be a visible fracture of the zygomatic buttress (lateral maxillary antral wall).

Management in A & E

The patient with the fractured zygoma may not present immediately after the injury if he does not realise that he has sustained a fracture. However, whenever the patient does present, a maxillofacial opinion should be sought, as there is a small possibility of retrobulbar haemorrhage following this fracture. This type of haemorrhage is a surgical emergency because, if it is left untreated, it may progress to blindness in the affected eye. The management of retrobulbar haemorrhage involves the judicious use of dexamethasone, acetazolamide and mannitol. Surgical drainage may be necessary (see Chapter 8). Simple analgesics are usually sufficient to control pain from a zygomatic fracture.

Ultimate management by maxillofacial surgery

If the patient has a straightforward fractured zygoma with no displacement and minimal symptoms, an expectant policy is pursued and the patient is reviewed weekly over a three to four week period until all the symptoms have resolved. With simple displacement, the zygoma may be elevated into the correct position by an incision in the temple and a sub-temporalis fascia approach from above. Alternatively, an incision can be made in the upper buccal sulcus in the mouth and an elevator passed underneath the zygomatic body through this intraoral approach. With markedly displaced or comminuted fractured zygomas, an open approach is used to fix the zygoma into its correct position with mini- or microplating systems. A bicoronal flap can be used to approach the zygomatic arch and the frontozygomatic region, whilst the subciliary or transconjunctival approach is used for the inferior orbital rim. For the frontozygomatic suture alone a small crow's foot or eyebrow incision suffices. With the subciliary incision there is a risk of late ectropion, particularly in the elderly. To avoid this, the incision must be carried immediately through the orbicularis oculi muscle and passed down between this muscle and the orbital septum. Alternatively, in the elderly, the transconjunctival or infraorbital incision should be used.

Isolated orbital wall fractures

By definition, fractured zygomas always involve the lateral orbital wall and orbital floor. Once the zygoma has been reduced into its correct position, the orbital walls usually need no specific management.

In contrast, an isolated orbital wall injury can occur without obvious damage to the surrounding orbital rim. The orbital floor is more commonly affected than the medial orbital wall, but both may occur in combination. Fractures of the orbital floor and medial orbital wall frequently result in herniation of the orbital contents and bleeding into the adjacent maxillary and ethmoid air sinuses respectively.

The lateral orbital wall is supported laterally by the temporalis muscle, and fractures of this wall without fractures of the orbital rim usually occur in conjunction with a fracture of the greater wing of the sphenoid. In this type of injury the lateral orbital wall may compress the lateral rectus muscle causing pain with abduction of the eye. It may even compress the optic canal and the optic nerve. In these cases the patient will complain of acute loss of vision at the time of the trauma or progressive visual deterioration over a few hours. The orbital roof fracture occurs in combination with frontal bone fractures and intracranial trauma.

Presentation

Signs of isolated orbital floor fractures include:

- pain in the affected eye
- diplopia
- limited elevation of the globe
- infraorbital paraesthesia
- ex- or enophthalmos
- eye pain
- fluid level in maxillary sinus
- "hanging drop" on x-ray.

The isolated orbital floor and medial orbital wall fracture are often missed because patients have very little in the way of symptoms initially. The patient has usually sustained a blow to the eye and may present with ipsilateral infraorbital anaesthesia, unilateral epistaxis, en- or exophthalmos, double vision, and limitation in eye movements (Figure 7.12). Where

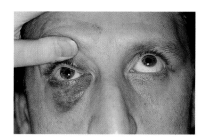

Figure 7.12 This patient has a right orbital floor fracture. He is unable to elevate the right eye effectively because of entrapment of orbital contents in the orbital floor defect (maxillary sinus roof).

a patient has any of these symptoms without an obviously fractured zygoma, the possibility of an orbital floor or medial wall fracture should be considered.

The orbital roof fracture is found in patients who sustain severe head injuries. The globe of the eye on the affected side is displaced downwards, there is an antimongoloid slant to the palpebral fissure and there may be proptosis of the affected eye.

Radiology

Occipitomental radiographs often show a fluid level (blood) in the affected maxillary sinus and, sometimes, the so-called "hanging drop" from the maxillary sinus roof (orbital floor), which is due to a combination of haematoma and periorbital contents herniating into the maxillary sinus (Figure 7.13).

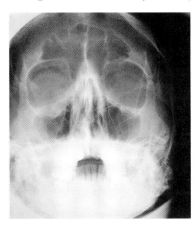

Figure 7.13 This straight OM shows a globular radiopacity in the right maxillary sinus roof caused by herniation of orbital contents through an orbital floor fracture (the "hanging-drop" sign). The patient has limitation of right eye elevation and numbness of the right cheek and upper lip.

Alternatively, there may be little to see other than some opacity of the maxillary sinus.

CT scans in the coronal plane demonstrate orbital floor, medial orbital wall, and orbital roof fractures clearly. The anteroposterior extent of the orbital floor fracture can be delineated more accurately with a CT scan in the sagittal plane. Axial CT scans are of little help in the management of these orbital wall fractures but are essential in optic canal trauma. The CT scan should be arranged approximately one week after the injury when the haematoma has settled, so that it is possible to get a true picture of the orbital defect and herniation of orbital contents.

Management in A & E

This fracture is frequently overlooked. With large defects there is often no immediate limitation of eye movement. The patient may have *no* en- or exophthalmos at presentation, because the post-traumatic periorbital oedema supports the globe of the eye in its correct position, despite large volumes of periorbital fat herniating into the maxillary antrum. It may take two or three months for the eye to sink back with these large orbital floor defects.

Conversely, a tiny slit-like defect in the orbital floor may trap orbital contents sufficiently to cause marked limitation of eye movements when the signs of the fracture will be obvious. Therefore, if the patient presents with unexplained infraorbital paraesthesia, or maxillary antral opacities and fluid levels, following a blow to the eye, a maxillofacial opinion should be sought immediately.

At worst, the patient simply has a dull ache in the affected eye. Simple analgesics usually control this pain.

Ultimate management by maxillofacial surgery

Approximately 50% of orbital floor and medial wall injuries will require surgical treatment. Orbital floors are approached through subciliary or transconjunctival approaches. This may need to be augmented by a Caldwell–Luc maxillary sinus approach. In extensive orbital floor and medial wall injuries a bicoronal flap approach, in conjunction with a subciliary incision, may be required.

The orbital roof injury is repaired in conjunction with neurosurgeons and the lateral orbital wall, if the optic canal is compressed, is also best managed with a combined intra- and extracranial approach. If the orbital floor and medial wall fracture is small, then the orbital contents can be readily supported in their correct position by a reinforced silastic sheet of approximately 1 mm thickness. With large medial wall and orbital floor defects, it may be necessary to use curved bone and cartilage grafts such as costochondral or iliac crest grafts. Orbital roof and lateral orbital walls require no support apart from direct fixation.

Mandible

The *mandible* can be fractured at different sites. Each of these presents with diverse symptoms but usually more than one fracture site is involved. For purposes of clarity, each fracture site will be described individually.

Mandibular condyle

Presentation

Signs of *condylar neck fractures* include:

- pain over TM joint
- swelling over TM joint
- pain and difficulty opening mouth
- blood from ipsilateral ear
- malocclusion occasionally.

The mandibular condyle articulates with the temporal bone to form the temporomandibular (TM) joint. There is a fibrocartilaginous meniscus between the head of the condyle and its fossa creating two joint spaces. Blows to any part of the mandible frequently cause an indirect fracture of the relatively weak neck of the mandibular condyle. The patient has pain with jaw movement and swelling over the joint in the preauricular region. There may also be bleeding from the external auditory meatus as its anterior wall forms the posterior surface of the temporomandibular joint. The patient rarely has a malocclusion, unless there is associated muscle spasm

or marked displacement of the fracture. The patient may experience ipsilateral deafness if the head of the condyle is forced into the external auditory meatus. The head of the condyle may very rarely be forced up into the middle cranial fossa.

The condylar head itself, within the capsule of the joint, may be fractured. When this occurs in young children, healing can cause later bony ankylosis and failure of effective mandibular growth on the affected side. This complication results in very small mandibles which are deviated to the affected side. The patient has marked limitation of mouth opening. Patients with acute intracapsular condylar head fractures present with pain, swelling, and limitation of jaw movement. Plain radiology is often unhelpful with condylar head fractures.

One or both condylar heads may dislocate anteriorly over the articular eminence. The patient presents with an open mouth which they are unable to close, pain over the jaw joint and the muscles of mastication (masseter and temporalis), and drooling of saliva. There is often a visible hollow just in front of the ear where the mandibular condyle should normally be sited.

The temporomandibular joint intra-articular meniscus can dislocate anteriorally. The patient feels a physical block to mouth opening over the affected temporomandibular joint and is unable to open the mouth fully. There may be pain in the muscles of mastication, and an antecedent history of clicking noises with jaw opening and closing. Plain radiology is unhelpful. Frequently, there is no obvious cause and no history of trauma. Occasionally though, the disc attachment may have been torn by previous trauma such as paralysed wide mouth opening in general anaesthetics, a whiplash injury, or blows to the jaw.

Radiology

The best radiographic view is the orthopantomogram (OPG) which shows the head of the condyle and the condylar neck extremely well (Figure 7.14). Failing this, the lateral oblique

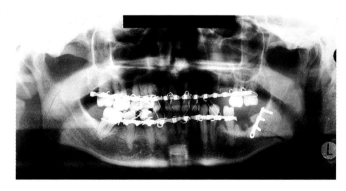

Figure 7.14 OPG radiograph showing fractures of the right condylar neck and left angle of the mandible after direct plate and indirect intermaxillary fixation.

view of the temporomandibular joint gives a reasonable view of the condylar neck as does the reverse Towne's view. The intracapsular condylar head fracture will not be seen clearly on these plain radiographs and tomography or CT scanning is necessary to confirm this diagnosis. The dislocated mandibular condyle will be visible as an empty fossa in front of the external auditory meatus. The dislocated fibrocartilaginous meniscus will not be seen by plain radiology, and arthrography or arthroscopy are necessary to confirm this diagnosis.

Management in A & E

Where there is an uncomplicated condylar neck fracture with no other mandibular fracture, or if there is suspicion of anterior dislocation of the temporomandibular joint meniscus, the patient should be referred to the next maxillofacial clinic. However, when the condylar fracture has resulted in more severe symptoms, or where it is suspected that a child has an intracapsular condylar head fracture, an urgent maxillofacial opinion should be sought.

In simple dislocations, when the mandibular condyles have been dislocated for less than two hours, it may be possible to reduce the condyle into its correct position without any specific medication. The index and second finger of both hands are placed over the lower molar teeth on either side and the thumbs are placed underneath the jaw on each side; the back of the mandible is pulled forwards and downwards on each side to distract the condyle from its position in front of the articular eminence; the condyle will then frequently fall back into the condylar fossa. If the mandible has been dislocated for more than three to four hours, this manoeuvre will probably not work because of spasm in the muscles of mastication. The patient should then be given an intravenous benzodiazepine such as 10 mg diazepam. This relaxes the jaw muscles and the patient may often relocate the mandibular condyles into the correct position spontaneously without any manipulation. After relocation has been completed successfully, it is wise to provide a support bandage running from under the jaw over the top of the head, to keep the mouth closed for a few hours.

If the patient redislocates immediately, the jaws may have to be wired together for a period of time. Occasionally, patients suffer with recurrent dislocation following traumatic damage to the capsule of the joint or in association with medication such as the phenothiazines or metoclopramide.

Ultimate management

Simple mandibular condylar neck fractures are usually managed conservatively with a soft diet. Occasionally, the patient may be put into intermaxillary fixation for two weeks to rest the joint. With marked displacement of the condylar neck it may be necessary to perform open reduction and fixation.

Intracapsular condylar head fractures are treated with aspiration of any haemarthrosis, early mobilisation, and close review of the development of the child to ensure that bony ankylosis does not supervene. If bony ankylosis does occur, this is best treated by reconstruction of the temporomandibular joint with a costochondral graft to replace the condyle, and temporalis fascia to reconstruct the fossa and intra-articular cartilaginous meniscus.

In recurrent or irreducible dislocation of the mandibular condyle, it may be necessary to explore the joint and remove the articular eminence.

Conservative measures, such as bite-raising appliances and small doses of tricyclic antidepressants, are used to treat dislocated fibrocartilaginous intra-articular discs initially. If there is no response, then the joint may be investigated with arthrography and arthroscopy and ultimately managed by open surgery to replace the fibrocartilaginous disc in its correct position over the condyle of the mandible.

Mandibular body fractures

Presentation

Signs of *mandibular body fractures* include:

- bloody saliva
- malocclusion
- limitation of jaw movement
- loose teeth
- tenderness and mobility at fracture site
- pain
- anaesthesia of lip
- sublingual haematoma.

Fractures of the angle, horizontal ramus or body of the mandible, midline, and para-midline (symphyseal and parasymphyseal) regions of the mandible all present with similar symptoms. The patient has a malocclusion, swelling over the fracture site, and drools blood-stained saliva from the mouth. There may be a sublingual haematoma and a laceration of the gingiva overlying the fracture (Figure 7.15). It is possible

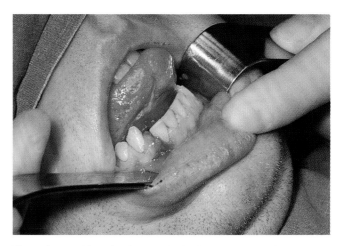

Figure 7.15 This patient has mandibular fractures at the right parasymphysis and left angle. The photograph shows torn gingiva and a step in the occlusion at the fracture site, and a sublingual haematoma.

to demonstrate mobility between the two segments of mandible adjacent to the fracture site. Teeth in the fracture line are mobile although this is often not due to intrinsic tooth mobility but simply represents the mobility of the fractured mandibular segment. The patient has pain with mouth movements and may have inability to open the mouth fully. When the fracture line passes through the inferior dental canal proximal (posterior) to the mental foramen there will be anaesthesia or paraesthesia of the ipsilateral lip from damage to the inferior dental nerve.

Radiology

The two best views to demonstrate mandibular fractures are the OPG used in conjunction with a PA radiograph of the jaws. Should the OPG not be available or the patient unfit to undergo this examination, then lateral oblique views of the jaws may be sufficient. Intraoral views are occasionally indicated.

Management in A & E

Simple analgesics or opiates should be administered to control pain, which is often severe if the fracture site is mobile. The mouth should be examined thoroughly and all loose debris, blood, saliva, and vomit should be aspirated. Ideally, the patient is nursed sitting up or on their side so that control of the airway is maintained. If there is any uncertainty over the tongue blocking the airway, then a large suture is passed through the tongue and taped to the side of the face. If the patient is unconscious, intubation is necessary. In addition, broad spectrum antibiotics such as cephalosporins, penicillins, and the more specific agent, metronidazole, are required.

Ultimate management

Ideally, the patient should be treated as rapidly as possible to relieve pain and minimise the risk of later complications such as infection, malunion, and non-union. The patient may be managed by inter-maxillary fixation whereby the lower jaw is

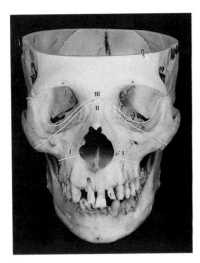

Figure 7.16 Le Fort I, II and III fracture lines marked on the skull.

Le Fort fractures
• lengthening of face
• epistaxis
• mobility of upper jaw
• bruising of upper anterior sulcus and palate
• posterior displacement of maxillary teeth producing malocclusion
• anterior open bite
• *Le Fort I*
• upper jaw mobile in relation to nose
• *Le Fort II*
• upper jaw and nose mobile on cheekbones and forehead
• telecanthus
• CSF leak
• *Le Fort III*
• bilateral black eyes
• CSF leak
• telecanthus
• upper jaw, nose and cheek bones mobile on forehead

---

fixed to the upper jaw with indirect wires placed around the teeth or around the jaws. Alternatively, open methods may be employed when the bone fragments are fixed with transosseous plates or wires.

Maxillary fractures

Fractures of the maxilla are usually caused by severe trauma to the middle third of the face. This has been associated with RTAs, but with the increasing use of blunt instruments in violent assault, such as baseball bats, severe maxillary fractures now occur with common assault. Any combination of fractures can occur which may be either united across the face as bilateral fractures or may be separated in the midline as unilateral fractures. They are classified, following the work of Rene Le Fort, into levels I, II and III fractures (Figure 7.16). Because of the severity of the originating trauma, concomitant damage to the globe of the eye and cranium are more common with Le Fort II and III fractures.

Le Fort I fracture

Presentation

This fracture occurs horizontally separating the tooth-bearing portion of the maxilla from the upper part of the face. The patient usually has bilateral epistaxis and posterior displacement of the tooth-bearing segment of the upper jaw so that the upper incisor teeth are placed behind the lower incisor teeth. There may be bruising visible in the sulcus between the upper jaw and the lips and cheeks, and on the palate. If there is a midline fracture, then a tear will be visible in the mucosa of the midline of the hard palate. Tapping on the upper teeth produces a brittle sound like the tapping of an empty egg shell. Furthermore, gentle traction on the upper anterior teeth, as described previously, will elicit movement of the upper jaw in relation to the rest of the face, particularly the nose and forehead.

Radiology

Lateral facial views and OPGs may show a fracture line extending horizontally backwards from the piriform aperture of the nose to the pterygoid plates. However, radiographs do not always show these fractures.

Management in A & E

Profound blood loss from the nose is very rare and, as with other maxillary fractures, nasal packing is usually not necessary. However, if there is significant haemorrhage, then anterior and posterior nasal packs should be used, and if there is a concomitant midline tear of the palate, this must also be sutured with a strong suture such as 2/0 or 3/0 silk on a cutting needle. The maxillofacial surgeon should be called as soon as a diagnosis has been made to aid in the emergency management of the patient.

Ultimate management by maxillofacial surgery

The Le Fort I fracture is reduced under general anaesthetic within the first 48 hours. After the upper jaw has been manipulated into its correct position, the maxilla may be fixed indirectly between the lower jaw and the rest of the facial bones (with Halo head frames or suspensions wires), or by direct methods such as titanium miniplate fixation.

Le Fort II fracture

Presentation

The Le Fort II fracture passes through the pterygoid plates and up through the suture between the zygoma and maxilla, and the nose and frontal bone. The nose and maxilla are therefore mobile in relation to the cheek bones and forehead. This sign can be elicited by gentle forward traction on the maxillary teeth with counter-pressure applied to the forehead or zygoma. Movement will be detectable at the sutures between the maxilla and zygoma at the inferior orbital rim and at the suture between the nose and the frontal bone in the glabella region. Tenderness is common over these sites. The patient has bilateral epistaxis and numbness of the cheeks. The middle third of the face appears long and there is a similar malocclusion to the Le Fort I fracture (Figure 7.17a,b). Patients

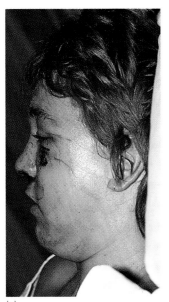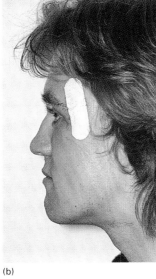

(a)

(b)

Figure 7.17 (a) This profile view shows a patient with a Le Fort II fracture. He has bilateral black eyes, epistaxis, and lengthening of the middle third of his face from the eyebrows to the lips. (b) After successful reduction of the fracture, the middle third of his face has been restored to normal proportions.

may feel that they are unable to open their mouths wide when in fact the maxilla has pushed the mandible open with its downward and backward movement. If the cribriform plate is damaged in Le Fort II and III fractures, there will be CSF rhinorrhoea.

If the medial canthi and lacrimal apparatus are damaged in this fracture, the patient will have traumatic telecanthus (that is increased width between the two medial canthi > 36 mm) and epiphora (leakage of tears onto the cheek).

Radiology

OM views show opacity of the maxillary sinus or fluid levels and separation at the zygomaticomaxillary sutures at the inferior orbital rim.

Management in A & E

Because of the potential for the cribriform plate damage in Le Fort II and III fractures with consequent disruption of the meninges, the patients are instructed not to blow their nose as this may cause contamination of the meninges with nasal secretions, and consequent meningitis. Prophylactic sulphonamides, such as co-trimoxazole, or alternatively chloramphenicol, may be used to prevent meningitis [6]. Once again, profound blood loss is unusual, but if bleeding is troublesome it should be managed with anterior and posterior nasal packs.

Ultimate management by maxillofacial surgery

Once again the fracture may be managed by indirect or direct means of fixation. With indirect methods, internal fixation wires may be used to suspend the maxilla from the frontal bone in the midline and the zygoma posteriorly. Alternatively, incisions can be made in the lower eyelid and over the

frontonasal suture and direct plating performed with micro- and miniplates.

Le Fort III fractures

Presentation

This fracture separates the zygoma, maxilla and nose (all the facial bones) from the base of the skull. The patient presents with a lengthened face, bilateral black eyes, and, if the separation of facial bones is severe, orbital dystopia (asymmetry of the position of the eyes). There is also bilateral epistaxis, malocclusion as before, and frequently inability to open the mouth wide because posterior displacement of the maxilla has already forced the mandible open. The face will be numb and palpation of the frontonasal and frontozygomatic sutures will demonstrate separation and tenderness.

Radiology

OM views show separation at the frontozygomatic, zygomaticomaxillary, and frontonasal sutures with fluid levels or complete opacity of the maxillary sinuses. A lateral brow-up facial view may show a fluid level in the sphenoid sinus.

Management in A & E

This is similar to the management of a Le Fort II fracture.

Ultimate management by maxillofacial surgery

Indirect fixation methods, such as a Halo metal head frame attached to splints on the upper and lower jaws by metal connecting rods, have long been in use. However, this apparatus is uncomfortable for the patient. Alternatively, the bicoronal flap provides access for direct fixation with titanium mini-or microplates at the frontozygomatic and frontonasal sutures, whilst lower eyelid and buccal sulcus incisions give access to the zygomaticomaxillary suture and Le Fort I level fracture respectively.

Anterior maxillary wall fractures

Presentation

This is a rare injury caused by a blow to the anterior maxillary wall. The patient will have numbness of the cheek, and palpation at the inferior orbital rim will elicit separation and tenderness at the fracture site. There may be associated medial canthal and lacrimal apparatus damage. OM radiographs show separation at the inferior orbital rim. A lower eyelid incision is used to approach the fracture, elevate it into the correct position and fix it with transosseous wires or plates.

Dentoalveolar fractures

Presentation

This problem affects children more frequently than adults and involves the incisor teeth more frequently than the molar teeth. It may be caused by direct blows to the teeth or indirect blows to the jaw when the lower jaw shuts rapidly causing the lower teeth to smash against the upper teeth.

It may affect one or more teeth and several distinct injuries are recognised. Fractures of the crown of the tooth occur horizontally or vertically. The fracture may involve the enamel of the crown alone, enamel and dentine, or extend into the pulp of the tooth. Alternatively, the root of the tooth may be fractured at different sites (Figure 7.18).

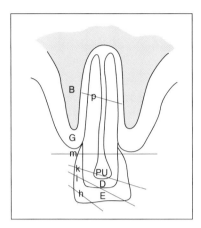

Figure 7.18 Diagram of an incisor tooth in its socket showing potential fracture sites: h: into enamel (E) only; l: into dentine (D); k: into the pulp (PU); m: decoronating the tooth to gum level; p: root fracture. The alveolar bone is shown as B and the gingival margin as G.

Teeth may be intruded or pushed into the bone, pushed out of position with fracture of the adjacent alveolar bone (subluxation), or completely extruded from the socket (avulsed).

The patient presents with pain, sensitivity of the affected tooth to touch and hot and cold drinks, bleeding gums around the tooth, malocclusion, and bloody saliva.

Alternatively, the patient may present with the tooth in their hand.

Radiology

Intraoral periapical radiographs are best. However, these may not be possible in a distressed child.

If tooth fragments have been lost and there is an associated soft tissue laceration, radiographs should be taken of these soft tissues to exclude implantation of the tooth fragment into the injured soft tissue. Similarly, chest x-rays may be necessary to exclude the possibility of inhalation of teeth or teeth fragments.

Management in A & E

In general, deciduous or primary teeth should be managed conservatively. If they have been avulsed, they should not be re-implanted. If they have been intruded they should be left alone. Fractures of deciduous teeth may be painful, in which case dental help is sought for application of a temporary dressing.

Permanent teeth usually require active intervention depending on the nature of the injury.

Root fractures of the teeth are managed with root canal therapy. Where the teeth have been avulsed or soft tissue lacerations have occurred, the patient will need antitetanus prophylaxis.

Avulsed teeth

Treatment for avulsed teeth
• Clean tooth with patient's saliva/milk
• Administer local anaesthesia
• Irrigate and clean socket
• Gently clean tooth
• Implant correctly
• Splint

These should be cleaned either by the patient sucking the tooth with their own saliva or by gently washing the tooth in milk. The ideal storage for medium avulsed teeth is saliva or milk. Normal saline is a reasonable substitute. The tooth should not be kept dry or soaked in tap water for any length of time. If the socket is full of blood clot, it should be gently irrigated with normal saline to clear the clot. The tooth is gripped by its crown the correct way round and re-implanted firmly into the socket. Local anaesthetic agents such as 2% lignocaine with 1 in 80 000 adrenaline or 3% prilocaine with octapressin may be needed for injection into the adjacent gingiva to achieve anaesthesia. Once the tooth has been re-implanted, it is supported with aluminium foil or lead foil obtained from an x-ray sheet until a more permanent splint is made. The patient may also have a mouth guard which can be used to hold the tooth in place.

Subluxed teeth

When radiographs have confirmed that there is no root fracture, local anaesthetic is instilled into the adjacent reflected gingiva in the sulcus. After a few minutes, when this has taken effect, the tooth is gripped firmly and pushed into its correct alignment. Splinting is not necessary unless the tooth is still very mobile. In the variant of subluxation when a permanent tooth is intruded into its socket, the tooth will be mobile after it is pulled into its correct position. In this case splintage is performed as for the avulsed tooth.

Fractured permanent teeth

Enamel fractures

If a substantial portion of the tooth crown has been fractured and is intact, it should be retained for later recementing. Alternatively, the sharp edges of the enamel fracture may be smoothed with a burr.

Enamel and dentine fractures

Again, the fragment of the fracture may be recemented later. The edges of the fracture may be smoothed and the raw dentine protected with a lining material such as zinc oxide/Eugenol paste.

Fractures into the pulp

Dental advice should be sought urgently for this fracture. The pink pulp chamber will be visible in the centre of the fractured crown.

Ultimate management by maxillofacial surgery

All avulsed, subluxed or intruded permanent teeth will be placed in their correct position in the dental arch. The opposing tooth in the opposite jaw may be smoothed to prevent regular trauma to the re-implanted tooth. Splints are fashioned to hold the tooth in place and some degree of movement of the tooth is acceptable to minimise the risk of later anklyosis. Subluxed teeth may be splinted for four days to four weeks and avulsed teeth are usually splinted for four weeks. If it is anticipated that the pulp of the tooth will ultimately necrose, root canal therapy is started within 7–14 days following injury.

Permanent teeth that have sustained fractures of the enamel or dentine are treated temporarily with sedative dressings placed over the exposed dentine. The patient is referred on to a specialist restorative dentist for reconstruction of the lost part of the tooth, with glass ionomer cements or with the tooth fragment that has been fractured off.

If the pulp of the tooth has been exposed, the pulp may be removed immediately. Alternatively, a sedative calcium hydroxide dressing is placed over the pulp with semipermanent restorations, prior to later root canal therapy and permanent restoration of the crown.

Lacerations

Lacerations are repaired as detailed in the box.

References

1. Shepherd JP, Gayford JJ, Leslie IJ, Scully C. Female victims of assault: a study of hospital attenders. *Journal Craniomaxillofacial Surgery* 1988;**16**:233.
2. Needleman HL. Orofacial trauma in child abuse: types, prevalence management and the dental profession's involvement. *Pediatric Dentistry* 1986;**8**:71–80.
3. Hill CM, Crosher RF, Carroll MJ, Mason DA. Facial fractures – the results of a prospective four-year study. *Journal Maxillofacial Surgery*. 1984;**12**:267–70.
4. Hutchison IL, Lawlor MG, Skinner DA. *ABC of major trauma: Major maxillofacial injuries.* British Medical Journal 1990;**301**:595–9.
5. Ellis E. Sequencing treatment for naso-orbito-ethmoid fractures. *Journal Oral Maxillofacial Surgery* 1993;**51**:543–58.
6. Leopard PJ. Dural tears in maxillofacial injuries. *British Journal Oral Surgery* 1971;**8**:222–30.

Further reading

Banks P (1987) *Killey's fractures of the middle third of the facial skeleton.* London, Boston: Wright Butterworth & Co. (Publishers) Ltd.
Banks P (1991) *Killey's fractures of the mandible*, 4th edn. Oxford, London, Boston: Wright an Imprint of Butterworth-Heinemann Ltd.
Rowe NL, Williams JLI, eds (1985). *Maxillofacial injuries*, Vols 1 & 2, Edinburgh, London, Melbourne, New York: Churchill Livingstone.

Facial lacerations: reparative steps

1. Clean the wound with topical antiseptic.
2. Take soft tissue radiographs if a foreign body is suspected in the wound.
3. If oil contamination has occurred, use acetone to clean wound.
4. Explore the wound carefully looking for through-and-through injuries.
5. Remove foreign bodies.
6. Do not discard any soft tissue.
7. Do not shave hair at sites such as eyebrow.
8. Repair tissues from deep to superficial and internal to external.
9. Ensure haemostasis.
10. Keep minimal tension on skin wounds.
11. Only excise wound edges if they are markedly black and ragged.
12. Avulsed fragments may be defatted and used as grafts.
13. Examine for associated injuries to the parotid duct and facial nerve and call maxillofacial surgeons to deal with these.
14. Approximate soft tissues accurately using land marks such as the vermilion border of the lip.
15. Drain subperichondral haematomas of the ear and nasal septum and apply pressure dressing.
16. Use fine nylon or prolene sutures of 4/0–6/0 thickness to close skin.
17. Use antirabies and antitetanus prophylaxis where appropriate.

8 Ophthalmic trauma

Ken K. Nischal
Senior Registrar, Oxford Eye Hospital

John S. Elston
Consultant Ophthalmologist, Oxford Eye Hospital

OBJECTIVES

■ To establish basic points of relevant anatomy and physiology of the ocular structures.

■ To correlate mechanism of injury to types of ocular trauma.

■ To describe a systematic approach to ocular examination in a trauma scenario.

■ To describe a mode of management which will minimise secondary trauma until the patient is seen by an ophthalmologist.

Opthalmologists' preoccupation with the eye does not release them from a medicolegal responsibility to detect, and manage appropriately, life-threatening conditions. Conversely, the trauma surgeon or emergency physician cannot be absolved of responsibility for failing to recognise sight-threatening injuries, and therefore they must have some idea of the likelihood of ocular involvement in specific trauma scenarios. For example, a retrospective study by Holt *et al.* in 1983 [1] of 1436 cases of maxillofacial trauma showed that 67% had ocular or periocular tissue involvement while Manfredi *et al.* in 1981 [2] reported a 6% incidence of blindness in patients who needed repair of facial fractures. Overall, eye injuries occur in 10% of cases of non-fatal trauma. Ocular trauma needs to be identified and then prioritised (Table 8.1), firstly in relation to the severity of systemic trauma (especially head trauma) and secondly in terms of urgency of management or referral. Early recognition of a sight-threatening condition such as a ruptured globe will allow appropriate safeguards to be taken while the patient is being stabilised, and thereby reduce the risk and/or amount of secondary ocular trauma.

Table 8.1 Prioritizing ocular trauma

Type of injury	*Action*
Eyelid trauma	Puncture wounds – treat with suspicion as the underlying globe may have been penetrated. If in doubt contact ophthalmologist Lid margin laceration – needs suturing by ophthalmologist/plastic surgeon
Laceration to cornea/sclera Ruptured globe with or without extrusion of ocular contents	Place clear cartella over affected eye. Contact ophthalmologist urgently. Avoid using depolarising muscle relaxants
Proptosis: retrobulbar haemorrhage	If external ophthalmoplegia with dilated pupil – contact ophthalmologist urgently. If no systemic contraindication, give i.v. acetazolamide 500 mg or i.v. mannitol 50–100 g
Enophthalmos Orbital floor fracture	Once systemically stabilised and appropriate scans of orbits performed, contact ophthalmologist
Orbital emphysema	Indicates medial orbital wall fracture most commonly; patient must avoid blowing nose. Needs antibiotic cover for five to seven days depending on severity. Call ophthalmologist once condition recognised for baseline examination. If there is rapid onset of proptosis with emphysema, call ophthalmologist urgently
Subconjunctival haemorrhage	If patient unconscious, ensure eye is kept closed to prevent secondary desiccation and chemosis. If posterior margins of haemorrhage not visible, exclude anterior cranial fossa floor fracture
Alkali chemical injury	Measure pH of conjunctiva, irrigate with minimum of 1 litre normal saline and repeat pH; repeat this until pH is neutral. Call ophthalmologist early **This is not the case for CS gas injury – see text**

Applied anatomy

Details of anatomy will not be discussed here but to fully appreciate the chapter a few terms and anatomical relations need to be clarified.

The orbit

The orbit is a pear-shaped cavity which connects with the intracranial cavity at its apex via the optic canal and superior orbital fissure. Relations (Figure 8.1) include:

- superior: anteriorly the frontal sinus and posteriorly the anterior cranial fossa containing the frontal lobe;
- inferior: maxillary sinus; the infraorbital nerve and vessels lie in the infraorbital groove in the floor of the orbit, hence orbital floor fracture invariably leads to infraorbital anaesthesia;
- lateral: anteriorly the temporal fossa and posteriorly the middle cranial fossa with the temporal lobe;
- medial: anteriorly the nasal cavity, and ethmoid sinuses and posteriorly the sphenoid sinus.

Structures entering/leaving the orbit

- Via the superior orbital fissure
  - lacrimal nerve*
  - frontal nerve*
  - superior ophthalmic vein
  - trochlear nerve
  - upper division of III nerve
  - nasociliary nerve*
  - VI nerve
  - lower division of III nerve
- Via the inferior orbital fissure
  - maxillary nerve (infraorbital nerve)
  - zygomatic nerve (branch of maxillary)
  - inferior ophthalmic vein
- Via optic canal
  - optic nerve
  - ophthalmic artery

*branches of the ophthalmic division of the V nerve

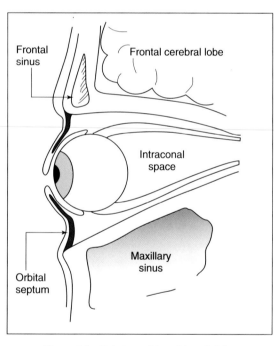

Figure 8.1 Relations of the orbit and globe.

Contents include:

- anteriorly and superotemporally – the lacrimal gland;
- anteriorly and medially: the lacrimal sac;
- centrally: the eyeball;
- arising posteriorly: the extraocular muscles (the four rectus muscles arise from the orbital apex to form a cone which contains the optic nerve);
- entering the orbit posteriorly: the orbital nerves and vessels, via the superior orbital fissure, optic canal and inferior orbital fissure (see box below); some are then intraconal and others extraconal in their course through the orbital cavity.

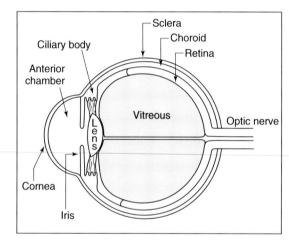

Figure 8.2 Anatomy of the eye (conjunctiva not shown).

The eyeball (see Figure 8.2)

- The conjunctiva is the outermost layer which covers the globe and is continuous with the conjunctival layer of the eyelids.
- The subconjunctival space separates the conjunctiva from the sclera (it is a potential space). A conjunctival laceration may or may not be associated with a scleral laceration; if it is, the scleral laceration may not lie directly beneath the conjunctival one because of the elasticity of the conjunctiva.
- The cornea lies centrally and is a continuation of the sclera; the junction of the two is called the limbus.
- Deep to the cornea/sclera lies the pigmented uveal layer, comprising:
  - anteriorly, the iris;
  - deep to the limbus, the ciliary body;
  - posteriorly, the choroid (a rich plexus of blood vessels and nerves lying deep to the sclera).
- Between the choroid and sclera lies the suprachoroidal space; if this fills with blood secondary to trauma, a choroidal detachment may develop causing elevation of the retina.

- The iris is a pigmented diaphragm with a central round aperture, the pupil.

> By definition, a penetrating injury of the globe is a perforating injury of the cornea or sclera.

Adnexae of the eye

- The *eyelids* provide protection to the cornea and conjunctiva when closed, preventing desiccation of these structures and the blink reflex also ensures adequate lubrication of the ocular surface; in unconscious patients both these functions need to be artificially replaced. Arising from the periosteum of the orbital margin is the fibrous framework of the eyelids, namely the orbital septum. Orbital fat lies behind this.

> Any eyelid laceration associated with prolapse of orbital fat indicates a breach of the orbital septum and necessitates thorough investigation to exclude orbitocranial injury.

- The *lacrimal gland* lies in the superotemporal quadrant of the orbit and produces serous secretions by reflex and emotional stimuli.
- The *lacrimal drainage system* comprises upper and lower canaliculi, a lacrimal sac just medial and deep to the medial canthus (inner corner of the eye), and the nasolacrimal duct which drains in the lower part of the lateral wall of the nose.

The cranial nerves (II, III, IV, V and VI) (see box below)

- The *optic nerve* is a CNS sensory fibre tract and therefore is surrounded by pia mater, arachnoid mater, and cerebrospinal fluid with a dural covering, the optic nerve sheath. Its length can be divided into four parts: intracranial, intracanalicular, intraorbital and intraocular. The intraorbital part is intraconal and lax to allow for eye movement. (The optic nerve is approximately 25 mm long in the orbit whilst the distance from the posterior globe to the optic canal is 18 mm.) As a result proptosis is rarely severe enough to cause a stretching injury. Instead traumatic optic neuropathy is usually due to a compressive injury, either bony injury in the canal with or without haemorrhage or contusion at the sclera–nerve junction.
- The upper and lower divisions of the *oculomotor nerve* pass through the superior orbital fissure and then lie intraconal; they supply the superior rectus/levator palpebrae superioris muscles and the medial and inferior rectus/inferior oblique muscles and the ciliary ganglion respectively.
- The *trochlear nerve* passes through the superior orbital fissure and lies extraconal to supply the superior oblique muscle.
- The *ophthalmic division of the trigeminal nerve* divides into three branches, lacrimal, frontal, and nasociliary, before it enters the orbit through the superior orbital fissure. The first two branches are extraconal and the last is intraconal for some of its course in the orbit. The *cornea* receives its sensory supply from branches of *the nasociliary nerve*.
- The *abducens nerve* enters via the superior orbital fissure and lies intraconal to supply the lateral rectus muscle.

Cranial nerves in the orbit

- Extraconal
  - trochlear nerve (IV)
  - lacrimal and frontal branches of the ophthalmic division of the trigeminal nerve (V)
  - maxillary nerve (V)
- Intraconal
  - oculomotor nerve (III)
  - nasociliary branch of the ophthalmic division of the trigeminal nerve (V)
  - abducens nerve (VI)

Pathophysiology of ophthalmic trauma (Table 8.2)

The mechanism of ophthalmic trauma is similar to that in other areas of the body, namely penetrating, blunt, and chemical. However, the frequency varies in different parts of the eye and its adnexae:

- eyeball: may suffer any three forms of injury or combinations;
- eyelids: usually suffer penetrating or blunt injury in the form of lacerations;
- bony orbit: usually damaged from blunt trauma;
- optic nerve: usually suffers contusion from blunt injury but may be transected as a result of a penetrating orbital injury.

Eyeball

Blunt trauma

If the eyeball itself is struck there is extreme deformation of the globe at the moment of impact (that is, a decrease in the anteroposterior diameter and an increase in the vertical height of the eyeball) with a concomitant but short-lived increase in the intraocular pressure. Damage occurs to the iris–lens complex as it is pushed back, and to the anterior chamber angle as it is forced open. The interface of different ocular constituents – retina/vitreous, choroid/sclera and optic nerve/ sclera – is also prone to injury. The possible results are:

- Iris–lens complex
  - gross tearing of iris root (iridodialysis) (Figure 8.3)
  - haemorrhage into anterior chamber (hyphaema) (Figures 8.4 and 8.5)
  - angle disruption with hyphaema
  - rupture of iris sphincter causing traumatic mydriasis (pupil irregularly dilated but still responds even if only slightly to bright light)
- Vitreoretinal interface
  - vitreous haemorrhage
  - retinal tear or dialysis/retinal detachment/retinal oedema (commotio retinae)
  - retinal haemorrhage
- Sclera–choroid interface
  - choroidal rupture/haemorrhage (Figure 8.6)
- Optic nerve–scleral junction
  - optic nerve contusion or rarely, avulsion, which usually occurs after sudden rotation of the globe.

Table 8.2 Ocular/adnexal signs and underlying pathology

Ophthalmic sign	*Possible correlating injury*
Bilateral periorbital ecchymoses ("panda bear" sign)	Basal skull fracture
Subconjunctival haemorrhage the posterior borders of which cannot be seen	Anterior cranial fossa floor fracture
Enopthalmos	Orbital floor fracture
Infraorbital anaesthesia	Orbital floor fracture
Orbital/periorbital emphysema	Usually medial wall of orbit fracture
Proptosis	Orbital haemorrhage
Pulsating proptosis	Caroticocavernous fistula/orbital roof defect
Pupils	
unilaterally fixed, dilated with afferent defect (that is, no consensual reflex either)	Orbital apex/superior orbital fissure syndrome (direct trauma may cause fixed dilated pupil but without an afferent defect)
bilaterally dilated with afferent defects	Tentorial herniation
bilaterally miosed	Pontine lesion
relative afferent pupillary defect	Optic nerve contusion or compression
Posterior segment	
subhyaloid/preretinal haemorrhage	Usually bilateral: indicator of subdural/intracerebral haemorrhage
diffuse multiple preretinal and retinal	Indicative of sudden and dramatic rise in intracranial venous pressure; in neonates and young children virtually diagnostic of non-accidental injury

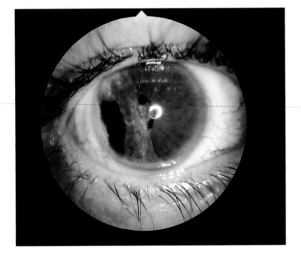

Figure 8.3 Iridodialysis in lateral half of iris.

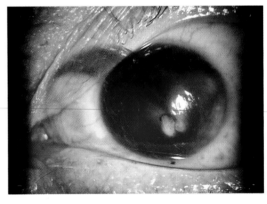

Figure 8.5 Full hyphaema with disruption of normal anterior chamber anatomy.

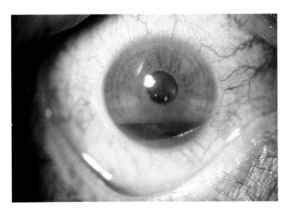

Figure 8.4 Small to moderate hyphaema.

If the force is great enough, the cornea or sclera or both may rupture, usually anteriorly at or near the corneoscleral junction, with prolapse of uveal tissue. It can, however, occur posteriorly with little damage to the anterior segment.

Penetrating trauma

Intraocular damage occurs along the track of the foreign body penetrating the eye. Evidence of external damage may be minimal and the history or circumstances of the injury are extremely important in excluding an intraocular foreign body. In addition to haemorrhage (anterior chamber, retina, choroid, or vitreous), retinal tear/detachment, lens capsule puncture with rapid onset lens opacity (Figure 8.7), and hypotony (lowered intraocular pressure) can occur.

Chemical trauma

Chemical burns of the eye are often bilateral and account for 7–10% of reported ocular trauma. Both alkalis and acids are capable of causing significant anterior segment damage. The degree of severity is directly proportional to the duration of contact, volume of chemical, chemical penetrability, and the

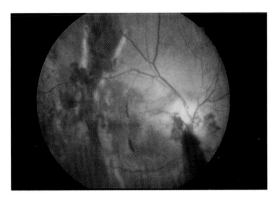

Figure 8.6 Choroidal rupture (there is also a subhyaloid haemorrhage near the optic disc).

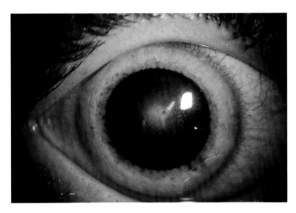

Figure 8.7 Focal lens opacity caused by a dart striking and penetrating the eye through the cornea.

pH of the solution. Alkalis cause more severe injuries because they penetrate ocular tissue very rapidly from saponification of cell membrane fatty acids. The hydroxyl ion (OH^-) causes collagen and glycosaminoglycans denaturation. In contrast acids cause coagulation of corneal epithelium proteins which act as a barrier to further penetration of the chemical.

The main tissues affected are the cornea and conjunctiva; these areas stain brilliantly with 5% fluorescein to show the epithelial defect caused by the injury. Around the limbus lie the pluripotent limbal stem cells which are responsible for re-epithelialisation; in severe injury there is limbal ischaemia

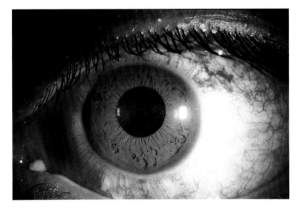

Figure 8.8 Area of localised ischaemia (blanched region) following an alkali injury.

(Figure 8.8) with subsequent loss of stem cells and lack of healing. Occasionally the periorbital skin may also be affected by the injury.

Ocular injuries with *O*-chlorobenzylidene malonitrile gas (CS gas) warrant a special mention. This compound is highly

soluble in water and irritates mucous membranes, causing an immediate pronounced local reaction on contact. The toxic basis of its actions is poorly understood but is thought to be due to the release of highly reactive chlorine atoms which form hydrochloric acid on contact with mucous membranes and skin. The patient describes a severe burning of the eyes and exhibits profuse lacrimation with blepharospasm and conjunctival oedema. In addition to a peculiar odour, many victims describe a burning, acidic taste. If inhaled it may cause sore throat, coughing, bronchospasm, and even apnoea. If swallowed in saliva, it usually invokes nausea and vomiting.

> An important difference between CS gas and an alkali such as ammonia, is that for the degree of symptomatic involvement with CS gas there is little or no staining of the corneal epithelium.

Although this compound can legally only be used during riot control by the police, it is still available to individuals [3]. Its use must be carefully looked for both from the history and the clinical signs and symptoms described, since its management is completely different from other alkali/acidic injuries.

Eyelids

Blunt trauma

This can give rise to a dramatic swelling of the lids due to their rich vascular supply and thin, distensible skin, which can

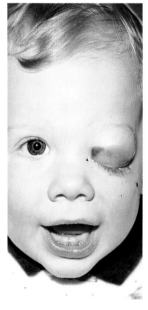

Figure 8.9 Ecchymosis following a fall; this was due to an orbital haemorrhage.

make examination of the eye extremely difficult (Figure 8.9). In severe cases the haematoma may spread to the other eyelid across the bridge of the nose. Spread elsewhere is limited by a subcutaneous fascial septum at the brow which prevents extension into the forehead, and by the orbital septum preventing extension into the orbit.

Penetrating trauma

Lid lacerations through the lid margin will heal irregularly if left untreated and this can lead to ocular surface damage and refractive irregularity from uneven spread of the tear film. Lacerations sited medially may disrupt the lacrimal canaliculi and lead to overflow of normal tear load. In addition all puncture wounds must be carefully examined as there may be an underlying perforation of the globe.

Bony orbit

Blunt trauma

Associated with deformity of the globe on blunt impact there is a sudden rise in the orbital pressure which can lead to a "blowout fracture" of the thin medial wall or more commonly, floor of the orbit. A "blowout fracture" can also occur with blunt ocular trauma caused by transmitted force from the orbital rim. Orbital floor and medial wall fractures reduce eye movements by compromising function of the adjacent extraocular muscle either by entrapment, haemorrhage, or interference with fascia; for example, there is restriction of

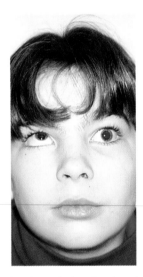

Figure 8.10 Patient is trying to look up but there is restriction of upgaze in the left eye due to inferior rectus entrapment secondary to orbital floor fracture.

upgaze (Figure 8.10) when the orbital floor is involved. Fractures of the orbital rim indicate a severe focal injury. Since the infraorbital nerve runs in the floor of the orbit, anaesthesia of the infraorbital skin is an important sign of orbital floor fracture. Enophthalmos, that is, the posterior displacement of the eye within the orbit, indicates that there is a large fracture. However, it is usually a late sign and becomes more obvious as the oedema and haemorrhage subside. Orbital emphysema usually occurs with a medial wall fracture that allows communication with sinuses. In these cases air enters the orbit from the nasal cavity but cannot leave as orbital fat acts as a one-way valve. Blunt trauma may affect the lacrimal gland directly by causing prolapse of the gland with or without haemorrhage. Injury causing orbital haemorrhage may threaten the optic nerve and eyeball secondary to raised intraorbital and intraocular pressure. Haemorrhage may develop in the subperiosteal, extraconal or intraconal spaces, or within the optic nerve sheath. Diffuse haemorrhage usually results in axial proptosis, whilst localised haemorrhage results in displacement of the globe away from the bleeding site. Visual loss in orbital haemorrhage is caused by compressive optic neuropathy from intrasheath or intraconal haemorrhages.

Penetrating trauma

This may also lead to haemorrhage as well as focal damage to the extraocular muscles or optic nerve. Penetration, for example by a blade or spike, may extend into the anterior cranial fossa via the superior orbital fissure. Important indicators of intracranial involvement include CSF rhinorrhoea, massive lid oedema disproportionate to the size of skin laceration caused by the CSF leak, and pulsating exophthalmos caused by orbital roof damage. Caroticocavernous fistula can occur after transorbital penetrating wounds.

The optic nerve

Each part of the optic nerve is vulnerable to different mechanisms of injury. The intraocular part may be damaged by penetrating injury or by avulsion/contusion; the intraorbital nerve may suffer penetrating injury or compression from orbital haemorrhage. The intracanalicular portion is fixed within the bony canal and is usually indirectly injured by acute compression transmitted through bone. Additionally the nerve is susceptible to ischaemia from disruption to its vascular supply and to secondary compression if it swells within the bony canal. The intracranial optic nerve is the portion least likely to suffer damage.

The cranial nerves

Traumatic damage to the cranial nerves supplying the extraocular muscles may be caused by laceration, tearing, contusion or compression of the nerves. Head trauma is a common cause of cranial neuropathies VI, III and IV (in that order of frequency).

Assessing the traumatised eye

History

Mode of injury

Road traffic accidents (RTA)

RTAs are a significant source of permanent visual impairment. About 40% of those who sustain ocular trauma in this way become blind in one or both eyes. RTA-related eye injuries are often bilateral, thus injury in one eye necessitates meticulous inspection of the other eye. If the windscreen has been shattered, patients need careful examination to exclude penetrating eye injury from glass. Although seatbelt legislation has reduced the rate of RTA penetrating injuries from 17 to 6%, the incidence of facial injuries (including orbital fractures) has increased because of contact with the steering wheel. Furthermore airbag-related eye injuries are being increasingly reported. This device relies on severe vehicle deceleration being detected by sensors which trigger the airbag inflators, usually by burning a substance such as sodium azide to produce nitrogen (96%), CO_2 (3%) and other gases and particles (sodium hydroxide, sodium carbonate, sodium bicarbonate, and metal oxides). Reported eye injuries include conjunctival alkali injury, anterior segment trauma (corneal abrasion, hyphaema), and posterior segment trauma (vitreous haemorrhage, retinal oedema, retinal detachment). In patients where airbag deployment is known to have occurred, thorough ocular examination is therefore necessary.

Alleged assault

This may be chemical, penetrating, or blunt in nature. It is important to establish the possibility of an alkali chemical injury as early as possible since delay in treatment leads to a poor visual prognosis. Use of a pH paper applied to the affected conjunctiva will help establish the degree of alkalinity/acidity present. Normal conjunctiva has a neutral pH. If a patient has been involved in public disorder situations, the use of CS gas should be established as soon as possible. CS gas is available illegally to the individual and therefore the use of a gas canister in an attack should be excluded in the history.

Where there is suspicion of penetrating injury it is important to establish whether an intraocular or orbital foreign body is likely to have been retained. For example, was a broken glass bottle used? Periocular lacerations in association with a history of alleged assault with a blade or knife should alert the examiner to the possibility of orbitocranial injury.

Blunt trauma is probably the most frequently encountered form of alleged assault and its mechanism may give a clue to the likelihood of ocular/orbital trauma. If fists were used then a direct blow to the eyeball is possible whereas objects with a larger surface area may not cause as much direct ocular damage because of protection from the brow and orbital rim.

Sport

Sports-related ocular injuries tend to be severe and occur particularly in hockey, squash, boxing, and rugby.

Falls

The elderly who fall accidentally may sustain lid lacerations, orbital haemorrhage, or blunt ocular trauma. Rupture of the globe at the site of previous cataract surgery is a recognised complication and therefore the patient should be asked about any previous ocular surgery. Nevertheless, children are more likely than adults to sustain sight-threatening injuries after ocular trauma in the home.

Foreign bodies

The composition of any possible foreign body is important to ascertain as it determines to some extent the severity of the tissue response and influences the decision to surgically intervene or not:

● iron, steel, aluminium, lead: relatively inert, unless accompanied by infection;
● brass, bronze: chronic inflammatory reaction;
● copper: purulent inflammatory reaction;
● stone, glass: inert unless accompanied by infection;
● organic foreign body: acute inflammatory reaction.

Establishing visual status before the accident

This is important but usually not immediately possible and may need the cooperation of a relative if the patient is comatosed or unconscious. Other important features of the ocular history include the presence of pre-existing ocular disease, for example glaucoma or squint, previous ocular surgery, the presence of a "lazy eye" due to amblyopia, and whether the patient normally wears spectacles for distance vision correction, for example driving glasses or glasses for watching television.

Examination

This is best divided into examination in:

● the emergency room
● the unconscious patient
● the conscious patient
● the intensive care/trauma unit.

In the emergency room: the unconscious patient

Symmetry of the eyes

Proptosis is usually obvious but may be difficult to detect if bilateral. Proptosis should be described as being *axial* or *non-axial*. Axial indicates that the proptosis is uniplanar and is usually associated with intraconal pathology while non-axial indicates that there is accompanying downward or upward displacement of the eye, usually associated with extraconal pathology. Post-traumatic axial proptosis is usually due to retrobulbar haemorrhage whilst a large subperiosteal orbital haemorrhage would produce a non-axial proptosis.

Occasionally post-traumatic proptosis may be *pulsatile*. This indicates either a traumatic caroticocavernous fistula (Figure

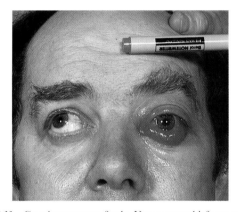

Figure 8.11 Caroticocavernous fistula. Note proposed left eye with marked conjunctival oedema (chemosis) and left ophthalmoplegia as the patient attempts to look up.

8.11) from rupture of the carotid artery within the cavernous sinus or an orbital roof fracture transmitting intracranial vascular pulsation to the globe. In post-traumatic caroticocavernous fistula the conjunctiva is oedematous with dilated vasculature. There is ophthalmoplegia and an afferent pupil defect.

In general, the proptotic eye can be gently retropulsed by placing a thumb on the upper lid and gently applying pressure. In this way the tension of the orbit can be judged. However, this procedure should only be carried out once the integrity of the globe is established. A tense eye indicates raised intra-orbital and intraocular pressure which may compromise the optic nerve and, more immediately, the central retinal artery.

Enophthalmos is usually a late feature of orbital fracture. It is uncommonly encountered as a presenting feature of acute trauma as it is masked by oedema and haemorrhage in and around the orbit. Although large orbital floor fractures may cause immediately apparent enophthalmos, these are usually associated with gross asymmetry of the face caused by facial

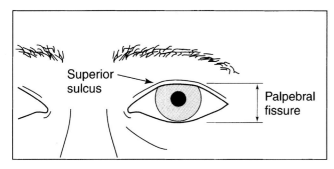

Figure 8.12 Superior sulcus and the palpebral fissure (see text).

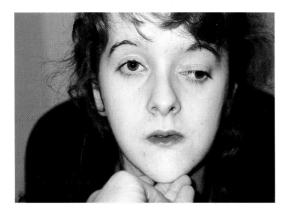

Figure 8.13 Gross left globe dystopia from orbital floor fracture.

fractures involving the zygoma. Signs suggestive of enophthalmos are a deep superior sulcus and a narrowed palpebral fissure (Figure 8.12).

Position of the eyes

- *Globe dystopia* is an inferior displacement of the affected orbit and can occur in gross orbital floor fractures (Figure 8.13).
- *Telecanthus* is increased tissue between the two eyes which may be a racially inherited feature, but secondary to trauma it is due to orbital fracture or fractures.
- *Tonic conjugate deviation* of the eyes to one side is indicative of damage to one frontal lobe. This can be due to stroke caused by traumatic occlusion of the carotid artery.
- An eye that is deviated laterally and inferiorly with ptosis, a dilated ipsilateral pupil and intact consensual reflex indicates a *III palsy* (Figure 8.14).

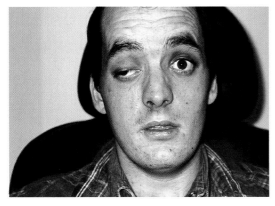

Figure 8.14 Right third nerve palsy.

- An eye that is turned in (esotropic) is suggestive of a *VI palsy* causing weakness of the lateral rectus muscle or due to avulsion/laceration of the lateral rectus (Figure 8.15).
- *Vertical misalignment* of the eyes (i.e. one eye looks up while the other looks down) is usually mechanical caused by muscle entrapment in an orbital floor fracture or damage to one of the vertically acting muscles (that is, superior and inferior rectus muscles or superior and inferior oblique muscles) (Figure 8.16).

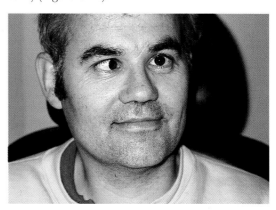

Figure 8.15 Left VI palsy; there is restriction of abduction of the left eye as the patient attempts to look to the left.

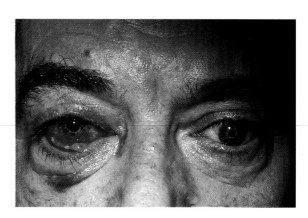

Figure 8.16 Laceration in the right infraorbital region with chemosis of the right conjunctiva. As the patient attempts to look down the right eye does not follow. This patient has had rupture and/or laceration affecting the right inferior rectus.

Note: In the absence of any evidence of muscle disruption, orbital haemorrhage and/or fracture, such a vertical misalignment may be caused by brainstem or cerebellar dysfunction producing skew deviation, which is a non-localising sign. However, in trauma the commonest site tends to be the pons and the lesion is usually but not always on the side of the eye that is higher (hypertropic).

Pupillary examination

- *Shape*: a tented/peaked pupil indicates a perforated globe with prolapse of uveal tissue; a large irregular pupil may be seen in traumatic mydriasis.
- *Size*: bilateral miosed pupils may indicate pontine damage. In contrast, large pupils are seen if the efferent supply to the pupil sphincter via the III nerve is disrupted, for example in the dorsal midbrain syndrome. **Note**: In the unconscious patient the only signs apparent in this condition are large pupils which react sluggishly to light.
- *Reflexes*: It is important to have a routine of examination of the pupil reflexes as the information gained can be vital.

Always perform the direct light test and the swinging light test (comparing the direct and consensual reflexes in the same eye). The direct light reflex tests the integrity of the ipsilateral reflex loop along the optic nerve (afferent) and oculomotor nerve (efferent). A bright focused light source is essential. In the swinging light test, one eye has a bright light shone into it along the visual axis. Both pupils (ipsi- and contralateral) should constrict equally. When the light is shone in the other eye, both pupils should again constrict to the same extent. This is repeated (the light is "swung" from eye to eye giving time for the response to be assessed). If the optic nerve is compromised in one eye, the pupil on that side will dilate as the light is shone directly into it, but constrict when the light is shone in the contralateral eye. This is termed an afferent, that is sensory pupillary defect, and may be absolute (no function at all in the optic nerve) or relative (some preserved function). There are certain physical signs which indicate specific diagnoses:

- *Unilateral dilated non-reactive pupil without afferent defect* (that is, the contralateral pupil constricts normally when the affected pupil has a bright light shone in it) indicates IIIrd nerve damage (that is, an efferent but not an afferent defect).
- *Unilateral dilated non-reactive pupil with afferent defect* indicates IIIrd nerve damage with traumatic optic neuropathy; if tense proptosis is also present, a retrobulbar haemorrhage is the most likely cause.
- *Unilateral or bilateral dilated pupils*, sluggish to direct light may indicate tentorial herniation.
- *A unilaterally miosed (constricted) pupil* with an ipsilateral partial ptosis indicates a traumatic Horner's syndrome (sympathetic denervation, Figure 8.17); neck trauma and ipsilateral carotid artery dissection need to be excluded urgently.

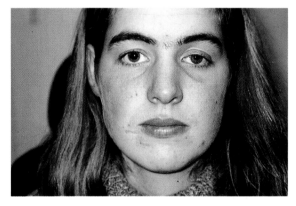

Figure 8.17 Left Horner's syndrome following a fall from a horse.

Integrity of the globe

It is very important to exclude a perforated globe as soon as possible so that adequate protective measures can be taken while the patient is being stabilised. The features which should make the examiner suspicious are:

- A history which makes a penetrating injury likely, for example RTA, where no seat belts were worn.
- Loss of normal corneal reflex – if a light is shone at a normal cornea the light reflected off the corneal surface has a sharp, bright quality to it whilst, if the globe is ruptured, the reflex is dull.
- Tented or peaked pupil (Figure 8.18).
- Shallow anterior chamber compared to the contralateral unaffected side. This is best assessed by shining a pen torch

at the lateral half of the cornea. Normally a crescentric shadow is seen on the medial side of the cornea. If the anterior chamber is shallow or flat, this crescentric shadow becomes barely discernible (Figure 8.19).

- Prolapsed uveal tissue. This appears as a brown mass adherent to the globe.
- Extrusion of other intraocular tissue, for example lens and vitreous (Figure 8.20).
- Chemosis (oedema of the conjunctiva) may be seen in a perforated globe but is more commonly associated with orbital haemorrhage, caroticocavernous fistula, retained foreign body, and chemical injury.

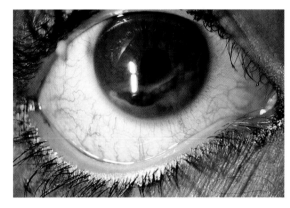

Figure 8.18 Penetrating injury of the cornea with prolapsed iris and resultant distortion of the pupil.

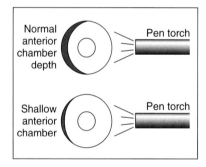

Figure 8.19 Examining for a shallow anterior chamber.

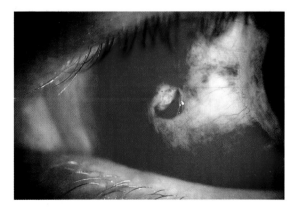

Figure 8.20 Perforation of the globe with prolapse of vitreous.

Ophthalmoscopy

Do not dilate the pupils pharmacologically in an unconscious patient in the emergency room as this may mask neurological signs. However, an attempt should be made to examine the following:

- *Red reflex* (see boxes). This is done by looking through the eyepiece of the ophthalmoscope with the dial on zero, from a distance of 20–30 cm, with the intrument's light source aimed at the pupil. Normally, the light is reflected back from the retina giving a red reflex. The red reflex may be partially or completely absent.

Causes of partial loss of red reflex

- Lens opacities induced by penetrating injury (see Figure 8.7)
- Vitreous haemorrhage
- Partial retinal detachment
- Partially dislocated lens

Causes of complete loss of red reflex

- Total hyphaema
- Vitreous haemorrhage
- Choroidal haemorrhage
- Choroidal detachments
- Complete retinal detachment

- *Anterior chamber.* The iris is normally clearly visible. It may be obscured by corneal opacity (for example from raised intraocular pressure causing corneal odema), a large corneal abrasion (with or without perforation of the cornea), or blood in the anterior chamber (hyphaema). A very large hyphaema is difficult to miss, as the anterior chamber appears red with no pupil or iris apparent (see Figure 8.5). When a hyphaema does not completely fill the anterior chamber, a fluid level of blood can be seen (see Figure 8.4). Fluorescein 5% solution should be instilled into the eyes. This stain fluoresces bright green when illuminated by cobalt blue filtered light – pen torches are readily avaliable to which an appropriate filter cap can be attached. Fluorescein stains the exposed corneal stroma if an abrasion is present (Figure 8.21). If a corneal perforation is present, aqueous leaks out of the eye, displacing the dye in the tear film at the site of the penetrating injury.

- *Vitreous.* Haemorrhage may occur in the vitreous (intragel) or behind its posterior face (subhyaloid or preretinal). A subhyaloid haemorrhage may be seen in association with subarachnoid haemorrhages and appears as well circumscribed deep red collections of blood close to the retina. If multiple preretinal and retinal haemorrhages are seen in neonates and young children, the possibility of non-accidental injury must be considered. An intragel haemorrhage is seen as a black "blob" against the red reflex. In penetrating trauma, a foreign body may be seen within the vitreous or retina usually surrounded by blood.
- *Retina.* Traumatic detachment of the retina may be partial or complete. If complete, an afferent pupillary defect (see above) will be present. The retina is out of focus, yellow-white and folded. Partial retinal detachment requires pupillary dilatation and ophthalmic expertise to diagnose. Retinal oedema (commotio retinae) often accompanies blunt trauma and appears as a localised patch of silvery white retina often with small haemorrhages. Haemorrhage may be seen with or without oedema. Purtscher's retinopathy due to fat emboli after fracture of long bones or after a crush injury of the chest can be recognised by widespread retinal haemorrhages in association with multiple cotton-wool spots.

  Sometimes, following severe blunt trauma, the choroid may rupture (see Figure 8.6) giving a very dark red streak-like haemorrhage under the retina.
- If the *optic nerve is avulsed*, haemorrhage localised to the papillary area occurs which partly obscures the view of the disc itself. A swollen disc implies either raised intracranial pressure or compression of the optic nerve and its sheath. A central retinal artery occlusion in association with a swollen disc is usually due to an orbital haemorrhage compressing the optic nerve and/or raising the intraocular pressure.

Eyelids

- *Ecchymosis* (haemorrhage into the lids). The accompanying swelling can make examination of the eye difficult. Bilateral ring eyelid haemorrhages ("panda bear" sign) may signify a basal skull fracture while even unilateral ecchymosis associated with a subconjunctival haemorrhage tracking forwards to the cornea is suggestive of an anterior cranial fossa floor fracture (Figure 8.22).

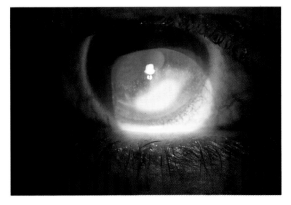

Figure 8.21 Corneal abrasion stained with fluorescein.

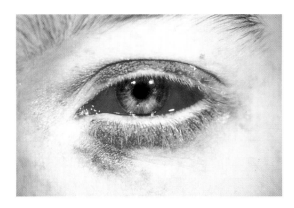

Figure 8.22 Ecchymosis with subconjunctival haemorrhage in a patient with skull fracture.

Occasionally an iridodialysis (disinsertion of the iris root, see Figure 8.3) may be seen and is recognised as a "second pupil" albeit distorted and displaced to one side of the central pupil.

All patients with ecchymosis should have the margins of the orbit palpated for bony defects, irregularities, and crepitations (indicating orbital emphysema). A localised upper lid haematoma may be indicative of an orbital roof fracture.

- *Lid laceration.* Penetrating wounds of the upper lid have a greater tendency for intracranial extension than those of the lower lid (see section below "In the intensive care unit").

Spontaneous eye movements in coma

- *Ocular bobbing* is a rapid downward deviation of the eyes with a slow drift up seen in destructive (haemorrhagic) pontine lesions.

In the emergency room: The conscious patient

In addition to the assessment detailed above, a number of additional tests should be carried out in the conscious and cooperative patient.

Assessment of vision

It is important to ascertain if there is a subjective reduction in vision in either eye. Visual acuity can be assessed in each eye separately with a reading test chart (with glasses, if worn). If acuity is reduced below the level of the largest print it should be recorded as ability to count fingers (CF), see hand movements (HM), perceive light (PL), or not perceive light (NPL). If a patient is able to count fingers then an assessment of visual field to confrontation may give valuable information with the test for a hemianopia.

Note: It is important to establish at the onset whether the patient usually wears spectacles or not since this will influence his acuity especially if they have been lost or broken.

Pupils

In the presence of a normal, intact light reflex, the accomodation reflex is always present. In contrast the converse is not true and light-near dissociation (that is absent or sluggish light reflex with intact accomodation reflex) can be a useful sign. To test for the accomodation reflex, first ask the patient to look at something in the distance (most easily done by asking the patient to look at a point on the ceiling), then place an accomodative target (most handy is the tip of a pen) about 5–10 cm from the tip of the patient's nose and ask the patient to look at the target. An intact accomodation reflex consists of slight convergence of the two eyes with constriction of the pupils. There are many causes of light-near dissociation of the pupillary reflex but post-trauma the commonest is damage to the dorsal midbrain in deceleration injury. The dorsal midbrain or Parinaud's syndrome consists of large pupils with light-near dissociation, lid retraction, limitation of upgaze, and convergence-retraction nystagmus induced by attempted upgaze.

Eye movements

These should only be tested once the integrity of the globe has been established. Abnormal extraocular movements may be due to mechanical limitation or a neural cause. The movements of the two eyes together (versions) should be tested for in nine positions of gaze with a bright focused light as the

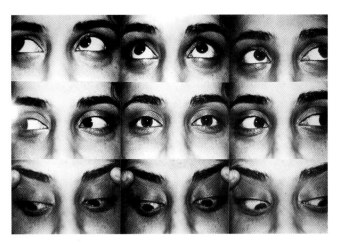

Figure 8.23 Examining eye movements in the nine positions of gaze.

target (Figure 8.23). Any restrictions should be noted as well as the positions in which double vision is seen. If double vision is present constantly, cover one eye at a time to establish whether it is monocular or binocular. Monocular diplopia in a trauma setting is most likely due to ipsilateral lens damage or dislocation while binocular diplopia is usually due to muscle imbalance. This may be mechanical or neural in origin and, if neural, supranuclear or infranuclear (peripheral).

The movements of one eye with the other eye covered (ductions) should then be tested. If on version testing there appears to be a restriction in one eye, then that eye should be tested in the same direction with the other eye covered. If the restriction is mechanical, for example muscle entrapment from orbital floor fracture, there will be no change on monocular testing, but if it is neural in origin the eye movement will be fuller.

The vestibulo-ocular reflexes (VOR) are helpful in diagnosing neural lesions which may be either supranuclear or infranuclear. Since the management of these two is different, they must be distinguished from each other. Supranuclear lesions causing abnormal eye movements usually involve the cerebral hemispheres or the brain-stem premotor centres and in such cases the VOR can be used to establish the integrity of the infranuclear pathways. The oculocephalic reflex is a VOR but must only be performed if cervical spine injury has been excluded. The patient is asked to fixate a target straight ahead while the head is rotated from side to side and up and down. A normal response consists of deviation of both eyes away from the direction of rotation of the head ("doll's eye movement"), and demonstrates integrity of nuclear and infranuclear ocular motor pathways and an intact vestibular

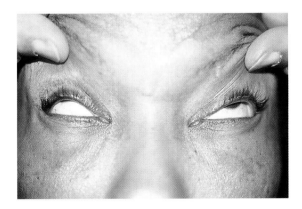

Figure 8.24 Bell's phenomenon. The eyeballs roll up as the patient tries to close the eyes.

Table 8.3 Eye movement disorders and localisation of intracranial injury

Eye movements	Likely area of injury
Tonic conjugate deviation to one side	Damage to ipsilateral frontal lobe (usually by stroke which may be caused by traumatic occlusion of the carotid artery)
Skew deviation (vertical misalignment of visual axes)	Non-localizing sign of posterior fossa damage
Conjugate horizontal gaze paresis	Ipsilateral pontine damage (may be bilateral)
Vertical gaze paresis	In trauma usually seen in association with other signs of doral midbrain damage, for example light-near dissociation of pupillary reaction, limited convergence, eyelid retraction, skew deviation, and convergence-retraction nystagmus (Parinaud's syndrome)
Complete ophthalmoplegia with dilated pupil with or without proptosis	Sphenocavernous or orbital apex syndrome
Internuclear ophthalmoplegia	Disruption of medial longitudinal fasciculus in brain stem
VI palsy	In isolation, can be a non-localising sign of raised intracranial pressure. Other signs usually present depending on site of injury
III palsy in isolation	If only pupillary fibres affected (that is, a dilated pupil) suggests damage to III in middle cranial fossa where these fibres lie peripherally in the nerve. With oculomotor weakness – of little localising value
with contralateral hemiplegia	Third nerve fascicle in the brain stem
unilaterally with bilateral ptosis	Characteristic of nuclear damage, that is tectum of midbrain anterior to the cerebral aqueduct
IV palsy	Usually bilateral in trauma. Since it is the longest and thinnest cranial nerve, localisation may be difficult and depends on other accompanying signs
Upbeat nystagmus	Posterior fossa injury
Downbeat nystagmus	Cervicomedullary junction injury
Horizontal nystagmus	Brain stem or cerebellar injury
Volitional gaze deficit	In the acute setting, deficits of voluntary gaze are likely to be due to a frontal or pontine haematoma

system. **Note**: In comatose patients the test is performed with the eyelids held open.

Bell's phenomenon is the upward rotation of the eyes on attempted closure of the eyelids against resistance (Figure 8.24). If normal, it implies that the supranuclear pathway is intact. It is a protective mechanism and is elicited by holding the eyelids open and asking the patient to try and close his or her eyes. This test is useful in patients with paralysis of upgaze. **Note**: 10% of normal patients have absence of this phenomenon.

The important abnormal eye movements are listed in Table 8.3.

> The degree to which eye movements are assessed depends on the systemic stability of the patient. Some of the above assessments may be best left until the patient is transferred to the ward or intensive care unit.

Periorbital sensation

If sensation to touch and pin-prick is intact in the infraorbital area served by the infraorbital nerve, an orbital floor fracture can be excluded.

In the intensive care unit

In addition to the assessment described above, once the patient is stabilised and transferred to ITU or a ward, further examination may be warranted. If the patient is conscious and has visual symptoms, the visual acuity must be recorded. If the patient usually wears spectacles which have been lost or broken, obtain a spare pair from a relative or friend so that the corrected acuity, and more importantly, that which the patient regards as "normal" is attained.

Eyelids

- *Lacerations*. The depth and location must be examined carefully. Through and through wounds should alert the examiner to the possibility of globe perforation. Lacerations near the medial aspect of the eyelids may have damaged the lacrimal drainage system. Dog bite-related lacerations often cause lacrimal canalicular disruption. It is important to recognise if any part of the eyeid is missing.
- *Ptosis*. In traumatic cases where a neurogenic aetiology has been excluded, the presence or absence of the eyelid crease on the affected side must be noted. Absence of the lid crease suggests damage to the levator palpebrae superioris usually with disinsertion of the levator aponeurosis. If this is associated with a laceration or puncture wound, early recognition increases the chance of accurate repair. Delayed recognition may lead to a heavy fibrous scar making repair difficult. A simple way of measuring the degree of ptosis is to use the marginal reflex distance (MRD): a light is shone into the eye along the visual axis in a conscious patient and the distance from the central corneal light reflex to the upper lid margin estimated. The normal MRD should be

4–4.5 mm, and if it is less, the difference is the size of the ptosis, for example, if the MRD in a patient is 2 mm, then the ptosis is approximately 2 mm.

Note: In a patient with ocular irritation or pain, it is always prudent to evert the upper lid to ensure there is no subtarsal foreign body present (Figure 8.25).

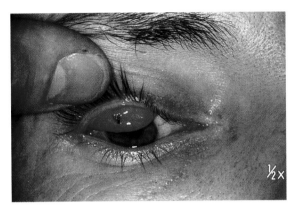

Figure 8.25 Subtarsal foreign body.

Cornea

● The use of fluorescein dye facilitates detection of *abrasions* as described previously. The normal corneal reflex when a light is shone in the eye is often lost when there is drying of the cornea secondary to exposure. This can be a problem in the unconscious patient but may also occur if blinking is compromised, for example in facial nerve palsy or loss of lid(s). This is especially so if Bell's phenomenon is absent, in which case the patient will need careful monitoring as the chances of exposure keratopathy developing are high.

● Removal of corneal *foreign bodies* should only be attempted once perforating injury has been excluded.

Conjunctiva

This is extremely elastic and lacerations must be carefully examined as there may be an underlying perforation of the globe which may not lie directly beneath the conjunctival laceration. The possibility of a retained foreign body must also be considered. In this context an eye movement disorder may indicate direct damage to extraocular muscles.

Conjunctival oedema (chemosis) may be an isolated finding but can also be seen in association with globe rupture, orbital fracture with or without haemorrhage, caroticocavernous fistula, and retained ocular foreign body. Haemorrhagic conjunctival oedema can be dangerous if the eyelids cannot close as this can lead to corneal exposure and ulceration.

Radiological interpretation

Indications for imaging

These include presence or suspicion of:

● a deep penetrating wound, to determine the extent of injury and whether any sinus or intracranial areas are involved;
● a foreign body, to localise it and in some instances determine its character;
● blunt trauma, to detect haemorrhage, orbital fracture and the state of the optic nerve and adjacent tissues.

Imaging modalities

Those available include plain x-ray, CT scan, MR scan, and ultrasonography.

Plain x-ray

This has been replaced by CT scan in the evaluation of facio-orbital injuries.

CT scan

CT provides good imaging of soft tissues, bone, acute haemorrhage, and foreign bodies. Facio-orbital injuries may be accompanied by intracranial trauma; thus both regions should be scanned at the same time. Scans can be taken in different planes (axial, sagittal, and coronal), and the resolution is best if these scans are taken directly rather than reconstructed by the computer. However, if a patient has a suspected cervical spine injury, the only direct scan plane taken is the axial one and the rest are reconstructed.

In *suspected orbital fractures*, a combination of oblique sagittal and coronal sections should be used as these display all the fracture margins, the fracture/inferior orbital rim relationship, and any displacement into the maxillary sinus, especially in orbital floor fractures [4]. The oblique sagittal section helps evaluate the inferior rectus in cases of orbital floor fractures (Figure 8.26) Bony window cuts should also be used as they allow subtle fractures to be detected.

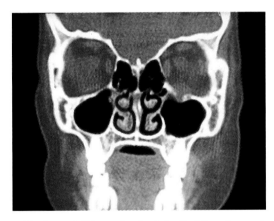

Figure 8.26 Coronal CT scan showing left orbital floor fracture (same patient as in Figure 8.10).

In suspected tramatic optic neuropathy, in addition to excluding fractures, coronal sections at the orbital apex are useful for determining the presence of compression.

In suspected intraocular or intraorbital foreign body, thin axial slices of 2 mm are needed; 2 mm slices can detect foreign bodies as small as 0.7 mm in one direction. Metal foreign bodies are easily detected but glass can also be seen and appears radiodense.

Note: Spiral CT can reduce scan times, motion artifact and the amount of contrast needed. If available this should be used for children and agitated adults. Three-dimensional CT reconstruction is only a complementary tool as small fractures may be missed if it is used alone.

MRI

MRI is less useful in the acute setting because bone is not visualised well and also it is contraindicated where a foreign body is suspected to be metallic. If the nature of the foreign body is in doubt, it must be assumed to be metal until proven otherwise. MR scanning plays an important role in secondary imaging:

- In cases of orbital haemorrhage where CT scan shows haemorrhage around the optic nerve, MRI with sections perpendicular to the course of the nerve is essential. This will differentiate between an intrasheath haematoma and one outside the optic nerve sheath. An intrasheath haemorrhage with visual loss may need urgent optic nerve sheath decompression.
- Wood and plastic foreign bodies are best imaged by MR.

Ultrasound

This can give information about the intraocular contents when the ocular media are opaque, in the case of anterior chamber or vitreous haemorrhage, or in the presence of tense closed lids. A 10 MHz ophthalmic probe is used for ocular examination or a 5 MHz probe for orbital examination. Scanning should be performed with a coupling agent such as methylcellulose with the eyelids closed in all cases. Dedicated ophthalmic probes facilitate examination as they are smaller than general probes used, for example in abdominal examination. Examination should not be performed in the presence of a ruptured/ perforated globe.

With ultrasound, foreign bodies can be detected and located. Intraocular air bubbles may also be imaged and indicate a ruptured or perforated globe which may not have been suspected.

Who should image the patient?

Ocular ultrasonography should be performed by the ophthalmologist. However, CT, and MR imaging may be performed by the referring emergency physician.

Interpretation

For the non-specialist, certain radiographic features are important:

- Air in the orbit (orbital emphysema) is usually due to medial wall fracture.
- Air inside the eye indicates a penetrating injury.
- The ocular coat on CT scan should be continuous in each eye. Loss of continuity suggests rupture or perforation of the globe.

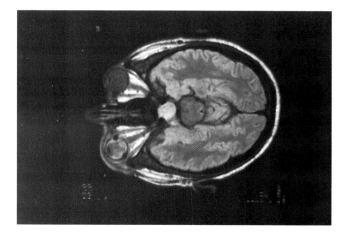

Figure 8.27 MR scan of patient with a pituitary tumour but who had previously had right retinal detachment surgery. The right eye shows the two ends of the plomb placed during ocular surgery on the outside of the globe; this should not be confused with air.

- Appearance of eyes which have had previous surgery. Figure 8.27 shows the MR scan of an eye which has had previous retinal detachment surgery.
- Dilated superior ophthalmic vein is characteristic of traumatic caroticocavernous fistula (Figure 8.28).

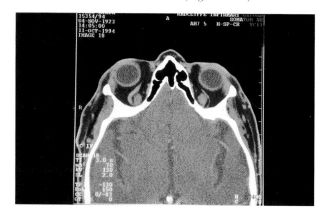

Figure 8.28 Prominent right superior ophthalmic vein in a case of caroticocavernous fistula.

Communication with the ophthalmic surgeons

The ophthalmologist usually first hears of serious ocular trauma from a referring emergency physician over the telephone. This initial contact is crucial in the continued management of the patient. The information that needs to be passed on to the ophthalmologist can be difficult to present logically especially when there are multiple ocular injuries. One way to organise the information is to follow a set routine of presentation:

- History
  - mode of injury
  - clues to type of foreign body if relevant
- Systemic assessment
  - vital signs including Glasgow coma scale
  - ATLS review including CT scan results
  - systemic problems
- Ocular assessment
  - visual acuity
  - pupils
  - anterior segment
  - fundoscopy
- Orbital assessment
  - eyelids and adnexa
  - extraocular motility
- Planned action by other teams
  - time of any surgery
  - if no other problems, time patient last ate.

Management

All ocular trauma should be prioritised (see Table 8.1, page 111). Ocular and orbital trauma may need ophthalmic input.

Immediately, as an emergency

Orbital haemorrhage

If a patient has reduced visual acuity, an afferent pupillary defect, proptosis, ophthalmoplegia, optic disc swelling, and/

or central retinal artery occlusion, immediate action is needed to maximise the chance of saving any sight. The ophthalmologist should be contacted and if one cannot attend within five minutes then the attending surgeon or emergency physician must take the following action:

1. Intravenous acetazolamide 500 mg or 50–100 g of mannitol by rapid i.v. infusion (250–500 ml of 20% mannitol).

2. Urgent lateral canthotomy in the emergency room (see Appendix 8A). This rapidly reduces the intraorbital pressure and may remove the immediate threat of central retinal artery occlusion and irreversible optic nerve damage in the presence of a large diffuse orbital haemorrhage.

3. Urgent CT scan to establish whether haemorrhage is diffuse in which case lateral canthotomy will suffice. If haemorrhage around the optic nerve is detected, an appropriate MR scan as detailed above should be performed immediately. Intrasheath haematomas will need optic nerve sheath decompression by the ophthalmologist. Most haemorrhages around the optic nerve are outside the optic nerve sheath and, although management of these is controversial, intravenous methylprednisolone is warranted after review by the ophthalmologist.

Note: Very rarely the clinical picture of proptosis, ophthalmoplegia, afferent pupillary defect, and decreased vision may be seen in orbital emphysema where there is intraconal air. The treatment outlined is exactly the same but the air needs to be drained by the ophthalmologist.

Chemical injury

If a patient is suspected of having such an injury, immediate treatment is irrigation of the conjunctival sac with at least one litre of normal saline via a drip-giving set. The pH of the conjunctiva should be taken first and irrigation repeated until normal pH has been reached. The conjunctiva should be anaesthetised with amethocaine 1% or benoxinate 0.4% before irrigation is commenced. Signs are listed in Table 8.4.

Note: **This is not the case for CS gas**. When CS gas injury is suspected the patient must be treated in a well-ventilated room. Dry air should be blown directly into the eyes. This encourages the dissolved gas to evaporate. Irrigating the eye without having done this first exacerbates the symptoms.

Urgently, within 1–2 h

Ruptured or perforated globe

The affected eye needs to be covered with a clear rigid cartella to prevent further damage. Depolarising muscle relaxants should be avoided during anaesthesia as their initial action is contraction of muscle. In a compromised globe sudden contraction of the extraocular muscles may cause extrusion of intraocular contents. However, the final decision regarding their use lies with the anaesthetist since certain circumstances may necessitate their use. Arrange for CT scan if foreign body suspected.

Note: All cases of ruptured globe should have parenteral broad spectrum antibiotics as soon as possible, such as ceftazidime or ciprofloxacin. The tetanus immunity state of the patient must also be determined and appropriate immunisation given if necessary.

Perforated globe where foreign body is still in situ, for example (glass fragment)

Do not remove the foreign body. Instead arrange for urgent CT scan to be done and contact the ophthalmologist.

Penetrating injury of the orbit with visual loss

Usually means damage to the optic nerve from the missile or a bony fragment, and a CT scan must be carried out (see also Traumatic optic neuropathy, below)

Orbital fracture with visual loss

A CT scan must be done to assess the optic nerve and detect any optic nerve sheath haemorrhage (see also Traumatic optic neuropathy below).

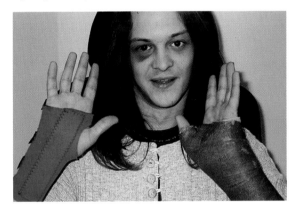

Figure 8.29   A patient with right traumatic optic neuropathy; bilateral wrist fractures were also sustained.

Traumatic optic neuropathy (Figure 8.29)

In this condition there is loss of vision without external or initial fundoscopic evidence of ocular or optic nerve injury. Treatment possibilities include endoscopic surgical decompression of the optic nerve in the canal, optic nerve sheath decompression (external approach), and high dose intravenous methylprednisolone (various regimens). None is of proven

Table 8.4 Signs of chemical injury

Chemical	Symptoms	Corneal staining	pH	Conjunctiva
CS gas	Severe burning of eyes, respiratory distress	Minimal, some punctate staining	Slightly acidic	Red, injected
Ammonia	Severe burning of eyes, respiratory distress	Corneal abrasion, may involve whole cornea	Highly alkaline	Red, injected but may also exhibit blanching of conjunctiva if severe

value but each may be indicated in individual cases. If there are no contraindications, a starting dose of methylprednisolone 30 mg/kg stat intravenously may be given and the patient then referred for an urgent ophthalmological consult.

Appropriate imaging (see above) should be arranged.

Soon, within 12–24 h

Anterior segment trauma (for example, hyphaema, iridodialysis)

Place a single eye pad over the eye if it is uncomfortable, until the ophthalmologist arrives.

Orbital emphysema

Prevent the patient from blowing his or her nose to stop further air entering the orbital soft tissue. Arrange CT scan to assess extent and other possible complications of orbital fracture. The patient will need a short course of systemic broad spectrum antibiotics to prevent orbital infection.

Lid lacerations

Provided the globe is intact, these need referral within 12 h. In the meantime systemic antibiotics should be started and the wound edges can be prevented from drying by placing a swab dampened with normal saline over the wound. Amoxicillin-clavulanic acid is the combination of choice for dog bites. However, if the patient is allergic to penicillin, erythromycin should be used.

Note: All patients must have their tetanus status checked and treated appropriately.

Orbital fractures

If there is no associated visual loss these can be referred any time within 24 h after admission. During this time appropriate CT scans as described earlier are essential. Furthermore, before any surgery is contemplated the patient's corrected visual acuity, extraocular movements, and colour vision must be recorded by an ophthalmologist.

Intraocular damage (for example, vitreous haemorrhage, retinal detachment)

This can be difficult to detect for the non-ophthalmologist so it is advisable to seek advice from the ophthalmologist whenever there is any uncertainty.

Routinely, within 24–48 h

Corneal abrasions

Referral for these is warranted only if intraocular damage is suspected or if after 24 h the abrasion is not healing at all. Otherwise treatment consists of immediate chloramphenicol ointment application to the affected eye. Obvious subtarsal (that is, under the upper lid) or conjunctival/corneal foreign bodies can be either irrigated away or removed with the tip of a cotton wool bud. If the foreign body does not come away easily the ophthalmologist should be informed within 3–4 h.

Conjunctival oedema (chemosis) ± haemorrhage

Simple subconjunctival haemorrhages do not need topical treatment or referral. When the conjunctiva is grossly haemorrhagic and oedematous, lid closure becomes problematic, especially in the unconscious patient. If this is not dealt with, there is secondary desiccation of the conjunctiva with further swelling. In these circumstances lid closure becomes impossible and exposure keratopathy develops. A lubricating agent such as lacrilube or simple eye ointment should be used up to six times daily and in the unconscious patient the eyes must be kept closed. If the lids cannot be taped *completely closed*, a 4/0 black silk suture will need to be passed through the margin of the upper lid and taped or sutured to the cheek.

Conjunctival lacerations

If a laceration is small and there is no evidence of retained foreign body, no treatment is required. If, however, the laceration is extensive, it may involve adjacent tissues, for example lacrimal drainage system, or deeper tissues, for example extraocular muscle(s), or it may be associated with a retained foreign body.

When this is the case exploration and suturing under either local or general anaesthetic is required.

Summary

Detection of ocular or orbital trauma is incumbent upon the attending emergency physician. Ophthalmic trauma may be blunt, penetrating or chemical. The traumatized eye should be assessed by the history (mode of injury, visual status before event, ocular history) and examination in the emergency room. In the *unconscious patient* this includes: symmetry of the eyes, position of the eyes, pupil examination, integrity of globe, ophthalmoscopy, eyelids, and spontaneous eye movements. In the *conscious patient* extra examinations will cover assessment of vision, pupils (accommodation), eye movements, and, periorbital sensation. Examination in the intensive care unit will also cover eyelids (ptosis), corneal, and conjunctival status.

Radiological investigation includes CT scan, MR scan, and ultrasound.

Discussion with the ophthalmologist should cover history, systemic assessment, ocular assessment, orbital assessment (including the lids), and planned action.

Management must cover prioritising ocular trauma and referring to an ophthalmologist as an emergency: urgent within 1–2 h, soon within 12–24 h, routine within 24–48 h.

References

1. Holt JE, Holt GR, Blodgett JM. Ocular injury sustained during blunt facial trauma. *Ophthalmology* 1983;**90**:14–18.
2. Manfredi SJ, Radi MR, Sprinkle DM *et al.* Computerised tomographic scan findings in facial fractures associated with blindness. *Plastic Reconst Surg* 1981;**68**:479–90.
3. Williams M. One minute wisdom. All you need to know about CS gas. *Nurs Stand* 1994;**8**:39.
4. Ball JB Jr. Direct oblique sagittal CT of orbital wall fractures. *Am J Radiol* 1987;**148**:601–8.

Further reading

Baker RS, Epstein AD. Ocular motor abnormalities from head trauma. *Survey Ophthalmol* 1991;**35**:245–67.

Eagling EM, Roper-Hall MJ. *Eye injuries: an illustrated guide*. London: Gower Medical Publishing, 1986.

Hunts JH, Patrinely JR, Holds JB, Anderson RL. Orbital emphysema: staging and acute management. *Ophthalmology* 1994;**101**:960–6.

Jakobiec FA, Navon SE, Rubin PAD. Trauma. *Int Ophthalmol Clinics* 1995;**35**(1).

Stensapir KD, Goldberg RA. Traumatic optic neuropathy. *Survey Ophthalmol* 1994;**38**:487–512.

Appendix 8A: performing a lateral canthotomy

The purpose is to relieve acutely raised orbital pressure caused by haemorrhage.

1. Inject 2% lignocaine or xylocaine with or without adrenaline into the lateral canthus; the shaded area shown should be raised by the resultant bleb of anaesthetic. (Right eye shown.)

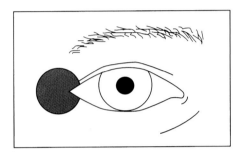

2. Using a heavy pair of sharp scissors, pass one blade between globe and canthal skin, with the sharp edge of the blade touching the inner surface of the lateral canthus. Make a cut 1–2 cm long towards the orbital margin. (Ideally this is preceded by this same manoeuvre but with a straight Spencer Wells forceps to crush the tissue prior to cutting it; practically this can prove difficult in a tense orbit.)

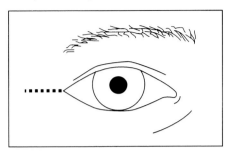

3. The lower cut edge of the wound is now turned out anteriorly and another cut made in this; the tip of the scissors should point away from the wound and towards the tip of the patient's nose. This manoeuvre is called an inferior cantholysis and will reduce considerably the intraorbital pressure.

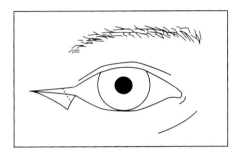

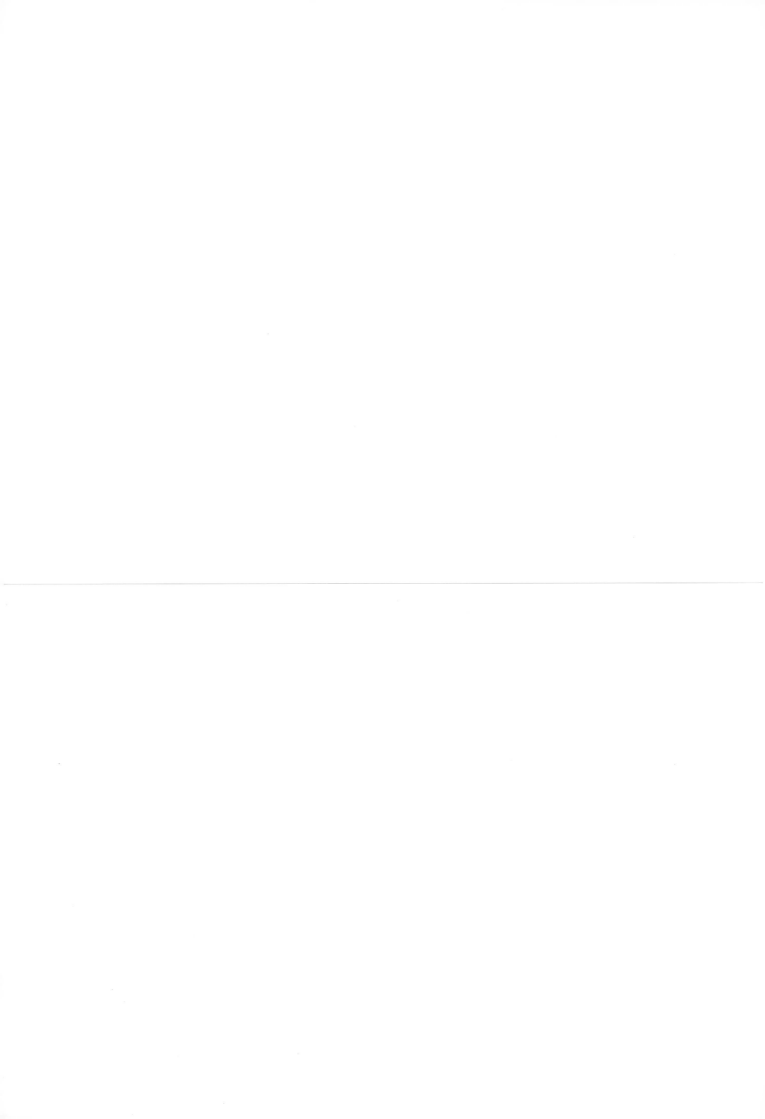

9 Otolaryngology

John H. Dempster
Consultant Otolaryngologist, Crosshouse Hospital, Kilmarnock

Iain R. C. Swan
Senior Lecturer, Department of Otolaryngology, Royal Infirmary, Glasgow

The management of trauma comprises a relatively small percentage of the overall workload of a typical otolaryngology department. The most common injury to present is a nasal

bone fracture and this will be discussed in detail. Numerous other potential problems may arise secondary to trauma, the most notable of which are listed in the box.

Nasal fracture

The bony nasal pyramid consists of a pair of nasal bones articulating with the frontal bone and maxilla. They are supported in the midline by the perpendicular plate of the ethmoid. The remainder of the external nose is comprised of cartilage and fibrofatty tissue. The nasal septum comprises the vomer and ethmoid bones posteriorly and the cartilagenous nasal septum anteriorly. Nasal anatomy is detailed in Figures 9.1 and 9.2.

Otolaryngological trauma

- Nose
  - soft tissue injury
  - nasal bone fracture
  - septal haematoma
- Ear/skull base
  - soft tissue injury
  - tympanic membrane perforation
  - disruption of ossicular chain
  - skull base fracture with labyrinthine injury and/or facial nerve injury
- Neck
  - penetrating injury
    - soft tissue injury
    - vascular damage
    - nerve damage
    - visceral injury
    - airway injury
  - blunt trauma
    - hyoid fracture
    - laryngeal fracture
    - cricoid fracture
    - cricotracheal separation.

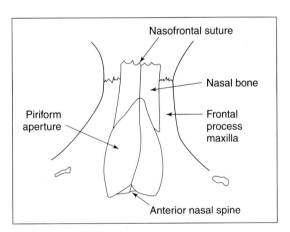

Figure 9.1 Nasal anatomy.

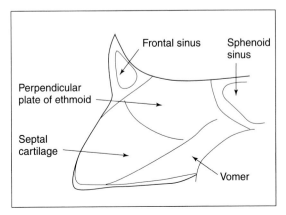

Figure 9.2 Anatomy of the nasal septum.

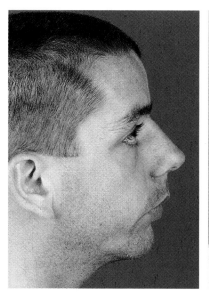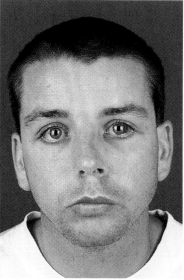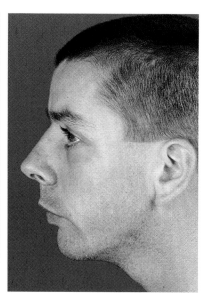

Figure 9.3 Classical signs of nasal fracture.

Nasal fractures (Figure 9.3) arise from two main types of trauma: a lateral blow, most commonly caused by collision with part of another body, and a frontal blow, usually occurring in road traffic or similar accidents.

Lateral injuries may produce lateral deviation of the nasal bones, often with depression of the bone on the side of injury. There may be an associated fracture of the nasal septum but complications other than epistaxis are rare.

Frontal injuries produce splaying of the nasal bones often with a comminuted fracture and significant flattening of the nasal pyramid. More severe injuries lead to impaction of the nasal bones into the ethmoidal complex often with disruption of the insertion of the medial palpebral ligament. There may be associated fractures involving other facial bones. CSF rhinorrhoea may occur from fracture of the cribriform plate.

A useful classification of typical injuries was reported in 1986 [1], the authors describing seven different types of injury, two of which were isolated fractures of the cartilagenous septum.

Assessment

Clinical assessment should aim to detect the classical symptoms and signs of any bony fracture:

● local tenderness
● crepitus
● oedema
● history of epistaxis
● haematoma
● change in shape of nose.

The other facial bones should be inspected and palpated. Examination of the nasal septum may reveal a dislocation, fracture, or haematoma. Orbital complications and CSF rhinorrhoea should be excluded in severe frontal injuries.

Investigations

The diagnosis of an uncomplicated nasal fracture is clinical. Routine radiology in the assessment of uncomplicated nasal fractures is unnecessary. Apart from the cost and radiation dose, the x-rays are often difficult to interpret and the results are most unlikely to affect clinical management. The clinical findings alone dictate the need for management. More complicated fractures involving other facial bones require radiological assessment, preferably by CT imaging.

The important points that need to be assessed and will dictate management are:

● Is there uncontrolled bleeding?
● Is there any alteration in the shape of the nose?
● Are there other associated facial bone injuries?
● Is there an associated CSF leak?
● Are there any open wounds that require closure?
● Is there a septal haematoma?

Management

Epistaxis

Immediate management is required to control bleeding. Nasal fractures are internally compound and bleeding can be profuse. The majority of bleeds associated with minor fractures will stop spontaneously and persistent bleeding, which can be life-threatening, may signify an ethmoid fracture with associated tear of the anterior ethmoid artery. Initial management is to pack the nose, preferably following local anaesthesia. A variety of materials can be used – Vaseline gauze, Vaseline with bismuth iodoform paraffin paste, Merocel/Caltostate dressings and balloons (Foley catheter, epistats). If the bleeding is uncontrolled by anterior nasal packing, the next stage is to insert anterior and posterior nasal packs under a general anaesthetic. Otolaryngological assistance should be sought at this stage. The nasal fracture should be reduced at the same time. Balloon catheters incorporating a posterior nasopharyngeal balloon are an option and can be inserted without the need for a general anesthetic. There is debate as to the duration that such packs should be left *in situ* – 48 hours is probably the minimum. The prescription of antibiotics to minimise the risk of sinus infection is generally recommended.

The majority of bleeds will be controlled by such methods but, for those that are not and for those that rebleed following removal, vessel ligation is indicated. As these severe, uncontrolled bleeds are usually secondary to disruption of the anterior ethmoid artery, ligation of this vessel via an inner canthal (Howarth's) approach is appropriate. Angiography followed by vessel embolisation with polyvinyl alcohol particles and microfibrillar collagen is a well-reported option although this technique requires appropriate radiological expertise and is not without complications.

The fracture

A simple nasal fracture only requires treatment if there is an associated cosmetic deformity. If the degree of deformity is unclear because of oedema and bruising, the nose can be reassessed in five to seven days when this has settled. It should be borne in mind that the group of individuals affected by facial trauma is likely to have had previous trauma and up to 30% may have suffered previous facial bone fractures. In many cases, therefore, the deformity will precede the recent injury and manipulation will be unsuccessful. Reduction should ideally be performed as early as possible.

Healing will have begun by approximately three weeks, earlier in children, and beyond this time simple manipulation will prove difficult. Simple digital reduction, under local or general anaesthetic, is usually sufficient. The majority of patients (up to 96%) find local anaesthetic satisfactory. This can be administered by blocking the infraorbital, infra-trochlear, and external nasal nerves, either intranasally or externally. Impacted fractures will need to be disimpacted with forceps (Walshams).

Postoperatively, external splinting with plaster of paris or thermoplastic devices is often advised but the literature would suggest this is unnecessary and unlikely to alter the eventual outcome. More severe fractures involving the ethmoid complex will require open reduction – via either an associated laceration or a bicoronal flap – and mini-plate fixation. The results following nasal manipulation have not been widely reported, but in one publication [2] 85% of patients who replied to a questionnaire expressed overall satisfaction. The response rate was poor, however, and it is likely that a significant percentage will require corrective rhinoplasty. As mentioned previously, an associated fracture of the nasal septum is a common occurrence. In the majority of cases this is not treated and it has been stated that the failure to do so is an important underlying reason for a failed nasal manipulation, because the bones are drawn out of position following the procedure. It may be worth performing a septal procedure, excising the overlapping edges of the bony and cartilagenous septum, at the time of manipulation to improve the eventual outcome.

Other facial bone injuries

These are dealt with in Chapter 7.

CSF leak

This indicates an associated fracture of the anterior skull base. Detection is based on awareness of the possibility (the patient may complain of a clear nasal discharge) and appropriate confirmatory tests, the best of which is high resolution CT cisternography with water-soluble contrast medium (me-trizamide). Accurate definition of the site of the leak is essential for successful surgical management. If a leak is suspected, prophylactic antibiotics are generally indicated although their value in preventing meningitis is debatable. The recent lit-erature [3] would suggest that the rate of meningitis may be similar in patients receiving antibiotics and those who do not. In the majority of cases, the fistula will close spontaneously but if this has not happened by seven days, surgery is indicated.

Various approaches are available – intracranial, extra-cranial, and endoscopic. The traditional method has been an *intracranial approach*. However, this is associated with the complications of a craniotomy, anosmia, and a reportedly high rate of fistula recurrence.

Extracranial repair, via an external ethmoidectomy approach for example, seems to have a high success rate (86% initial success rate) without the complications of a craniotomy. The management of choice nowadays is *endoscopic repair* if the appropriate surgical skills are available. This allows excellent visualisation of the leak and accurate closure with mucosal grafts from the septum or turbinates along with a very low complication rate.

In all methods, the use of fibrin sealants appears to be a significant advance.

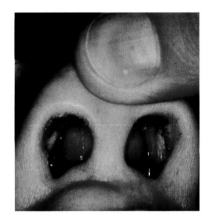

Figure 9.4 Post-traumatic nasal septal haematoma.

Septal haematoma (Figure 9.4)

The exact incidence of a septal haematoma, a collection between the cartilage and the mucoperichondrium, in as-sociation with nasal fractures is not known. Septal haematoma is associated with fracture of the nasal septum and therefore presents with swelling in both nostrils. If detected immediately the haematoma can be aspirated. This procedure may need to be repeated. Later detection, by which time the haematoma may have organised, will generally require incision and drain-age, if the clot is to be satisfactorily evacuated. Following drainage, nasal packing or a quilting stitch should be employed to prevent re-accumulation. Antibiotics are probably indicated to prevent infection and abscess formation. An alternative strategy in late detection is simply to prescibe antibiotics and await resolution of the haematoma.

Haematoma formation is submucoperichondrial and can lead to an avascular necrosis of the cartilage. This is more likely in the presence of abscess formation. Necrosis of cartilage will lead to collapse and loss of the cartilagenous support of the nose with a cosmetic deformity consisting of a supratip depression and columella retraction. This can be corrected at a later stage by an augmentation rhinoplasty, although the results are often unsatisfactory.

Ear/skull base trauma

Soft tissue injuries to the ear may involve lacerations to the pinna or auricular haematoma. The pinna has an excellent blood supply and extensive lacerations heal well after ap-propriate debridement. Similarly, pieces of the pinna which have been avulsed can usually be re-attached successfully.

The cosmetic results following auricular haematomas are rarely good with varying degrees of "cauliflower ear" as the outcome. Exploration under general anaesthesia is best with avoidance of topical vasoconstrictors. The skin and muco-perichondrium should be incised inside the rim of the helix. All haematoma should be carefully removed followed by meticulous haemostasis with fine bipolar diathermy. The skin flap is replaced and the concha carefully packed with acriflavine gauze. A pressure bandage is then applied.

In addition to local soft tissue injuries, the ear is frequently affected by head injuries and skull base fractures. The symptoms and signs of significant injury that need to be evaluated are listed in the box.

Symptoms and signs of significant otological or skull base injury

- Bleeding from the external auditory canal
- Loss of hearing
- Disturbance of balance
- Otoscopic evidence of temporal bone fracture
- Facial nerve weakness/paralysis
- CSF leak from the ear

Investigations

Radiology is aimed at confirming an underlying skull base fracture, in particular of the temporal bone. The diagnosis of a skull base fracture is made clinically and although high resolution CT scanning will be useful in defining the exact site of the fracture, management can proceed without it. Plain radiological screening will frequently miss clinically detectable temporal bone fractures. A CT scan will usually be indicated to assess any intracranial pathology secondary to the trauma. Managament of otological trauma or the otological consequences of a skull base fracture is seldom an emergency, but early assessment of facial nerve function and detection of a CSF leak (a clear discharge which may present as otorrhoea, a middle ear effusion, or rhinorrhoea) are important. The otolaryngologist will also wish to know if there is any active bleeding and whether the patient has noticed a reduction in hearing.

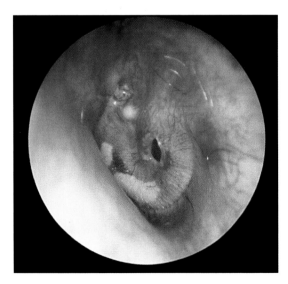

Figure 9.5 Traumatic tympanic membrane perforation.

Management

Tympanic membrane perforation (Figure 9.5)

This is probably the most common otological injury and can be secondary to a penetrating injury, a direct blow to the ear, or a skull base fracture. The patient will complain of pain, bleeding, a decrease in hearing, and possibly tinnitus. The vast majority of these (over 90%) will heal spontaneously and no immediate management is required. It is usual, however, to instruct the patient to keep the ear dry to minimise the possibility of infection. Otological follow-up is necessary to ensure healing and that there is no residual hearing deficit. At initial presentation, the external auditory canal may be full of blood clot; this should generally be left to resolve. Attempted removal is likely to be painful, may introduce infection, is unnecessary, and unlikely to alter the provisional diagnosis.

Petrous bone fracture

A fracture involving the temporal bone is classically described as being either transverse or longitudinal. In practice, most are comminuted with elements of both. It must be remembered that a petrous bone fracture is a compound skull fracture and should be managed accordingly. Such a fracture is likely to present with symptoms and signs relating to the ear and to the head injury – 25% of all severe head injuries will have otoscopic evidence of a skull base fracture. Otological symptoms include deafness, tinnitus, vertigo, and facial nerve paralysis. Otoscopy may reveal a fracture line in the external auditory canal, a tear at the margin of the tympanic membrane, or a haemotympanum (Figure 9.6). There may be CSF in the

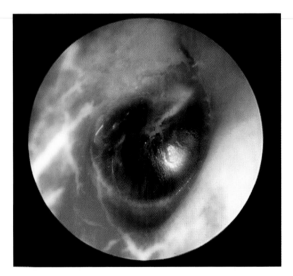

Figure 9.6 Haemotympanum.

external auditory canal and bruising over the mastoid process (Battle's sign). If the fracture line involves the bony labyrinth, the hearing impairment is typically sensorineural and likely to be permanent. A conductive loss may arise secondary to ossicular disruption or a haemotympanum. Any disequilibrium should be treated conservatively because, in the majority of cases, resolution will take place with time. Management of a CSF leak, reported to occur in 16.5% of petrous bone fractures [4], is initially conservative, and as many as 85% of these leaks will close spontaneously. If this fails, surgical repair is indicated. Persistence beyond 7–10 days is generally considered an indication for surgery.

Perilymph leak through the fracture site

This presents as a fluctuating sensorineural hearing impairment plus vertigo, and may also close spontaneously but, if not, surgical exploration via a tympanotomy is indicated to seal the leak and prevent further symptoms.

Facial nerve damage

The facial nerve is reported to be injured in 20% of longitudinal fractures and 50% of transverse fractures of the petrous temporal bone (Figure 9.7 and 9.8). As mentioned earlier,

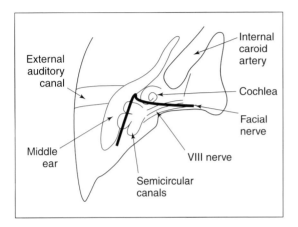

Figure 9.7 Relationship of VII and VIII cranial nerves with temporal bone.

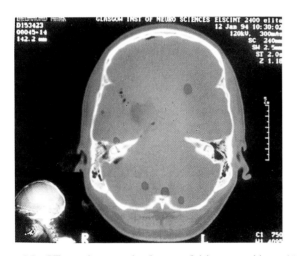

Figure 9.8 CT scan demonstrating fracture of right temporal bone, CSF in middle ear, and intracranial air.

most fractures are a mixture of the two. A total transection of the nerve is uncommon, and nerve injury is typically related to intraneural haematoma, oedema, or compression with a bony fragment. The typical site is reported to be in the tympanic segment, distal to the geniculate ganglion. Patients are often seriously ill and the VII nerve injury may have to be dealt with when the general condition has improved. Immediate onset of complete paralysis is generally regarded as an indication for surgical exploration. This is usually a transmastoid procedure with decompression, anastomosis, or grafting as indicated. Frequently, an intact oedematous nerve will be all that is found, with no recognisable nerve interruption.

If the paralysis is partial or delayed, the outlook with non-operative management is reasonable: it is reported that up to 93% of cases will have some degree of recovery five months following the incident [5]. However, if the facial nerve paralysis

continues to progress, surgical exploration with decompression may still be indicated.

Neck trauma

Minor wounds to the soft tissues of the neck are common and the general principles of wound management apply. More major trauma, either blunt or penetrating, is relatively uncommon but can lead to life-threatening consequences from severe bleeding or airway obstruction. Laryngeal anatomy is detailed in Figure 9.9.

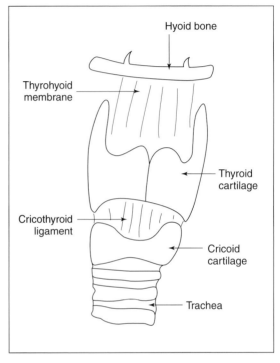

Figure 9.9 Laryngeal anatomy.

Assessment

Initial assessment aims to identify the mechanism and force of the injury. Penetrating wounds should be readily detected and careful assessment for any visceral injury, major vessel damage, or neurological injury, especially to the VII nerve, is required. As with such wounds elsewhere, it is important to remember that they may penetrate much more deeply than they initially appear to do. If the wound is closed and the trauma blunt, the main concern surrounds the patency of the airway. The box lists the main symptoms and signs of concern.

Symptoms and signs indicating significant blunt trauma to neck	
• Hoarseness	• Loss of thyroid prominence
• Dysphagia	• Tenderness
• Dyspnoea	• Crepitus
• Haemoptysis	• Surgical emphysema
• Bruising	• Stridor
• Oedema	• Vocal cord paralysis

The otolaryngologist needs to know:

- Is the trauma blunt or penetrating? What was the mechanism involved (knife wound, gunshot injury) and likely force involved?
- Has there been significant bleeding suggestive of major vascular damage? Is the patient still bleeding?
- Is the airway satisfactory? Is there marked tenderness or crepitus surrounding the laryngeal framework that would suggest a major injury with cartilage fracture?

Stridor may not initially be present but can develop rapidly owing to oedema.

Laryngotracheal trauma is relatively uncommon because the structures receive a degree of protection from the mandible, sternum, and sternomastoid muscles. Indeed, those patients with severe injuries are likely to die before medical attention arrives at the scene of the accident. Blunt trauma is usually secondary to road traffic accidents (60%), the neck being hyperextended causing the laryngeal cartilages to be compressed against the cervical spine. Sporting injuries are less common (20%). The resultant pathology depends on the power and direction of the force plus the nature of the laryngeal cartilages. In the younger age group, the laryngeal cartilages are likely to be pliable, and the framework will therefore tend to spring back producing a fracture of the thyroid cartilage but maintainance of the external profile. If calcified, as happens with ageing, the larynx will be flattened, resulting in loss of profile. In both, there can be widespread disruption to the internal structure of the larynx with displacement of the arytenoids and epiglottis. In addition there can be extensive oedema and haematoma formation, as well as damage to the hypopharynx and cervical oesophagus. Penetrating injuries to the neck in the UK are typically due to knife wounds, gunshot injuries being uncommon.

Investigation

In the acute stage, radiology of the neck is often performed, but the information obtained is unlikely to alter initial management, which should be based on a clinical assessment of the patient. Radiology may well be required at a later stage prior to any reconstruction that may be considered; CT scanning is the investigation of choice.

Management

Considerable debate centres on whether there should be mandatory surgical exploration of all wounds that penetrate the platysma versus a more conservative policy of exploration only for wounds where symptoms or signs of damage to important structures exist (that is, bleeding, expanding haematoma, surgical emphysema, dysphagia, or neurological injury). The two main causes of morbidity and mortality following blunt or penetrating trauma are bleeding and airway obstruction.

Bleeding

External compression will control bleeding but if the history suggests the possibility of major vessel damage, even if the bleeding has stopped, the wound should be explored and vascular defects repaired. Conservative management may appear superficially to be satisfactory, but aneurysm formation and A–V fistula formation may occur at a later date.

Airway

Management has essentially two aims:

- to secure and maintain an airway.
- to minimise long-term morbidity associated with stenosis of the airway or vocal dysfunction.

Tracheostomy is the favoured method of securing the airway. Endotracheal intubation may prove impossible because of the grossly deranged anatomy, and is dangerous: it may cause further disruption of the larynx with loss of an already compromised airway. Once the airway has been assessed and dealt with, further evaluation can take place and surgical intervention planned (that is, repair of mucosal lacerations, reduction and fixation of laryngeal fractures, intraluminal stenting).

Facial nerve injury

Extracranial injury to the facial nerve, typically by a stab wound, requires exploration and repair. After identification of the nerve endings, damaged tissue and fat should be removed. Epineurial suture using micro-instruments to obtain a tension free anastomosis are the aims – the sutures should produce contact between the stumps without buckling or bulging the nerve. If there is loss of nerve tissue, interpositional grafts with the great auricular or sural nerve are required.

References

1. Murray JAM, Maran AGD. A pathological classification of nasal fractures. *Injury* 1986;**17**:338–44.
2. Crowther JA, O'Donoghue GM. The broken nose: does familiarity breed neglect? *Ann Royal Coll Surgeons Engl* 1987;**69**:259–60.
3. El Jamal MS. Antibiotic prophylaxis in unrepaired CSF fistulae. *Br J Neurosurg* 1993;**7**:501–5.
4. Glarner H, Meuli M, Hof E *et al*. Management of petrous bone fractures in children: analysis of 127 cases. *J Trauma* 1994;**36**:198–201.
5. Adegbite AB, Khan MI, Tan L. Predicting recovery of facial nerve function following injury from a basilar skull fracture. *J Neurosurg* 1991;**75**:759–62.

Acknowledgement

Mr Brian O'Reilly is thanked for supplying the clinical photographs.

10 Trauma of the spine and spinal cord

James R. S. Leggate
Consultant Neurosurgeon, Hope Hospital, Salford

Peter A. Driscoll
Accident and Emergency Department, Hope Hospital, Salford

Carl L. Gwinnutt
Consultant Anaesthetist, Hope Hospital, Salford

Catherine A. Sweby
Senior Physiotherapist, Hope Hospital, Salford

OBJECTIVES

- To understand the epidemiology of spinal cord injury.

- To understand the anatomy of the spinal column.

- To know the types of forces responsible for spinal injury.

- To realise the differences between primary, secondary and partial neurological damage.

- To realise the differences between neurogenic and spinal shock.

- To understand the assessment and management of the patient with a suspected spinal injury following resuscitation.

- To know how to communicate with a spinal centre.

Epidemiology

In the United Kingdom, between 10 and 15 cases of spinal cord injury occur per year per million population. Many are the result of trauma on the road or on the sports ground. Road traffic accidents account for almost half of the 700 patients admitted to spinal injury units each year. Sports such as trampolining, gymnastics, rugby, diving, skiing, hang-gliding and, more recently, bungie jumping are also associated with spinal cord injury. It is therefore not surprising that 60% of spinal injured patients are between the ages of 16 and 30, and 85% are less than 45 years old. Penetrating spinal trauma from knife or gunshot remains much less common in the UK than North America. The incidence is increasing, however, and is most likely to be seen in young males.

Over the past quarter of a century, advances in the management of spinal cord injured patients have resulted in an improvement in overall survival and quality of life. In the first quarter of the twentieth century approximately 90% of spinal cord injured patients died each year, whereas currently less than 5% of these patients are expected to die annually. There is, however, scope for improvement.

> Nearly one-fifth of patients will have a deterioration in spinal cord function between their arrival at the primary receiving hospital and admission to the specialist spinal unit.

Anatomy of the spinal column

Vertebral column

The spinal column is made up of separate vertebrae which provide protection and support for the spinal cord whilst allowing mobility. These vertebrae are held together by a series of ligaments, upon which the stability of the vertebral column primarily depends (Figure 10.1). The anterior longitudinal ligament runs from the anterior arch of the atlas to

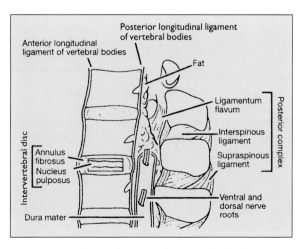

Figure 10.1 Lateral view of the cervical column showing the important ligaments.

the sacrum and is very important in maintaining vertebral alignment. The posterior longitudinal ligament connects the posterior aspect of the vertebral bodies, and the intertransverse ligament connects the transverse processes. The latter constitutes the lateral column.

Schematically, these ligamental complexes can be divided into three vertical complexes. The front one consists of the anterior longitudinal ligaments and the anterior half of the intervertebral discs. The middle complex is made up from the posterior longitudinal ligaments and the posterior half of the intervertebral discs. The posterior complex is structurally the most important and consists of the ligamentum flavum along with the interspinous and supraspinous ligaments.

> If any two of these complexes are torn the vertebral column is rendered unstable.

Stability in the thoracic and lumbar regions is also dependent upon the alignment of the facet joints. These have a steeper inclination than in the cervical spine and this reduces the chances of subluxation and dislocation (Figure 10.2). In the

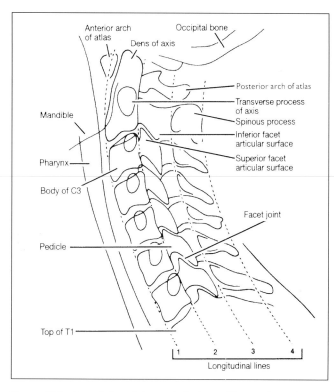

Figure 10.2 Lateral view of the cervical column. The anterior and posterior borders of the spinal canal are demarcated by the second and third longitudinal line.

thoracic region the facet joints face outwards and backwards allowing flexion, extension, and abduction as well as rotation of one vertebra on another. In the lumbar region, the vertical alignment of the facet joints permits flexion, extension, and abduction but prevents any rotation. The fifth lumbar vertebra is normally prevented from slipping forward on the sacrum by the direction of the articular facets and the intervertebral disc. As a result of these stabilising features, vertebral disruption in the thoracic or lumbar areas will result only when a significant force has been applied – usually with a rotatory element. This is particularly true in the case of the thoracic vertebrae, which have additional support from the ribs.

Nevertheless, the vertebral column is vulnerable at the points where the direction of curvature of the spine changes.

At the cervicothoracic and thoracolumbar junctions, the mechanical stresses which result from this change in direction are amplified by the contrast in mobility. This is because the attachments to the skeletal structure of the chest by the ribs make the thoracic vertebrae relatively immobile compared to the cervical and lumbar vertebrae. As a result, when the vertebral column is subjected to abnormal forces, injury usually occurs at C5/C6/C7 or T12/L1. Two-thirds of the fractures in the thoracic and lumbar region occur between T12 and L2. Similarly, at the lumbosacral junction, the sacrum's attachment to the pelvis makes it much less mobile than the lumbar vertebrae. As a consequence, the lumbosacral junction is also a common site for injury.

Spinal canal

The spinal cord, and its meningeal coverings, run through the spinal canal to the level of the L1/2 disc (adult) or L2/3 lumbar vertebrae (newborn). Injuries at this level can lead to pressure on the distal spinal cord (conus) and the lumbar and sacral nerve roots below the termination of the cord (cauda equina). This may cause bladder and bowel symptoms along with both upper and lower motor neurone signs in both legs.

Between the bony canal and the dura mater is a potential space which is normally filled with extradural fat and blood vessels. The size of the space varies with the region of the vertebral column and the presence of degenerative disease processes. In the thoracic area, the space is small and therefore has a limited capacity to adapt to injuries which impinge into the spinal canal (see later). In contrast, at the level of C2 there is a large potential space behind the odontoid (dens). Consequently injuries in this area are not automatically fatal. This has been described in Steel's rule of three (see box).

Steel's rule of three

One-third of C1's spinal canal area is occupied by the odontoid, one-third by the intervening space and one-third by the spinal cord.

Spinal cord

This consists of bundles of nerve fibres transmitting impulses to and from the higher centres (Figure 10.3a). The posterior columns carry sensory fibres transmitting vibration, fine touch, and proprioception. The corticospinal tracts carry motor fibres which cross over to the contralateral side in the medulla. In contrast, the spinothalamic tracts carrying pain, temperature, and coarse touch fibres cross over to the contralateral side within two vertebral bodies' height (Figure 10.3b). This feature, of certain fibres crossing the spinal cord, is important in interpreting the clinical signs after spinal injury (see below).

In the cervical region the spinal cord is supplied by the anterior and posterior spinal arteries. The anterior spinal artery is formed by a branch from each of the vertebral arteries, and runs down the midline in the anterior median fissure of the spinal cord. It supplies the whole cord from the spinomedullary junction down to the conus. Branches run posteriorly at segmental levels to supply the portion of the cord anterior to the posterior grey columns.

The posterior spinal arteries comprise one or two vessels on either side of the midline formed from branches of the posterior inferior cerebellar artery or from the vertebral artery itself at the spinomedullary junction. Perforating branches of

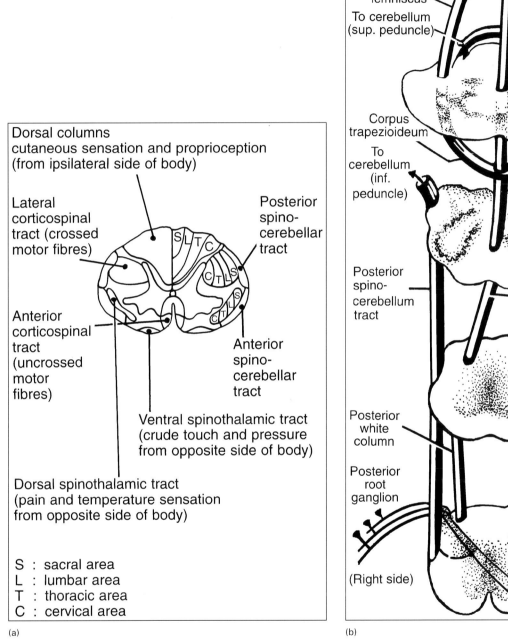

Dorsal columns
cutaneous sensation and proprioception
(from ipsilateral side of body)

Lateral corticospinal tract (crossed motor fibres)

Posterior spino-cerebellar tract

Anterior corticospinal tract (uncrossed motor fibres)

Anterior spino-cerebellar tract

Ventral spinothalamic tract (crude touch and pressure from opposite side of body)

Dorsal spinothalamic tract (pain and temperature sensation from opposite side of body)

S : sacral area
L : lumbar area
T : thoracic area
C : cervical area

(a)

To medial geniculate body

To thalamus

Midbrain

Lateral lemniscus

Spinal lemniscus

To cerebellum (sup. peduncle)

Medial lemniscus

Pons

Corpus trapezioideum

To cerebellum (inf. peduncle)

Spiral ganglion

(left cochlea)

Upper medulla

Posterior spino-cerebellum tract

Decussation of medial lemnisci

Lower medulla

Posterior white column

Anterior spinocerebellum tract

Posterior root ganglion

Spino-thalamic tract

(Right side)

Spinal cord

(b)

Figure 10.3 (a) Cross-section of the spinal column showing the long tracts; (b) longitudinal diagram of the spine showing cross-over of spinothalamic tract fibres.

these vessels supply the grey and white matter of the posterior columns. Lower down, over the back of the spinal cord, there is an anastomotic plexus formed by the terminal branches of the anterior and posterior spinal arteries.

Spinal branches of trunk arteries supply the cord after entering the spinal canal through the intervertebral foramen. These sizeable vessels at the T1 and lower thoracic level are known as the arteries of Adamkiewicz. The lower spinal branch may arise from the T9–T11 intercostal artery. The first thoracic intercostal vessel supplies a radicular branch to the spinal cord. This augments the descending anterior spinal artery in its blood supply of the cervical cord.

Damage to the anterior spinal artery may result from the retropulsion of a disc or bony fragment following acute flexion or impaction injuries. This artery is particularly vulnerable in areas where the canal diameter is compromised by the presence of posterior osteophytes. Such injuries lead to cord signs, typically in the "watershed" area of the cervical cord, namely at the C6/7 level.

Mechanisms of injury

The box below lists the aetiology of spinal injury. The level at which the spinal cord is injured is related to the mechanism of injury. Victims of penetrating trauma and motor cyclists are more likely to injure their thoracic and lumbar spines. In contrast, car occupants and victims of falls and diving tend to sustain cervical damage.

Aetiology of spinal injury	
● Road traffic accidents	48%
● Falls from a height	21%
● Sporting accidents	14%
● Violent acts	14%
● Other	3%

Road traffic accidents

RTAs produce approximately 50% of the spinal injuries in the UK. They can result from side, rear or front collision. Inspection of the windscreen may reveal a bulls-eye' pattern due to the patient's face or head hitting the glass. This is associated with neck and head injuries. Ejection from the car increases the chance of a spinal injury to approximately 1 in 13. Rear end collisions can produce hyperextension of the neck followed by hyperflexion (the "whiplash phenomenon"). Unprotected victims such as pedestrians hit by cars, or motor-cyclists, have a high chance of sustaining a spinal injury.

Sporting activities

Those infamous for producing spinal trauma are rugby, especially after collapse of a scrum, gymnastics, trampolining, horse riding, skiing and hang-gliding. Diving is a common cause of neck injuries during the spring and summer months, particularly in young males who have recently drunk alcohol. The victim usually misjudges the depth of the water or dives from too steep an angle and hits his/her head on a solid surface.

The common feature of all the mechanisms leading to spinal injury is that the vertebral column is subjected to a series of abnormal forces. These can act either singly or in combination to produce flexion, extension, rotation, lateral flexion, compression, and distraction. The commonest movements are:

● hyperflexion
● hyperflexion with rotation
● hyperextension
● rotation
● compression.

Pure hyperflexion injuries

In the adult these frequently occur at the T12–L2 levels and in children at the T4–5 levels. They may be caused by flexion over a lap belt in a vehicle following a forward impact, falling

in a bent position or a weight falling on to the top of the lower back. The actual pattern of damage resulting is dependent on:

● the position of the fulcrum of the motion
● the relative strength of the bones and ligaments
● the degree of force.

When the fulcrum is positioned inside the vertebral body, a compression (wedge) fracture results (Figure 10.4). The amount of force needed to produce such a fracture depends on the strength of the underlying bone. In cases of reduced bone density such as osteomalacia, osteoporosis, and metastatic bone deposits, the force may be so trivial that the patient cannot remember it.

Wedge fractures are the commonest type of fracture of the lumbar and thoracic vertebral bodies and are usually stable because the posterior ligaments remain intact. However, if the force is sufficient to compress the anterior part of the vertebral body to 50% of the height of the back part, the posterior ligaments are torn. This results in an unstable condition. If the back part of the body is compressed at the same time, further collapse of the anterior surface is possible before the posterior ligaments are torn.

Determining instability is important because of the potential for further neurological injury (see box).

Stability and instability
A spinal injury is stable when controlled movements will not cause a neurological deficit. With an unstable injury, controlled movements can lead to, or aggravate, neurological damage.

When a person is restrained anteriorly (for example by a lap belt) the fulcrum of the motion is at the anterior abdominal wall. This leads to stretching of both the anterior and posterior aspects of the vertebral column. Initially the posterior longitudinal ligaments tear and the spinous processes fan out. Simultaneously part of the spinous process can be avulsed. With further stretching the facet joints can sublux or dislocate and the posterior aspects of the intervertebral discs can tear. The typical bony lesion associated with this condition is a horizontal fracture extending through the body, pedicle and posterior elements of the vertebra. This is known as a *chance fracture*. L1–3 are most prone to this type of injury.

If the direction of force is such that lateral flexion occurs, a compression fracture of the lateral part of the vertebral column can result.

Pure hyperflexion can occur in the cervical vertebrae but is less common because the forward movement is limited by the chin hitting the sternum. Extreme hyperflexion (e.g. diving accidents) can result in all the cervical ligaments being torn. In addition, the violent contact between two adjacent cervical vertebral bodies may be sufficient to fracture the anterior superior corner of the inferior vertebrae. This is known as a *tear drop fracture* and it is commonly found in the C5/6 region. In view of the associated ligamentus damage, this condition leaves the patient's neck mechanically unstable.

Hyperflexion with rotation

This is responsible for 50–80% of cervical injuries and is also the commonest cause of thoracolumbar injuries. It often follows road traffic accidents or direct trauma, causing significant disruption of the posterior elements of the vertebral column.

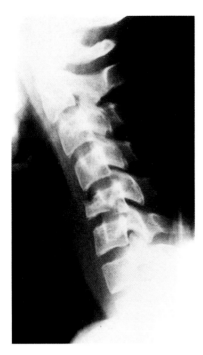

Figure 10.4 Lateral radiograph showing compression fracture of C5. The cortical surface is disrupted, the height of the vertebral body is reduced, and trabecular pattern is lost. Part of the posterior inferior corner of the vertebral body is projected backwards into the spinal canal.

In less serious injuries the stabilizing elements are stretched but in severe cases they can tear and the facet joints, lamina, transverse processes, and vertebral bodies may fracture. In the cervical region the relatively flat facets may dislocate. At the same time the spinous processes of C6/7 can be avulsed by the taut interspinous ligaments (*clay shoveller's fracture*). A *shearing injury* may also occur as the force attempts to slide the vertebra either anteriorly or posteriorly with respect to one below. In doing so it tears all the intervertebral ligaments and displaces the vertebral body by 25%. In the case of anterior displacement, the superior facet is often fractured.

Hyperextension

This tears the anterior stabilizing elements and can produce an avulsion fracture of the anterior inferior aspect of the vertebral body. Occasionally the posterior aspect of the vertebral body is crushed with fragments of bone being pushed into the vertebral canal. When an extension force is associated with rotation, fractures can occur in the lamina, pedicles, and articular surfaces of the vertebral bodies. Due to the stabilising effect of the rib cage, hyperextension injuries are usually only found in the cervical and, to a lesser extent, in the lumbar region.

A special type of hyperextension fracture occurs through the pars interarticularis of C2 following hyperextension with distraction or compression. This is known as the "*hangman's fracture*", as it is the cause of death following judicial executions. In extreme cases the fracture gap widens and extends into the C2/3 intervertebral disc. If there is a distraction component to the mechanism of injury, the vertebral body of C2 is displaced anteriorly and, ultimately, there is bilateral facet dislocation of C2 on C3.

Rotational forces

These can tear the posterior longitudinal ligamental complex and so have a higher chance of producing instability. This

may be associated with a unifacet dislocation. A common site for this type of injury is the T12/L1 junction.

Compression forces

These can only be applied to straight parts of the vertebral column. Therefore the cervical and lumbar parts are affected with the commonest site being L1. These forces are occasionally severe enough to fracture the vertebral bodies and project bone fragments and soft tissue into the spinal canal. It may also be seen at C5 after diving accidents. In *Jefferson's fracture* the lamina and pedicles of C1 fracture when they are subjected to a compressive force between the occipital condyle and C2. In addition, the transverse atlantal ligament holding the dens in position can be torn. This will allow the skull and C1 to slide forward on C2. This lesion is not automatically fatal because of the potential space behind the odontoid (remember Steel's rule).

Pathophysiology of spinal injuries

Primary neurological damage

This is a neurological injury resulting directly from the initial insult. It usually results from blunt trauma causing abnormal movement in the vertebral column. This leads to a transient or permanent reduction in spinal canal volume by bone or soft tissue and possibly direct impingement on the spinal cord (Table 10.1). If the potential space around the spinal cord is

Table 10.1 Neurological injury in relation to the site of trauma

Fractures or dislocations	Frequency (%) of neurological injury
Any	14
Cervical spine	40 (50–60% if unstable)
Thoracic spine	10
Thoracolumbar spine	35
Lumbar	3

already reduced, for example by osteophytes, the chance of neurological damage is increased.

Less commonly, the primary spinal damage is caused by penetrating trauma. Stabbings cause only a localized area of injury. In contrast a much more extensive area of destruction and oedema occurs when the spinal cord is subjected to a large force such as a gunshot (see Chapter 22).

Secondary neurological damage

This is deterioration of the spinal cord after the initial insult. The three common causes are mechanical disturbance of the back, hypoxia, and poor spinal perfusion. These effects are additive.

As described above, the vertebral column may be mechanically unstable following injury. In these cases the spinal cord could be further damaged by direct pressure or ischaemia if the vertebral column is moved inappropriately.

> Secondary neurological damage is not caused by careful, coordinated log rolling of the patient.

Hypoxia can result from any of the causes mentioned in Chapter 5, but significant spinal injury on its own can also cause hypoxia (Table 10.2). The common underlying problem

Table 10.2 Respiratory failure in spinal injury

Tetraplegic	Paraplegic
Intercostal paralysis	Intercostal paralysis
Phrenic nerve palsy	
Inability to expectorate	
V/Q mismatch (see Chapter 3)	

is usually a lack of respiratory muscle power following a high spinal lesion. Lesions above T12 will progressively involve the intercostal muscles, whilst injuries above C5 will cause phrenic nerve palsies, paralysing the diaphragm.

A lesion at C3 or C4 will result in a weak diaphragm, with only partial contraction occurring. Alternatively, a lesion at C5 will allow normal innervation of the diaphragm. Therefore any lesion above C4 will usually result in the patient requiring mechanical ventilation, as only the accessory muscles will be left to produce minimal inspiration. A lesion at C4 or C5 will allow partial or complete diaphragmatic activity.

With only the diaphragm and upper accessory muscles working, a paradoxical breathing pattern will appear, and apical expansion will be limited. Some stability of the rib cage is gained by the action of scaleni in lesions above C8. Furthermore innervation of the intercostals occurs between T1 and 11. Consequently the effect on inspiration and expiration is dependent upon the level of injury between C5 and T11. The abdominals are innervated between T6 and L1, therefore the stability of the abdominal wall and the effectiveness of a cough will also depend on the level of the spinal lesion.

Inadequate spinal perfusion results from either general hypovolaemia or a failure of the spinal cord to regulate its own blood supply. This failure in autoregulation can occur after cord injury. A fall in mean arterial pressure will therefore produce a reduction in spinal perfusion. Conversely, if the pressure is increased too much, a spinal haemorrhagic infarct could develop.

Secondary damage leads to interstitial and intracellular oedema, which may further aggravate any deficiency in spinal perfusion. As this oedema spreads, neurones are squeezed and an ascending level of clinical deterioration will be produced. With high spinal injuries, this process can lead to secondary respiratory deterioration.

Partial spinal cord injury

This is becoming more common. Consequently there is an increase in the number of spinal victims who have the scope for significant improvement (and deterioration!) following medical intervention.

Anterior

This injury is due to direct compression or obstruction of the anterior spinal artery. It affects the spinothalamic and corticospinal tracts (Figure 10.5), resulting in a loss of coarse

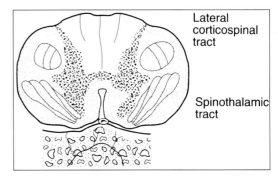

Figure 10.5 The anterior cord syndrome.

touch, pain, and temperature sensation and flaccid weakness. This type of injury is associated with fractures or dislocations in the vertebral column.

Central

Central injuries are usually found in elderly patients with cervical spondylosis. Following a vascular event, the cortico-spinal tracts are damaged with flaccid weakness in the upper limbs and a spastic upper motor neurone type weakness in the lower limbs. This is due to the more centrally situated cervical pyramidal tracts supplying the arms being the most severely affected (Figure 10.6). In view of this anatomical

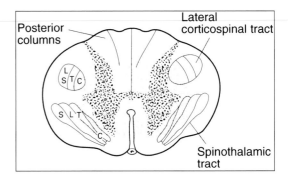

Figure 10.6 The central cord syndrome.

arrangement in the centre of the cord, sphincter function is maintained and the upper limbs are affected more than the lower limbs.

Sacral fibres in the spinothalamic tract are positioned laterally to corresponding fibres from other regions of the body (Figure 10.6). It follows that anterior and central injuries, which are primarily affecting the midline of the spinal cord, may not affect the sacral fibres. This leads to the phenomenon of "sacral sparing" in which sensation is lost below a certain level on the trunk but pinprick appreciation is retained over the sacral and perineal area (Figure 10.7).

Lateral (Brown–Séquard syndrome)

This condition results from penetrating trauma. All sensory and motor modalities are disrupted on the side of the wound at the level of the lesion. Below this level, however, there is a

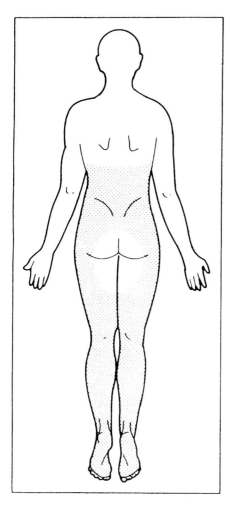

Figure 10.7   Sacral sparing.

contralateral loss of pain and temperature sensation and an ipsilateral loss of muscle power and tone (Figure 10.8).

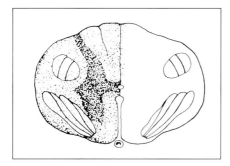

Figure 10.8   Brown–Séquard syndrome. (Speckled area = site of damage.)

Posterior

This is a rare condition. It results in a loss of vibration sensation and proprioception (Figure 10.9).

Special types of shock

Neurogenic shock

Following significant injuries at or above T6 there will be loss of the adrenergic outflow from the sympathetic nervous system. Consequently the vasomotor tone is lost and, if the lesion is high enough, sympathetic innervation of the heart ceases. The

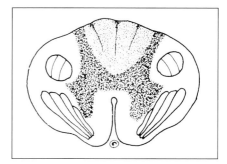

Figure 10.9   Posterior cord syndrome. (Speckled area = site of damage.)

result is vasodilatation, hypotension, bradycardia, and the loss of temperature control. This is called neurogenic shock. It is important to detect this cause of shock, because the hypotension is not due to true hypovolaemia. Furthermore its presence may also mask the normal response to hypovolaemia caused by other injuries. With incomplete spinal injury, some sympathetic control will remain, thereby allowing a normal response. The onset of neurogenic shock can take minutes to hours to develop. This is because spinal injury can initially result in a pressor response owing to the release of catecholamines into the circulation. Such a situation may persist for up to 24 hours before levels of catecholamines fall, unmasking neurogenic shock.

The lack of sympathetic tone also enhances the vagal effect produced by stimulation of the pharynx, for example during laryngoscopy. This can lead to profound bradycardia requiring treatment with atropine (see later).

Spinal shock

This refers to the neurological condition occasionally seen after spinal injury. It consists of complete loss of sensory, motor and segmental reflex activity with flaccidity below the level of the spinal cord injury. Beevor's sign, that is movement of the umbilicus when the abdomen is stroked, may be present.

This state can last for days or weeks but areas of the cord are still capable of a full recovery. Parts which are permanently damaged give rise to spasticity once the flaccid state has resolved. If there has been a complete transection of the cord, lower motor nerve reflexes will return below the level of the lesion. This is seen as exaggerated responses to stimuli; however, there will be no sensation.

Management of the patient with suspected spinal cord damage

It may appear surprising, but spinal injuries are often missed initially. There are several causes for this (see box) but a common reason is the failure of the clinician to consider the possibility of spinal trauma.

Causes of missing a spinal injury
• Not considering the possibility
• Unconsciousness
• No obvious spinal deformity
• Distraction by other injuries
• Poor interpretation of radiographs
• Assuming a normal radiograph excludes a spinal injury

A further difficulty faced by these patients is that the basic rules of trauma management may be forgotten because they are labelled as requiring specialist care. Consequently, deterioration is frequently looked upon as an urgent need to transfer the patient rather than an incentive to manage the problems causing secondary spinal injuries. It is essential that the clinician does not allow this to happen. To prevent any further neurological damage, therefore, the possibility of spinal injury must be considered where there is an appropriate mechanism of injury.

> **Fifty per cent of patients with damage to the spinal cord have other injuries as well.**

Primary survey and resuscitation

Before the patient with a proven or suspected spinal injury leaves the resuscitation room, the airway must be cleared and secured. The unconscious spinal injury patient should have the airway secured by intubation as the risk of regurgitation and aspiration is increased owing to the presence of a paralytic ileus, a full stomach, and an incompetent gastro-oesophageal sphincter. As close to 100% oxygen should be being administered, not least because the damaged spinal cord is very

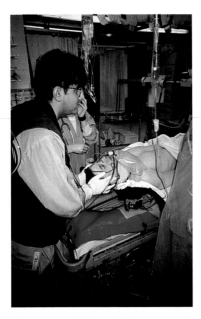

Figure 10.10   Doctor manually immobilising a patient's head and neck.

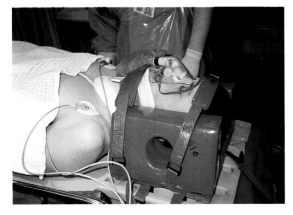

Figure 10.11   Patient's head and neck immobilised with a semirigid collar and head block.

sensitive to hypoxia. During these activities the spine must be immobilised. With respect to the neck, this can be achieved by an assistant holding the head (Figure 10.10) or by the use of a commercially available apparatus (Figure 10.11).

> Intubation is not contraindicated in the presence of cervical spine injury.

In patients exhibiting signs of a high spinal cord injury, for example tetraplegia, neurogenic shock, diaphragmatic breathing, or isolated forearm flexion, consideration must be given to intubation and ventilation before the patient is moved.

Persistent signs or symptoms of shock must not be attributed to the presence of spinal cord injury, particularly if there is penetrating trauma. Correction of any bleeding source is still relevant in cases of spinal injury because of the risks of hypoperfusion of the spinal cord. In the presence of an isolated spinal cord injury, a systolic blood pressure of 80–90 mmHg is initially acceptable and usually achieved with a fluid challenge of 0.5–1 litre. Patients with an enduring bradycardia of less than 50 beats per minute should be given atropine 0.5–1 mg intravenously, and repeated if the heart rate remains low. If this fails, inotropes may be required, but this will involve the use of invasive haemodynamic monitoring to ensure that the patient does not develop pulmonary complications from inappropriate fluid management.

The loss of vascular tone in patients with high spinal injuries causes them to be prone to postural hypotension. This can occur when the patient is tipped or lifted suddenly, as well as when the trolleys are turned at speed. As a result, there can be underperfusion of areas of the body and episodes of ventilatory–perfusion mismatch. It is therefore essential that these potential problems be prevented by the careful and coordinated movement of these patients.

During the initial neurological assessment, an asymmetrical weakness may become apparent or a lack of response to peripheral stimulation. These should be noted and a definitive neurological examination be performed in the secondary survey.

Finally, remember to keep the patient covered by warm sheets and blankets. This not only avoids embarrassment but also prevents heat loss from vasodilatation.

Secondary survey

All patients must be examined, in detail, from head to toe irrespective of whether they have a spinal injury (see Chapter 1). This may be delayed until after the patient arrives in an intensive care unit or until after urgent surgery for the management of other injuries. It is important to remember that an intra-abdominal injury may be masked in a patient with spinal injuries because of the reduction in sensation. Ultrasound, CT scanning, or diagnostic peritoneal lavage can be helpful in detecting intra-abdominal injury in such cases.

The remainder of this section will concentrate on identifying the presence of spinal cord injury in order to plan the patient's care to achieve the best possible outcome. All neurological signs are to be taken seriously, and the clinician should never assume that they are a result of an old injury.

Most conscious patients with spinal injury will complain of pain in the region of the injury, which radiates on movement. In addition, it is essential to enquire whether there is absent or abnormal sensation in the limbs or areas of the trunk. If there is no vertebral pain, patients should be asked to cough and then have their heels tapped. This can occasionally reveal a painful area in the back. Patients are then requested to move each limb in turn provided there is no pain or discomfort in the limb or spinal column.

A full neurological examination must be carried out including the cranial nerves and the higher functions. Each dermatome (Figure 10.12) is tested for sensitivity to a broken

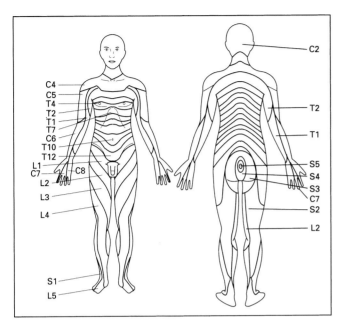

Figure 10.12 Sensory neurological assessment.

"orange stick" (sharp/painful sensation) and cottonwool (fine touch). Ideally this should be carried out on both sides of the patient simultaneously so that the doctor can detect any asymmetry. The tone, power, coordination, and reflexes should then be tested and any asymmetry noted. Muscular power can be classified (see box) to facilitate temporal comparison as well as variation between the right and left, and upper and lower limbs.

The MRC scale for muscle power

0 = total paralysis
1 = a flicker of contraction but no movement
2 = movement but not against gravity
3 = movement against gravity
4 = movement against resistance
5 = normal power

Partial spinal injury

A complex situation can arise where there is partial spinal damage. As the presence of early spinal activity (Table 10.3) is very important in predicting recovery, care must be taken to detect these findings in the trauma patient.

Table 10.3 Spinal activity predicting recovery

Activity at 72 hours	% walking after 1 year
None	0
Partial sensory function	47
Motor activity present	87

In the unconscious patient, important signs can be detected which increase the chances of there being a spinal injury (see box).

Signs of spinal injury in the unconscious patient

- Diaphragmatic breathing
- Hypotension with bradycardia
- Flaccid areflexia (especially a flaccid anal sphincter)
- Loss of reflexes below the level of the lesion
- Loss of response to pain below the level of the lesion
- Priapism (a full erection is not required)

If there is any spontaneous movement it must be noted and the following questions asked:

(1) Is the movement truly spontaneous or is it secondary to painful stimuli?
(2) Are all the limbs moving equally?

All trauma patients must have a rectal examination. During this, the sphincter tone can be assessed and the bulbocavernosus reflex tested if spinal injury is suspected. This test involves squeezing the glans penis and detecting digitally any increase in tone of the anal sphincter. There is a negative response if there is no spinal injury, or if the state of spinal shock exists.

Following this peripheral examination, the vertebral column can be examined. Whilst in-line stabilisation is maintained manually, the immobilisation device can be removed and the neck checked for any overt deformities, tenderness, malalignment, bogginess, or spasm.

Examination of the whole of the back should then be carried out by log-rolling the patient and removing the long spinal board if still in place. A minimum of four people are needed (Figure 10.13), with care being taken to ensure the

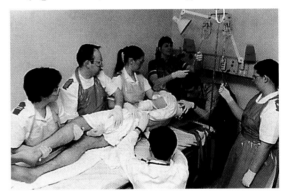

Figure 10.13 Log-rolling a patient to enable examination of the back.

vertebral column is not subjected to any twisting forces. This requires all the personnel to move the patient simultaneously and by the same amount. In addition to checking the vertebral column, the pressure areas should also be assessed at this stage and any debris removed. This is especially important if the patient is potentially going to be in the same position for several hours as further tests are carried out.

A patient can develop pressure sores within 45 minutes of lying on a long spinal board.

It is important to be aware that the classic signs of vertebral injury, such as pain, bruising, bogginess, deformity, and tenderness, are unreliable. Woodring *et al* showed that 13% of patients with cervical injury were asymptomatic and 5% did not have a reduced level of consciousness to explain this.

The secondary survey finishes with completion of the patient's history (see Chapter 1). It is important that any previous medical problems affecting the spinal cord or vertebral column are accurately recorded. This must include information on conditions that increase the risk of spinal cord injury following trauma. Examples include Down's syndrome and rheumatoid arthritis. The doctor should also get as much information as possible about the mechanism of injury, the presence of neurological impairment post incident, and the treatment provided. This will come from the ambulance personnel, witnesses, and the patient.

By the completion of the secondary survey, the trauma victim should have a naso- or orogastric tube and urinary catheter *in situ*. These tubes can help prevent bladder and gastrointestinal distension developing after spinal injury. Urinary catheterisation must be performed under strictly aseptic conditions and the tube secured with tape to the abdominal wall or thigh. These actions will help reduce the incidence of infection.

Investigations

Plain radiography

As described in Chapter 1, a lateral cervical spine x-ray will have been taken during, or shortly after, the resuscitation. Errors in interpreting this film can lead to missed spinal injuries. Such mistakes are often the result of any combination of the following reasons:

- Failure to appreciate that an innocuous abnormality on a plain film can in fact represent an extensive injury as seen on CT.
- A normal plain cervical spine series does not exclude a cervical injury.
- Patients with spinal injury have damage at more than one level in 3–16% of cases.
- There can be a spinal cord injury due to vascular compromise without any skeletal injury. This is known as SCIWRA (**s**pinal **c**ord **i**njury **w**ithout **r**adiological **ab**normalities) and is most frequently seen in children who are less than 8 years old.
- Failure to systematically examine the whole film.

One way of avoiding this problem is to use the "AABCS" system (see box).

The AABCS system of radiological interpretation

- **A**dequacy
- **A**lignment
- **B**one
- **C**artilage and joints
- **S**oft tissue

The lateral cervical spine radiograph

Adequacy of the film

An adequate lateral cervical spine radiograph will detect approximately 80–90% of cervical injuries. However it is only "adequate" when all the cervical vertebrae, as well as the

C7–T1 joint, are visible. This may be achieved either by the doctor pulling down on the upper limbs as the x-ray is being taken (Figure 10.14), or a "swimmer's view" or oblique views being taken. If these fail to show the required area then a CT scan of this area must be carried out.

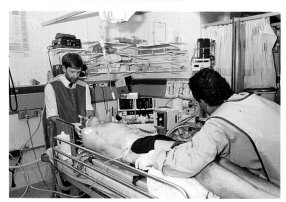

Figure 10.14 Radiograph being taken with the arms pulled down and the head immobilised.

> Most of the diagnostic difficulties occur at the atlanto-axial and cervicothoracic junctions. The latter is also the place where the majority of the missed lesions occur.

Alignment

The anterior and posterior longitudinal lines as well as the posterior facet margins should trace out a smooth contour from T1 to the base of the skull. The spinolaminar line should also be a smooth curve except at C2, which can be posterior to the line by up to 3 mm. Normally, the spinous processes are nearly equidistant and converge to a general point behind the neck of the patient. Divergence is an abnormal sign.

A break in the contour of these lines may be due to displacement or fracture of a vertebra. The commonest sites are C1/2 and C6/7. The maximum displacement allowed is

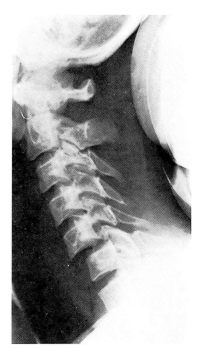

Figure 10.15 Unilateral facet dislocation between C5 and C6.

3.5 mm. Slippage greater than this is associated with cervical spine instability because it implies that the posterior longitudinal ligament is torn.

If the vertebra has slipped less than a half of the width of a vertebral body, then a unifacet dislocation is usually responsible (Figure 10.15). If the displacement is greater, then bilateral facet dislocation is present (Figure 10.16).

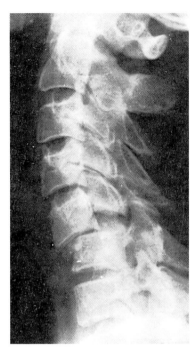

Figure 10.16 Bilateral facet dislocation between C5 and C6.

With hyperflexion injuries there can be an associated "tear drop" fracture of the anterior superior corner of the vertebral body, a flexed posture, widening of the interspinous gap and narrowing of the intervertebral space anteriorly and widening posteriorly (see Figure 10.4). In contrast, hyperextension of the neck can lead to avulsion of the anterior inferior corner of the vertebral body along with opening of the intervertebral space anteriorly and narrowing posteriorly.

The simple loss of the normal cervical lordosis may be due to a variety of conditions (see box) and therefore only indicates that the patient may have sustained a cervical injury.

Loss of cervical lordosis
● Muscular spasm
● Age
● Previous injury
● Radiographic positioning
● Hard collar

Bones

If C1 is examined carefully on the lateral view a fracture of the lamina and pedicles may be seen. This is produced by a compressive injury and is known as a Jefferson fracture. It is structurally unstable and a third of these injuries are associated with fractures of C2.

Fractures of the pars interarticularis of C2 (hangman's fracture) can be quite subtle. Only in extreme cases is there anterior displacement of C2 on C3, opening of the posterior

disc intervertebral space and bilateral facet dislocation (Figure 10.17). This condition produces cervical instability.

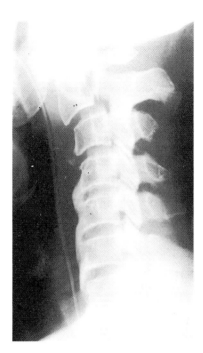

Figure 10.17 Lateral radiograph showing a hangman's fracture, anterior displacement of C2 on C3, and opening of the posterior intervertebral disc space. Soft tissue swelling is present along with signs of ankylosing spondylitis.

With regard to C3–T1, the heights of the anterior and posterior aspects of each vertebral body should be the same. A disparity of greater than 2 mm is significant and implies there is a compression fracture (Figure 10.18). A disparity

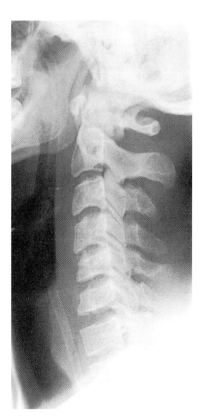

Figure 10.18 Diving injury with compression fractures of the bodies of C5 and C6 and an associated Jefferson fracture, not obvious on this lateral view.

greater than 25% can only occur if the middle and posterior ligamental complexes have been torn; it is therefore a sign of mechanical instability.

A "tear drop" fracture often results from a hyperflexing force and is located in the anterior superior corner of the vertebral body of C5/6 and T12/L1/L2 in adults or T4/5 in children. As it is associated with a significant rupture of the ligamental complexes, the radiograph shows interspinous widening and marked soft tissue swelling. This can be used to distinguish it from a simple avulsion fracture. A further clue is that the height of the fragment of bone in a tear drop fracture is greater than its width. With avulsion fragments the width is usually greater than its height.

The spinal canal should be over 13 mm wide and is measured from the posterior surface of the vertebral body to the spinolaminar line (see Figure 10.2). Narrowing of the canal occurs following dislocations and compression fractures which displace segments of bone posteriorly (see Figure 10.4). Pre-existing disease and degeneration may also lead to a narrowing of the canal. In these situations there is a higher chance of the spinal cord being damaged following any bone displacement.

Cartilage and joints

Narrowing of the anterior disc space, with widening posteriorly, indicates there has been a hyperflexion injury. Conversely, hyperextension produces widening of the anterior disc space with narrowing posteriorly.

Normally the facet joint has parallel articular surfaces with a gap of less than 2 mm. Following a unifacet dislocation there is usually soft tissue swelling and the vertebrae above the lesion are rotated so that both facet surfaces are seen on the lateral view. This feature is called the "bow tie" sign. Below this level the vertebrae are normally aligned. A bifacet dislocation is associated with forward displacement of the vertebral body (over 50%), widening of the interspinous processes, disc space narrowing, and soft tissue swelling. However, there is no rotation of the vertebrae (see Figure 10.16).

It is important to remember that the transverse ligament may rupture without there being any bony injury. Therefore the gap between the anterior surface of the dens and the posterior surface of the anterior arch of C1 should be checked in all cases. It is normally less than 3 mm in the adult and less than 5 mm in the child.

Soft tissue

The "rule of thumb" is that the gap between C1–3 and the air shadow, caused by the oro/nasopharynx, should be less than 7 mm (Figure 10.2). Below the level of the larynx the trachea is separated from the vertebrae by the oesophagus. Consequently the gap between the air shadow (trachea) and the bones is increased to 21 mm in the adult (one vertebral body width) and 14 mm in the child. In children this gap can be wider due to crying, neck flexion, and presphenoidal adenoidal enlargement. The latter leads to an increase in the prevertebral soft tissue gap at C1/C2.

The stability of the vertebral column is dependent on ligaments which cannot be seen on plain x-rays. Consequently, the lateral cervical radiograph is checked for radiological clues of ligamentous injury (see box). It is important to note that even with major spinal injury there could be little abnormal on the plane lateral radiograph.

Radiological clues of cervical instability
• Facet joint overriding
• Facet joint widening
• Interspinous fanning
• Greater than 25% compression of the vertebral body
• Greater than 10 degree angulation between vertebral bodies
• More than 3.5 mm vertebral body overriding with fracture

Additional radiography

When a spinal cord injury is suspected further radiographs will need to be taken (see box). However, in most cases the patient will have to be taken to the x-ray department. Therefore, these are only requested once the patient is haemodynamically stable.

Additional spinal radiographs taken after resuscitation	
• Cervical	Anteroposterior
	Open mouth
• Thoracic	Lateral
	Anteroposterior
• Lumbar	Lateral
	Anteroposterior

The anterior/posterior and open mouth cervical radiograph

These detect a further 10–15% of the cervical abnormalities. In most cases the patient will have to be taken to the x-ray department when resuscitation is complete. They should be examined using the same principles described for the lateral view. Therefore once the adequacy of the film has been assessed the ABCs are inspected.

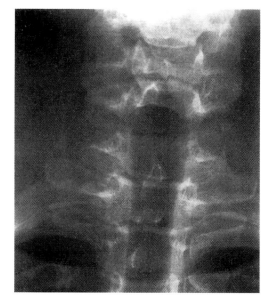

Figure 10.19 Anteroposterior radiograph showing unifacet dislocation of C6 (arrow). The spinous process of C6 is rotated to the right compared with the spinous processes of C5, C7, T1. The C6/7 intervertebral space is widened.

Alignment

Malalignment of spinous processes and pedicles may indicate a unifacet dislocation or a fracture of the lateral articular surface (Figure 10.19). These injuries are associated with the spinous processes rotating to the side of the injury.

Bones

The vertebral bodies should be rectangular with a regular internal trabecular pattern. A careful inspection will therefore reveal any compression, vertical fissures, and steps in the end plates.

Cartilage and joints

Irregularity in height of the articulating surfaces indicates disruption of the joint.

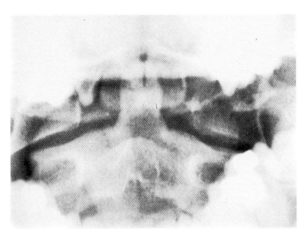

Figure 10.21 Open mouth odontoid view showing a Jefferson fracture of the atlas with outward displacement of the right lateral mass.

Soft tissues

The paravertebral tissue must be assessed as disruption of the normal air shadow can indicate that there is an underlying fracture or dislocation.

The open mouth view

Alignment

This view demonstrates the C1/C2 articulation. The distances between the lateral masses of the atlas and the odontoid peg (dens) are normally symmetrical. In adults there should be less than 2 mm lateral overriding between C1 and C2 (Figure 10.20). Jefferson fractures are often seen clearly in this view (Figure 10.21).

Bones

The dens must be carefully examined. Fractures can, rarely, occur in the peg itself (Type 1), at its base (Type 2), or extend into the body of C2 (Type 3). Type 2 is the commonest and it leads to cervical spine instability (Figure 10.22). A common

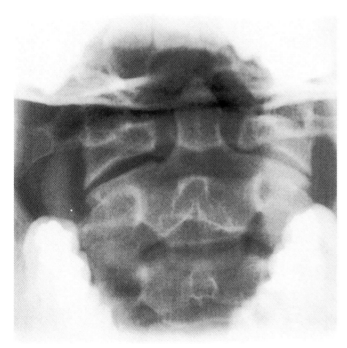

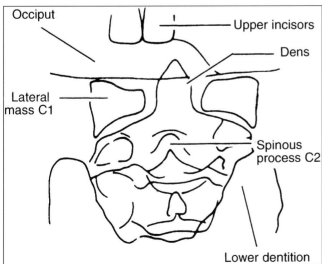

Figure 10.20 Open mouth radiograph showing normal alignment of the dens and the spinous processes of C2. There is no lateral overriding of C1 on C2, and the dens is symmetrically placed between the two lateral masses of C1. Notice the artefact created by the occiput overlying the dens. This can be mistaken for a fracture.

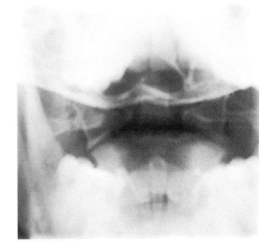

Figure 10.22 Open mouth view showing a Type 2 fracture of the dens.

error is to misread the dark shadow of either the overlying teeth or the epiphyseal plate as a fracture. The epiphysis is V-shaped and should have fused by 12 years of age. Non-union of this secondary ossification centre leads to formation of an os odontoideum. This is seen as a characteristic smooth convex border at the tip of the dens.

Cartilage and joints

The articulating surfaces should be parallel to one another.

Soft tissues

Soft tissue shadows are not usually evident on this view.

Lateral thoracic and lumbar radiographs

The same system as previously described is used to interpret these two radiographs. Once the adequacy of the films has been determined, the "ABCS" is carried out.

Adequacy

Check the adequacy and quality of the films. Count the vertebrae and make sure that all five lumbar vertebrae can be clearly seen along with the lumbar–sacral junction and the thoracic vertebrae under investigation.

Alignment

The anterior and posterior longitudinal lines, as well as the spinolaminar line should trace out smooth curves (Figure 10.23). These change from kyphotic to lordotic at the T1/L1 junction. In the lumbar region, a line running through the facet joints should also trace out a smooth curve. This is difficult to see in the thoracic region because of the overlying ribs.

An anterior displacement greater than 25% is usually due to a shearing injury. It is associated with fractures of the facets and tearing of all three ligamental complexes. The spine is therefore mechanically unstable. Hyperflexion with rotation can also produce anterior displacement due to subluxation or dislocation of the facet joints once the ligaments have been torn. There are not necessarily any fractures to the vertebral bodies in contrast to the pure hyperflexion injury which leads to the fractures described previously.

Fractures of the pedicles can occur in areas of the lumbar spine. In these cases the vertebral column can move anteriorly or posteriorly depending on the direction of the initiating force.

Bones

Each vertebra must be assessed individually. The cortical surface is inspected first for steps, breaks, or abnormal angulations. An inability to trace out the cortical margins indicates that there is an overlap of bone. In the upper thoracic region the facet joints, spinous processes, and transverse processes normally cannot be seen because of overlying ribs, soft tissues, and the alignment of the facet joints. Elsewhere in the vertebral column this loss of cortical margin usually results from a fracture or dislocation.

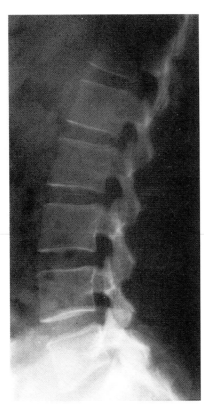

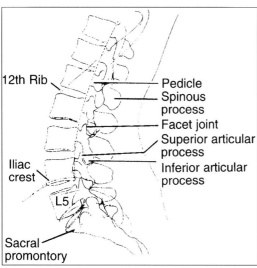

Figure 10.23 Lateral radiograph showing the normal alignment of the lumbar vertebrae and the sacrolumbar junction.

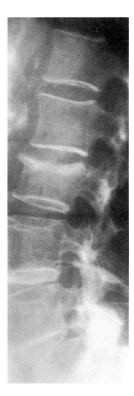

Figure 10.24 Lateral radiograph of the lumbar vertebrae showing an axial compression fracture with disruption of the superior articular surface of L3.

The rest of the bone is then inspected for alterations in the internal trabecular pattern, lucencies, and increases in density. A reduction in the height of the anterior and posterior surface, relative to that found in the adjacent vertebra, indicates that the patient has been subjected to an axial compression force (Figure 10.24). This is commonly associated with soft tissue swelling, anterior wedging, vertical fractures of the spinolaminae junctions, and posterior displacement of fragments into the spinal canal.

A discrepancy greater than or equal to 2 mm between the anterior and posterior height of the vertebral body indicates that there is a fracture. However, this rule of thumb does not apply to T11–L1, where these dimensions can exist normally. A 50% discrepancy is always abnormal and implies there has been significant ligamental damage (Figure 10.25). This is

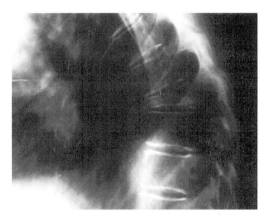

Figure 10.25 Lateral radiograph of the thoracic vertebrae showing wedge fracture which is greater than 50% of the vertebral height. The adjacent vertebral disc spaces are narrowed.

usually associated with soft tissue swelling and, in extreme situations, subluxation of the facet joint and widening of the interspinous gaps.

Hyperextension injuries can lead to widening of the anterior disc space with fracture and posterior displacement of the posterior aspects of the vertebrae. Chance fractures of the vertebral bodies are best seen on the lateral view and can extend into the laminae and pedicles. Occasionally there is also an increase in posterior vertebral height with widening of the posterior disc space.

Fractures involving the pedicles and lamina are potentially unstable because there may be associated tearing of the intervertebral ligaments. Isolated fractures of the transverse and spinous processes can result from direct trauma. More commonly, however, they are associated with other fractures. Damage to the spinous processes in particular may be part of a hyperflexion or hyperextension pattern of injury.

Cartilage and joints

The intervertebral discs should be similar and even throughout. In addition their height usually increases progressively down the spine to L4/L5. Commonly the disc at L5-S1 is narrower than that at L4/L5. Following chronic stress the disc will shrink even further. This is associated with dense sclerosis of the underlying cortical surfaces and the development of marginal osteophytes.

Unilateral or bilateral facet dislocation can occur in the lumbar region and it is usually associated with widening of the interspinous gaps, fractures of the articular surface (best seen on the AP view) and soft tissue swelling. Subluxation occurs when the upper articular surface is riding high on the

one below but they are still in contact with one another. This is also associated with widening of the interspinous gaps.

Soft tissue

The soft tissue shadows around the vertebral column needs to be assessed because disruption indicates that there may be an underlying bony or ligamental injury.

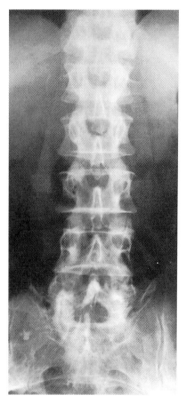

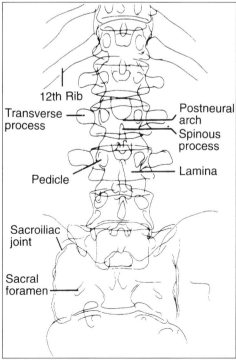

Figure 10.26 Anteroposterior radiograph and line diagram showing vertical alignment of the spinous processes and the gradual increase in width of the lumbar vertebrae and the interpedicular distance.

Anteroposterior (AP) thoracic and lumbar views

Alignment

The AP radiograph should be examined in the same systematic fashion described for the lateral view. After the adequacy and quality of the film has been assessed, the vertical alignment of the spinous processes should be checked. The distance between the two lateral borders of the vertebra, the pedicles, and the facet joints increases progressively down the vertebral column (Figure 10.26).

Malalignment may indicate a unifacet dislocation or a fracture of the lateral articular surface (Figure 10.27). In these

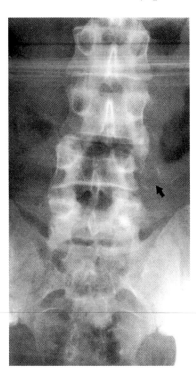

Figure 10.27 Anteroposterior radiograph of the lumbar vertebrae showing a crush fracture of L4 with rotation of the spinous processes of L4 and L5 to the right. There is also a fracture of the transverse process of L4.

cases, the spinous process rotates to the side of the injury. A lateral compression fracture will produce scoliosis on the AP view.

Bones

Each vertebra must be checked separately for deformity. The superior and inferior surface of the vertebral body should be parallel. A crush fracture may be detected on the AP view by noting loss of trabecular pattern, overlapping of bone fragments, and widening of the interpedicular distance. An anterior/superior wedge fracture indicates the spine has been subjected to either a hyperflexion or hyperextension injury. With hyperflexion there is associated soft tissue swelling, anterior disc space narrowing, widening of the posterior disc space, loss of the anterior vertebral height, and, in extreme situations, subluxation of the facet joints. Rarely there is lateral wedging of the vertebral bodies from lateral flexion and rotation.

Isolated fractures of the transverse and spinous processes can occur following direct trauma as well as be part of the pattern of injuries resulting from hyperflexion and hyperextension mechanisms. Gross disruption of the vertebral body usually indicates that there has been axial compression. This

is associated with soft tissue swelling, retropropulsion of bone fragments into the spinal canal, and anterior wedging.

Cartilage and joints

The intervertebral disc spaces and facet joints must be checked in the manner described previously for the cervical spine.

Soft tissue

Examination of the soft tissues is carried out once the skeletal system has been assessed. Soft tissue swelling can indicate the presence of an underlying bony or ligamental injury. Beware that soft tissue changes following fractures of the upper thoracic vertebrae can mimic a ruptured thoracic aorta.

Special Investigations

Obliques

These enable the clinician to assess the intervertebral formina, the pedicles, and the facet joints. They may also be requested when spondylolisthesis or unifacet dislocation is suspected on the routine films. However, with the advent of CT scanning these radiographs are rarely required in the emergency situation. Consequently they should only be requested following consultation with the specialist who will be in charge of the patient's long-term management.

The shape traced out by the pedicle, transverse process, and the superior and inferior facet on an oblique view of the lumbar vertebrae has been likened to that of a "Scotty dog". A break in the "dog's" neck indicates a fracture of the pars interarticularis. This can result from traumatic spondylolisthesis.

Sternum and ribs

An injury causing damage to the upper eight thoracic vertebrae may also fracture the sternum or ribs and thereby increase the chances of the thoracic injury being unstable. Radiographs of the sternum and relevant ribs should therefore be taken in this case.

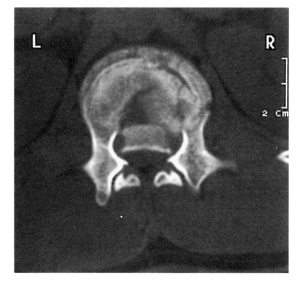

Figure 10.28 CT of fractured lumbar vertebral body with fragments extending posteriorly into the spinal canal. (Courtesy of Dr D. Nicholson.)

Computerised tomography (CT)

Following plain x-rays, CT scanning has become the mainstay for investigation of spinal cord injuries. Its axial slices and reconstructive capabilities give CT scanning the ability to visualise middle and posterior column fractures (Figure 10.28). In addition, the degree of canal compromise can be accurately determined to within 1 mm or less. By adding CT scanning to plain films, detection of spinal fractures in patients with multiple injuries has been reported as increasing from 85 to 96%. However, it is not without its own pitfalls. Fractures which parallel the plane of the scan and typically involve the facets or pedicles can be missed on axial sections. Though three-dimensional images can be reconstructed they usually add little that changes the neurosurgeon's management of the particular spinal injury from the plain axial and sagittal CT images.

Plain CT does not demonstrate the intraspinal contents other than bone fragments. For this reason contrast enhancement is required and has been superseded by MR scanning. Nevertheless, there is still an indication for CT myelography in units without MR scanning facilities and where there is unexplained deterioration in spinal cord function following resuscitation or after the development of an anterior or partial cord syndrome. In these cases deformation of the intrathecal contrast by an extradural mass lesion may suggest the development of a haematoma with resultant cord compression.

Magnetic resonance imaging (MRI)

This is now the investigation of choice where visualisation of the contents of the spinal canal is required. However, resuscitation equipment must be MRI-compatible. In addition to imaging the spinal canal contents (Figure 10.29), MR scans are ideal for detecting ligamentous and intervertebral disc damage. Clearly the ability to evaluate soft tissue injury is of enormous benefit to the surgeon in planning a stabilising or decompressive procedure. It is often used in conjunction with CT scanning as this provides better views of the bony structures than MRI.

> Both MRI and CT scanning have removed the radiological "blind" area at the craniocervical junction and at the cervicodorsal junction.

Definitive management

Caution is needed before declaring a patient free from a spinal injury because palpation of the vertebral column is not a foolproof way of detecting vertebral damage. Furthermore, cervical injuries can be present with no radiological evidence of damage. Therefore, spinal stabilization must be maintained until specialist advice is obtained if a spinal injury is suspected from either the mechanism of the injury or examination.

Published work has shown the advantage of giving high doses of methylprednisolone in the first 24 hours after blunt spinal injury (see box). The reason for this improvement is not known but workers have postulated that it could be due to a decrease in lipid peroxidation, protein degradation, catabolic activity, or an increased impulse conduction by activation of ion pumps.

The early use of methylprednisolone following blunt spinal injury

- 30 mg/kg i.v. over 15 minutes immediately
- Then 5.4 mg/kg/h for 23 hours

Immobility of the skeletal system is associated with severe osteoporosis in patients with major spinal cord injury. The use of steroids can complicate this. Gastrointestinal tract paralysis can also result in ulcerations and haemorrhage, and these effects again can be complicated by the side effects of steroids. As in trauma to the central nervous system following head injury, the presence of hyperglycaemia can be detrimental to CNS function. In this respect, the addition of steroids and the production of secondary hypoglycaemia can produce some deterioration in spinal cord function. In addition to these effects, high-dose or long-term steroid therapy is also associated with the occurrence of pancreatitis. This is often seen in patients without steroid therapy but with a severe spinal cord injury where an elevated serum amylase is associated with an ileus, abdominal distension and intermittent pyrexia.

Penetrating trauma (especially gunshot wounds) increases the risk of infection. This has been used as an explanation for the higher mortality Figures in these patients when they are given steroids.

Surgical care

Following evaluation of the spinal cord injury by plain radiography, CT, and MR scanning, a decision as to the need for surgical stabilisation can be made more accurately. The degree of urgency used to be related to the question

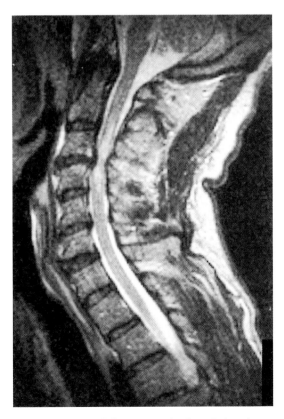

Figure 10.29 C3/4 central disc prolapse showing spinal cord compression and an area of high signal in the cord indicating oedema. (Courtesy of Dr D. Nicholson.)

of stability versus instability. Nowadays it is recognised that even relatively stable injuries to the spine may be associated with significant cord compression. This can follow pre-existing narrowed spinal canal dimensions or associated soft tissue compromise, such as prolapsed discs or developing epidural haematomas. In these circumstances early surgery is indicated to optimise neurological outcome. In addition to the above reasons, delayed surgery allows physiological stabilisation of a patient when imaging techniques have failed to demonstrate an obviously recoverable lesion amenable to surgical intervention.

In the early hours of management following cervical spine injury, sufficient protection to the nervous system can be afforded by in-line traction and log-rolling with the patient's neck fixed in a hard collar. With radiological control, skull traction can be applied using increasing weights as necessary to maintain alignment without overdistraction. The pins are usually placed in the coronal plane in line with the external auditory meatus approximately 1.5 cm above the pinna. The technique of surgical decompression of the spinal cord injury usually renders the spine unstable. It is therefore never carried out in isolation, but is instead performed in conjunction with some form of stabilisation. In the cervical spine this may take the form of anterior fusion with the use of bone grafts in association commonly with plating systems. This is usually combined with a posterior stabilisation technique with bone grafts applied either to the lamina of the cervical vertebra or between the spinous processes and held in place with wire. The use of metal (either titanium or stainless steel) plates wired into position over the lamina is also widely used to stabilise the cervical spine posteriorly. More recently lateral mass screw techniques, combined with either plates or bar fixation techniques, have been widely developed. The use of screw techniques for odontoid peg fracture fixation is also an accepted part of the armamentarium for cervical fracture stabilisation.

In the thoracic and lumbar spine, anterior and anterolateral techniques for vertebral body stabilisation and for vertebral body replacement (for example the Moss cage) are now routinely practised in specialised units handling patients with spinal cord injuries. These latter techniques involve considerable blood loss and should only be practised in those units experienced in such techniques, with anaesthetic staff aware of all of the physiological impacts that such techniques have on patients with compromised spinal cord function.

With surgical stabilisation, long-term sequelae can be avoided, for example by early mobilisation of patients with partial or insignificant spinal cord injury. In the thoracolumbar spine the correction of kyphus deformity following compression fractures is associated with reduction of chronic or relapsing back pain. This is in comparison to a conservatively treated group where evidence of such symptoms may be as high as 30% or more.

Management on the ward

The development of specialist spinal centres and rehabilitation centres for patients with spinal cord injuries has undoubtedly allowed expertise to develop in certain areas. However, owing to sheer numbers and distances involved, many patients will not go directly to these units. More commonly patients are admitted, at least initially, to the local hospital under the care of the orthopaedic surgeons. It is therefore essential that these clinicians manage the patient appropriately and communicate with the specialist when necessary.

Patient movement

Personnel need to be made aware of the situation if there is a chance that the spine could be injured. Extra care should be taken to work in a coordinated fashion and not, inadvertently, to move or twist any part of the vertebral column.

Transfer of patient from/to trolley

A minimum of six people will be required to transfer the patient if he or she is not already on a back board. One team member must stabilise the head and cervical spine with hands and forearms. On this person's command, four of the team lift the patient vertically while keeping the spine perfectly level. The sixth member then removes what the patient was lying on, and inserts the new surface. The team then lowers the patients. At no time should the patient be subjected to a bending or twisting force

Complications

In addition to pressure sores and urinary tract infection (Table 10.3), cardiopulmonary complications are the major cause of death in the acute phase of care of patients with spinal cord injuries. Atelectasis and difficulty with clearance of respiratory secretions accounts for most of the respiratory complications noted. The combination of stasis and cardiovascular embarrassment may account for an incidence of pulmonary embolus of between 3 and 13%.

The development of contractures in the soft tissues is best managed by prevention and to this extent the role of the physiotherapist in the spinal cord-injured patient is paramount.

Table 10.3 Complications in patients with spinal cord injury on a general ward

	Thoracic lesion (%)	Lumbar lesion (%)
Pressure sore	61	40
Urinary tract infection	80	62

Respiratory physiotherapy

In addition to these vital activities, the physiotherapist plays an important part in providing respiratory care.

The non-ventilated patient

Initial assessment should be carried out as soon as possible, so that any future deterioration or improvement can easily be monitored (see box). This is particularly important for management of respiratory function in cervical and high thoracic lesions. In these cases the level of the lesion may rise owing to ascending oedema in the spinal cord, causing increasing paralysis of respiratory muscles in the first few days after admission.

Important parts of the respiratory assessment

- Previous respiratory history
- Current oxygenation
- Respiratory rate. An increasing rate may indicate respiratory fatigue or presence of secretions. A decrease may indicate neurological deterioration
- Assessment of expansion and alterations in breathing pattern
- Lung function tests. If the vital capacity falls below 500 ml mechanical ventilation may be indicated
- Neurological and sensory levels
- Psychological state
- Results of chest x-ray, ABGs and auscultation

In the non-ventilated patient treatment aims at prophylaxis as well as being directed towards particular respiratory problems.

(1) *Positioning and postural drainage.* Positioning can be used to maximise ventilation to dependent areas of the lung, particularly when there is traumatic quadriplegia. In such cases maximum oxygenation and functional residual volume is achieved in the 60–90° head-up position. However, the best position for coughing and deep breathing is a 0–35° head-up position.

Positioning may also be used with postural drainage where there is established lung infection. However, in acute spinal injury this may need modification in order not to inflict any further mechanical injury to the spinal cord. Furthermore, gravity may also cause the abdominal contents to splint an inactive diaphragm. As a result lung volume can be reduced.

(2) *Breathing exercises.* The patient is taught breathing exercises aimed at increasing expansion of the lateral, apical and basal areas of lung fields, as well as improving diaphragmatic activity. An incentive spirometer can be used to facilitate expansion by providing the patient with visual feedback. It can also provide an early indication of change in respiratory function.

(3) *Intermittent positive pressure breathing (IPPB).* This is a form of assisted breathing using intermittent positive pressure which is triggered by even a minimal inspiration. Ventilation can be improved during its use. Nevertheless, for continued improvement in lung volumes, careful selection of patient and positioning should be used. The main benefit of IPPB appears to be its assistance in clearance of secretions in patients with sputum retention. The IPPB device can also be used to administer nebulised drugs which may be beneficial in patients with poor inspiratory effort.

(4) *Breathing exercises.* The high tetraplegic patient may be unable to perform localised breathing exercises and instead may be taught glossopharyngeal breathing. This is a method where boluses of air are gulped in and out of the lungs. Lung volumes can be increased with between five and eight mouthfuls and the technique may also assist secretion clearance.

(5) *Assisted coughing.* This is essential for the patient with respiratory insufficiency from spinal cord injury. Secretions need to be moved from the small to large airways and an effective cough is required for efficient expectoration. It is assisted by an application of a compression in an inwards and upwards direction against the thorax. This creates a push against the diaphragm and takes the place of abdominal activity. Various methods of assisted cough may be used but the compression should be synchronised with the expiratory effort of the patient. Once completed, the pressure should be lifted to allow the diaphragm movement for the next inspiration. Care should also be taken if the cervical spine is unstable, with extra stability being provided by additional personnel controlling the shoulders and upper ribcage. Pressure through the abdomen should be avoided at all times and extreme care should be taken if paralytic ileus is present.

(6) *Suction.* If the assisted cough is insufficient to clear secretions, nasopharyngeal suction may be considered. This should be undertaken with extreme caution as vagal stimulation is unopposed and may result in bradycardia or asystole. Therefore atropine should be available for intravenous use if needed and preoxygenation with 100% oxygen should always be performed.

In the case of deteriorating respiratory function, mechanical ventilation, bronchoscopy, or tracheostomy need to be considered.

The ventilated patient

Patients who are being mechanically ventilated are deprived of the normal mechanisms by which debris and secretions are cleared from the respiratory tract. This is the result of paralysis of the respiratory muscles either as a result of sedative or neuromuscular blocking drugs or the spinal cord injury itself. The role of the physiotherapist is, therefore, to replace these mechanisms in order to prevent the development of hypoxia, which itself may further damage the spinal cord and other organs.

(1) *Positioning.* As before.

(2) *Manual hyperinflation (MHI).* MHI or "bagging" involves delivery of a volume of gas by a manual inflation bag to hyperinflate the lungs, promoting collateral air flow. It is commonly used in the treatment of ventilated patients in an attempt to re-inflate areas of atelectasis and promote removal of excess bronchial secretions. The technique commonly consists of a slow deep inspiration, an inspiratory hold to utilise collateral ventilation, followed by a quick release of the inflation bag to improve the expiratory flow rate.

MHI is a form of positive pressure ventilation and has a number of haemodynamic effects which may be detrimental to the patient with a spinal injury. Common problems include impairment of venous return, a reduction in cardiac output, and hypotension. The cardiac output may also be reduced as a result of vagal stimulation causing a reflex bradycardia. As these effects are normally compensated for by the sympathetic nervous system, patients with a high spinal cord lesion may not have this ability. Therefore during MHI the patient's cardiovascular parameters must be observed for adverse effects. Prolonged bagging must not be undertaken in patients who are haemodynamically unstable, or when there is an acute spinal cord injury or head injury.

(3) *Manual techniques – percussion, shaking and suction.* *Percussion* is a technique of slow rhythmic clapping using relaxed, slightly cupped hands over the lung fields. This creates an energy wave which is transmitted to the airways. It enhances the clearance of secretions and should be used only if indicated by the presence of excessive bronchial secretions or retained secretions causing atelectasis. It should not be performed routinely on ventilated patients. Care must be taken as percussion can cause dysrhythmias and bronchospasm. However, it does not appear to significantly alter blood pressure or ICP, and therefore may be suitable for use in those with head injury or spinal cord injury.

Shaking uses the hands placed over the appropriate lung fields. At the point of maximum inspiration the therapist starts to shake the chest using body weight to assist. This continues throughout the period of expiration. It cannot be used effectively in patients with rib fractures and should be used cautiously in spinal cord injuries because of the degree of movement caused.

Suction is performed only if indicated by the presence of retained secretions which cannot otherwise be removed. Acutely, these may cause a sudden drop in minute volume, a rise in airway pressure or profound hypoxia. Suction is only successful if the secretions are accessible to a catheter. Haemodynamic disturbances are common during suction and include dysrhythmias, hypotension, hypoxia, and even cardiac arrest. During suction the patient's oxygen supply is dramatically reduced, whilst the stimulation of the procedure may increase oxygen demand resulting in profound hypoxia. A number of precautions must be taken to reduce this, including pre-oxygenation with 100% oxygen either via the ventilator or by MHI. A closed line suction system can be used so disconnection from the ventilator is avoided; this may enable Fi_{O_2} and PEEP to be maintained. A maximum of 10 seconds should elapse during the suction procedure. If sympathetic reflexes are absent a bradycardia may occur. In some patients an instillation of saline (10–20 ml prior to suction) may be beneficial to assist the procedure.

Transport

The arrangements for transfer of patients into specialist spinal units are best managed by strict local protocols. These regimens need to include agreement on analgesia, as well as on such things as fluid resuscitation regimens. The mechanism of transport for such patients will vary according to the geographical location of the primary hospital. Slow road transport may be more appropriate for certain situations rather than more rapid air transfer.

Summary

In summary, whilst the management of patients with spinal cord injury has improved dramatically in the last quarter of the twentieth century, there is no reason to suspect that further improvement cannot be achieved in the first quarter of the next. Initial recognition and safe management of the patient with spinal cord injury is paramount. Definition of the injury in each particular case is more easily ascertained with up-to-date imaging techniques such as CT scanning and MR imaging. The development of basic science research techniques examining the potential for axonal regeneration will inevitably need to be associated with intensive rehabilitative techniques in order to optimise recovery of patients with spinal cord injury in the future.

Further reading

Agarwal A, Peppleman W, Kraus D, Eisenberg C. The cervical spine in rheumatoid arthritis. *Br Med J* 1993;**306**:79–80.

Ali J, Qi W. Pulmonary function and posture in traumatic quadriplegia. *J Trauma* 1995;**39**:334–7.

Baker J. The initial hospital management and resuscitation of patients with spinal cord injuries. *Semin Orthop* 1989;**4**:15–27.

Baker J. The first aid management of spinal cord injuries. *Semin Orthop* 1989;**4**:2–14.

Benzel E, Hart B, Ball P. Magnetic response imaging for the evaluation of patients with occult cervical spine injury. *J Neurosurg* 1996;**85**:824–8.

Bott J, Keilty S, Noone L. Intermittent positive pressure breathing: a dying art? *Physiotherapy* 1992;**78**:656–60.

Bracken M, Shepard M, Collins W *et al*. A randomized controlled trial of methyprednislone or naloxone in the treatment of acute spinal cord injury. *N Engl J Med* 1990;**322**:1405–11.

Donovan W, Bedbrook G. Clinical Symposia: Comprehensive management of spinal cord injury. New Jersey: CIBA Pharmaceutical Company, 1982.

Cohen A, Bosshard R, Yeo J. A new device for the care of acute spinal injuries: the Russell extraction device (RED). *Paraplegia* 1990;**28**:151–7.

Cooper C, Dunham M, Rodriguez A. Falls and major injuries are risk factors for thoracolumbar fractures: cognitive impairment and multiple injuries impede the detection of back pain and tenderness. *J Trauma* 1995;**38**:692–6.

Driscoll P, Ross R, Nicholson D. The cervical spine. In: Nicholson D, Driscoll P (eds). *ABC of emergency radiology*. London: BMJ, 1995.

Driscoll P, Ross R, Nicholson D. The thoraco and lumbar spine. In: Nicholson D, Driscoll P (eds). *ABC of emergency radiology*. London: BMJ, 1995.

Flanders A, Schaefer D, Doan H, Mishkin M, Gonzales C, Northrup B. Acute cervical spine trauma: correlation of MR findings with degree of neurological deficit. *Radiology* 1990;**177**:25–33.

Folman Y, Masri W. Spinal cord injury: prognostic indicators. *Injury* 1989;**20**:92–3.

Gallon A. The use of percussion. *Physiotherapy* 1992;**78**:85–9.

Grundy D, Penny P, Graham L. Diving into the unknown. *Br Med J* 1991;**302**:670–1.

Grundy D, Swain A. *ABC of spinal cord injury* (3rd edn). London: BMJ, 1996.

Hinds C, Watson D. *Intensive care. A concise textbook* (2nd edn). London: WB Saunders Ltd, 1996.

Kendall L, Jackson S. (1987) Intensive therapy physiotherapy management of the adult patient. In: Downie R (ed.) *Cash's textbook of chest, heart and vascular disorders for physiotherapists* (4th edn). London: Faber and Faber, 1987.

King D, Morrell A. A survey on manual hyperinflation as a physiotherapy technique in intensive care units. *Physiotherapy* 1992;**78**:747–50.

Majernick *et al*. Cervical spine movement during oro-tracheal intubation. *Ann Emerg Med* 1986;**15**:417–20.

Oller D. The relationship between face or skull fractures and cervical spine and spinal cord injuries: a review of 13,834 patients. *34th Ann Proc AAAM*;1990:315–27.

Peach F, Grundy D. How preventable are spinal injuries? *Health Trends* 1991;**23**:62–6.

Paratz J. Haemodynamic stability of the ventilated intensive care patient: a review. *Aust Physio* 1992;**38**:167–71.

Prendergast M, Saxe J, Ledgerwood A, Lucas C, Lucas W. Massive steroids do not reduce the zone of injury after spinal cord injury. *J Trauma* 1994;**37**:576–9.

Shaffer M, Doris P. Limitations of crosstable lateral views in detecting cervical spine injury: a retrospective analysis. *Ann Emerg Med* 1981;**10**:508–13.

Sims A. Atlantoaxial instability in Down's syndrome. *Br Med J* 1987;**294**:988–9.

Swain A, Dove J, Baker H. Spine and spinal cord. In: Skinner D, Driscoll P, Earlam R (eds). *ABC of major trauma* (2nd edn). London: BMJ, 1996.

Toscano J. Prevention of neurological deterioration before admission to a spinal cord injury unit. *Paraplegia* 1988;**26**:143–50.

Ward T. Spinal injuries. In: Webber B and Pryor J (eds) *Physiotherapy for respiratory and cardiac problems*. London: Churchill Livingstone, 1993.

Webber B. *The Brompton Hospital guide to chest physiotherapy* (5th edn). London: Blackwell, 1988.

Wood M. Respiratory therapy. In: Whiteneck G, Addler C, Edwards-Carter R, Lammertse D, Manley S, Menter R. (eds). *Comprehensive neurologic rehabilitation vol. 1: The management of high quadriplegia.* New York: Demos Publications, 1989.

Woodring J, Lee C. Limitations of cervical radiography in the evaluation of acute cervical trauma. *J Trauma* 1993;**34**:32–9.

Zipnick R, Scalea T, Trooskin S, *et al*. Hemodynamic responses to penetrating spinal cord injuries. *J Trauma* 1993;**35**:578–82.

11 Abdominal trauma

David J. Jones
Consultant Surgeon, Department of Surgery, Wythenshawe Hospital, Manchester

Sir Miles H. Irving
Professor of Surgery, University of Manchester, Department of Surgery, Hope Hospital, Salford

OBJECTIVES

- To describe the various types of abdominal trauma.
- To discuss patient assessment.
- To describe the investigations required.
- To discuss management and treatment for specific injuries.

This chapter covers the specific management of abdominal trauma and assumes that the victim is being resuscitated and that the primary survey has been performed. The surgeon called to assess a trauma victim must ascertain if a significant intra-abdominal injury has occurred and decide whether surgical intervention is indicated. The management of an abdominal trauma victim inevitably depends on the clinical expertise and resources available. The priority is to identify those patients with injuries which require immediate life-saving surgical intervention, from those with less severe injuries who can be observed and investigated. Growing experience with improved methods of assessment and investigation, has enabled patients with appropriate injuries, for whom surgery would once have been considered mandatory, to be managed conservatively.

In the United Kingdom most abdominal injuries occur following blunt trauma sustained in road traffic accidents; penetrating trauma from stabbing and gunshot wounds is less common.

Types of abdominal injury

Blunt trauma

Blunt trauma (Figure 11.1) causes damage from a combination of compressive, shearing, and bursting forces. Compression occurs when direct pressure is applied, such as in a seatbelt injury. Oblique forces and deceleration injuries cause shearing of viscera where anchored, such as at the duodenojejunal flexure and peritoneal attachments of the bowel. A sudden increase of pressure within a segment of bowel may result in bursting which usually occurs away from the point of direct pressure. The liver, spleen, and kidneys are the organs most vulnerable to blunt trauma.

The presence of an intra-abdominal injury after blunt trauma is not always immediately apparent, as clinical findings are sometimes difficult to interpret. This is particularly true if the patient has other major injuries, is unconscious, or is already ventilator-dependent. However, certain physical signs are highly reliable indicators of major intra-abdominal injury and should provoke a high index of suspicion.

Penetrating trauma

This is an increasing problem in the UK, especially in inner city areas, but is less common than in the USA. Penetrating wounds are usually obvious (Figure 11.2), but peritoneal cavity involvement may not be. The latter should be considered if there is a wound lying anywhere on the trunk below the fourth

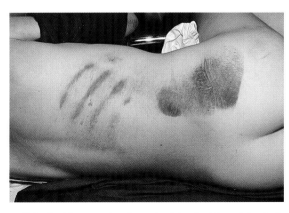

Figure 11.1 Bruising over the ribs and pelvis after blunt abdominal trauma; there is a high risk of major intra-abdominal and chest injury.

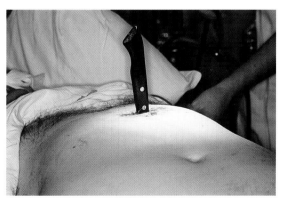

Figure 11.2 Upper abdominal stab wound. The knife had passed through the short gastric vessels and its tip was lying between the intra-abdominal oesophagus and upper pole of the spleen. The weapon should not be removed prior to surgery.

intercostal space. The consequences of a gunshot wound depend on the velocity of the bullet or missile (see Chapter 22). Energy is dissipated into the surrounding tissues perpendicular to the trajectory causing a varying amount of damage proportional to the degree of energy transfer. For example, low velocity bullets cause damage confined to the tissues immediately adjacent to the track, and the bullet usually comes to a halt in the body. In contrast, high velocity weapons are capable of causing more extensive tissue damage, over a wider area. In these circumstances the bullet usually passes through the body leaving both entry and exit wounds. If the peritoneal cavity is breached by a gunshot wound, there are almost invariably significant visceral injuries, so a laparotomy is considered mandatory for such patients. Tangential gunshot wounds are exceptions to this rule, as the peritoneal cavity may be spared, so selected patients can be managed conservatively. Stab wounds tend to be less serious than gunshot wounds, with a lower incidence of visceral injury. Consequently surgery is no longer considered mandatory for all these patients.

Assessment of patients with abdominal trauma

History and clinical features

It is important to obtain as much information as possible about the nature of the accident from the victim, witnesses, and paramedical personnel involved at the scene of the incident. The mechanism of the injury, the time elapsed following the injury, and the nature of any penetrating weapon must be ascertained.

The abdomen needs to be inspected for abrasions, lacerations, and penetrating wounds. Note is taken of imprinting of clothing on to the abdominal wall; especially at the site of seatbelt restraint. Embedded weapons or penetrating objects should not be removed as this may precipitate further bleeding if a major vessel has been transected. The abdomen is palpated to detect muscular defects and areas of guarding and tenderness. Rebound tenderness should be elicited by gentle percussion, rather than by suddenly removing a deeply palpating hand, which is always uncomfortable and gives false-positive signs of peritonism. It is customary to listen for bowel sounds, although their presence or absence soon after major trauma is of little clinical value when deciding whether or not to operate. To complete the examination the back and perineum need to be inspected. This will require the patient to be log-rolled if any spinal injury is suspected (see Chapter 10).

A rectal examination is mandatory because it can provide essential information (see box below). In females, a vaginal examination should also be performed.

A rectal examination is performed and the gloved finger inspected for blood which suggests rupture of the rectum or sigmoid colon. Anal sphincter tone is assessed and the wall of the rectum carefully palpated; bony fragments from pelvic fractures which could penetrate the rectum should be felt for. In females a vaginal examination should also be performed.

A nasogastric tube must be passed in all major trauma victims, to aspirate the stomach and minimise the risk of vomiting and pulmonary aspiration. If blood is aspirated, the possibility of a gastric or duodenal perforation should be considered. The urethral meatus is examined for the presence of blood and the perineum examined for bruising and swelling. In the presence of the former signs, or if it is not possible to

pass a catheter, and the patient has a major pelvic injury, rupture of the urethra should be suspected and a suprapubic approach considered (see Chapter 2).

The findings on abdominal examination are difficult to interpret if the patient has adjacent soft tissue, rib, back, and pelvic injuries, as these may also give rise to muscular guarding and tenderness. Furthermore, if the patient is unconscious, or ventilator-dependent, abdominal examination rarely yields useful findings in the absence of an intra-abdominal catastrophe with marked progressive distension from massive haemorrhage.

If abdominal trauma is suspected, but an immediate laparotomy is not indicated, the abdominal examination should be repeated at frequent intervals, in case the need for surgery arises.

Investigation of abdominal trauma

The investigation of an abdominal trauma victim depends on the clinical condition and the risks entailed in moving the patient away from the resuscitation room or intensive care unit. For example, if there is an obvious intra-abdominal catastrophe, it is dangerous to waste time performing detailed investigations. In these cases an immediate laparotomy is indicated. However, if a patient remains stable after resuscitation, further investigation is appropriate. An erect (if possible) chest x-ray is examined for evidence of a pneumoperitoneum, and the pelvic x-ray for major pelvic fractures. Plain abdominal radiographs are of little value after blunt trauma, but may reveal embedded bullets or missile fragments after penetrating injuries.

Diagnostic peritoneal lavage (DPL)

If the clinical signs on abdominal examination after blunt or penetrating trauma are difficult to interpret, and there is not an indication for an immediate laparotomy, a diagnostic peritoneal lavage (DPL) may provide evidence of intra-abdominal haemorrhage or perforation [1]. The reasons for performing a DPL are given in the box.

DPL carries a low but real risk of complications, so the procedure should be performed by an experienced surgeon. Whilst the only absolute contraindication to DPL is a clear indication for an immediate laparotomy, there are relative contraindications (see box).

DPL has an excellent sensitivity for abdominal trauma, although diaphragmatic and retroperitoneal injuries may give false-negative results. In experienced hands the technique has very low false-positive and false-negative rates of 1% or less [2].

A positive DPL indicating bleeding was initially deemed to be an indication to perform a laparotomy. However, if the patient remains stable after resuscitation, the demonstration of intra-abdominal haemorrhage by DPL is no longer considered an absolute indication for surgery. A trial of conservative management may be appropriate, provided there are facilities for intensive observation and immediate surgery should the need arise. If the DPL is only positive, on account of the microscopic examination of the effluent, and the patient has other serious injuries that demand urgent surgery, a laparotomy or abdominal imaging can be deferred until after these more urgent injuries have been treated. In those cases where DPL shows evidence of faecal debris or intestinal organisms, laparotomy is of course mandatory.

Diagnostic peritoneal lavage

Technique

1. Insert a urinary catheter and a nasogastric tube.

2. Prepare the abdomen using antiseptic solution.

3. Inject local anaesthetic in the midline below the umbilicus.

4. Make a 4 cm midline incision down to the fascia.

5. Incise the fascia and peritoneum and grasp the edges with clips.

6. Insert a peritoneal dialysis catheter.

7. Aspirate with a syringe looking for blood or bowel contents.

8. Instill 10 ml/kg of warm saline (700 ml for a 70 kg man) and distribute by gentle agitation of the abdomen.

9. Drain off after 5–10 min depending on the degree of urgency.

Analyse the effluent in the laboratory

Positive result

- > 5 ml blood on immediate aspiration
- Obvious intestinal contents
- > 100 000 RBC/mm^3 or 500 WBC/mm^3 in the drained lavage fluid
- Elevated amylase.

Complications

- Haemorrhage
- Visceral injury.

Reasons for performing a DPL

- Signs that are equivocal or obscured by adjacent soft tissue injuries
- Unreliable signs owing to head injury, intoxication or paraplegia
- Signs that are difficult to assess because the patient is undergoing lengthy radiological or extra-abdominal surgical procedures
- Unexplained hypotension or blood loss, even if abdominal examination is normal

---

Relative contraindications for DPL

- Previous surgery
- Gross obesity
- Advanced pregnancy
- Cirrhosis
- Established coagulopathies

Imaging

A positive DPL confirms haemorrhage but does not identify the source of bleeding. If the patient is haemodynamically stable after resuscitation and remains so for at least 30 minutes, it is reasonable to carry out more detailed investigations. These may necessitate moving the patient to the x-ray department. Imaging with either ultrasound (Figure 11.3) or CT scanning

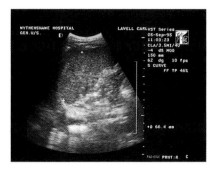

Figure 11.3 Abdominal ultrasound scan, showing a non-expanding splenic haematoma.

may be used to identify the likely source of bleeding [3]. If the patient has suffered major intra-abdominal bleeding, free fluid will be seen on the scan. The site of bleeding may be suggested by demonstrating specific organ damage and CT is particularly useful for the assessment of liver, splenic (Figure 11.4), renal, and retroperitoneal injuries. The decision whether

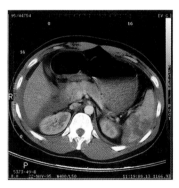

Figure 11.4 CT scan showing multiple splenic haematomas.

to perform a CT or ultrasound scan will depend on the available resources and expertise. Ultrasound scanning is operator-dependent and less accurate than CT scanning but has the advantage of being mobile so the patient does not have to be moved out of the resuscitation room. Recent studies have demonstrated that once trained to perform ultrasound, surgeons can be as accurate as radiologists in detecting the presence of intraperitoneal blood.

There was some optimism that ultrasound and CT imaging would obviate the need for DPL; however, scanning does not reveal the nature of any free fluid, so does not distinguish between blood and intestinal contents. If the clinical signs are difficult to interpret, intestinal perforation may be overlooked if a DPL is not performed. DPL and imaging should therefore be considered as complementary techniques. The findings of both ultrasound and CT scanning are more easily interpreted if performed prior to DPL, if the clinical circumstances permit.

Laparoscopy

It seems likely that diagnostic laparoscopy will be used increasingly in the assessment of abdominal trauma, as surgeons become more experienced in this technique [4,5]. The indications for laparoscopy are essentially the same as for DPL, namely a haemodynamically stable patient with equivocal clinical signs, unexplained blood loss, or neurological impairment following blunt or penetrating trauma.

In most centres, diagnostic laparoscopy would be performed under a general anaesthetic in the operating theatre, where it is easy to position the patient and proceed to laparotomy if the need arises. The procedure can also be performed in the resuscitation room, under local anaesthetic and sedation, with the use of small 5 mm laparoscopes, but the facilities and expertise are not widely available at present. Prolonged laparoscopic procedures are inappropriate in unstable patients and insufflation with CO_2 is unwise in patients likely to have raised intracranial pressure secondary to head injuries.

A thorough laparoscopic assessment entails manipulating and inspecting bowel loops, so that intestinal injuries are not overlooked. The confident identification and assessment of retroperitoneal, duodenal, and pancreatic injuries is extremely difficult. Nevertheless, it is proving to be useful in the diagnosis of diaphragmatic tears after upper abdominal stab wounds. Laparoscopy may also reveal whether a tangential gunshot wound has breached the peritoneal cavity and identify those for whom conservative treatment might be appropriate.

Laparoscopy should therefore be viewed as complementary to DPL and CT or ultrasound. If these investigations suggest intra-abdominal injuries, laparoscopy might help clarify the need for surgery.

Patients with a need for immediate surgical intervention

Some trauma victims have obvious life-threatening intra-abdominal injuries or bleeding when first examined and fail to respond to resuscitation. They require immediate life-saving surgery, without any further investigation.

The success of surgery under these conditions is dependent on rapid control of haemorrhage. The abdomen is opened via a long midline incision and blood and clots are evacuated by hand, swabs, and suction. Obvious bleeding points can then be controlled by direct finger pressure and by applying haemostatic forceps to any clearly identified spurting vessels. A more common scenario is to encounter continuing bleeding of imprecise origin. Under such circumstances it is best to pack off the bleeding areas to obtain temporary control of the haemorrhage, whilst the anaesthetist continues to resuscitate the patient. This minimises the risks of progressive hypothermia and irreversible shock. Once the patient is more stable, it is safer to perform a more detailed laparotomy and control the bleeding points. Specific visceral injuries are managed as discussed later in this chapter.

Patients with a definite indication for surgery

There are significant visceral injuries in 95% of patients with abdominal gunshot wounds, so a laparotomy should be considered as mandatory for such patients. The exception to this rule is after a tangential abdominal gunshot wound when the peritoneal cavity may be spared, and further investigation to look for intra-abdominal injuries is indicated. The clinical

status of the patient will determine whether preoperative investigations are appropriate.

Patients who present with embedded penetrating weapons and objects also have a definite need for surgical intervention. The object should be left undisturbed until surgery, as removal may cause further bleeding if a major vessel has been transected (Figure 11.2). If bowel or omentum has herniated through a penetrating wound, it should be covered with moist swabs to prevent desiccation, and reduced at laparotomy.

Surgery for patients with stab wounds

Victims who have been stabbed and have obvious continuing intra-abdominal haemorrhage, peritonitis, and embedded weapons require surgical intervention. Those who only have localised tenderness around the wound with no evidence of peritonitis or continuing bleeding can be managed conservatively with close observation of the pulse rate and blood pressure, and frequent re-examination of the abdomen [6]. If they remain well after 48 hours they can be discharged. Some authorities advocate exploration of stab wounds under local anaesthesia to ascertain whether or not the peritoneal cavity has been breached. In practice, this can be difficult and the premature discharge of a patient with a false-negative exploration may have serious consequences. If the peritoneal cavity is breached and the clinical signs are difficult to interpret, a DPL may be useful. DPL, however, has a higher false-negative rate in patients with stab wounds compared to those with blunt trauma. Visceral perforations are also easily overlooked on CT scanning, hence there is a need for close clinical observation of patients managed conservatively after penetrating trauma. It is possible to damage any abdominal organ following trauma, but certain visceral injuries are more common than others.

Hepatic trauma

The liver is particularly vulnerable to trauma [7], despite being partially protected from injury by the rib cage. One-fifth of victims of blunt trauma coming to laparotomy and two-fifths with penetrating abdominal injuries have liver damage.

Liver injuries may be classified according to the presence of haematomas, lacerations, and vascular injuries to the major hepatic veins or the inferior vena cava. Although there are several classifications of liver injury to facilitate the comparison of different management strategies, they are of less use to the surgeon who only occasionally has to deal with hepatic trauma. The American Association for Surgery of Trauma, Liver Injury Scale is the most widely accepted (Table 11.1). A more simple grading of liver injuries based on the liver segments involved and the magnitude of surgical intervention required is probably of more practical use (see box).

Grade of liver injury [9]
• Grade I: Injuries which do not require operative intervention, or any injury requiring surgery limited to one hepatic segment
• Grade II: Any injury that requires surgical intervention involving two or more segments
• Grade III: Any injury with associated juxta- or retro-hepatic vein injury

Table 11.1 Liver Injury Scale [11]

Grade	Type	Description
I	Haematoma	Subcapsular, non-expanding, < 10% surface area
	Laceration	Capsular tear, non-bleeding, 1 cm depth
II	Haematoma	Subcapsular, non-expanding, 10–50% surface area intraparenchymal, non-expanding < 2 cm in diameter
	Laceration	Capsular tear, active bleeding, 1–3 cm depth, < 10 cm in length
III	Haematoma	Subcapsular, > 50% surface area or expanding, ruptured subcapsular haematoma with active bleeding; intraparenchymal haematoma > 2 cm or expanding
	Laceration	> 3 cm depth
IV	Haematoma	Ruptured intraparenchymal haematoma with active bleeding
	Laceration	Parenchymal disruption involving 25–50% of hepatic lobe
V	Haematoma	Parenchymal disruption involving > 50% of lobe
	Vascular	Juxtahepatic venous injuries
VI	Vascular	Hepatic avulsion

Some patients with major hepatic injuries remain unstable despite resuscitation and require an immediate laparotomy. Diagnostic procedures under these circumstances only delay effective treatment. Many patients with a positive DPL from liver trauma, have injuries which stop bleeding spontaneously. They do not need an immediate laparotomy and many will settle on conservative treatment. Those patients who remain stable after resuscitation can be investigated further to assess the presence and extent of any suspected hepatic injury.

Ultrasound and CT scanning provide an estimate of the amount of blood within the peritoneal cavity and may confirm and delineate the nature of the liver injury and the segments involved. Dynamic intravenous contrast-enhanced CT scans give the most detailed information, whereas ultrasound is portable and more practicable. The clinical value of imaging is uncertain, as neither CT nor ultrasound scanning predict with sufficient confidence those patients in need of surgical intervention. The haemodynamic status of the patient remains of paramount importance in deciding when to operate. The information gleaned from a scan does, however, give the responsible surgeon a greater subjective awareness of the presence and nature of any liver injury.

Surgery for hepatic trauma

Performing a laparotomy on a patient with liver trauma decreases the intra-abdominal pressure. This decompresses any tamponading effect and increases the risk of precipitating further haemorrhage. The effective control of such bleeding is a challenge to any surgeon's skills. A bilateral subcostal incision gives the best exposure, although most major trauma victims found to have liver injuries will have been opened with a long midline incision. If there are significant injuries to the suprahepatic vena cava, the incision can be extended into a median sternotomy.

Pringle described a useful technique in 1908 to reduce bleeding from the liver, by occluding the portal vein and hepatic artery in the free edge of the lesser omentum at the foramen of Winslow, using a finger and thumb or vascular clamp. This does not, however, control back bleeding from the hepatic veins which can still be profuse. When there is bleeding coming from behind the liver it is important not to lift the liver forward, as this may precipitate torrential haemorrhage from torn hepatic veins. Additional control of bleeding from the liver may be obtained by clamping the inferior vena cava above and below the liver. This results in complete vascular occlusion of the liver which can be tolerated for about an hour at normal body temperature. If there are major injuries to the hepatic veins or inferior vena cava itself, internal shunting between the cava and right atrium may be necessary. Clearly such complex techniques are only likely to be successful in the hands of an experienced liver surgeon.

Standard suturing techniques to control profuse haemorrhage from major liver wounds often fail, as the sutures just cut through the soft pulpy parenchyma. Minor liver wounds which have stopped bleeding and non-expanding haematomas are best left alone and the area drained. Minor wounds which continue to bleed may be controlled with sutures mounted on blunt atraumatic needles. These can then be tied so as to oppose the edges of the laceration without cutting through the parenchyma. Tying the suture over a pack of an absorbable haemostatic gauze improves the chances of success.

Intrahepatic packing of larger liver wounds with gauze was introduced by Halsted prior to World War I. Whilst this is sometimes effective, secondary infection and bile leakage were common amongst survivors. Intrahepatic packing frequently fails as rents in major vessels in the liver wound are splinted open rather than closed. Towards the end of World War II improvements in perioperative and postoperative care, enabled hepatic haemorrhage to be treated surgically. Unfortunately, this did not reduce mortality, as more complicated surgery in critically ill patients still carried a high morbidity and mortality because of bleeding, secondary sepsis, and liver failure.

It is now appreciated that inappropriate attempts to control bleeding by opening up any tears in the major hepatic veins and inferior vena cava, increases the severity of haemorrhage. A conservative surgical approach with temporary extrahepatic gauze packing is therefore the favoured option for unstable patients with active bleeding from the liver. The packing should be placed around the liver so as to close the lacerations. The packs should be removed or changed after 48 hours. Packing may be life-saving and buy time to transfer the patient to a unit with expertise in the management of complex liver injuries, with a view to definitive debridement or liver resection once the patient is stable.

A useful technique to control bleeding from severe parenchymal injuries is to wrap the liver in an envelope of absorbable mesh that is sutured so as to close and tamponade bleeding wounds. Mesh hepatorrhaphy has the advantage that, if the bleeding is controlled, a second laparotomy to remove packs is avoided.

If the liver wounds continue to bleed despite surgical intervention and packing, selective angiography of the coeliac axis and superior mesenteric artery should be performed. This allows selective embolisation with coils or gelfoam. These techniques are also useful for patients with delayed bleeding who present with haemobilia.

Injuries to the major hepatic ducts are usually due to penetrating trauma and are easily overlooked at laparotomy. Small bile duct injuries may be repaired over a T-tube. More complex injuries, require reconstruction with a Roux-en-Y hepaticojejunostomy. Injuries to normal sized ducts carry a significant risk of stricture formation which predisposes the patient to cholangitis and secondary biliary cirrhosis.

In view of the risk of continued oozing of blood and bile from liver injuries the area should be drained with either a closed or open drainage systems.

Conservative treatment of liver injuries

Patients with intra-abdominal trauma who are stable after resuscitation may be discovered to have liver injuries on ultrasound or CT scanning. The associated bleeding may stop spontaneously. Therefore provided they remain stable, a non-operative approach is reasonable.

Splenic trauma

The spleen is vulnerable to both blunt and penetrating abdominal trauma (Figures 11.5, 11.6). The management

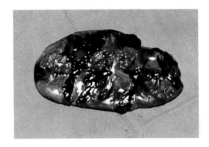

Figure 11.5 Multiple splenic haematomas. The patient had other major intra-abdominal injuries, so conservative treatment was not appropriate and a splenectomy was performed.

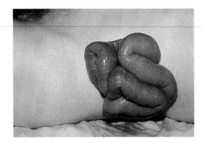

Figure 11.6 Spontaneous small bowel eviscerat through a wound in the left loin following a stabbing injury with a knife.

of splenic trauma is changing with a trend towards conservation of the spleen, where appropriate and safe. The spleen has an important immunological function, and splenectomy is associated with a small risk of subsequent overwhelming postsplenectomy infection (OPSI), which may occur many years later. This occurs in less than 1% of patients needing a splenectomy, but carries a very high mortality rate. OPSI is most common after splenectomy in childhood. Splenectomy is therefore no longer considered mandatory for all patients with ruptured spleens especially children [10]. It is not sensible, however, for a surgeon to strive to conserve a spleen because of the small risk of OPSI, when an expeditious splenectomy is needed to control the bleeding and save the patient's life.

Injuries to the spleen can be classified according to the presence of haematomas, lacerations, and vascular injuries to the splenic pedicle (Table 11.2). Splenic trauma is a common finding in patients with obvious overwhelming intra-abdominal bleeding who require an immediate laparotomy. Less severe injuries may result in localised pain and tenderness in the left upper abdomen. The clinical findings may be difficult to

Table 11.2 Splenic Injury Scale [11]

Grade	Type	Description
I	Haematoma	Subcapsular, non-expanding, < 10% surface area
	Laceration	Capsular tear, non-bleeding, < 1 cm deep
II	Haematoma	Subcapsular, non-expanding, 10–50% surface area; intraparenchymal non-expanding, < 5 cm
	Laceration	Capsular tear, 1–3 cm deep, not involving a trabecular vessel
III	Haematoma	Subcapsular, > 50% surface area or expanding; ruptured subcapsular haematoma with active bleeding; intraparenchymal haematoma, > 5 cm or expanding
	Laceration	> 3 cm deep or involving trabecular vessels
IV	Haematoma	Ruptured intraparenchymal haematoma with active bleeding
	Laceration	Involving segmental or hilar vessels with major devascularisation (> 25% of spleen)
V	Laceration	Completely shattered spleen
	Vascular	Hilar vascular injury which devascularises the spleen

interpret if there are rib fractures, a feature commonly associated with blunt splenic trauma.

Virtually all patients with splenic trauma will have a positive DPL. Ultrasound and CT scanning may demonstrate intra-abdominal fluid and reveal definite damage to the spleen (Figures 11.3 and 11.4). The nature and extent of these injuries can be assessed and graded, although the information obtained does not predict with confidence whether conservative treatment, splenorrhaphy, or splenectomy is appropriate. The haemodynamic status of the patient remains of paramount importance when deciding to operate.

If splenic trauma is confirmed on investigation conservative treatment is sometimes justified (see box). Conservative treatment is feasible in about one-fifth of adults and three-quarters of children with splenic trauma. Surgical intervention is indicated if the blood transfusion requirements exceed two units in adults or 20 ml/kg in children. A non-operative approach is successful in about 90% of children and three-quarters of adults managed conservatively. It should be remembered that blood transfusions are not without risk, so it is inappropriate to give massive transfusions just to save a spleen.

Requirements for conservative management of splenic trauma

- Haemodynamic stability after resuscitation with no evidence of progressive intra-abdominal haemorrhage
- No requirement for laparotomy
- Facilities available for intensive observation and repeated scanning as necessary
- Immediate availability of surgical staff and an operating theatre should an urgent splenectomy be needed

---

Operative strategy for splenic trauma

The key to success in surgery on the injured spleen is good exposure and retraction. If a laparotomy is performed and there is no active bleeding from the spleen, adherent clot should not be disturbed. Under these circumstances, the spleen must be carefully inspected, with judicious retraction of the abdominal wall. The lesser sac should be opened to exclude concomitant pancreatic and retroperitoneal injuries. The left subphrenic space should be drained and the abdomen closed. If there is active bleeding from the spleen, clots and fresh blood should be quickly evacuated and aspirated from the area to provide the best possible view of the spleen. In the presence of overwhelming bleeding, the blood loss can be partially controlled by grasping the vessels in the splenic hilum between finger and thumb, whilst resuscitation of the patient continues. Adequate examination of the spleen necessitates dividing its lateral and inferior attachments; this allows the spleen to be delivered up into the wound.

Conventional surgical techniques for controlling haemorrhage are often unsuccessful, as sutures cut through the spleen with ease. In addition, handling the spleen, however careful the surgeon, tends to aggravate the bleeding, and it may be further exacerbated by unsuccessful attempts at suturing. Under these circumstances, the safest option is to perform a prompt life-saving splenectomy.

If the spleen is damaged but the haemorrhage is not severe and the patient is otherwise stable, it is reasonable to attempt to repair the spleen. The chance of success is dependent on the experience and skills of the operating surgeon who must judge what is feasible and safe. If there is continuing bleeding from an accessible laceration an attempt at suture control is reasonable. However, this should be abandoned if it is not successful immediately. The sutures should be inserted through the splenic capsule, with good margins from the wound edges, which are opposed as the suture is tied.

Expanding splenic haematomas should be opened in order to evacuate the clot, and the bleeding vessel sutured whenever possible. For more severe injuries, the spleen should be mobilised, devitalised tissues debrided, and an attempt made to control the bleeding point. The cut edges should be carefully oversewn and defects closed with mattress sutures if feasible. If oozing continues, haemostasis may be improved by packing the bleeding surface with haemostatic gauze or fibrin glue, and by suturing the omentum over the raw surface. A useful technique for controlling haemorrhage is to wrap the spleen in an envelope of absorbable mesh, to tamponade the bleeding.

Following splenorrhaphy or splenectomy, the splenic bed is drained and the patient closely monitored postoperatively for signs of continuing haemorrhage in case further surgical intervention is needed.

Patients who require a splenectomy should be vaccinated against pneumococcal and *Haemophilus influenzae* type b (Hib) infection and receive prophylactic benzyl penicillin for two years.

Colonic injuries

The large bowel is injured in only 5% of patients with severe blunt abdominal trauma and rarely occurs in the absence of other visceral injuries. The transverse colon is the most vulnerable segment of the large bowel followed by the sigmoid and right colon. Blunt trauma may result in haemorrhagic contusions, partial lacerations, perforation, transection, or ischaemic necrosis (Table 11.3). Most abdominal stab wounds

Table 11.3 Colon Injury Scale [10]

Grade	Type	Description
I	Haematoma	Contusion or haematoma without devascularisation
	Laceration	Partial thickness, no perforation
II	Laceration	Laceration < 50% of circumference
III	Laceration	Laceration > 50% of circumference without transection
IV	Laceration	Transection of colon
V	Laceration	Transection with segmental loss

are inflicted in the upper abdomen and left hypochondrium, where the transverse and sigmoid colon are at greatest risk. Isolated colonic injuries are not uncommon after stabbings and carry a low mortality if treated early. The colon is involved in about 50% of patients with abdominal gunshot wounds, most of whom have sustained damage to other intra-abdominal organs.

The prognosis and management for colonic injuries depends on their severity and the extent and duration of any faecal contamination of the peritoneal cavity. A delay in diagnosis carries a risk of severe faecal peritonitis and overwhelming intra-abdominal sepsis. The site of the injury, whether proximal or distal is also important.

Surgical treatment of colonic injuries

It is important to avoid inappropriate repair of damaged bowel, especially if there is severe faecal contamination, because of the risks of anastomotic breakdown and intra-abdominal sepsis. If there is any doubt about the wisdom of a primary repair or anastomosis, they are best avoided.

Haemorrhagic contusions do not usually require specific attention as bowel viability is rarely affected. Minor isolated colonic injuries with minimal contamination may be treated by primary closure, following a thorough peritoneal lavage.

If the patient has more severe large bowel damage, with gross faecal contamination and other associated major injuries, the safest option is to resect the devitalised colon and exteriorise the bowel ends as a proximal stoma (ileostomy or colostomy) and distal mucous fistula. Some severe injuries of the right colon may be treated by resection and primary anastomosis, if there is little contamination and there are no associated major injuries. A repair or resection and primary anastomosis for more distal injuries, after performing on table colonic lavage and creating a covering defunctioning stoma, may seem attractive. However, there is still a risk of sepsis, if the repair fails, as faeces may spill over into the distal bowel.

An alternative option for large bowel trauma, is to repair the injury and exteriorise the affected segment of colon, and then cover with saline soaked swabs. Once the patient has recovered, the healed segment is returned to the peritoneal cavity. If the repair fails, the peritoneal cavity is not contaminated, and the defect is easily converted to a loop stoma. This can be resected and the colon reanastomosed once the patient has fully recovered. Although exteriorisation is commonly described in surgical texts, it is rarely performed, perhaps because of the frequency of conversion to a colostomy.

Trauma services are improving and patients are seen and treated at an early stage before progressive intra-abdominal sepsis has taken hold. In trauma centres where early surgical intervention is common practice, there is a tendency towards primary repair of large bowel injuries.

Rectal injury

Injuries affecting the upper part of the rectum, within the peritoneal cavity are managed as for colonic injuries. The middle and lower thirds of the rectum are below the peritoneal reflection, in a closed space, where disruption of the bowel carries a risk of major pelvic sepsis. The morbidity and mortality of injuries to the extraperitoneal rectum is greater than for other large bowel injuries because of the consequences of such infection. Rectal injuries may be classified according to the presence of haematomas, lacerations, and devascularisation of the bowel (Table 11.4). Rectal trauma often

Table 11.4 Rectum Injury Scale [10]

Grade	Type	Description
I	Haematoma	Contusion or haematoma without devascularisation
	Laceration	Partial thickness laceration
II	Laceration	Laceration < 50% of circumference
III	Laceration	Laceration > 50% of circumference
IV	Laceration	Full thickness laceration with extension into the perineum
V	Vascular	Devascularised segment

occurs in patients with major pelvic trauma when there are likely to be associated bony, vascular, and urological injuries. In the UK most penetrating rectal injuries are due to impalement or are self-inflicted wounds (Figure 11.7), whilst gunshot wounds and stabbings affecting this area are uncommon.

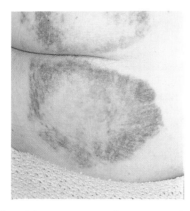

Figure 11.7 Buttock haematomas secondary to extraperitoneal rupture of the rectum, owing to the vigorous insertion of a foreign object for sexual gratification.

The perineum should be carefully inspected if penetrating trauma is suspected. In the case of self-inflicted rectal injury there may be no external evidence of trauma on perineal examination. The vagina and rectum should be carefully assessed by digital examination, sigmoidoscopy, and speculum examination.

Management of rectal trauma

If the rectum is sufficiently damaged to necessitate resection, a primary anastomosis is not advisable. The rectal stump should be stapled or oversewn and the proximal colon exteriorised as an end colostomy. If the rectum is amenable to repair it should be defunctioned by creating a colostomy as close to the rectum as is feasible. Loop colostomies are quick to create but allow faeces to spill over into the distal colon and rectum. It is safer to divide the colon and completely defunction the rectum. This can be achieved by mobilising the colon, which is then divided using a linear stapler cutter. The closed distal colon is left beneath the abdominal wall and the proximal colon is opened as an end stoma. This completely defunctions the rectum, whilst the bowel ends remain in close proximity, thus facilitating their eventual reanastomosis.

The presacral space is a potential site for infection and should be drained in all patients with major rectal injuries. Necrotic tissue and perineal wounds should be carefully debrided and left open to heal by secondary intention. Residual faeces in the rectum may propagate infection, even if the bowel has been defunctioned, so faeces should always be washed out.

Rectal trauma due to foreign bodies

An endless list of objects have been inserted into the rectum, and the history of the event may not be forthcoming. Serious injury is unusual as the rectum is rarely perforated. The anal sphincters may be damaged but subsequent incontinence is rare. The size and position of the object may be revealed by a plain x-ray. Most objects are easily removed, although this may necessitate sedation or a general anaesthetic and bimanual manipulation of the object from above and below. Once the object has been extracted, the rectum must be inspected for evidence of perforation, which can be confirmed by a water-soluble contrast study, if suspected.

Gastric injuries

Most gastric injuries occur following penetrating rather than blunt trauma. Gastric rupture is a rare consequence of a direct blow to the upper abdomen, for example from a steering wheel in a head-on collision. It is more common if the stomach is distended, with alcoholic beverages for example. If the stomach ruptures, the risk of sepsis depends on the time elapsed since the victim last ate. The stomach is usually empty between meals when the bacterial count is low, compared to soon after a meal when the bacterial count is much higher. The stomach is sometimes affected by traumatic rupture of the diaphragm when it may herniate into the chest. Gastric injuries should be suspected if blood is aspirated from a nasogastric tube. If the patient does not need surgery for other injuries, a Gastrograffin contrast study helps to demonstrate the presence or absence of a gastric injury, if suspected.

When the stomach is assessed at operation, the lesser sac should be opened (while the gastroepiploic arch is preserved), in order that the posterior wall of the stomach can be inspected. Stab wounds are usually paired with opposing wounds on the anterior and posterior walls. As the stomach is well vascularised its blood supply is rarely compromised and it heals well. Therefore the majority of gastric wounds, even long stab wounds, can be safely closed with sutures, so resection is rarely necessary.

Duodenal injuries

Injuries to the duodenum are easily overlooked, especially after blunt trauma and when the retroperitoneal portion is

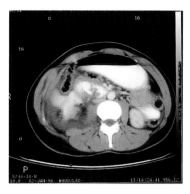

Figure 11.8 Double contrast CT scan showing rupture of the third part of the duodenum with extravasation of contrast into the retroperitoneal space.

affected (Figures 11.8 and 11.9). The duodenum is susceptible to haematomas and lacerations and the consequences depend on the portions of the duodenum that have been damaged (Table 11.5). A high index of suspicion for duodenal injury

Table 11.5 Duodenum Injury Scale [10]

Grade	Type	Description
I	Haematoma	Involving single portion of duodenum
	Laceration	Partial thickness, no perforation
II	Haematoma	Involving more than one portion
	Laceration	Disruption, < 50% of circumference
III	Laceration	Disruption of 50–75% circumference of D2
		Disruption of 50–100% of D1, D3, D4
IV	Laceration	Disruption > 75% circumference of D2 involving ampulla or distal bile duct
V	Laceration	Massive disruption of duodenopancreatic complex
	Vascular	Devascularisation of duodenum

should be associated with certain mechanisms of injury, for example seatbelt constraint, or handle bar abdominal injuries in cyclists. Many duodenal injuries are only discovered at the time of surgery. DPL will often be negative, but a duodenal injury should be considered if blood is aspirated from the nasogastric tube or the patient has an elevated serum amylase. A plain abdominal radiograph may show paraduodenal gas shadows. If a duodenal injury is suspected in a stable patient, a water-soluble contrast study or contrast-enhanced CT scan may provide useful information (Figure 11.8).

If a laparotomy has been performed, a duodenal injury should be suspected, particularly if there is an adjacent retroperitoneal haematoma or bile collection. Under these circumstances the duodenum is carefully mobilised and inspected. Small wounds can be closed with simple suture techniques and they usually heal well, because of the good vascularity of the duodenum. More extensive wounds of the third and fourth parts of the duodenum may necessitate resection and reanastomosis. Complex injuries to the second part of the duodenum are especially difficult to manage because of the proximity of the ampulla. There is much debate over the management of these injuries which are relatively rare in UK practice. Repair of the injured duodenum by protective decompression with gastrostomy, duodenostomy, and jejunostomy tubes is often feasible. The duodenum can be isolated as an end loop, by performing an antrectomy and oversewing

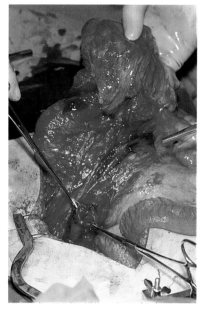

Figure 11.9 Rupture of the third part of the duodenum in a driver of a car involved in a head-on collision. The defect has been held open by the forceps. Note the bile staining beneath the ileocolic mesentery which has been mobilised and reflected upwards to expose the duodenum. The injury had been demonstrated on CT scan. The patient underwent early surgical intervention and primary closure of the defect.

or stapling the apex of the duodenum, with a roux-en-Y anastomosis of the stomach to the jejunum and drainage of the bile duct when appropriate. Any leak from the duodenum then becomes an end fistula which is easier to manage than a side fistula if the duodenum remains in normal continuity. An alternative is to repair and then "defunction" the damaged duodenum by occluding the pylorus with a pursestring suture and performing a gastrojejunostomy. The pursestring eventually breaks down restoring normal continuity, by which time the duodenal injuries should have healed. In some large duodenal defects an end-to-side roux-en-Y loop can be used for repair.

It is prudent to insert a feeding jejunostomy tube into any patient undergoing repair of complex upper gastrointestinal injuries. This allows the early reintroduction of enteral nutrition, in case complications preclude an early resumption of oral feeding.

Pancreatic injuries

The pancreas is to some extent protected from trauma, being a deep retroperitoneal structure, and is damaged in only a small proportion of patients with major abdominal trauma. Isolated pancreatic injuries are uncommon and they are usually associated with injuries to the adjacent duodenum, vessels, liver, spleen, and major vessels. This largely accounts for the high morbidity and mortality in patients with pancreatic injuries. In the UK most pancreatic injuries arise after rapid deceleration type injuries and high speed collisions when the epigastrum impacts on a steering wheel. In the USA most arise following penetrating stab and gunshot wounds. Pancreatic injuries vary from simple contusions, to fractures, lacerations, and occasionally complete disruption (Table 11.6).

Table 11.6 Pancreas Injury Scale [10]

Grade	Type	Description
I	Haematoma	Minor contusion without duct injury
	Laceration	Superficial laceration without duct injury
II	Haematoma	Major contusion without duct injury or tissue loss
	Laceration	Major laceration without duct injury or tissue loss
III	Laceration	Distal transection or parenchymal injury without duct injury
IV	Laceration	Proximal transection or parenchymal injury involving ampulla
V	Laceration	Massive disruption of pancreatic head

Diagnosing a significant pancreatic injury in the absence of a clear indication for a laparotomy is difficult. Isolated injuries may take weeks or months to manifest. An elevated serum amylase raises the possibility of pancreatic trauma, although a slight elevation is very common after upper abdominal injury and many patients with significant pancreatic injuries have a normal serum amylase.

If a pancreatic injury is likely, the most useful information is obtained by contrast-enhanced CT scanning. For patients with missed injuries or delayed presentation, an ERCP is useful, although this is rarely practicable in the emergency situation.

Many pancreatic injuries are discovered when a laparotomy is performed for other indications. A pancreatic injury should be suspected if there is oedema, haematoma, or retroperitoneal bile staining around the pancreas, and when it is directly affected by a penetrating wound. The pancreas should be fully exposed, by opening the lesser sac and mobilising the stomach and duodenum. If a penetrating pancreatic wound is discovered, it is important to ascertain whether or not the main duct has been damaged. For wounds of the body and tail, this is best accomplished by transection and distal pancreatectomy.

If an injury to the pancreatic duct seems likely, but cannot be confirmed on inspection, a pancreatogram should be obtained. The duct may fill if contrast is injected into the gallbladder. If this fails, the alternatives are to cannulate a pancreatic duct if visible, open the duodenum and cannulate the ampulla, or to transect the distal pancreas and cannulate the divided duct.

Pancreatic tissue which is clearly devitalised should be debrided. Simple contusions and minor lacerations require control of bleeding, and adequate drainage of the area. Capsular tears should be left open as closure increases the risk of pseudocyst formation.

Transection or disruption of the body and distal pancreas are best treated by completing a formal distal pancreatectomy. The duct and pancreas at the level of resection are oversewn or stapled. Approximately 80% of the pancreas can be resected before a patient is at risk of endocrine insufficiency and diabetes.

Injuries to the head or neck which do not involve the pancreatic duct are simply drained. Complex injuries with damage to the proximal duct warrant a distal pancreatectomy and roux-en-Y reconstruction to provide adequate drainage of the proximal pancreas.

Severe injuries affecting both the duodenum and pancreas are difficult to manage. Their treatment has to be tailored to the individual patient and it is difficult to make generalisations

(see "Duodenal injuries", earlier in chapter). However, it is prudent to insert a feeding jejunostomy at the end of a laparotomy for pancreatic trauma, to allow early enteral feeding even if complications arise.

About one-third of patients with pancreatic injuries develop fistulas; most are low volume and heal spontaneously with conservative treatment and parenteral or jejunostomy feeding. If the fistula persists, an ERCP should be performed to delineate the anatomy. The other main complication is the development of a pancreatic abscess, which is best drained by further open surgery.

Small bowel injuries

The small bowel is vulnerable to penetrating trauma and occasionally bursts following blunt trauma. Injuries vary from contusions and haematomas to lacerations and segmental loss (Table 11.7). These injuries are easily overlooked and leakage

Table 11.7 Small Bowel Injury Scale [10]

Grade	Type	Description
I	Haematoma	Contusion or haematoma without devascularisation
	Laceration	Partial thickness, no perforation
II	Laceration	< 50% of circumference
III	Laceration	> 50% of circumference without transection
IV	Laceration	Transection of small bowel
V	Laceration	Transection with segmental tissue loss
	Vascular	Devascularised segment

of small bowel contents can cause serious intra-abdominal sepsis if not controlled. The demonstration of visceral disruption is one of the main advantages of performing a DPL as these injuries are easily overlooked with imaging techniques.

If the intestinal blood supply is not compromised, small defects can be safely repaired. If there is doubt about the viability of the injured segment or there is more severe disruption, it should be resected and it will usually be safe to perform a primary anastomosis (Figure 11.10). Mesenteric

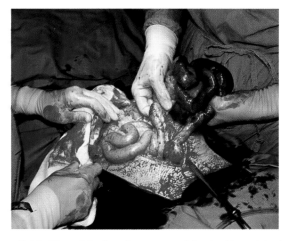

Figure 11.10 Tear of the ileocolic mesentery following blunt abdominal trauma sustained by a driver of a car involved in a head-on collision. The patient had major intra-abdominal haemorrhage and the associated ileum was ischaemic and had to be resected. He underwent early intervention and a primary anastomosis.

tears often lead to haematomas, such that it can be difficult to be certain of the small bowel viability. Any expanding mesenteric haematomas should be opened to identify and control the bleeding vessels. If the bowel appears viable, but there is some doubt, it can be preserved and a second look laparotomy performed after 24–48 hours, to exclude progressive ischaemia.

Wound management

There is a high risk of wound infection in trauma victims who have severe faecal contamination of the peritoneal cavity and established intra-abdominal sepsis. A thorough peritoneal lavage should be performed in all trauma patients coming to laparotomy, with saline or a solution of tetracycline. If there is overwhelming sepsis, the peritoneum and muscle are closed and the skin left open to allow the wound to drain. If there is little faecal contamination and no established intra-abdominal sepsis, primary closure is performed provided the patient undergoes early surgical intervention.

Antibiotics

Infection is a major cause of morbidity and mortality in patients who do not succumb to early haemorrhagic complications. The key to minimising severe sepsis is early surgical intervention, a thorough peritoneal lavage, and the prevention of further contamination by appropriate treatment of any visceral injuries. The risk of infective complications is reduced if all patients with major penetrating and blunt abdominal trauma receive early prophylaxis with broad spectrum antibiotics. There is much debate regarding the ideal duration of antibiotic treatment and the decision will be influenced by the degree of contamination encountered.

Summary

Faced with an abdominal trauma victim, a clinician must first decide whether the patient has sustained severe intra-abdominal injuries that necessitate an immediate laparotomy. Those who remain stable after initial resuscitation can be investigated further, by diagnostic peritoneal lavage, ultrasound, and CT scanning. All patients with abdominal gunshot wounds, embedded penetrating weapons, and perforated bowel will require surgery. Many patients with liver and splenic trauma can be managed conservatively provided they are haemodynamically stable. There is a growing trend towards splenic conservation for injured spleens, especially in children, because of the risk of subsequent sepsis.

References

1. Root HD, Hauser CW, McKinley CR *et al.*. Diagnostic peritoneal lavage. *Surgery* 1965;**57**:633–7.
2. Fischer RP, Beverlin BC, Engrav LH *et al.* Diagnostic peritoneal lavage fourteen years and 2586 patients later. *Am J Surg* 1978;**136**:701–4.
3. Feliciano DV. Diagnostic modalities in abdominal trauma. *Surg Clinics N Amer* 1991;**71**:241–56.
4. Crist DW, Shapiro MB, Gadacz TR. Emergency laparoscopy in trauma, acute abdomen and intensive care patients. *Clin Gastroenterol* 1993;**7**:779–84.
5. Simon RJ, Ivatury RR. Current concepts in the use of cavitary endoscopy in the evaluation and treatment of blunt and penetrating truncal injuries. *Surg Clinics N Amer* 1995;**75**:157–74.
6. Nance FC, Wennar MH, Johnson LW, Ingram JC Jr, Cohn I Jr. Surgical judgement in the management of penetrating wounds of the abdomen; experience with 2212 patients. *Ann Surg* 1974;**179**:639–46.
7. Reed RL, Merrell RC, Meyers WC, Fischer RP. Continuing evolution in the approach to severe liver trauma. *Ann Surg* 1992;**216**:524–38.
8. Shackford SR, Molin M. Management of splenic injuries. *Surg Clinics N Amer* 1990;**70**:595–620.
9. Buechter KJ, Zeppa R, Gomez G. The use of segmental anatomy for an operative classification of liver injuries. *Ann Surg* 1990;**211**:669–73.
10. Moore EE, Cogbill TH, Malangoni MA *et al.* Organ injury scaling II: Pancreas, duodenum, small bowel, colon and rectum. *J Trauma* 1990;**30**:1427.
11. Moore EE, Shackford SR, Pachter HL *et al.* Organ injury scaling; spleen, liver and kidney. *J Trauma* 1989;**29**:1664.

12 Urinary tract trauma

Simon A. V. Holmes
Consultant Urologist, St Marys Hospital, Portsmouth

Roger S. Kirby
Consultant Urologist, St George's Hospital, London

OBJECTIVES

- To appreciate and understand the regional anatomy in order to define the likelihood and type of injury sustained.

- To understand that careful examination of the patient can help localise the site of injury but to be aware that other parts of the urinary tract may be involved.

- To realise that prompt and thorough radiological investigation is necessary to identify those patients who require early intervention.

- To understand that expertise may be required from the outset to plan and interpret investigations so that inappropriate early management can be avoided, as these injuries can have devastating long-term complications.

The urinary tract is susceptible to damage from injuries to the chest, abdomen, and pelvis. Although fortunately uncommon, these injuries can be potentially dangerous owing to the consequences that can follow, namely severe haemorrhage and/or urinary extravasation. Haemorrhage more likely follows injury to the upper urinary tract because of its high vascularity in that it receives 25% of the entire cardiac output, whilst urinary extravasation more commonly follows lower urinary tract injury. If either or both of these circumstances are to be avoided, prompt and effective investigation, diagnosis, and treatment must be initiated. In this way the short- and long-term complications can be minimised and the normal function of the urinary tract preserved.

Applied anatomy

The kidneys lie high up in the retroperitoneum alongside the vertebrae T12 to L3. They are relatively well protected from minor trauma anteriorly by the abdominal viscera within the peritoneal cavity, and posteriorly by the lowest ribs and the muscles psoas and quadratus lumborum. It should thus be remembered that they can potentially be damaged by lower thoracic injuries. As additional protection, they are surrounded by the cushioning effects of the perinephric fat that lies within Gerota's fascia. Although the body of the kidney moves with normal respiration the renal hilum remains relatively fixed in position by the attachments of the vessels at the renal pedicle. This differential mobility of the renal pedicle and the renal body can lead to vascular damage during rapid deceleration injuries. The renal pelvis is an uncommon site for injury as it lies medially but it can rupture if it is already dilated as a result of a pre-existing congenital pelviureteric junction obstruction or any other congenital anatomical variant [1] (Figure 12.1). This is particularly so in children.

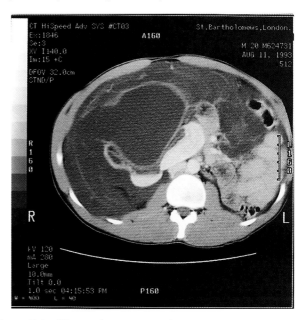

Figure 12.1 CT scan of a young man after abdominal trauma. Note the congenitally absent left kidney and the large pelvi-ureteric junction obstruction which had perforated leading to urinary extravasation. The right kidney remnant is marked on the scan.

The ureter is rarely injured other than iatrogenically. It runs down on the psoas muscle behind the posterior peritoneum and it is thus well protected from blunt trauma. It is also highly mobile throughout its length, further reducing vulnerability to injury. As a result of these features there were only 24 isolated ureteric injuries recorded during the whole of World War II.

The urinary bladder is a more common site of injury. In children it is predominantly an abdominal structure and only assumes its position in the pelvis after about the eighth year of life. It is then surrounded by the bony pelvic ring and the other pelvic contents protecting it from most blunt trauma.

In males the bladder neck is contiguous with the prostate and this is firmly fixed to the symphysis pubis by the puboprostatic ligaments. In women the pubovesical ligaments attach to the back of the symphysis. Posteriorly the base of the bladder is supported by the rectum and the rectovesical ligaments, and in females by the uterus and vagina. Inferiorly it is supported by the pelvic floor. As a consequence of these attachments the bladder neck and trigone remain fixed whilst the remainder of the bladder is free to expand during bladder filling, up and out of the pelvis where it is exposed to lower abdominal injuries. The superior surface of the bladder is the only portion covered by peritoneum. As a consequence it is the weakest and least well supported part of the bladder.

The *male urethra* is anatomically divided into four portions (Figure 12.2). The membranous urethra is surrounded by the

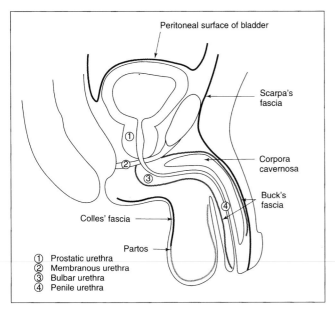

Figure 12.2 Anatomical arrangement of pelvic fascia and the male urethra.

urogenital diaphragm which forms a single anatomical unit with the prostate at the time of injury. Thus, if urinary extravasation from a urethral rupture at this point occurs, urine spreads within the confines of the Colles' perineal fascia. Colles' perineal fascia is a continuation of Scarpa's abdominal fascia and the scrotal dartos muscle. Extravasated urine and blood can thus extend posteriorly into the perineum and scrotum, yielding the typical "butterfly" haematoma (Figure 12.3), and superiorly up to the clavicle, which is its superior

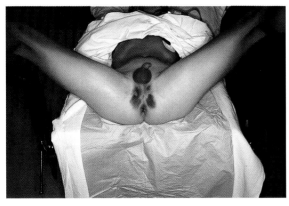

Figure 12.3 The typical "butterfly haematoma" from bruising confined within Colles' fascia.

attachment. However, it does not extend into the buttocks or thighs because of the attachments to the fascia lata.

The bulbar and penile urethra are confined within Buck's fascia and, thus, bruising after injury to these parts of the urethra may be confined to the shaft of the penis, assuming that the fascia remains intact after the injury. This is often not so with bulbar urethral injuries, in which case any extravasation again spreads within the confines of Colles' fascia.

The corpus spongiosum and corpora cavernosa are confined within Buck's fascia and any injury to the erectile tissues will lead to extravasation of blood within this space (Figure 12.4).

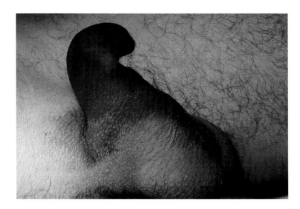

Figure 12.4 Bruising confined to Buck's fascia and the penile shaft. This injury was due to a fractured penis.

The *female urethra* is about 4 cm long, has a muscular wall throughout its length, and represents the external sphincter mechanism for the bladder. It is an uncommon site of injury, save in direct penetrating injuries to the perineum.

Mechanism of injury

Mechanism of injury is either blunt or penetrating. Penetrating injuries, most commonly affecting the kidney, are fortunately still fairly rare in the UK. They are usually due to stab wounds or gunshot injuries, but associated serious injuries are almost invariably also present (in over 80% of cases). Gunshot wounds are divided into those which give rise to high or low energy transfer. High energy transfer usually destroys the soft tissue organs directly in its path. Low energy transfer leads to cleaner injuries and, if these injuries are confined to a renal pole, the kidney can often be preserved. Penetrating injuries of the lower urinary tract are less common but can affect the bladder or urethra, and, once again, are often associated with other injuries.

Blunt injury to the urinary tract comes from sporting injuries, road traffic accidents, and industrial and domestic accidents. Renal injuries are typically caused by the kidney being crushed between the mobile ends of the lower ribs and the lumbar spine. This is often found in association with retroperitoneal bruising and fracture of the ribs, or the transverse processes of the lumbar spines. Indirect injuries to the kidney can follow a rapid deceleration such as falling from a height or a road traffic injury. In these cases either the arterial intima of the renal artery or one of its branches tears, and the flap occludes the vessel lumen. Occasionally the whole vessel avulses from the pedicle.

For the sake of description and also management policy renal injuries can be classified as either minor or major (see box).

Classification

• Minor: 80% of cases
  • contusion of the kidney
  • shallow cortical laceration
  • calyceal disruption
• Major: 20% of cases
  • renal pedicle injury
  • deep cortical laceration
  • shattered kidney
  • collecting system injury

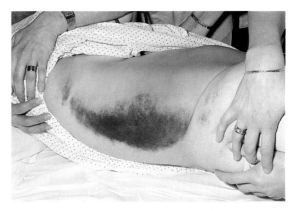

Figure 12.5 Loin bruising from a renal injury.

Lower urinary tract injury arises almost exclusively from blunt trauma. Rupture of the bladder can be intraperitoneal, which occurs after a blow to the full bladder through the weakest part of the bladder, or extraperitoneal, which usually follows a fracture of the pelvis from perforation by one of the bony fragments. In fact 75% of all the bladder ruptures are associated with pelvic fractures, and are thus extraperitoneal.

Likewise, posterior urethral disruption injuries result from delivery of a severe external force and are nearly always associated with a pelvic fracture. In all, about 10% of pelvic fractures are associated with some degree of urethral injury, the mechanism being the differential movement of the prostatic urethra, which is attached to the pubis by the puboprostatic ligaments, and the membranous urethra. These injuries are thus far more likely to occur in the male patient but can follow disruption of the anterior pelvic ring in females. Once the urethra is disrupted the prostate then rides up owing to the interposition of haematoma, and the two urethral ends separate.

Bulbar urethral injuries occur from trauma to the perineum, typically from a "fall astride" injury, such as onto a bicycle crossbar, or a kick in the perineum. Other parts of the anterior urethra are uncommonly injured, except iatrogenically, owing to its great mobility, but penetrating wounds do occur and foreign bodies inserted into the urethra may be a source of trauma. Penetrating injuries in the perineum also occur, but are uncommon.

Injury to the erectile tissue can follow any penetrating injury to the penis or may result from rupture of the corpora by blunt trauma, such as that which can occur after violent movements during sexual intercourse, giving rise to the fractured penis (Figure 12.4). Other penile injuries, such as amputation and skin degloving, usually result from the penis or nearby clothing being caught in some form of machinery.

Assessment

As previously mentioned urinary tract trauma is commonly associated with injury to other organs. Therefore the primary survey and resuscitation must be carried out initially as described in Chapter 1. Following this, a precise history of the mechanism of the injury must be obtained.

Once this has been completed attention can be directed towards the urinary tract during the secondary survey. A careful examination should be made: look for areas of bruising or swelling, possible penetrating wounds, crepitus or fractured ribs, and deformation of the pelvis (Figure 12.5). Renal injuries

cause tenderness on the affected side and a loin swelling may be palpated. The single most important indication of urinary tract trauma is the presence of blood in the urine or at the urethral meatus. A sample of urine should be obtained, if possible, by spontaneous micturition, or if this is not possible by bladder catheterisation, except when there is visible blood at the urethral meatus, or anything else to suggest a urethral injury. The amount of blood in the urine does not necessarily correlate with the severity of the injury, nor does its absence preclude significant trauma. A rectal examination should always be performed, not only to look for elevation of the prostate following urethral disruption, but also to check for any concomitant rectal and/or pelvic injury [2].

Radiological investigations and their interpretation

At the end of the secondary survey a more accurate diagnosis of the site and extent of injuries will need to be made. This may be part of a multidisciplinary effort depending on the other injuries incurred. If a renal injury is suspected, an intravenous urogram should be performed early in the course of evaluation, although, if available immediately, a CT scan is often more valuable.

If intravenous urography alone is available, a number of features should be looked for during the sequence of films (see box).

Radiological features of i.v. urography

• Control film
  • pneumothorax
  • rib fractures
  • fractures of transverse spinous processes
  • loss of psoas shadow
  • free peritoneal gas
  • soft tissue displacement by haematoma
  • spinal scoliosis away from injury
• sequential films
  • absent nephrogram
  • cortical tears
  • contrast extravasation

The absence of any nephrogram, even on delayed films, suggests severe renal pedicle injury (or an absent kidney). Cortical tears, extravasation of contrast, and ureteric injuries can usually be established on later films as the contrast moves down the urinary tract.

With the increased availability of CT scanning, this investigation has become the investigation of choice in large trauma centres in the USA. Contrast CT scanning is able not only to assess more accurately the severity of any renal injury and the depth of a cortical laceration, and to quantify the degree of perirenal haematoma formation or extravasated urine, but also to assess the integrity of other organs such as the liver and spleen. Segmental devascularisation may also be visible after contrast injection, and be distinguishable from simple haematoma. These findings are important because they can be an indication for earlier surgical intervention [3].

Should a renal vascular disruption be suspected, arteriography should follow immediately if some form of reconstructive surgery to the kidney is planned [4]. Arteriography is able to demonstrate occlusion of the renal artery or one of its branches (Figure 12.6); alternatively, it may define an intrarenal haematoma by demonstrating displacement of

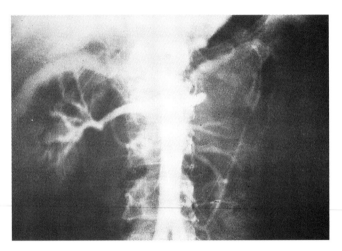

Figure 12.6 Renal arteriogram after rapid deceleration injury showing complete occlusion of the left renal artery from an intimal flap or avulsion.

renal vasculature and the collecting system. Perirenal collections and subcapsular haematomas that do not compromise the cardiovascular system can be diagnosed and followed with serial ultrasounds [5].

Ureteric injury should be suspected if the intravenous urogram shows a normal renal collecting system anatomy, with some delay of excretion on the affected side, extravasation of contrast into the retroperitoneum, and a normal bladder outline (from excretion from the contralateral kidney). If necessary, a cystoscopy and retrograde ureterogram (Figure 12.7) will identify the site and extent of damage, and simultaneous insertion of a ureteric stent can be attempted. This can be achieved under general or local anaesthesia, or sedation, as the clinical situation dictates.

Lower urinary tract injury may be more difficult to locate clinically and one is often faced with a differential diagnosis of ruptured bladder and/or ruptured urethra. In these circumstances the initial contrast study should be a retrograde urethrogram which, if necessary, can be performed in the emergency room. This study must include an oblique film so that the integrity of the urethra can be established. Extravasation of contrast without filling of the bladder is diagnostic of a complete urethral disruption, whilst a partial disruption is indicated by extravasation and filling of the bladder. If this study is normal the same catheter can be advanced into the bladder and a cystogram performed to look for an intraperitoneal rupture of the bladder. This investigation must involve injection of at least 250 ml sterile contrast material in order to distend the bladder, otherwise small holes will be missed [6]. When there is an extraperitoneal perforation the bladder typically has a teardrop shape secondary to compression by pelvic haematoma with contrast leakage confined to the pelvis (Figures 12.8 and 12.9). An intraperitoneal perforation leads to diffuse extravasation of contrast medium throughout the peritoneal cavity.

These indications for investigation are valid when any part of the urethra is suspected of being injured, and not just when a pelvic injury is present. In particular, bulbar urethral injuries,

Figure 12.7 Retrograde ureterogram showing ureteric injury and extravasation of contrast.

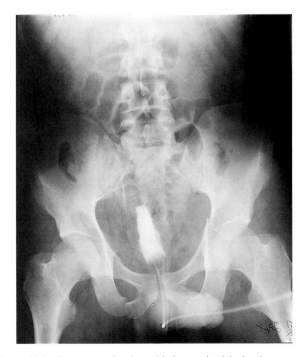

Figure 12.8 Cystogram of patient with fractured pelvis showing "teardrop" shape from compression by pelvic haematoma. There is no evidence of rupture of the bladder, although the patient had a ruptured urethra.

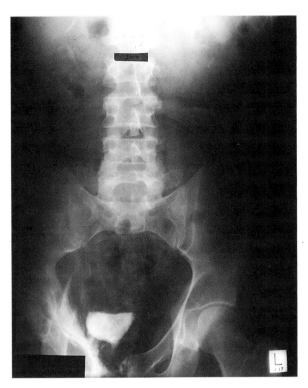

Figure 12.9 Cystogram of patient with pelvic fracture showing extraperitoneal rupture of the bladder and extravasation of contrast.

which are more common than posterior urethral injuries, can be partial or complete tears, and urethrography should be used to determine their presence and extent prior to further management.

In practice, when patients are severely injured, it is often necessary to perform both an intravenous urogram (or CT scan) and cystourethrography in order to delineate the anatomy of the entire urinary tract and to identify or exclude any significant injury.

Communication with a urologist

There can be no doubt that early diagnosis and management of urinary tract injuries will reduce the short- and long-term morbidity of patients. It is known, for example, that the need for a nephrectomy after renal or ureteric injury is greatly reduced if prompt and appropriate treatment is able to minimise urinary extravasation. The timing and need for urological assistance in the emergency room situation depends on the experience of the medical team in charge of the patient. Generally, however, as a urinary tract injury is suspected, a urologist should at least be informed. This allows planning of any necessary investigations to be coordinated with other specialities, depending on the range of injuries sustained. In fact, numerically, the majority of urological injuries are renal contusions and are managed non-operatively but the decision to take this course must be an informed one. Lower urinary tract injuries are potentially serious and can be exacerbated by inexperienced intervention. The passage of a urethral catheter in the presence of a pelvic fracture can convert a partial urethral tear to a complete disruption and should not be attempted without urological confirmation of urethral patency or at least without some previous experience. It is thus appropriate to involve specialist help with these cases even before radiological investigation is commenced.

Treatment

Renal injuries

Penetrating abdominal and thoracic injuries usually require surgical exploration, in part so that the full extent of the associated injuries can be established and dealt with. If present, isolated renal polar injuries can be repaired or, if this is not possible, a partial nephrectomy can be undertaken. Any more extensive injuries will necessitate a nephrectomy. All renal explorations for traumatic injuries should be undertaken through a generous intraperitoneal incision. The first objective of the operation is to gain control of the main renal vessels and this needs to be achieved before Gerota's fascia is opened and the kidney inspected.

Blunt renal trauma comprises about 90% of renal injuries and the majority of these (over 80%) are classified as minor, and early surgical intervention is not required. In these circumstances the patient is confined to bed until the haematuria resolves and is given prophylactic antibiotics and appropriate analgesia. Serial clinical observations of vital signs are made, together with, if necessary, ultrasound evaluation of the renal fossa.

The option of surgical exploration of major renal injuries is the subject of some controversy [7]. Life-threatening haemorrhage, renal pedicle injuries, and disruption of the pelviureteric junction with urinary extravasation undoubtedly benefit from early exploration and reconstruction, although a nephrectomy may be required. The remainder of major renal injuries are probably best managed by careful observation and follow-up with ultrasound or CT scanning. In an extensive review of blunt renal trauma Carlton found that 85% required no surgery, 5–10% required judgement and then surgical exploration, and 5% were non-salvageable and required an immediate nephrectomy [8].

The long-term management of all of these types of injuries involves a regular assessment of blood pressure and renal function, and a watch should be made for the development of hydronephrosis or arteriovenous fistulae.

Ureteric trauma

As previously mentioned isolated ureteric injuries are rare but if they do occur some form of surgical intervention will be necessary. The eventual surgical option depends on a number of features:

- site of injury (upper or lower ureter);
- nature of injury (blunt injury with avulsion or penetrating injury);
- timing of diagnosis after injury;
- associated injuries.

If the injury is complicated by one of the above features, that is the diagnosis is made very late or the wound is contaminated, a nephrectomy may be the best solution. If not, the two ureteric ends can be approximated and the spatulated ends anastamosed over a ureteric stent. If this is not possible for any reason, the options for upper ureteric injuries include transuretero-ureterostomy and ileal neoureter. In contrast, with lower ureteric injuries, the ureter should be reimplanted into the bladder with the help of either a psoas hitch or a Boari flap [9].

Bladder injuries

When diagnosed, an intraperitoneal rupture of the bladder usually requires surgical repair. In fact, it is an injury that is often associated with other abdominal injuries, and repair is frequently performed at the time of an exploratory laporotomy because of the symptoms of peritoneal irritation. The defect in the bladder is closed in two layers with an absorbable suture, and a large suprapubic catheter and a urethral catheter are left on free drainage. At 10 days a cystogram is peformed and, if there is no leakage, the catheters can be separately withdrawn.

Extraperitoneal perforations can nearly always be managed by urethral catheter drainage alone. A 20F catheter is left *in situ* for 10 days and healing is confirmed by cystography prior to catheter removal. The temptation to operate on these patients with pelvic trauma should be resisted if possible, because of the risks of encountering uncontrollable haemorrhage. Blood loss following a pelvic fracture can be considerable and, if this pelvic haematoma is disturbed during surgery, the tamponade is removed and further bleeding may be catastrophic.

Posterior urethral injuries

Of all urinary tract injuries there is perhaps the greatest controversy regarding the management of urethral trauma following a pelvic fracture. The aim of treatment immediately after such an injury should be to reduce the length and hence severity of subsequent stricture formation that follows these injuries, without compromising the chances of successful repair later. Such an uncomplicated stricture is amenable to a simple anastamotic urethroplasty and this reduces the risks of subsequent impotence and incontinence. A major posterior urethral and bladder neck reconstruction, however, is associated with a higher long-term complication rate.

Upon a diagnosis of a posterior urethral disruption injury, the initial treatment option lies between early surgical repair and delayed reconstruction. The majority of opinion currently favours performing a suprapubic cystotomy at the time of presentation, accepting the inevitable stricture that follows, and then reconstructing the urethra three months or more later [10]. If the problems of early surgery and operating in a pelvis full of haematoma and bone fragments are avoided, the risks of causing inadvertent incontinence or impotence are reduced. The technique of the subsequent delayed repair is variable but the operation can usually be achieved using a one-stage perineal stricture excision, combined with a urethral end-to-end anastomosis. Occasionally substitution urethroplasty, with the use of skin from the scrotum or penis, or even a transpubic repair, is necessary for particularly complex strictures.

Immediate urethral repair is a technically difficult procedure on friable, traumatised tissues. As an alternative, some authors have advocated alignment and approximation of the urethral ends by dividing the puboprostatic ligaments to allow the prostate to drop down into the pelvis from its elevated position. Alternatively, with a combination of open cystoplasty and urethral endoscopy, a catheter can be introduced to bridge the defect which will facilitate subsequent urethroplasty.

Anterior urethral injuries

The concepts of management for anterior urethral injuries are the same as those for the posterior variety: namely, urinary diversion proximal to the injury (by suprapubic cystotomy) and delayed anastamotic urethral repair. However, the differences in the modality of the injury and mode of presentation of anterior injuries mean that there are a few variations to this theme. Penetrating injuries by a knife wound or blunt injury from a confined blow to the perineum can be explored immediately, via the perineum, and the spatulated urethral ends anastomosed over a Foley catheter. More devastating perineal trauma, or those patients with associated pelvic or other injuries, should have a proximal diversion, and delayed assessment and reconstruction. Some bulbar urethral injuries will only be identified when the stricture develops some months after injury and these patients can undergo a simple anastomotic urethroplasty on diagnosis.

Urethral injuries in the female

Usually caused by a penetrating injury, these injuries are uncommonly isolated, and radiological imaging and subsequent surgical exploration of the bladder is often required. If isolated, early repair combined with bladder drainage is advocated, if urethral stenosis and/or incontinence are to be avoided. Injuries can also occur during traumatic childbirth, although these are uncommon and often unrecognised immediately.

Penile and scrotal injuries

Injuries to the erectile tissues can often be diagnosed from a combination of the history and the palpable defect in the corpora. Prompt repair minimises the deviations that result from subsequent fibrosis, especially during erection. Degloving injuries to the penis or scrotum should be thoroughly debrided of all non-viable tissue as they are often contaminated wounds. At the time of this exploration the viability of the testes should be assessed and the integrity of the urethra confirmed.

Summary

Urinary tract trauma is fortunately relatively uncommon. The consequences of it can, however, be devastating. Once the bones and soft tissues from other injuries have healed, a patient may be left with the long-term sequelae of urinary tract damage, such as incontinence, impotence, or recurrent stricture formation. The fact that these injuries most often affect young people makes them all the more destructive.

The principles behind the management of these injuries is simple:

- *Awareness.* Patients with thoracic, abdominal, pelvic, and perineal injuries may have urinary tract damage and the diagnosis should be considered from the outset.
- *Accurate diagnosis.* Radiological imaging of the urinary tract must be used to confirm or exclude injuries. This should, if necessary, delineate the entire urinary tract and it should be remembered that there may be more than one site of injury.
- *Prompt treatment.* Upper urinary tract injuries are mostly treated non-operatively but a proportion of cases require surgical exploration and it is these patients that need to be identified promptly. Lower urinary tract injuries likewise require careful evaluation so that those who need intervention can be selected. In these cases the general principle of diverting urine proximal to the site of injury is nearly always valid and it is often the only immediate treatment required. The overall management strategy should be to

provide an optimal functional result to the urinary tract with minimal long-term complications to the patient.

References

1. Presti JC. Ureteral and renal pelvic injuries from external trauma: diagnosis and management. *J Trauma* 1989;**29**:370.
2. Franko ER. Combined penetrating rectal and genitourinary injuries: a challenge in management. *J Trauma* 1993;**34**:347.
3. Peters PC, Sagalowsky AJ.Genito-urinary trauma, in *Cambell's urology*, (Walsh PC, Retik AB, Stamey TA, Darracott Vaughan E, eds). Philadelphia: Saunders WB, 1993, pp. 1057–68.
4. Guerriero WG. Management of renal trauma. *Urol Clin N Amer* 1988;**68**:1071.
5. Goletti O. The role of ultrasonography in blunt abdominal trauma: results in 250 consecutive cases. *J Trauma* 1994;**36**:178.
6. Cass AS, Luxenberg M. Features of 164 bladder ruptures. *J Urol* 1987;**138**:743.
7. Cass AS, Luxenberg M. Management of renal artery injuries from external trauma. *J Urol*, 1987;**138**:266.
8. Carlton CE Injuries of the kidney and ureter, In *Cambells urology*, 4th edn, Harrison JV, Gittes R, Perlmutter A, Stamey TA, Walsh PC, eds, Philadelphia: WB Saunders, 1978.
9. Hendry WF. Ureteric injuries, in *Textbook of genito-urinary surgery*, Whitfield HN, Hendry WF, eds. London: Churchill Livingstone, 1985; pp. 849–58.
10. Spirnak JP. Pelvic fracture and injury to the lower urinary tract. *Urol Clin N Amer* 1988;**68**:1057.

13 Pelvic injuries

Fergal P. Monsell
Consultant Orthopaedic Surgeon, Great Ormond Street Hospital for Children NHS Trust, London

E. Raymond S. Ross
Consultant Orthopaedic Surgeon, Salford Royal Hospitals NHS Trust, Salford, Manchester

OBJECTIVES

■ To provide on overview of the epidemiology, applied anatomy, and biomechanics of injuries to the bony pelvis.

■ To outline the assessment of the patient in general and the pelvis in detail following such injury.

■ To summarise the special investigations required to evaluate this type of injury accurately.

■ To describe details of the immediate and definitive surgical care of such patients.

Pelvic fractures are a diverse group of injuries that include fractures of the pubic ramus in the elderly, avulsion fractures in athletic individuals, and high energy fractures resulting from road traffic accidents. The latter group commonly have major disruptions to the integrity of the pelvic ring, a high incidence of concomitant injuries, and a high mortality.

> The mortality associated with major pelvic fracture ranges from 4–50%.

Whilst recognising that the low energy injuries can also have an impact on health care resources and may lead to long-term morbidity, this chapter deals specifically with high energy pelvic fractures. Acetabular and proximal femoral fractures will only be considered where they are in association with major pelvic disruption. As the definitive management of this type of injury is best performed in a central specialist unit, we will concentrate on the first 24 hours following injury.

Epidemiology

Major trauma to the pelvic girdle is relatively uncommon and accounts for approximately 3% of all skeletal injuries [1]. These injuries are more common in an urban environment and typically involve males aged between 20 and 40 years of age [2]. They are frequently caused by road traffic accidents and affect both the vehicle occupant and pedestrian. In the United Kingdom the annual incidence is estimated at approximately 1 per 50 000 population, which means that a regional population of two to three million will generate between 40–50 cases per year.

> In a survey of blunt trauma in the Mersey Region, 157 major pelvic injuries were recorded in a calendar year, with an overall mortality of 50% [3].

Recent advances in the management of these patients have involved a more precise understanding of the mechanism and pattern of injury. This has led to an appreciation of the need for immediate stabilisation in selected cases, adequate fluid resuscitation, and appropriate management of associated injuries. Nevertheless, the mortality associated with this type of injury remains between 4–50% [3,4].

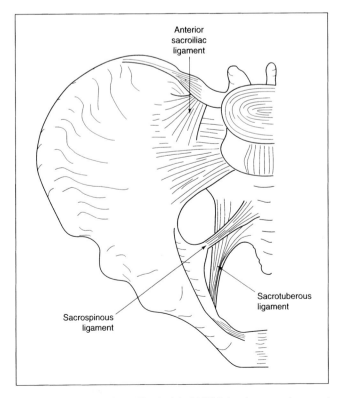

Figure 13.1 Lateral view of hemipelvis, highlighting the sacrospinous and sacrotuberous ligaments.

Applied anatomy

A working knowledge of the functional anatomy of this region is necessary to understand the fracture patterns which are commonly seen (Figures 13.1–13.3).

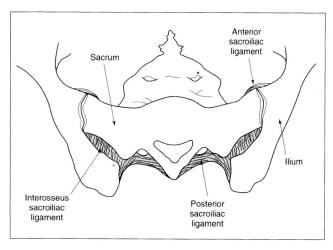

Figure 13.2 Axial view of sacroiliac complex. (Redrawn with permission from *Fractures of the pelvis and acetabulum* (ed. M Tile), 2nd edn, Baltimore: Williams and Wilkins, 1984.)

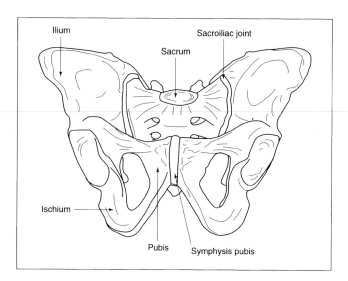

Figure 13.3 Anterior aspect of the pelvis, highlighting the pubis, iliopubic eminence and pubic symphysis. (Redrawn with permission from *Grant's Atlas*, 9th edn, Baltimore: Williams and Wilkins, 1991, p. 148.)

The bony pelvis is formed from the paired innominate bones which articulate posteriorly with the sacrum and anteriorly with each other at the pubic symphysis. This ring configuration is essentially unstable, and relies almost entirely on the intervening ligaments for structural integrity. The sacroiliac complex posteriorly and the pubic symphysis anteriorly are most important in this respect. The sacroiliac complex consisting of the sacroiliac joint, sacrospinous, and sacrotuberous ligaments, is of primary importance in maintaining the overall stability of the bony ring. The symphysis pubis is a secondary cartilaginous joint that completes the ring anteriorly.

The articulated pelvis forms a bony skeleton which surrounds the caudal part of the peritoneal cavity and the perineum. It contains the distal sigmoid colon, anorectum, bladder, posterior urethra, uterus and ovaries in the female, and prostate in the male. The proximity and arrangement of these structures accounts for the frequent occurrence of major

visceral injuries that are associated with pelvic girdle disruption. The pelvic walls and viscera are supplied by branches of the internal iliac artery and drain into tributaries of the internal iliac vein via the visceral venous plexuses that surround the rectum, uterus, and prostate. Haemorrhage from these structures into an unrestricted retroperitoneal space can be torrential and is associated, in part, with the high mortality that accompanies this type of injury.

Pathomechanics

The hemipelvis may be subjected to force in three primary directions. Each produces a predictable pattern of injury and will be considered individually.

> Instability may be defined as the potential for increasing displacement of the fracture with loading.

External rotation

This results from direct anteroposterior compression, a direct blow to the posterior iliac spines, or forced external rotation to the lower limb (Figure 13.4). This initially causes rupture

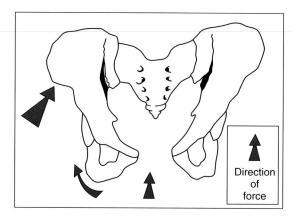

Figure 13.4 External rotation type injury. (Redrawn with permission from *Rob and Smith's Operative Surgery. Trauma Surgery, Part 1*, London: Butterworth-Heinemann, 1989, p. 495.)

of the interpubic ligaments and disruption of the symphysis pubis. With increasing force, the anterior sacroiliac and sacrospinous ligaments fail or avulsion fractures occur at their origin or insertion. The situation eventually reaches an endpoint with the posterior ilium abutting onto the sacrum such that any further force could lead to traumatic dislocation of the hemipelvis.

Internal rotation

The most common type of pelvic fracture results from lateral compression resulting from a force transmitted either directly by a blow to the iliac crest or indirectly via the femoral head (Figure 13.5). In either case the force can lead to compression

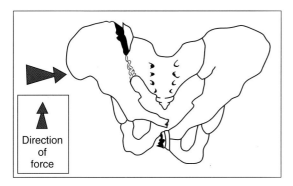

Figure 13.5 Internal rotation type injury. (Redrawn with permission from *Rob and Smith's Operative Surgery. Trauma Surgery, Part 1*, London: Butterworth-Heinemann, 1989, p. 495.)

fractures of the posterior sacroiliac complex and pubic rami on either the same or opposite side of the hemipelvis. The latter is termed a bucket-handle injury and, in this situation, the hemipelvis is typically rotated superiorly and medially.

Vertical shear

This type of injury was originally described by Malgaigne in 1855 [5] and is essentially a fracture dislocation of the hemipelvis. There is massive posterior disruption through the sacrum, sacroiliac joint, or ilium, in association with anterior disruption through both pubic rami or the symphysis pubis (Figure 13.6). The hemipelvis is usually displaced postero-superiorly and is accompanied by massive bone and soft tissue

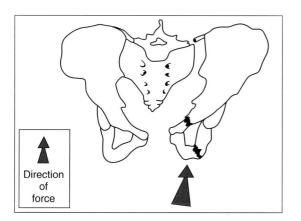

Figure 13.6 Vertical shear injury. (Redrawn with permission from *Rob and Smith's Operative Surgery. Trauma Surgery, Part 1*, London: Butterworth-Heinemann, 1989, p. 495.)

damage. This can lead to a high mortality or morbidity in those who survive.

> Vertical shear type pelvic fractures are always unstable.

It is important to understand how these forces disrupt the pelvis and produce the varying degrees of skeletal instability which will dictate the patient's optimum management. The

classification described by Tile [6] (Table 13.1) is useful, as it describes the fracture pattern according to likely instability.

Table 13.1 Classification of pelvic fractures [6]

Type	Pelvic fracture degree
A	*Stable*
A1	Fractures of the pelvis not involving the ring
A2	Stable, minimally displaced fractures of the ring
B	*Rotationally unstable, vertically stable*
B1	Open book
B2	Lateral compression: ipsilateral
B3	Lateral compression: contralateral (bucket-handle)
C	*Rotationally and vertically unstable*
C1	Unilateral
C2	Bilateral
C3	Associated with an acetabular fracture

In addition to the forces applied to bone, studies suggest that both venous and arterial bleeding following pelvic fracture occurs as a consequence of tensile forces on the retroperitoneal vessels [4]. The loss of skeletal stability associated with the ligament/bony disruption permits expansion of the pelvis beyond its normal dimensions and abolishes effective tamponade. Continuing haemorrhage into an unrestricted retroperitoneal space can therefore be torrential and is associated with the high mortality seen in these injuries.

Assessment

As with any clinical situation, a detailed history from the patient or from a reliable witness is crucial (see box).

Assessment in pelvic trauma

- Motor vehicle accident
  - time and mechanism of injury
  - seating position and seatbelt use
  - vehicle speed, entrapment, or ejection
- Pedestrian injury
  - speed and direction of impact
- Falls
  - height and body position on impact

The ABC of basic lifesaving in a trauma victim is the starting point for all patients. Once the airway has been secured, the cervical spine stabilised, and effective breathing ensured, then circulation must be considered (see Chapter 1).

> Major pelvic fractures are immediately life-threatening. Rapid, accurate diagnosis and treatment is critical if unnecessary mortality is to be avoided.

If the patient does not achieve haemodynamic stability, a cause of hidden bleeding must be sought and, where possible, stopped. In the past, immediate consideration has been given to intrathoracic and intraperitoneal bleeding, with little notice being taken of the blood loss from a pelvic injury. The dilemma that has been described by clinicians in this situation, where the site of blood loss is uncertain, must cease. If a patient has clinical or radiological evidence of pelvic ring disruption and obvious continuing blood loss, restoration of the pelvic ring should be equal in importance to the control of hepatic or splenic haemorrhage. In this situation, application of an external fixator, in the emergency room if necessary, will often prevent death by exsanguination. There should be no hesitation in applying such a device as part of the immediate management, and this should be performed before other diagnostic and therapeutic manoeuvres. The techniques used in applying this device are described in detail on pages 181–3.

> Restoration of the pelvic ring should be equal in importance to the control of hepatic or splenic haemorrhage.

> Application of an external fixator, in the emergency room if necessary, will often prevent death by exsanguination.

When the patient has been stabilised by immediate fluid transfusion, with or without an external fixator, further detailed examination is required to localise any associated injuries. The major cause of death during the early phase of treatment is decompensated shock. Consequently, vital signs including pulse, blood pressure, respiratory rate, and oxygen saturation should be continuously recorded to augment the clinical assessment.

External marks, pattern bruising, visible compound wounds and sensory abnormalities should be looked for as part of the general examination. This helps to evaluate the mechanism of injury as well as localising the underlying injuries. Scrotal, buttock, or diffuse bruising along the line of the inguinal ligament, suggesting major retroperitoneal haemorrhage, and limb swelling and deformity, indicating long bone fracture or hip dislocation, should be noted. In the conscious patient, pain should be localised, thus identifying concealed injury. The presence of limb paraesthesia suggesting neurological damage at cord or root level may be seen. Suprapubic tenderness is invariable, but generalised peritonitic abdominal tenderness may indicate a haemoperitoneum or perforated abdominal viscus. Inability to void despite a full bladder, fresh blood at the external meatus and an abnormally mobile, high-riding prostate on rectal examination suggest urethral rupture. *These physical signs will only be detected if they are sought.* Rectal examination is mandatory in the assessment of these patients and will reveal the presence of blood and palpable bony fragments in a transrectal compound fracture and alterations in sphincter tone associated with neurological injury.

> Failure to perform rectal examination in a patient with a major pelvic fracture is negligent.

Clinical assessment of pelvic stability involves direct manipulation by gentle compression of the iliac wings and traction on the leg. Severe displacement, extensive posterior bruising, associated neurovascular injury, and the presence of an open wound are all valuable clinical signs of instability and indicate the need for pelvic stabilisation to prevent further soft tissue damage. Furthermore, the mortality associated with this type of trauma is substantially increased in the presence of an open wound, and therefore a thorough evaluation of the surrounding skin and anorectal mucosa is essential.

Radiological assessment

Plain radiography

Anteroposterior radiographs of the pelvis identify the presence of a fracture in up to 94% of cases [7]; however, complete assessment requires further images, including inlet and outlet views of the pelvis. This simple radiographic series, coupled with careful clinical examination, provides a rapid and inexpensive assessment of the fracture pattern and stability. It can be performed in the context of any District General Hospital, without the need for specialised imaging techniques, and allows immediate decisions regarding external pelvic stabilisation to be made.

> Anteroposterior radiographs of the pelvis identify the presence of a fracture in up to 94% of cases.

The plain anteroposterior radiograph, obtained as part of the primary survey should be scrutinised for fracture lines, particularly at the pubic rami, posterior ilium, and sacral body.

The integrity of the pubic symphysis and sacroiliac joints should be assessed and the presence of associated injuries including proximal femoral fractures, hip dislocation, and iliac wing fractures noted. If there is evidence of injury to the pelvic ring, inlet and outlet views are required.

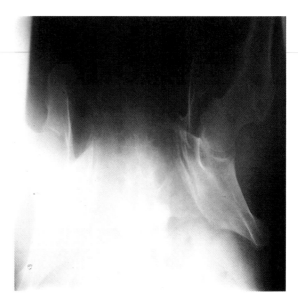

Figure 13.7 Pelvic inlet view. Note pubic symphysis diastasis and right acetabular fracture.

Pelvic inlet views (Figure 13.7) are obtained with the beam directed towards the feet, centred on the anterior superior iliac spine at an angle of approximately 50–60° to the x-ray plate in a supine patient. This projection demonstrates subtle compression of the ring, the coronal nature of pubic rami fractures, and evidence of posterior displacement of the hemipelvis.

Pelvic outlet views (Figure 13.8), in contrast, are obtained with the beam directed towards the patient's head at approximately 45° to the x-ray plate and are used to demonstrate superior migration and displacement of fracture fragments in a vertical shear injury.

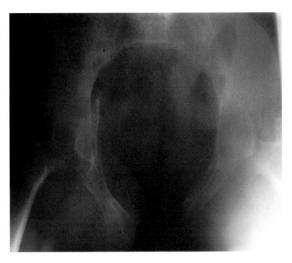

Figure 13.8 Pelvic outlet view. Note pubic symphysis diastasis and right acetabular fracture.

Computerised tomography (CT)

CT scanning has a major role in determining the integrity of the sacroiliac complex, and provides details of the exact configuration of a fracture. This information is valuable if internal fixation is contemplated, particularly of the sacrum and sacroiliac joints (Figure 13.9). CT scanning is not, however,

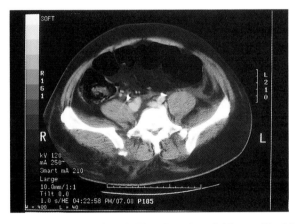

Figure 13.9 CT scan of pelvis. Note disruption of right sacroiliac joint.

essential in defining the optimum immediate management of a patient with a pelvic fracture, as plain radiographs, with careful interpretation, are usually sufficiently accurate.

Urethrography

Urethral rupture frequently accompanies this type of trauma and, if suspected clinically, is best evaluated by immediate ascending urethrography, prior to attempts at catheterisation (see Chapter 12). Ideally, a dynamic urethrogram should be performed, as this best visualises the posterior urethra, the most common site of injury. Occasionally it will be necessary to perform this investigation in the resuscitation room and this is best achieved with a 14G Foley catheter, inserted into the fossa navicularis, and inflated by 1–2 ml of water. After an initial injection of 5–10 ml of 30% Hypaque, a spot film is obtained so that extravasation from a partial or complete rupture can be demonstrated. If the posterior urethra is normal, a further 50 ml can be introduced into the bladder

to obtain a cystogram. Evidence of urethral injury is a relative contraindication to urethral catheterisation and in this circumstance the bladder should be drained by the suprapubic route.

Angiography

A patient with evidence of arterial compromise or continuing major blood loss, in spite of adequate fluid resuscitation and pelvic stabilisation, requires arteriography and occasionally venography as part of the early evaluation. Although this requires transfer to a radiography department the majority of patients will be sufficiently stable following initial resuscitation to allow this to be performed safely. Angiography is performed with a Seldinger technique, via a percutaneous, transfemoral approach from the less injured side. Once the cannula is in place, contrast is injected proximal to the site of suspected injury. Often multiple bleeding points from branches of the internal iliac artery are demonstrated that are amenable to transcatheter embolisation. If, however, embolisation is unsuccessful or there is evidence of major arterial occlusion, open exploration of the injured vessel is indicated.

Haemodynamic instability

Severe pelvic injuries rarely occur in isolation. Consequently, there are usually several potential causes for any haemodynamic instability. These include injuries to intra-abdominal or retroperitoneal organs, pelvic vascular, or thoracic injuries. Supra-umbilical peritoneal lavage may provide useful information, with the presence of fresh blood indicating an intraperitoneal injury that requires emergency laparotomy. The presence of a blood-stained effluent following peritoneal lavage must be interpreted cautiously as approximately 15% occur without major intra-abdominal injury [8]. However, the absence of blood staining following a properly performed peritoneal lavage reliably excludes intraperitoneal injury. Major thoracic injuries should be evaluated by physical examination and chest x-ray; occasionally further imaging including thoracic CT scanning and arch aortography may be required.

Management

External pelvic stabilisation

Indications

Immediate stabilisation is required for patients with uncontrolled hypotension, in spite of adequate resuscitation, for patients with obvious clinical instability or patients in whom instability is likely in view of the pattern of their pelvic injury.

Tile [9] has considered the biomechanical properties of a variety of fixation devices and concluded that an externally placed device is incapable of restoring sufficient stability to the pelvic ring to allow its definitive use. External fixation, however, does allow reduction of a displaced pelvic fracture and restore sufficient stability in the short term to arrest severe haemorrhage, and allow other life-saving procedures to be accomplished in safety. Furthermore, the application of an external fixator to the pelvis is a straightforward procedure which can be accomplished, where necessary, under local anaesthesia in the resuscitation room of an A & E department.

External rotation injuries to the pelvic girdle, with disruption of the pubic symphysis and unstable vertical shear injuries, should be stabilised early in the resuscitation phase of management. Internal rotation injuries of the pelvis with injury to ipsilateral anterior and posterior elements tend to be stable and usually do not require stabilisation.

If there is any doubt regarding the stability of a particular fracture, careful clinical assessment of pelvic ring stability should be performed in the manner described above. Immediate stabilisation is required for patients with uncontrolled hypotension in spite of adequate resuscitation, for patients with obvious clinical instability, or patients in whom instability is likely in view of the pattern of their pelvic injury.

Choice of equipment

There are many commercially available pelvic external fixator systems and the following description is intended as an overview of the principles and techniques involved. As the exact type of fixator may vary between hospitals, it is essential that any clinician responsible for the primary management of trauma should be familiar with the location and application of all available equipment.

Anterior external fixator

In essence, this technique involves insertion of threaded pins into the iliac blade and construction of an interconnecting, rigid frame. The frame can be assembled in a number of ways but this discussion will focus on a simple, effective configuration (Figure 13.10). Insertion of pins into the anterior border of

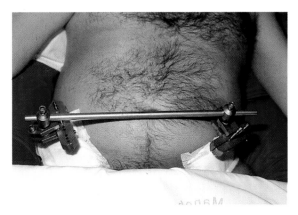

Figure 13.10 Simple anterior external fixator.

> It is essential that any clinician responsible for the primary management of trauma should be familiar with the location and application of all available equipment.

the ilium, between the anterior superior iliac spine (ASIS) and anterior inferior iliac spine (AIIS) provides a better mechanical environment [10]; however, in view of the potential for iatrogenic neurovascular damage, this should be performed only by individuals with experience of surgical approaches in this region.

Depending on the condition of the patient, this procedure can be performed in the operating theatre or receiving room of the A & E Department with general anaesthesia or field block using 1% lignocaine with 1:200 000 adrenaline solution. The skin must be prepared with antiseptic solution and the operative field isolated with sterile surgical towels. The optimum site for pin placement is immediately posterior to the anterior superior iliac spine and at the level of the iliac tubercle. The skin is incised transversely to allow subsequent compression of the frame if required, and the superior border of the iliac wing is exposed. The oblique orientation of the iliac wing may lead to incorrect pin placement. Consequently, it is recommended that a guidewire is inserted along both iliac surfaces to define the correct alignment prior to pin placement. Most pins are self-tapping and can be inserted with a brace without predrilling. However, it is possible to insert the pins with a powered drill, but this is not recommended as it may increase the incidence of damage to the deep neurovascular structures. When two pins have been inserted into each ilium, the pelvis is reduced by compression of the iliac wings in an external rotation injury, or traction on the leg in a vertical shear injury. The external frame is attached by a series of clamps and the construction secured by tightening of the intervening bolts.

The pin sites are cleaned with antiseptic and covered with a porous dressing; infection at the pin sites can be avoided provided regular cleaning and dressing changes are performed. It is important to exercise meticulous pin-site care, because infection may interfere with surgical approaches required for definitive internal fixation.

Posterior external fixator

In patients with sacral fractures or sacroiliac disruption, an anteriorly placed external fixator will be inadequate in establishing stability, and a posterior compression clamp has

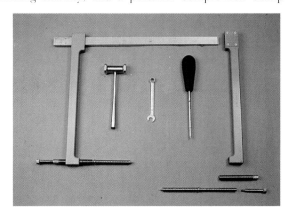

Figure 13.11 Pelvic compression clamp; component parts.

been developed for use in these circumstances (Figure 13.11).

This device is also suitable for insertion in the emergency department and has the advantage of being more straightforward to apply. In essence it consists of a clamp that delivers a compressive force, via two nails, to the posterior aspect of the pelvic ring. The patient is prepared as described previously and the anterior and posterior superior iliac spines are located by palpation. The optimum point of insertion in an average individual is three to four finger breadths anterolateral to the posterior superior iliac spine along the line that connects the ASIS and PSIS (Figure 13.12).

The potential problems associated with incorrect pin placement are listed in the box. When the site of insertion has been confidently localised, the skin is incised and the

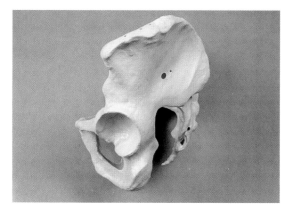

Figure 13.12 Pelvic compression clamp; insertion point.

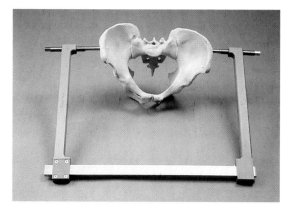

Figure 13.13 Pelvic compression clamp; inserted onto model pelvis.

nails are introduced through threaded tubes until they engage the outer cortex of the ilium; the clamp is then inserted over the nails. The pelvis can then be reduced as previously described and stabilised by means of tightening up the clamp (Figure 13.13). This device is recommended for short-term use only and should be replaced as soon as possible with definitive fixation. The same principles of wound management previously described are employed to prevent infection.

Potential problems of incorrect pin placement

- Damage to neurovascular structures emerging from the greater sciatic notch in a caudally placed pin
- Fracture to iliac blade in a cranially placed pin
- Displacement of hemipelvis in a cranially placed pin

Internal fixation

> It should be possible for a specialist to review the case history and radiographs within 24 hours of injury.

While the application of an external fixator is an excellent technique in the short term, the long-term results of this treatment in isolation are frequently unsatisfactory, particularly in patients with displaced sacroiliac complex injuries. Late complications of pelvic fractures are listed in the box. These

---

Late complications of pelvic fracture

- Malunion
- Non-union
- Leg length discrepancy
- Low back pain

---

may be disabling in up to 52% of patients [12]. This has led to recommendations for aggressive, early stabilisation by internal fixation in selected cases [13]. However, there are potential disadvantages associated with this management plan including loss of tamponade leading to increased bleeding, deep sepsis, and wound breakdown, especially following a crush injury. As these risks may be outweighed by potential benefits, any procedure should be considered on a patient-to-patient basis. Usually surgery is delayed for five to seven days so that the patient's overall condition can achieve its optimum level [6]. Where an early laparotomy gives access to the public symphysis or sacroiliac complex or when a posterior open fracture exposes the sacroiliac area, immediate plating may be indicated. When this situation arises, communication with a colleague with a special interest in complex trauma may be appropriate in the immediate post-injury period. In any event, with modern communications, it should be possible for a specialist to review the case history and the radiographs within 24 hours of injury, allowing careful planning of the early management and the delivery of optimum patient care.

Summary

Major fractures of the pelvis are still associated with a high mortality rate. It is therefore essential that doctors dealing with this type of trauma have the appropriate skills and equipment to deal effectively with such patients.

Aggressive fluid resuscitation must begin immediately and other potentially life-threatening injuries must be identified and controlled. In addition there must be restoration of pelvic stability so that massive bleeding can be controlled. The choice of external fixator device is dependent on an understanding of the basic pathomechanics and recognition of specific fracture patterns. Immediate stabilisation is required for patients with uncontrolled hypotension in spite of adequate resuscitation, for patients with obvious clinical instability, or in patients in whom instability is likely in view of the pattern of their pelvic injury. The definitive management of this type of patient is becoming centralised to specific units, and immediate discussion with and early transfer of these patients to such a unit is recommended.

References

1. Brooker AF, Edwards CC (eds). *External fixation: the current state of the art.* Baltimore: Williams and Wilkins, 1979.
2. Monahan PRW, Taylor RG. Dislocation and fracture dislocation of the pelvis. *Injury* 1981;**6**:325–33.
3. Muir L, Boot D, Gorman DS, Teanby DN. Epidemiology of pelvic fractures in the Mersey region. *Injury* 1996;**27**:199–204.
4. McMurtry R, Walton D, Dickinson D, Kellam J. Pelvic disruption in the polytraumatised patient. *Clin Orthop* 1980;**151**:22–30.
5. Malgaigne JF. *Treatise on fractures.* Philadelphia: J.B. Lippincott, 1859.
6. Tile M. Pelvic ring fractures: Should they be fixed? *J Bone Joint Surg* 1988;**70-B**:1–12.

7. Young JWR, Burgess AR, Brumback RJ, Pola A. Pelvic fractures: The value of plain radiography in early assessment and management. *Radiology* 1986;**160**:445–51.
8. ACS. *Advanced Trauma Life Support® Student Manual.* American College of Surgeons, 1993
9. Tile M (ed.). *Fractures of the pelvis and acetabulum.* Baltimore: Williams and Wilkins, 1984.
10. Mears D, Fu FH. Modern concepts of external fixation of the pelvis. *Clin Orthop* 1980;**151**:65–72.
11. Ganz R, Krushell RJ, Jackob RP, Küffer J. The anti-shock C clamp. *Clin Orthop* 1991;**267**:71–8.
12. Räf L. Double vertical fractures of the pelvis. *Acta Chir Scand* 1966;**202**:283–95.
13. Goldstein A, Phillips T, Sclafani SJA. Early open reduction and internal fixation of the disrupted pelvic ring. *J Trauma* 1986;**26**:325–33.

14 Limb injuries

Malcolm Smith

Consultant Trauma and Orthopaedic Surgeon, St James' University Hospital, Leeds

OBJECTIVES

■ To consolidate the priorities in trauma management.

■ To understand the importance of the mechanism and energy of injury.

■ To be able to assess and treat limb injuries.

■ To be able to communicate with the orthopaedic trauma team according to commonly understood basic principles.

Role of orthopaedic trauma surgeon

In the United Kingdom blunt trauma predominates. The MTOS (UK) Figures indicate that about 50% of such UK patients have extremity trauma. Though the majority of these injuries are isolated and not a threat to life, musculoskeletal injuries also provide the majority of the problems in polytrauma patients. As these multiply injured patients benefit enormously from early skeletal stabilisation, it is essential that orthopaedic surgeons are involved from the initial assessment. The old idea that they simply "set the bones" is outdated. Instead the Orthopaedic Traumatologist should be considered a key team member who can appreciate the global problems of the injured patient as well as providing a clear vision of the management priorities (see box).

The priorities of trauma management
● To save life
● To save limb
● To limit disability

It is therefore useful to further consider the importance of limb injuries and the role of the orthopaedic trauma surgeon in these respects.

Management

The overall management of the patient follows the basic guidelines described in Chapter 1.

With regards to the limb itself, the aims of treatment after assessment are to reduce and hold the fracture, and rehabilitate the limb and patient. Different forms of treatment are available depending on the fracture's degree of displacement, the need for reduction, the degree of instability, and likely healing process. The decision with regard to the form of treatment of more complex injuries is clearly one for the orthopaedic surgeon who will then take on responsibility for the patient's further care.

In all situations the general aim of the rehabilitation of the whole patient and limb should be at the forefront of the surgeon's mind so that appropriate treatment can be planned. On occasion bone injuries that are usually treated conservatively are treated operatively to facilitate early rehabilitation, such as the fracture of the humerus in a patient with lower limb injuries that may be fixed in order to allow the use of crutches and aid the patient's functional rehabilitation.

Whilst today the stable fracture is still treated nonoperatively unstable and displaced injuries are often reduced and held by operative means. The variety of specific implants available has now increased our ability to stabilise any aspect of the skeleton. Despite the improved technology, the overall aim of fracture stabilisation is to use the most minimally invasive implant that will facilitate bone healing and allow early return of joint function. This is most commonly seen these days with the femur. An intramedullary nail can be passed via a minimal buttock incision across the fracture and locked by transverse screws to provide bony stability along the whole length of the bone. The fixation needs to be stable enough to reduce pain, allow free nursing care, early limb rehabilitation, and facilitate bone healing.

After immediate ABC resuscitation the vast majority of patients require care of the limb injuries. This should be prioritised in the order of life saving, limb salvage, and disability limiting procedures.

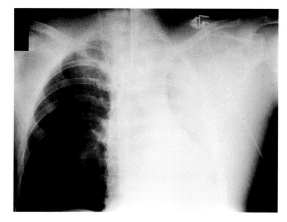

Figure 14.1 High energy injury to left shoulder with the scapulothoracic disassociation.

Saving life

With regard to saving life, the most obvious action is limiting haemorrhage from injuries to the pelvis (see Chapter 13) or from limb injuries where profuse blood loss can occur from single high energy injuries to the proximal skeleton such as the shoulder girdle (Figure 14.1), or femur (Figure 14.2), or

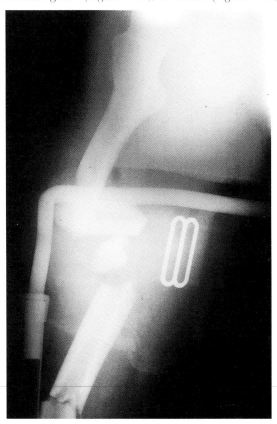

Figure 14.2 High energy fracture of the femur.

from multiple smaller injuries. Of greater numerical importance is the effect of early skeletal stabilisation on the general care of the polytrauma patient. Some years ago orthopaedic surgeons would consider a complex multiply injured patient "too sick to operate on". This led to long-term care on traction, considerable difficulties with nursing, and a situation which has been termed "horizontal crucifixation". Through the early 1980s it was shown that [1,2] the early stabilisation of proximal long bone fractures (particularly the femur) led to a significant reduction in mortality from multisystem organ failure (MOF) and the shock lung syndrome (ARDS). This improvement is thought to be due to the role of skeletal stabilisation in facilitating nursing care and enabling early patient mobilisation. Overall, this has resulted in a dramatic change in management and to a philosophy that "the patient is too sick not to operate on". Today early fracture stabilisation has become the norm throughout the developed world and the improvement in survival confirmed. Today our understanding of the complex immunological processes involved in the pathophysiology of MOF and ARDS is rapidly improving [3, 4]. Despite some cautionary work [3] there is strong evidence for aggressive early skeletal stabilisation in the vast majority of polytrauma patients. This philosophy forms the backbone of modern orthopaedic trauma management.

Saving the limb

Severe open limb injuries are a threat to both life and limb. Aggressive modern management includes wound debridement,

copious lavage, early skeletal stabilisation, and subsequently healthy (usually delayed) soft tissue cover. Close teamwork between the orthopaedic trauma surgeon and plastic surgeons who can reliably import fresh viable tissue from a remote area is essential. This has immensely improved the survival of limbs under threat [5] and such combined care is now the recommended treatment in the United Kingdom, endorsed by both the British Orthopaedic Association and the British Association of Plastic Surgeons [6].

Limiting disability

Despite the emphasis on life- and limb-saving surgery, the vast majority of an orthopaedic surgeon's time is spent trying to limit medium- and long-term disability by the treatment of fractures. Modern fixation has significantly reduced the disability time leading to rapid rehabilitation into the community wherever possible.

Anatomy

It is important to consider that limb injuries always have soft tissue and bony components. A cross-section through the lower leg is shown in Figure 14.3. This illustrates the outside skin,

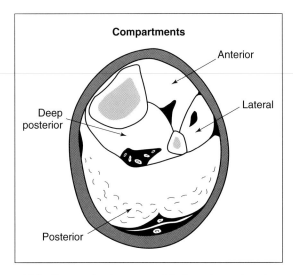

Figure 14.3 Cross-sectional anatomy of the lower leg to show the relevant deep muscle compartments enclosing neurovascular bundles.

bones, and layers of fascia enclosing the muscle compartments with their associated vessels and nerves. In the lower limb, the tibia and femur are the major weightbearing bones. In many situations nerves and vessels are anchored near bony surfaces and therefore at risk after local injury. In the leg this is particularly so behind the knee where the popliteal vessels are anchored as they enter the fascial compartments and around the neck of the fibula where the common peroneal nerve is subcutaneous. In the lower leg there are four compartments which are non-distensible. In addition to enclosing muscle groups these tether the tibia and fibula together and have an important structural role. This pattern is reflected in all of the limbs where the details of the compartmental anatomy may be different but the principles are similar.

A diagram representing a long bone (tibia) appears in Figure 14.4. The bone, consists of three areas: proximal

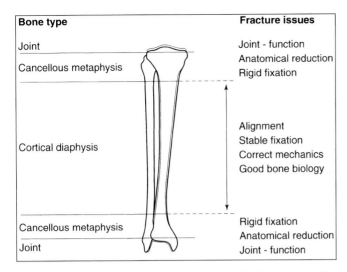

Bone type	Fracture issues
Joint	Joint - function
Cancellous metaphysis	Anatomical reduction
	Rigid fixation
Cortical diaphysis	Alignment
	Stable fixation
	Correct mechanics
	Good bone biology
Cancellous metaphysis	Rigid fixation
	Anatomical reduction
Joint	Joint - function

Figure 14.4 The principles of fracture treatment related to the area of bone injured.

metaphysis, diaphysis (or shaft), and distal metaphysis. Both the metaphyseal areas support the articular surface of the joint above and below. Here the trabecular pattern within the cancellous bone is aligned to transmit the lines of force and support the articular cartilage. Articular cartilage is hyaline, it has no blood supply, and it is nourished by the flow of articular fluid during joint motion. In both the knee and ankle, the articular cartilage is quite thick (2–3 mm), highly specialised in its microstructure, and essential to weightbearing and joint motion. In contrast the cancellous metaphyseal bone has many blood spaces and is highly cellular. In the diaphysis the cortex thickens as it becomes a strong weightbearing tubular structure. Here it is composed of dense lamellar bone with imprisoned osteophytes nourished through the haversian canal system. Whilst this bone is living and as such does contribute towards healing, its cellular activity is limited. Consequently the majority of healing is from the periosteum and endosteum. It is essential that treatment of diaphyseal fractures facilitates healing and therefore maintains bone vascularity, allows appropriate mechanical stress, and maintains fracture position whilst the healing process occurs.

Pathology

In principle it is convenient to consider two types of fractures: those that affect the shafts (diaphysis) of the long bones and those that involve the ends (metaphysis and joint). In diaphyseal fractures the problem is one of holding the reduction with a stabilisation device that will facilitate normal bone healing. The healing process in the relatively inert cortical bone of diaphysis can be slow. The patient's rehabilitation and early discharge is aided by appropriate stabilisation (today most lower limb diaphyseal fractures are stabilised with intramedullary nails). Furthermore, skeletal stabilisation allows early recovery of muscle function, joint movement, and functional rehabilitation of the patient. Recent knowledge has shown that micromovement [7] and good blood supply [8] to the bone fragments are essential for healing to take place.

Fractures of joints occur through the articular cartilage and underlying metaphyseal (cancellous) bone. Here the bone is more cellular and bone healing less of a problem. However displacement of an articular fracture leads to early degenerate change, stiffness, pain, and deformity [9]. The management in these circumstances aims to restore and maintain the normal

anatomy by stable internal fixation [10]. This enables joint movement and thereby facilitates articular cartilage nourishment by the flow of synovial fluid.

Energy of injury

The concept of energy of injury is important with regard to both the whole patient and the limb injury. Low energy injuries tend to be isolated, uncomplicated, and associated with more minor soft tissue damage (Figure 14.5). Often

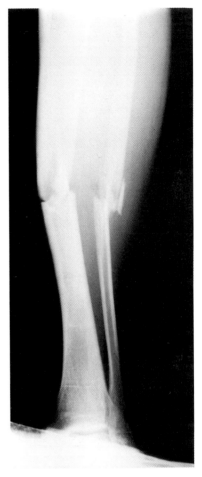

Figure 14.5 Low energy fracture of the tibia.

the bony injury is relatively stable and only requires simple treatment although some, because of an unstable fracture pattern, may require operative care in order to maintain alignment during healing. As the transfer of energy at the time of the injury increases then so does the degree of local tissue disruption [4] and the chances of associated injuries (see Chapter 22). With regard to the limb itself, the energy of injury is the main factor associated with the severity of injury, the treatment required, and long-term prognosis. High energy transfers are commonly associated with a more severe soft tissue injury, often a breach in the skin (open fractures), and commonly a multifragmentary, unstable bone injury that requires fixation. However, a more simple fracture pattern may also be present in a high energy injury. This general rule is the same for penetrating trauma. For example, knives produce less damage than low velocity projectiles, whereas high energy projectiles cause massive energy transfer with cavitation and bone destruction.

Pathophysiology

After a fracture, a haematoma forms, diaphyseal bone ends die back, and subsequent cellular repair material from periosteum and endosteum envelopes the fracture and eventually provides early bone union. Later this enveloping material converts to fibrous tissue, callus, and immature woven bone. Subsequent remodelling into lamellar bone takes a considerable time but eventually a true cortical tube reforms.

Compartment syndrome

This condition results from haematoma or soft tissue (muscle) swelling after injury. The injury can occasionally be minor and does not have to include bone injury. The pathophysiology of this syndrome is that after injury, progressive muscle swelling occurs such that the pressure within the muscle compartment exceeds venous pressure; this prevents venous drainage and further swelling, and then occludes the local arterial supply causing muscle infarction. In the acute phase the muscle infarction can cause a threat to the limb and to life owing to infection or myoglobinuria. If the infection is avoided the final result is fibrotic contraction of muscle which appears white and does not contract. This muscle fibrosis produces contracture and poor joint function.

Assessment

The assessment of the majority of limb injuries will take place during the secondary survey, after initial resuscitation is underway (see Chapter 1). With regard to extremity trauma the only exception is of profuse bleeding where control of haemorrhage by direct pressure may be necessary during the primary survey for circulatory resuscitation.

Indentification of fractures can be difficult (see box) particularly when there is a thick overlying muscle or obvious coexisting trauma. Limb assessment therefore requires a methodical approach incorporating clinical suspicion and radiology.

Sites of occult fractures which can be commonly missed

- Shoulder girdle
- Whole spine
- Pelvis/acetabulum
- Femoral neck
- Femoral condyles
- Wrist and fingers
- Feet and toes

Symptoms and signs of bony injury

- Pain and tenderness
- Swelling
- Deformity
- Abnormal posture or movement
- Crepitus
- Obvious bony ends

Simple clinical assessment of the limb for symptoms and signs as shown in the box should be performed looking for swelling, tenderness or deformity, abnormal movement, or crepitus. Whenever an injury to the limb is suspected the distal neurovascular status must be assessed and recorded. The neurological status is important for treatment planning although the prognosis is usually determined by the injury. Assessment of the vascular status is essential as the presence of a vascular injury converts a more straightforward injury into a major surgical emergency (see box).

Signs of vascular insufficiency

- Pain (severe and unremitting)
- Perishing cold
- Paraesthesia
- Pallor or purple colouring
- Paralysis
- Pulse reduced or absent
- Poor capillary refill

If the patient is conscious, the clinical history and mechanism of injury provides the major clue to the pattern of injury, aided of course, by complaints of pain or tenderness. If the patient is unconscious valuable information will be provided by the paramedics and a careful systemic examination is essential. Assessment is always easier as early as possible; the orthopaedic trauma surgeon should be involved during the resuscitation of all seriously injured patients. If the patient has an isolated injury he or she should be informed as soon as a significant muscular skeletal injury is suspected.

In open fractures the initial assessment in A & E should grade the injury with regard to gross severity as minor, moderate, or severe, and note the degree of contamination. Formal grading (Table 14.1) is only possible after surgical

Table 14.1 Open fracture classification (Guistillo)

Grade	Description
I	Low energy, minimal soft tissue damage, wound < 1 cm
II	Higher energy, laceration > 1 cm, no flaps or crushing minimal contamination, slight comminution
IIIa	High energy, adequate soft tissue cover despite flaps or lacerations, comminuted or segmental fracture
IIIb	High energy, extensive soft tissue stripping, massive contamination, inadequate soft tissue cover
IIIc	Vascular injury requiring repair, any open fracture

debridement. The open fracture is a surgical emergency because of the possible risk to life, certain risk to limb, and high chance of late soft tissue and bone infection. The neurovascular status must be recorded. The patient's next wound assessment will be in the operating room prior to definitive treatment. The presence of a vascular injury in association with an open fracture carries the worst possible prognosis and must be identified immediately. A white limb below the level of injury with empty veins and cool skin will be easy to identify. However, on many occasions a serious vascular injury may not be so obvious and a high index of suspicion should lead to further investigation which requires specialist referral and may need angiography.

The absence of an open wound does not mean that the fracture is low energy; a severe soft tissue injury can exist within a closed skin envelope and carry the same serious poor prognosis for limb salvage, bone healing, and subsequent function as a serious open injury. Accordingly a general assessment of the degree of soft tissue damage (Table 14.2)

Table 14.2 Soft tissue injury in closed fractures

Grade	Example
Minor	Greenstick fracture of the forearm of a child
Moderate	The generalised swelling and haematoma often seen around a fractured tibia
Severe	The generalised swelling of a massive haematoma formation and stripping of skin from its underlying fascia, or with a compartment syndrome

inside a closed skin envelope should be attempted and recorded by an assessment of the swelling, bruising, and condition of the muscle compartments. A serious vascular injury can also be present in a closed fracture.

Compartment syndrome

The pathognomic clinical sign of a compartment syndrome is *pain*. This occurs initially on stretching the involved muscles but is subsequently severe and unremitting if the pressure is not relieved as an emergency.

Radiological interpretation

An x-ray of bone defines the majority of fracture patterns but can only provide clues to the degree of soft tissue damage and cannot provide any information with regard to the viability of bone fragments. The essential test for bone injuries are two plain x-ray views at right angles to one another and incorporating the joint above and below the injury. A number of additional films may be required to satisfy this (Figure 14.6). In some situations it is appropriate to obtain oblique views (for example, acetabulum, pelvis, scaphoid) as these bones do not lie in the neutral plane to the x-ray beam. If a fracture extends into a joint then radiographs of the joint itself are essential.

Sometimes simple x-ray examinations alone will not adequately define the fracture and further radiological investigations by CT scan (Figure 14.7), tomography, or bone scanning (Figure 14.8) may be required. However, complex investigations should only be initiated after specialist advice and never delay essential initial treatment. The majority of more complex investigations are used to confirm the diagnosis

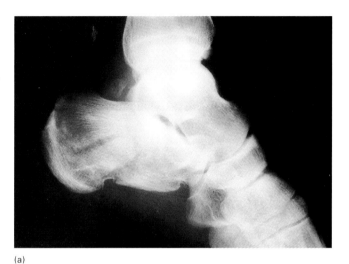

(a)

(b)

Figure 14.7 A multifragmentary os calcis fracture (a) involving the subtalar joint whose anatomy is illustrated best by CT scanning at right angles in the plane of the joint (b). A clear step in the subtalar joint can be seen.

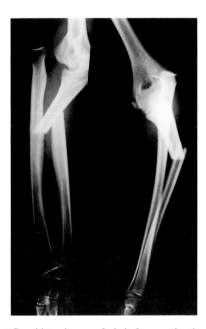

Figure 14.6 AP and lateral x-ray of whole forearm showing an ulna fracture with a dislocation of the radial head (Monteggia fracture). It is essential to show the whole bone in two planes including the joint above and joint below to define the injury fully.

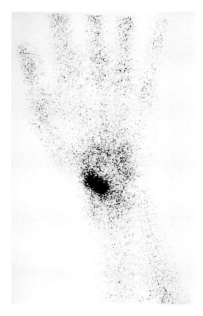

Figure 14.8 A positive technetium bone scan taken two weeks after the scaphoid fracture.

of fracture or performed preoperatively to identify complex fracture patterns and to help plan reconstructive surgery. Obvious fracture dislocations (usually of the ankle) should be reduced before x-ray, if possible, to relieve the pressure on the skin.

Bone scanning is often used to show occult fractures which are not visible on normal x-ray and where bone formation is occurring. This was popular in the scaphoid where fractures can be difficult to see on routine x-ray views. More recently MRI scanning is being used for the same reason. Inspection of the soft tissues on limb x-rays is often ignored. This is unfortunate as it can provide clues to the presence of underlying fractures and the degree of energy transfer. The presence of significant soft tissue swelling and local air should be identified.

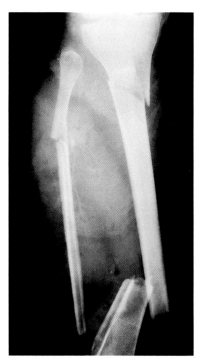

Figure 14.9 High energy fracture of the tibia.

In some areas, such as in the knee or elbow, an effusion can easily be seen. Wide separation of the bony fragments as shown in Figure 14.9 indicates high energy transfer.

Communication with orthopaedic surgeons

The orthopaedic trauma surgeon is a key member of the trauma team who can only contribute to the patient's care when there has been good early communication. The character of the orthopaedic service and the specialist services that it provides will depend on the hospital involved and in some situations early communication with a regional specialist centre (for example, reparding injuries to the spine, pelvis or hand, or complex open injuries) may be required from the outset (see box).

Essential information required
• Clear history indicating the mechanism and energy of injury
• Isolated injury or polytrauma
• General patient condition
• Bony injury
• fracture site
• pattern
• displacement
• Neurovascular status
• pre-injury
• post-injury
• after any intervention
• Soft tissues
• open (minimal, moderate or severe, and degree of contamination)
• closed (bruising, degloving, potential compartment syndrome)
• Treatment and response

Good communication requires a clear history with a mechanism of injury, followed by a description of the specific injury and the general condition of the patient. With regard to the limb, information is required on the bone, soft tissue, distal neurovascular status, and any intervention that has taken place. It is essential to know about the presence or absence of the distal pulse and neurological function as the former changes the situation to one of an extreme emergency. With regard to soft tissue injuries in open fractures, a simple grading is initially all that is required as formal assessment is only possible in theatre and after debridement. Despite the numerous complex fracture classification systems, a simple description is first required. This should include an assessment of the fracture pattern (either transverse, oblique, spiral, or multifragmentary), displacement (describing the position of the distal part relative to the proximal part in terms of the proportion of the bone width itself that is displaced), the angulation, and rotation. These descriptive terms are important for assessing stability and the requirement for further treatment.

An assessment of the energy transfer at the time of injury is essential for prediction of the extent of hard and soft tissue damage, and subsequent prognosis. In addition an understanding of the mechanism of injury will guide the initial assessment to occult injuries that would otherwise be unsuspected.

Injuries to the soft tissues are a fundamental part of limb injuries, and no fracture can be considered without its soft tissue envelope. Whilst open fractures allow for contamination of the fracture haematoma, some closed fractures can be equally serious, particularly when they result from high energy transfer. Accordingly closed fractures must not be considered less of a problem than open fractures. Severe open fractures require expert combined orthopaedic and plastic surgical care. A compartment syndrome can be a threat to life, limb, and long-term function.

General assessment of the limb incorporates an accurate history, a methodical clinical examination and a radiological assessment. The routine plain x-rays should be in two planes and show the whole bone including the joint above and the joint below. Occasionally more complex investigations are required.

Given the frequency of limb injury, orthopaedic surgeons should be involved in the initial assessment of all polytrauma patients and be informed rapidly of the presence of a patient with a significant isolated limb injury. Management of trauma patients is multidisciplinary. There are many pitfalls but good communication and preplanning solves the majority of problems.

References

1. Bone LB, Johnson KD, Weigech J et al. Early versus delayed stabilization of femur fractures. J Bone Joint Surgery 1989;71-A: 336-40.
2. Johnson KD, Cadambi A, Siebert GB. Incidence of adult respiratory distress syndrome in patients with multiple musculoskeletal injuries: Effect of early operative stabilization of fractures. J Trauma 1985;25:375-84.
3. Pape HC, Giannoudis PV, Smith RA. Influence of thoracic trauma and primary femoral intramedullary nailing on the incidence of ARDS in multiple trauma patients. Injury 1993;24:82-103.
4. Giannoudis P et al. Molecular mediations in trauma. British Trauma Society Meeting, Leeds. Oct 6-7,1995.
5. Green AR. The courage to co-operate: the team approach to open fractures of the lower limb. Ann R Coll Surg Engl 1994;76:365-6.
6. British Orthopaedic Assoc & British Assoc of Plastic Surgeons. The early management of severe tibial fractures: the need for combined plastic and orthopaedic management. Report of the BOA/BAPS Working party on Severe Tibial Injuries, Journal 1993.
7. Sarmiento A. A functional below-the-knee cast for tibial fractures. J Bone Joint Surgery 1967;49-A:855-75.
8. Perren SH, Cordey J, Rahn BA, Gautier E, Schneider E. Early temporary porosis of bone induced by internal fixation implants. A reaction to necrosis not to stress protection? Clin Orthop 1988;232:139-51.
9. Schatzker J. Changes in the AO/ASIF principles and methods. Injury 1995;26: (Suppl 2):S-B51-S-B56.
10. Linas A et al. Healing and remodelling of articular incongruities in a rabbit fracture model. J Bone Joint Surgery 1993;75-A:1508-23.

Further reading

Hansen ST Jr, Swintowski MF. Protocols into orthopaedic trauma. London: Raven Press, 1992.
Rockwood CA, Green DP. Rockwood and Green's fractures, vols 1, 2 & 3. Philadelphia: Lippincott & Co., 1991.

15 Soft tissue injury

Stewart Watson

Consultant Plastic, Hand and Microsurgeon, Withington Hospital, Manchester

David J. Coleman

Consultant Plastic Surgeon, The Radcliffe Infirmary, Oxford

OBJECTIVES

- To understand early radical excision of the wound.

- To discuss collaborative planned reconstructive programme with other specialties.

- To be alert to presence of compartmental compression.

- To understand early definitive reconstruction of all injured tissues where possible, including tendons and nerves.

- To attempt wound closure by fifth day if not before.

Soft tissue management: aims and primary considerations

It is the aim of modern reconstructive plastic surgery to get all soft tissue injuries fully debrided, reconstructed, and closed by the end of the fifth day and this process starts with the first operation on the evening of injury. It is usually possible to get them treated by the end of the third day, but it is recognised that there is a window of five days in which closure can be safely and satisfactorily performed. This applies just as much to the *multiply injured patient* as to the patient with a *single limb injury*. The importance of this cannot be overemphasised when the final morbidity following injury is estimated. A closed well-vascularised soft tissue envelope gives the best chance for the deeper tissues to heal and considerably reduces the risk of infection. Soft tissue injuries, although seldom life-threatening, will often be the cause of long-term morbidity if they are badly managed, and can be the factor that prevents the patient returning to work or to their leisure activities.

If there is tendon or nerve damage, this also has to be properly assessed in the first five days and either repaired or reconstructed at this time or a plan made for future repair and reconstruction. Long-term morbidity results from a missed nerve or flexor tendon injury because the window of opportunity for repair has not been fulfilled.

Methods of achieving this aim

Modern reconstructive plastic surgery has advanced so much in the past 20 years that we now have methods of flap transfer which can heal very large wounds, often using microsurgical techniques. The application of these wound healing techniques now allows us to do a very thorough and extensive debridement without the worry of how the wound is going to be reconstructed and closed. All wound debridements must be extremely thorough; there is no place for the preservation of any soft tissue which is poorly vascularised, damaged, or degloved. Damaged soft tissue is radically debrided in one, two, or occasionally three separate operations, followed by definitive reconstruction and wound closure.

Communication between other disciplines and plastic surgeons

Soft tissue injuries need to be managed by reconstructive plastic surgeons with an interest in trauma, and the facilities necessary to manage it. They need to be involved on the day of admission and present at the first operations [1].

Tissue response to injury

The response of soft tissues to injury is determined by the mechanism of injury, the energy exerted on the tissues, the mechanical arrangement of the tissues and their blood supply. In recent years there has been a rediscovery of the vascular anatomy of soft tissues [2,3]. This knowledge has allowed developments in flap design and increased the power of flap reconstruction, but has also enabled us to better predict tissue response to injury.

Mechanisms of soft tissue injury

Most injuries are associated with a combination of mechanisms and a composite of injured tissues. The history will often supply the most useful information regarding the mechanism and energy of injury. It is particularly important to recognise patients with high energy injuries (see box).

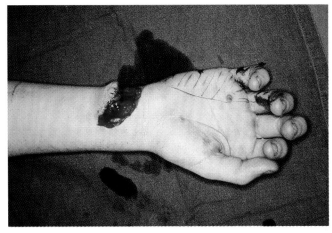

(a)

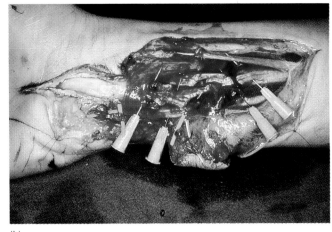

(b)

Figure 15.1 (a) Cut wrist; (b) tendons and nerves prepared for direct primary repair.

Recognition of high energy injuries

History

- Any road traffic accident: drivers, passengers or pedestrian
- Falls from a significant height
- Any injury mechanism involving extensive or localised crushing
- Missile wounds
- Contamination from the scene of the accident
- A history of entrapment or lying immobile on the injured limb for a prolonged period
- Any suggestion of possible limb ischaemia

Examination

- Large or multiple wounds
- Imprints or tattooing from dirt or tyres
- Crush or burst wounds
- Closed degloving. Skin is intact but with no blood supply due to shearing between the deep fascia and subcutaneous tissues. It can be difficult to diagnose but may be suspected from the boggy feel of the skin or the abnormal looseness of the skin when it is pinched

X-ray

- The fracture pattern can often give clues to the degree of energy transfer through the bone. Important features include:
  - Multiple bone fragments
  - Wide displacement of fracture fragments
  - Any segmental injury
  - Air in the tissues
  - More than one fracture in the same limb

Laceration

Lacerations are usually relatively low energy injuries, with a narrow zone of injury. They may involve nerve, vascular, or tendon injury, but rarely are associated with fractures. Lacerations from a machete attack may involve fractures. They may involve specialised skin features such as eyelids, lips, fingertips etc. (Figures 15.1 and 15.2). They may be accompanied by loss of tissue. There is usually little non-viable tissue in the wound. Primary healing of such wounds can be expected.

Abrasion

Abrasions are friction injuries of skin and are associated with varying degrees of burn and tattooing of foreign bodies into the skin. The burn component of the injury is assessed in the same way as a thermal burn. A partial thickness abrasion can be expected to heal spontaneously by epithelialisation, a full thickness abrasion will not. Tattooing of the skin with grit, soot, or other particulate matter is important to recognise because, if it is not removed, such particles cause permanent tattooing (Figure 15.3). Abrasions are an indication of friction and may be a sign of shearing forces exerted on deeper layers of the soft tissue envelope.

Traction/avulsion

These injuries are more likely where greater energy has been exerted on the tissues, and are often a reflection of a blunt mechanism of injury. There will be a wide zone of injury, with much non-viable tissue in the wound. There may be extensive lacerations. Fractures are common. Nerves and tendons may be exposed, but are often not divided. Vascular injuries may occur and their presence may worsen the ischaemia of marginally viable tissue (Figures 15.4 and 15.5). *Degloving* is common in such injuries. Degloving is caused by shearing forces which separate tissue planes, rupturing their vascular interconnections, and causing tissue ischaemia. This most frequently occurs between the subcutaneous fat and deep fascia (Figure 15.6), resulting in skin degloving and ischaemia. Degloving injuries can be open or closed, localised or circumferential. Degloving may occur only in the single, subcutaneous plane, but where present in multiple planes, such as between muscles and fascia and between muscles and bone, it is an indication of a severe high energy injury with a limited potential for primary healing. Compartment syndromes should be anticipated in traction/avulsion injuries. These injuries, if mismanaged, carry the potential for, at best, poor healing and poor functional outcome and, at worst, gas gangrene and

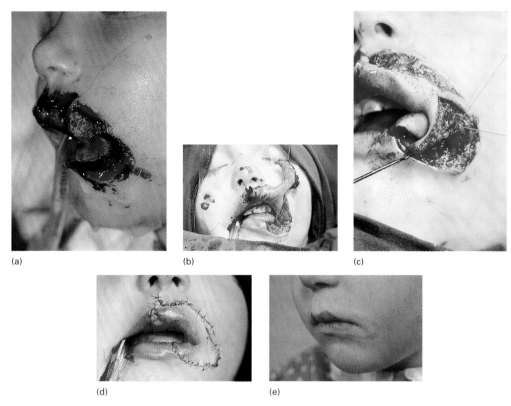

(a)　　　　　　　　(b)　　　　　　　　(c)

(d)　　　　　　　　(e)

Figure 15.2　(a) and (b) Dog bite to lips; (c) wound edges debrided (see later); (d) wound closed in layers; (e) result 3 years later.

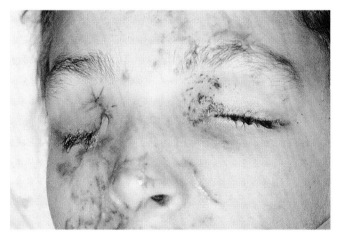

Figure 15.3　Tattooed scars from inadequate removal of ingrained dirt at time of initial wound management.

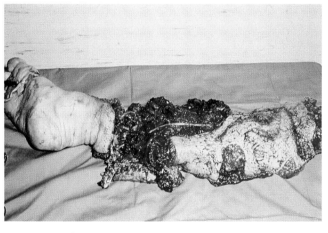

Figure 15.4　Severe traction/avulsion injury.

amputation or death. Such injuries require careful wound assessment and wound excision by surgeons experienced in such problems. Primary wound healing will often only be achieved with reconstructive surgery.

Crush and compartment syndrome

Crush injuries are a further variant of blunt injury and are often accompanied by degloving and *compartment syndrome*. Injury to tissues within a closed fascial compartment leads to bleeding, exudate and swelling of these tissues, and increased interstitial pressure. As the interstitial pressure rises above capillary perfusion pressure, the blood supply to the viable tissues is reduced, resulting in further ischaemic tissue injury and swelling. This cycle causes a worsening compartment syndrome with muscle ischaemia and nerve ischaemia pro-

gressing to muscle necrosis, skin necrosis, and limb loss. The consequences of non-recognised compartment syndrome and muscle death are very severe (Figure 15.7a and b). There is marked loss of function, and muscle necrosis may result in renal failure. This process can be arrested by early recognition and decompression of the affected compartment(s) by fasciotomy. The most reliable early clinical sign of compartment syndrome is pain worsened by passive stretching of affected muscles. The pain will usually be inappropriately severe for the apparent injury. Any patient with severe pain must be carefully assessed for compartment compression before being given opiate or other strong analgesia. There is a particular problem in recognising compartment pressure in unconscious patients. In unconscious patients there is no alternative but to either monitor compartment pressure continuously or decompress all muscle compartments. Where doubt exists com-

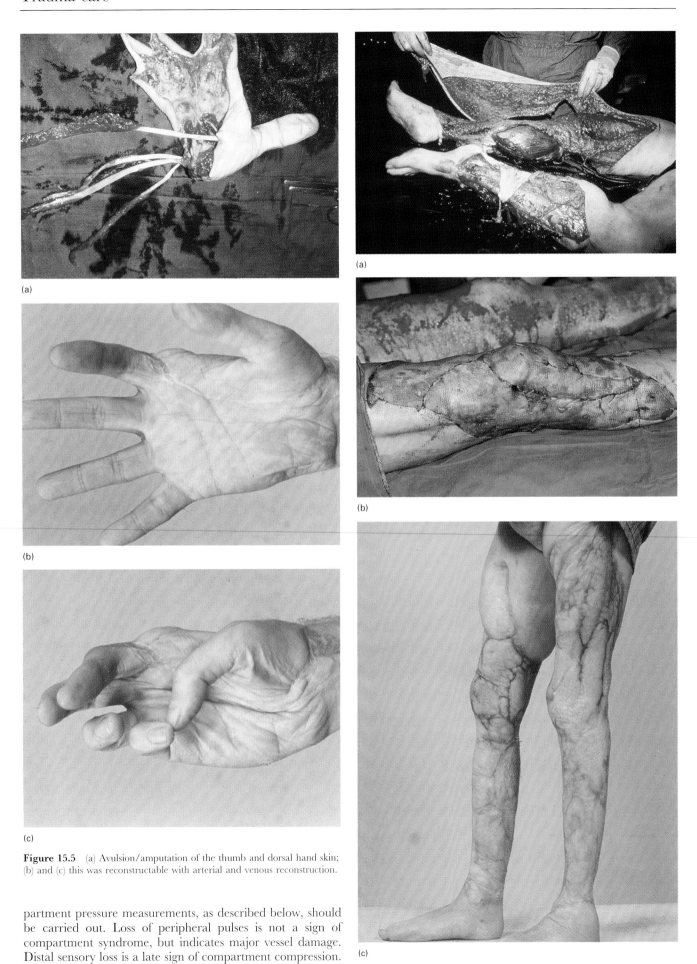

Figure 15.5 (a) Avulsion/amputation of the thumb and dorsal hand skin; (b) and (c) this was reconstructable with arterial and venous reconstruction.

partment pressure measurements, as described below, should be carried out. Loss of peripheral pulses is not a sign of compartment syndrome, but indicates major vessel damage. Distal sensory loss is a late sign of compartment compression. Where the crush is localised and affecting a periphery, it may still be possible to excise all non-viable tissue and obtain primary wound healing (Figure 15.8).

Figure 15.6 (a) Bilateral degloved legs; (b) reconstructed by reapplying the degloved skin after defatting and using additional meshed skin grafts; (c) later result.

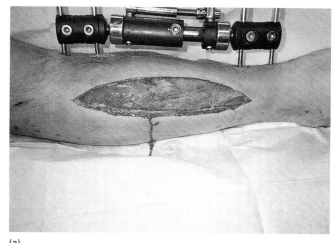

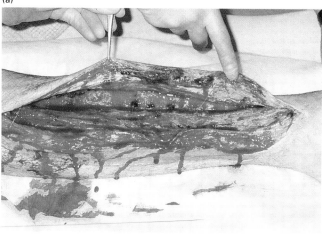

Figure 15.7 (a) A late fasciotomy reveals dead anterior compartment muscle; (b) after debridement of dead anterior compartment muscle.

Burn

Burn injuries may occur in isolation or in association with multiple injuries. Their pathogenesis and management is described elsewhere in this book (Chapter 19).

Anatomy of soft tissue injury

Different soft tissues respond to injury in different ways. In any wound it is important to assess and record each tissue which has been injured or exposed by the injury.

Skin

The skin provides a robust, waterproof integument with important temperature control, infection limitation, and sensory functions. It has a rich blood supply with an abundant subdermal plexus. The vascular pattern by which blood vessels reach the skin is important in predicting how skin will respond to degloving. There are four patterns by which vessels pass from the deep vascular axes to the skin (Figure 15.9) [4,5]. Blood vessels passing from a fascial compartment to the skin are called perforators. The density of perforators varies between areas of the body; they are most numerous in fixed-skin areas of the body, such as the palms and soles. These areas tend to resist degloving, but when it occurs, skin necrosis is likely. In mobile-skinned areas, such as the trunk, perforators pass obliquely through the subcutaneous fat and subdermal areas for long distances. Degloving can readily occur between the fat and deep fascia, but because of the elongated course of the cutaneous vessels, degloved flaps on the trunk will usually survive. The limbs usually have several large septocutaneous or fasciocutaneous perforators which then run along the deep fascia before entering the skin. Where these major perforators are divided or where degloving occurs in a plane superficial to them, skin necrosis is likely.

Fat

Adipose tissue is much less resistant to ischaemia than skin. Fat is arranged in compartments in tissue; fat necrosis is often more extensive than skin necrosis. It is not usually possible to salvage skin overlying areas of extensive fat necrosis. Viable skin overhanging areas of fat necrosis often has to be sacrificed in order to achieve thorough wound debridement and primary healing.

Muscles

Muscles also have a variety of patterns of vascular anatomy. Some have major, dominant vascular axes, others have multiple segmental vessels. These patterns determine their utility as muscle flaps for reconstruction. The response of muscle to injury is determined more by the presence of direct muscle laceration and compartmental compression. Some muscles, such as gastrocnemius, have a major vascular axis from the popliteal artery above the knee outside the posterior compartment of the lower leg. This renders it relatively resistant to injuries of the lower limb, and can often provide useful reconstruction about the knee.

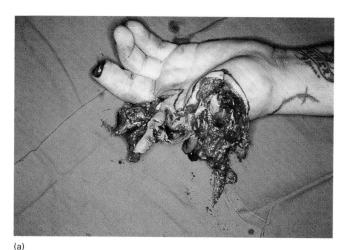

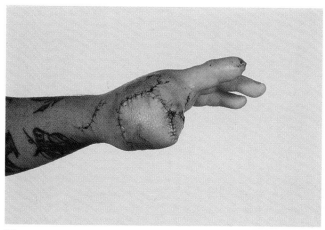

Figure 15.8 (a) Crushed thumb not salvageable; (b) after debridement 1° closure using dorsal skin.

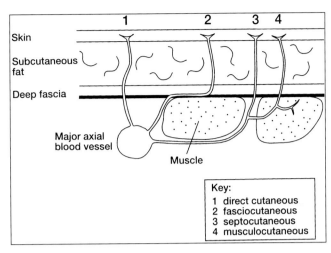

Figure 15.9 Deep vascular access to the skin.

- skin
- subcutaneous fat
- fascia
- muscle compartments
- tendons, nerves, and blood vessels.

The size and shape of the skin defect is recorded and whether there are multiple wounds. It is valuable to take a Polaroid photograph at this stage. This provides very useful information when the case is reviewed later on in the management. It also allows the wound to be dressed or covered after the initial inspection so that other doctors can review the Polaroids without having to take the dressing off repeatedly. The first dressing should be a simple sterile dressing or saline-soaked sterile dressing.

An estimate is made of whether there is circulation to the skin. In a good light, do the capillary refill test using a sterile finger but beware that in pale skin this might not be conclusive or reliable. The best assessment of blood flow in the skin is to see if the skin bleeds pink blood on pin prick not blue blood. The vascularity of the leg must be assessed by examination of the major pulses by palpation and with a Doppler.

There must then be a specific examination to look for signs of nerve damage and tendon damage: test sensation in the skin and muscle movement, as far as this is possible, depending on the patient's general state.

If there is going to be a delay getting to theatre, the **muscle compartment pressures need to be recorded at this stage.**

Nerves

The three grades of nerve injury are well known and the pathophysiology of injury and recovery is described elsewhere. Neurotmesis is usually associated with sharp trauma and, where primary repair can be performed, a satisfactory functional outcome might be expected. Neuropraxia and axonotmesis, associated with blunt trauma, will give similar clinical signs, but may have differing outcomes, depending on the length of the damaged nerve segments and the extent of the damage. It is important to document the neurological findings on clinical examination at an early stage if at all possible. Where nerve injury is suspected, inspection of the relevant injured nerve trunk should be part of the initial wound exploration.

Tendons

Tendons gain their nutrition from synovial fluid, vincula blood supply and vessels from their muscular origins, and bony insertions. They will desiccate and necrose if exposed and devoid of paratenon, so every attempt should be made to provide soft tissue cover for tendons at an early stage. Tendons do have an intrinsic ability to heal provided some source of nutrition is preserved.

Wound healing

There have been major advances in the understanding of the biology of wound repair, but as yet these have not provided a means of manipulating wound healing. The priority, as always in trauma, remains the preservation of life and appropriate resuscitation to allow early surgery. The path to the goal of primary healing, which restores function and allows early rehabilitation, remains a close adherence to the principles of wound exploration, debridement and early wound closure with appropriate well-vascularised tissue.

Assessment

It is assumed that adequate resuscitation has taken place, or is taking place.

A careful history of the injury is taken as far as possible, to determine the mechanism of soft tissue injury, as outlined above. In assessing soft tissue injury the surgeon needs to consider the different soft tissues individually:

Classification of soft tissue injury

Classification of the soft tissue injury can only be made under general anaesthetic. The Gustillo Classification is usually used [5]. It must be emphasised that the state of the soft tissue injury cannot be fully evaluated without a general anaesthetic and any attempt to classify soft tissue injury does not help with the initial management. The initial management can only be done by evaluation of each layer of soft tissue individually. Classifications are useful for retrospective case review and audit but any initial classification needs to be reviewed and updated over the first few days.

Muscle compartment pressure measurements

Surgeons must be aware that muscle compartment pressures have to be monitored in the first five days. The signs and symptoms are outlined above. The importance of this cannot be overemphasised. With the pressure transducers which are available in Intensive Care Units and on anaesthetic trolleys in the operating theatre, the measurement of pressure in muscle compartments is now easy to perform. It must be remembered that a muscle compartment which is partly open or partly decompressed can still develop a compartmental compression in the rest of the compartment. A muscle compartment has to be fully released before it is properly decompressed [6–8].

Management of soft tissue injury

When initial life-saving measures have been instituted and the patient is stabilised, the soft tissues are assessed along with the other systems and a plan is made for their treatment, integrated with the other treatment that the patient requires. At the first operation the soft tissue is evaluated and fully debrided by a surgeon familiar with the management of soft tissues. The aim, which has been outlined above, is to remove all devascularised, crushed, or degloved soft tissues completely so that reconstruction can take place with the expectation of primary healing. This will minimise any chance of infection and, with the provision of a well vascularised soft tissue envelope, the deeper structures are given the best environment in which to heal.

The first 4 hours

1. Thoroughly explore the wounds, clean and debride each soft tissue layer specifically (details below).
2. Restore arterial blood supply if interrupted.
3. Ensure skeletal stabilisation.
4. Decompress muscle compartments if required.
5. Carry out estimation and possible repair of nerve and tendon damage.
6. Salvage skin grafts from skin which is to be excised.

Clean and debride

Techniques of soft tissue cleaning include the following.

Irrigation

The wounds are irrigated with copious quantities of Hartmann's solution. This does not, however, remove devitalised tissue or particulate matter.

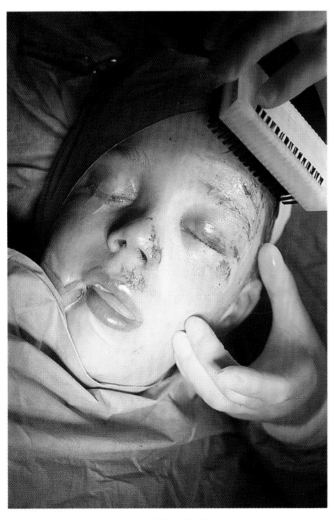

Figure 15.10 Scrubbing dirt from abrasions.

Scrubbing

The skin surface is scrubbed (Figure 15.10) with swabs or a soft brush, with the use of Betadine or solvents for grease. This is particularly important for abrasion injuries of the skin in which there is dirt in the abraded dermis. This dirt can be removed from the skin only in the first few days before epithelialisation has taken place.

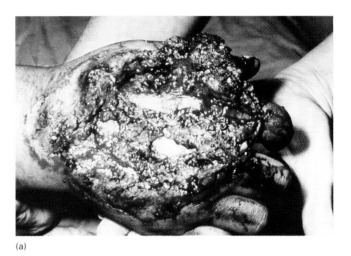

(a)

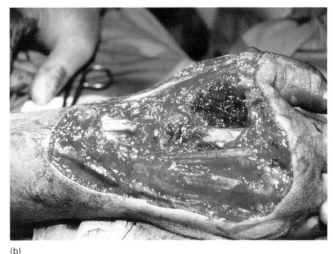

(b)

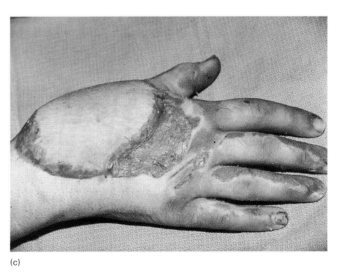

(c)

Figure 15.11 (a) A grossly contaminated wound on dorsum of hand; (b) after debridement; (c) reconstructed with free groin flap and skin graft.

Picking

Particulate matter is picked from the wound and from all tissues, including joints, often with loop magnification for greater clarity.

Wound excision

The above three methods of wound cleaning are only suitable for relatively minor degrees of soft tissue injury, where there is no question of any reduced blood supply, crush injury, or degloving, and where there is no heavy impregnation of the soft tissues by dirt or particulate matter (Figure 15.11). In these more severe injuries, wound excision with a scalpel is the only definitive way to debride soft tissue back to healthy, undamaged tissue. Each layer of soft tissue is specifically and individually excised, the tissues cut back until they bleed pink blood and not ooze blue blood.

There is a big debate about whether wound cleaning, debridement, and excision should be performed under tourniquet control or without tourniquet. The argument for not using a tourniquet is that the surgeon can readily see which tissues bleed pink blood and which do not. The disadvantage, however, is that it does lead to blood loss and it is difficult to keep the wounds free of blood so the view is not so good. In the absence of any major vascular injury which has been reconstructed, we would recommend debriding the wound under tourniquet control and letting the tourniquet down when the surgeon wishes to assess the blood supply.

Skin

This is cut back until there is brisk, pink dermal bleeding with no gross contusion or deep skin abrasion. The presence of dermal bleeding will not be seen with a tourniquet up, but excision is made to what is thought to be the proper level and then it is checked for pink dermal bleeding.

Subcutaneous tissue

As stated above, this is more susceptible to injury than the skin itself. The zone of subcutaneous damage is invariably larger than the zone of skin damage, so in this respect trauma is similar to a pressure sore. There is a bigger zone of subcutaneous damage than skin damage, thus undermining is produced. It can be difficult to judge how much subcutaneous fat has been damaged in the first 24 hours. A decision is made on appearance and bleeding. The typical changes of dead fat to a greyish pink discoloration are not apparent until about 24–36 hours.

It is important to appreciate the mechanism of degloving. This is where the subcutaneous fat shears off the deep fascia. It will be seen from the section on the blood supply to the skin that this will inevitably shear the blood supply to the subcutaneous tissue and skin. In certain areas of the body it is possible to get degloved skin which is still well vascularised, but this is the exception and all degloved skin must be assumed to be devascularised and examined carefully. It is only preserved if it is obvious that there is pink dermal bleeding and the subcutaneous fat proves to be fully viable on the second wound exploration. Viable degloved skin with dead subcutaneous fat will not heal primarily and may well become infected. In severe injuries, for instance limbs that have been run over, it is common for there to be circumferential degloving over a long length of the limb (see Figure 15.6). In less severe injuries it is common to get localised areas of degloving with

non-vascularised skin intermingled with areas where there is skin vascularity (Figure 15.12). This presents the surgeon with a dilemma about whether to preserve small islands of vascularised skin among large areas of non-vascularised skin. The non-reconstructive plastic surgeon is often tempted to preserve as much skin as seems viable, but the experienced reconstructive plastic surgeon will not preserve small areas of vascularised skin and would rather debride the whole area, opting for a primary flap reconstruction so that there can be no compromise about getting good primary healing.

Muscle

Muscle again is debrided until it looks healthy and there is pink bleeding. It is not always possible to be sure about the viability of muscle from its appearance at the first operation. Muscle can look sick but still be vascularised and recover. In these cases it is acceptable to do a cautious debridement of muscle with a definite plan to re-examine under general anaesthetic at 24–36 hours, when it is usually more obvious which muscle is dead and needs to be resected. It is very important, because of the risk of infection, not to leave dead muscle beyond this period.

Major arterial damage reconstruction/skeletal stabilisation

Neither of these will be the subject of this chapter except to say that this obviously requires the cooperation of trauma-orientated specialist surgeons in the same operative procedure; the order of repair will vary, depending on techniques.

Release of deep fascia to decompress muscle compartments

If there is compartmental compression or it cannot be certainly excluded, then the muscle compartments are thoroughly released by full length fascial releases. If there is only one muscle compartment with raised pressure all compartments in that part of the limb must be released, never just the one muscle compartment. For instance, in the leg, below the knee, if there is compartment syndrome in just the anterior compartment all four compartments of the calf are released. In the upper arm, forearm and thigh both the anterior and posterior compartments are released by long linear incisions over the muscle compartments. In the leg two incisions are required [1,5]. Figure 15.13 shows the exposure lines for fascia release in the lower limb [1]. The lateral incision is called the safe lateral incision and is placed anterior to the peroneal artery perforators. It gives access to the anterior and peroneal muscle compartments. The medial incision is called the safe medial incision and is placed anterior to the posterior tibial perforators. It gives access to the superficial and deep posterior muscle compartments. Release of the deep posterior compartment is not an easy dissection and requires careful dissecting anterior to the posterior tibial neurovascular bundle. The soleus and deep fascia is released off the back of the tibia, preserving segmental arteries from the posterior tibial artery to the tibia.

In the hand five incisions are required: two linear dorsal incisions to release the four interosseous muscle compartments; on the volar surface a carpal tunnel incision is extended to the mid-palm to release the carpal tunnel and the central compartment; a linear incision is made over the radial border to decompress the thenar muscles and over the ulnar border to decompress the hypothenar muscles.

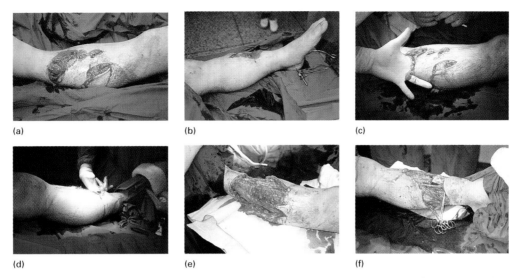

Figure 15.12 (a) and (b) Medial and lateral views of crushed leg; (c) and (d) the surgeon demonstrating the area of localised degloving; (e) and (f) the defect after debridement of non-viable degloved skin and degloved skin bridged to give a wound ready for reconstruction.

In the foot a medial plantar incision on the non-weight-bearing skin is used to release the medial and central compartments. A lateral incision, again not on the weightbearing skin, allows access to the lateral compartment. On the dorsum one or two incisions are required to release the four interosseous compartments.

Estimation of nerve and tendon damage

It may be possible to do a primary repair of nerve and tendon damage at the first operation if everything is favourable. Otherwise a plan is made for the future reconstruction.

Skin salvage

In degloved skin which is to be excised and discarded, either a split skin graft is taken from the skin or the skin itself is excised as a full thickness graft. Full thickness grafts need to be reapplied to the limb on the day, but split skin grafts can be stored in the refrigerator at 4°C for application over the ensuing week.

Second operation after 24–36 hours

At this second-look operation bony fixation is checked and compartmental compression is checked. All the different layers of the soft tissues are then specifically re-examined and debrided.

1. Repeat clean and debridement of each soft tissue layer specifically. At this stage the extent of the subcutaneous fat damage is usually more apparent. In complex limb injuries, where primary healing is paramount to a good outcome, it is not usual to leave skin which is undermined. It is usual to debride the skin to the same extent as the subcutaneous fat, even though this means discarding viable dermis. Reconstruction is more satisfactory after this type of radical debridement than leaving undermined skin. Check muscle compartment pressures.
2. Consider repair or make a plan for the management of any tendon and nerve division.
3. If the wounds are relatively simple and thoroughly debrided and if the reconstruction is easy – for instance, a skin graft or simple flap – proceed with definitive cover at this time.

4. In more complicated reconstructions, an integrated plan of the management of all tissues is made for the next two days. This may involve transferring the patient to a Plastic Unit if a complex microvascular reconstruction is required.

At 48–60 hours

A third-look operation may be required in difficult cases, to be absolutely sure of the soft tissue debridement and to check muscle compartment pressures. Definitive cover may be performed at this stage, or planned over the next twodays.

Fluorescein tests

Intravenous fluorescein is given and after 10 minutes in a darkened operating theatre an ultraviolet light is shone at the skin. Areas that do not fluoresce yellow do not have a blood supply. This is a reliable technique except for the palms of the hands and soles of the feet, but anaphylactic reactions to the fluorescein have been recorded. This test is now seldom performed as it is thought to have little advantage over the experienced judgement of clinical tissue viability.

Wound reconstruction

There is a reconstructive 'ladder' for the closure of wounds, described by Court-Brown *et al.* in their chapter 15 [5].

- delayed direct closure occasionally with dynamic wound closure techniques;
- skin graft;
- local flap;
- free flap transfer.

It is important that the reconstructive surgeon is fully conversant with all methods in order to choose the method that is most appropriate to reconstruct the soft tissue injury. There should be no compromise by choosing a simpler method of wound closure which does not produce the best chance of primary healing and a well vascularised soft tissue envelope.

In *delayed primary closure*, simple wounds may be closed at 3–5 days, when the oedema settles. In *split skin graft* or *mesh grafting techniques*, if the wound bed is well vascularised and there is no exposure or bare cortical bone, fractures, joints,

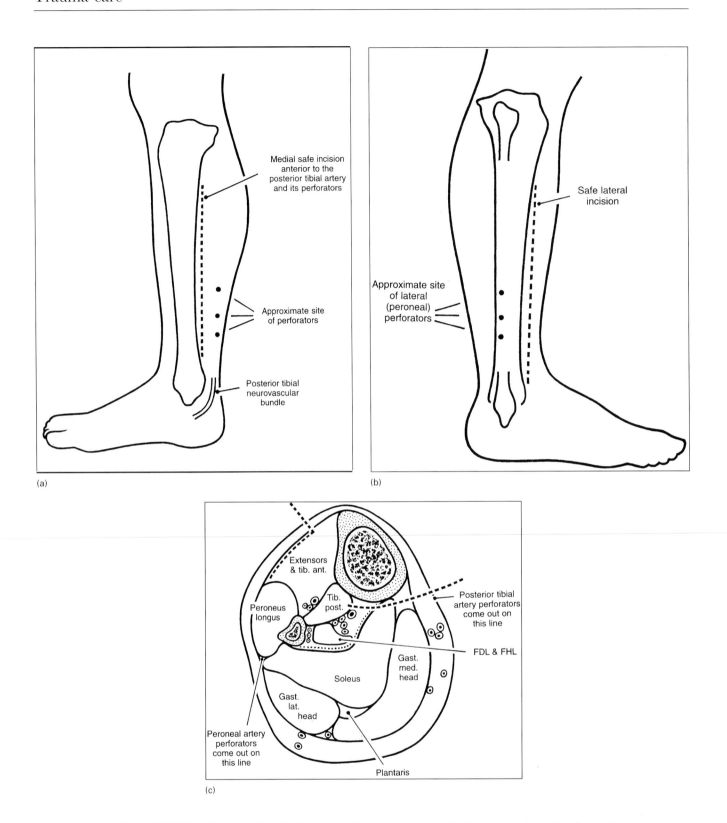

Figure 15.13 (a) and (b) Medial and lateral incisions for fasciotomies; (c) transverse section of the leg showing the incisions for muscle compartment release.

nerves or tendons, a simple skin graft may close the wound satisfactorily.

There are two types of *local flap* available [5]: fasciocutaneous flaps either proximally or distally based, and muscle flaps. These are suitable forms of reconstruction for the majority of limb defects. These flaps are simple in concept but difficult to plan and perform in damaged limbs. They should be performed by surgeons familiar with their use.

Free tissue transfer is a powerful reconstructive technique that brings in new, well-vascularised tissue to the injured limb. It can reconstruct very large defects. It is a technique that needs to be practised by units which do a lot of microvascular surgery, where a team of anaesthetists and nurses is available to ensure a good outcome. The workhorse of free tissue transfer for big defects in the limbs is the latissimus dorsi myocutaneous flap (Figure 15.14).

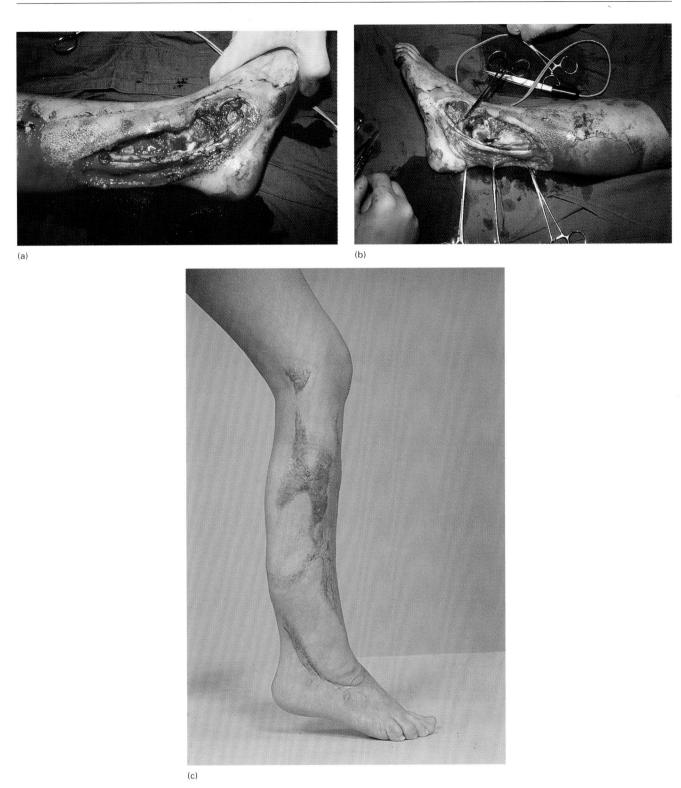

(a)

(b)

(c)

Figure 15.14 (a) Compound leg injury before debridement; (b) after debridement and ready for latissimus dorsi flap resurfacing; (c) latissimus dorsi flap in place 6 months later.

Specialised areas

Hand

The reconstruction of a severely damaged hand is a very complex and specialised field [9]. It requires surgeons experienced in all aspects of hand reconstruction, supported by a specialist team of physiotherapists and occupational therapists. In the multiply injured patient, perhaps with life-threatening injuries, it can be very difficult to devote enough care and attention to non-life-threatening areas like the hand. Badly managed hand injuries, however, can be a considerable source of morbidity in the long term, so, if at all possible, every effort must be made to do the optimal hand reconstruction in the first few days, along with managing all the patient's other problems. One of the main problems with hand injuries is that divided tendons and nerves can only be primarily repaired in the first few days. After this time retraction of the nerves and tendons makes it unlikely that direct repair can be performed. For this

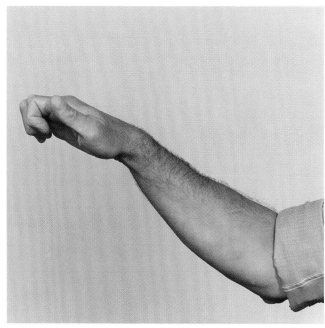

(a)

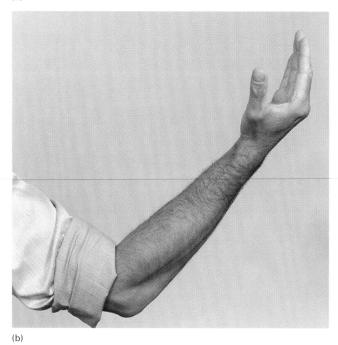

(b)

Figure 15.15 (a) Correct positioning of an injured hand: interphalangeal joints straight, metacarpophalangeal joints flexed to 60–80°, the wrist in neutral or comfortably extended, the thumb comfortably abducted; (b) forearm in a supinated position, not left in a pronated position.

reason, even in complex injuries, injury to tendons and nerves needs to be properly assessed at the first and second operations and either definitive reconstruction performed at this time, if everything is favourable, or a plan made for future management. The deferring of the repair of a divided tendon or nerve because it seems a much more trivial injury than the other injuries is not acceptable. We do not want the patient to be in the position of making a full recovery from life-threatening conditions (head, chest or abdominal injuries), but because the flexor tendon was not repaired the patient cannot go back to work or leisure activities because there is no finger flexion. Reconstruction of flexor tendons at a late stage can be very difficult.

It is worth emphasising two important factors in the management of the hand:

1. The injured hand should be elevated above the heart and monitored for compartment compression.
2. The injured hand should be correctly positioned and splinted (Figure 15.15) with:
   - interphalangeal joints straight;
   - metacarpophalangeal joints flexed to 60–80°;
   - the wrist in neutral or comfortably extended;
   - the thumb comfortably abducted;
   - forearm in a supinated position not left in a pronated position.

Face

All types of soft tissue injuries are seen in the face. The face has an extremely good blood supply; adequate wound excision and early closure can be expected to achieve primary healing in most situations. The face has several areas of highly specialised soft tissues, notably eyelids, nose, lips, hair-bearing areas and pinnae. Where lacerations and tissue loss involve these structures, it is particularly important to repair each layer accurately in its correct anatomical position. For example, it is essential to align the vermilion border of the lips and the repair the eyelid structures accurately. Even in extensive lacerations such as a severe dog bite injury (Figure 15.3), there was no significant tissue loss and, after excision of all wound edges, the lacerations were closed primarily with accurate alignment of the lip margin, and healing was achieved without infection. Careful repair of such wounds at the primary procedure will reduce the need for later scar revisional surgery.

Small amounts of tissue loss can usually be dealt with by wound excision and closure with little distortion of the facial features. Where there is massive tissue loss, it is necessary to import tissues to obtain closure. Simple grafts from scalp, postauricular sites or the neck are best where possible. Primary flaps in facial trauma are rarely indicated. However, in severe injury a free tissue transfer may be needed to obtain healing.

Scalp lacerations can result in significant haemorrhage and emergency suturing for haemostasis may be needed. Scalp loss can be repaired with skin grafts if the pericranium is preserved; however, if there is bare cranial bone, flap repair will be needed. The *facial nerve* should always be repaired primarily where circumstances allow. Isolated lacerations of the *lower lacrimal canaliculus* rarely cause epiphora; complex attempts at repair with stents may damage previously uninjured parts of the lacrimal apparatus and should be avoided.

References

1. BOA/BAPS. *The management of open tibial fractures.* Booklet published by the British Orthopaedic Association and the British Association of Plastic Surgeons, London, September 1997.
2. Cormack GC, Lamberty BGH. *The arterial anatomy of skin flaps.* Edinburgh: Churchill Livingstone, 1994.
3. Taylor GI, Palmer JH. The vascular territories (anglosomes) of the body: experimental study and clinical applications. *Br J Plast Surg* 1987;**40**:113–41.
4. Ruberg LR, Smith DJ. *Plastic surgery. A core curriculum.* Mosby: St Louis/Year Book, 1994, esp. p. 610.
5. Court-Brown Charles M, McQueen Margaret M, Quaba Awf A. *The management of open fractures.* London: Martin Dunitz, 1996.
6. McQueen MM, Christie J, Court-Brown CM. Acute compartment syndrome in tibial diaphyseal fracture. *J Bone Joint Surg* 1996;**78**: 95–8.
7. McQueen MM, Christie J and Court-Brown CM. Compartmental monitoring of tibial fractures. *J Bone Joint Surg* 1996;**78**:99–103.
8. McQueen MM. How to monitor compartment pressures. *Techn Orthop* 1996;**11(1)**:99–101.
9. Lister G. *The hand: diagnosis and indications.* Edinburgh: Churchill Livingstone, 1993.

16 Psychological trauma

Martin P. Deahl

Consultant and Senior Lecturer in Psychological Medicine, St Bartholomew's Hospital, West Smithfield, London and Consultant Psychiatrist, 256(L) Field Hospital, RAMC (V).

OBJECTIVES

- To highlight the importance of psychological factors in the management of the trauma patient.

- To describe the normal psychological response and the stages of adjustment following trauma.

- To emphasise the contribution of pretrauma patient characteristics in the aetiology of abnormal psychological reactions following trauma.

- To describe the nature and prevelence of psychiatric disturbance following trauma.

- To consider the effects of trauma and its psychological sequelae on relatives and staff.

- To consider the management of psychological problems in the trauma unit; when to refer to a psychiatrist.

- Preventing long-term psychiatric disability.

Distressing psychological reactions are a universal and normal part of the response to injury and trauma. Unlike a physical injury, however, the psychological aftermath of accidents and disasters alike remains unseen and often passes unnoticed on a surgical ward or in the busy A & E Department. Nevertheless, its sequelae can be as disabling as any physical injury. Following trauma all individuals undergo a process of adaptation and adjustment to their circumstances. The psychological reactions that follow are predictable and are a normal part of the stress response. They only become pathological when they become excessive in duration or intensity.

The psychological consequences of injury should concern everyone involved in trauma management and should not be marginalised as a peripheral issue delegated to specialist mental health professionals. Failure to recognise and respond appropriately to psychological problems in the early stages following trauma increases the likelihood of long-term sequelae that may be as disabling as any physical handicap and cause untold suffering to patients and relatives, who themselves become secondary victims. A disturbed mental state may distort considerably the perception and description of physical symptoms giving rise to an inaccurate and misleading medical history, diagnostic errors, and incorrect management. Staff must be able to distinguish normal reactions from the abnormal

and identify those individuals in need of specialist psychiatric help. Psychological problems may lead to behavioral disturbances which cause disruption and potentially can seriously interfere with the work of a busy department. The trauma team must know how to manage disruptive patients, particularly as immediate intervention may be required when specialist psychiatric help is unavailable. Changes in behaviour may also have diagnostic significance and may be the only sign of undiagnosed head trauma or causes of cerebral hypoxia.

Broadly speaking, there is a reciprocal relationship between the physical and psychological needs of any trauma patient. Although the psychological welfare of trauma victims is necessarily subordinate to immediate life-saving physical treatment, rehabilitation begins in the A & E Department. A good therapeutic relationship established between the trauma team, a patient and his family, lays the foundations for a successful long-term psychological outcome. All trauma staff, nursing and medical, should be able to provide reassurance, support, and simple counselling for their patients as they pass through the stages of psychological trauma.

The nature and extent of the psychological response of any trauma patient is strongly influenced by a variety of premorbid factors (see box) [1]. In general, these interact with the immediate psychological impact of trauma in a reciprocal fashion to influence the clinical picture following injury. In the early stages following injury, the patient's immediate response is determined primarily by the psychological impact of the incident and the subsequent injury. Premorbid factors are of relatively minor importance. As time passes, however, the significance of premorbid disposition increases and ultimately has a major role in determining the patient's long-term psychological outcome.

A previous history of psychiatric disorder is perhaps the most important vulnerability factor. Indeed, as many as one-third of adults admitted following traumatic injury suffer from a diagnosable psychiatric disorder at the time of the accident, and a further fifth suffer from a personality disorder. Substance misuse (drugs and alcohol) and personality disorders are the most commonly diagnosed conditions and may themselves have been contributory to the trauma. Other premorbid variables that predict a poor psychological outcome include poor general physical health and a "neurotic" worrying personality. Previous experience of accidents and trauma may be a powerful influence for good or bad. History tends to repeat itself: many accident victims develop positive coping strategies that they can mobilise and which are protective following subsequent trauma. Conversely, an inability to cope following previous trauma is strongly predictive of a poor psychological outcome.

Vulnerability factors predisposing to psychiatric morbidity following trauma

- Anxiety-prone "worrying" personality
- Previous history of psychiatric disorder
- Previous psychological trauma (including childhood abuse)
- Drug and alcohol misuse
- Poor general physical health

Following trauma, the victim passes through a series of well-defined and fairly predictable psychological stages. (Table 16.1) With the passage of each stage, not only do the patient's emotional reactions vary, but so do the psychological needs and those of the relatives. As time passes the patient becomes less passive and the relationship between staff and patient becomes less directive and more receptive.

Normal responses following psychological trauma

Primary (acute) post-trauma phase

The immediate behavioural and emotional reaction following trauma is primarily determined by the emotional impact of the accident and the impact of the injury. The perceived threat to life and the significance of an accident or disaster are the most important variables for predicting acute responses. This phase generally lasts from minutes to hours but may occasionally last longer. Premorbid factors are of relatively minor importance. Apart from traumatic brain damage and those injuries giving rise to organic delirium, the type and location of any trauma only plays a minor role in determining the immediate psychological response.

The typical primary response is one of emotional numbness or denial. This reaction may be seen as a psychological defence against an intolerable reality and represents an expression of the primitive biological response to acute danger and injury, namely fight (aggression), flight (panic) or freezing (apathy). In the A & E Department, or at an accident site, the patient may appear apathetic and bewildered. Aimless wandering can hamper the work of the emergency services and endanger life. Victims may fail to take life-saving action, and deny the need for medical attention despite obvious injuries.

An awareness of the immediate emotional response to injury is important even if a patient appears calm and compliant. It can distort the perception of symptoms and even severe injuries may be denied in the first minutes following trauma. Levels of anxiety and physiological arousal are often low, although depersonalisation may be seen. Occasionally, underlying emotions may be so strong that a dissociative state occurs, and the patient may suffer from complete amnesia as the psychological impact of the trauma completely overwhelms the patient's cognitive processes.

However, gross behavioural disturbances or obvious emotional distress are uncommon during this stage and disturbed behaviour immediately following trauma is more likely to be the result of organic factors such as intoxication with alcohol and drugs, head injury, and cerebral hypoxia.

Secondary (subacute) phase

The secondary phase usually begins hours after the trauma and lasts a few days but may occasionally last several weeks. It is accompanied by the realisation that the unthinkable has become a reality. Psychologically, the secondary phase is characterised by unwanted intrusive thoughts and repetition of the trauma. The clinical picture is influenced by the physiological and psychological effects of the physical injury, and the psychosocial effects of treatment. Behavioural abnormalities and observable emotional reactions are common and about 45% of injured adults will experience periods of marked emotional and behavioural change [2].

Analgesia

Abnormal behaviour and disturbances of mental state are potentiated by pain, and the provision of adequate analgesia during this stage is an essential adjunct to psychological well-being. *Pro re nate* (PRN) analgesia should be avoided wherever possible because patients often feel guilty and are reluctant to request analgesia. Furthermore busy nursing staff may be equally reluctant to administer analgesia frequently. Instead continuous infusion pumps or patient-controlled analgesia (PCA) should be employed whenever possible to minimise the initial euphoriant effect of opiates (which can further compromise mental state) and the inevitable "clock-watching" as the analgesic effect diminishes and the patient awaits further medication.

Subjective distress

Appearances are often misleading and at least 40% of patients are subjectively emotionally very distressed, despite the lack of any abnormal behaviour. Shivering or shaking is often seen and may be the only clinical sign. Sympathetic overactivity is present, and the sensation of pain may be exaggerated as a result, increasing demands for analgesia. Subjective distress impairs cognitive function, and may interfere with a patient's ability to understand instructions or impart accurate information. Reliability of the medical history, police statements,

Table 16.1 Stages of psychological response to trauma

Stage	Time	Reaction	Importance of premorbid factors
Primary	Minutes/hours	Numbing/denial	+
Secondary	Hours/days	Emotional distress/anxiety/intrusive thoughts and repetition of trauma	+ +
Long-term reactions	Months/years	Depression/anxiety-states/PTSD*	+ + +

* PTSD: Post-traumatic stress disorder

and any other factual information cannot be assumed, even in a cooperative patient, during this stage and should always be reviewed later. Following disasters in particular, patients must cope with a number of secondary events which can perpetuate and exacerbate psychological distress, lead to a deterioration in mental state; and further delay recovery. As time passes secondary events such as family attitudes, police, and insurance investigations and the attentions of the press, assume increasing importance, and influence the clinical picture. These include media attention, visits from VIPs, memorial services, inquests, and public inquiries.

Anxiety

During the secondary phase anxiety is extremely common, and often comprises worrying, obsessive thoughts about the accident, an exaggerated startle response, inattention, and poor concentration. Nightmares are infrequent initially and usually only begin several days following trauma. Anxiety may be aggravated by the fear of police or press enquiries, particularly if a patient feels responsible for an accident. Extreme reactions, such as panic or a complete absence of psychomotor and affective responses, are unusual and occur in less than 1% of the injured, although more frequently following disasters.

Depression

Depressed mood days and weeks following an accident are common and may be due to guilt, shame, or grief owing to real or imagined loss. "Survivor guilt" is particularly common following disasters. It is important not to overlook the influence of a pre-existing affective disorder. A patient whose lifestyle is centred around physical activities is likely to sustain a more severe depressive reaction and have greater difficulty adjusting when real or imagined physical disability occurs. Depression is particularly common following severe burns and spinal cord injuries.

Elevated mood

Elevated mood and occasionally frank hypomania may be seen during the secondary phase. Some patients become floridly euphoric (the survivor syndrome). Less frequently hypomanic and even manic behaviour may occur as a defence against feelings of guilt related to an accident. Disruptive behaviour frequently occurs in patients threatened by a perceived loss of autonomy and independence, who may feel weak or ashamed at being a victim.

Aggression

Following trauma, aggressive behaviour in an injured person is seen in about 5% of individuals. Pre-existing personality problems and alcohol or drug misuse increase the likelihood of aggression. Aggressive behaviour may be the manifestation of underlying anxiety but, occasionally, it may be secondary to a more serious abnormality of mental state such as mania or delirium. Aggression is often directed towards helpers, family, and the reminders of reality. Aggressive reactions are less frequent amongst injured disaster victims compared to injured victims of accidents and, when they do occur, are more likely to be provoked by the emotional impact of the accident or trauma. It cannot be emphasised too strongly that behavioural abnormalities may be the only sign of brain

damage or cerebral hypoxia, which are all too easily overlooked.

Denial

Some patients somatise their distress and show little obvious emotional or behavioural disturbance. They may deny any emotional symptoms but report severe pain out of proportion to the severity of injury. These individuals, typically males with rigid, well-defended personalities (the "stiff upper-lip" type) and obsessive-compulsive personality traits, are threatened by a perceived lack of control associated with their injury. Tactful supportive counselling to legitimise and facilitate the expression of feelings and emotions may not only help the patient but reduce the need for analgesia.

Delirium

Delirium is an acute organic brain disorder, characterised by clouding of consciousness, cognitive impairment, and disorientation. The patient's mental state often fluctuates and is typically worse at night ("sundowning"). Lesser degrees of clouding of consciousness may be manifest as inattention and inability to attend to external stimuli, and may be easily missed. Almost any psychiatric symptom such as panic, paranoid ideation, hallucinations, as well as aggressive and disruptive behaviour, may all be secondary to delirium. The risks are increased in the very young and very old, and disruptive, manic, or rude behaviour in middle-aged or elderly people should always raise the suspicion of an underlying organic disorder. Delirium should also be suspected if a patient does not recognise the severity of injury or denies emotion, despite having sustained serious injury. During delirium a patient may experience vivid dreams and nightmares which may merge with hallucinations to produce behavioral disturbance. Subtle changes in mental state owing to delirium may not be noticed by staff but detected by relatives, whose perception of the patient's mental state should always be sought. The family may not spontaneously volunteer their concerns for fear of stigmatising their relative as "mad".

Delirium may be provoked or exacerbated by the use of a variety of drugs including those with anticholinergic activity, strong analgesic sedatives, and other psychotropic agents. It is also more common in individuals with pre-existing cognitive impairment (for example, owing to substance misuse), and among those with severe physical injuries. Almost all patients requiring artificial ventilation experience periods of delirium, especially when they have concurrent severe physical injuries.

Two-thirds of patients showing these diverse reactions do not justify a psychiatric diagnosis. They are, nevertheless, crucial to the eventual outcome. Although distressing psychological symptoms frequently spontaneously resolve they may occasionally persist and develop into more prolonged adjustment disorders requiring formal psychiatric intervention. In the short term these symptoms may interfere with medical treatment, physical recovery, and the increasing likelihood of surgical and other long-term physical complications. As a consequence the length of stay of surgical patients with psychiatric co-morbidity is significantly longer than that of other patients.

Long-term psychological reactions

About 50% of injured adults report some permanent distressing physical symptoms or complaints two to three years after their injury. For the majority, reduced quality of life is the major problem. Despite this, long-term psychiatric disorders occur in less than 20%. Mayou [3] studied 188 RTA victims aged 18 to 70 years: 20% developed acute stress reactions. At one year 10% suffered from affective disorders (mostly depressive illness) and a further 10% experienced phobic travel anxiety.

In a random sample of accidentally injured adults the long-term incidence of psychiatric disorder was 17% during the first year and 9% after two years; 6% suffered from an organic mental disorder alone [2] and one-third also suffered organic mental disorders, in addition, two years after the trauma.

There is considerable evidence that the incidence of long-term psychological and psychiatric disorder following disasters and accidents is proportional to the severity of sustained physical injuries, unrelieved pain, and the extent of permanent physical disability. This is particularly evident following head injuries [4] and burns patients [5]. Victims of disasters appear to suffer from a higher rate of subsequent psychiatric disorder that is also related to the extent of any physical injury. Despite this association, severity of injury alone is not in itself a good predictor of outcome and will only identify a quarter of those patients who go on to develop long-term psychiatric difficulties. Premorbid vulnerability factors as well as psychosocial variables subsequent to the accident all influence long-term psychiatric morbidity. A strong emotional reaction during the first few weeks after an accident will predict 50% of patients who go on to develop long-term psychiatric problems. A few patients will not have shown any abnormal behaviour or adjustment reactions during their hospital stay.

The majority of injured persons involved in accidents sustain minor injuries. In these cases it is premorbid factors, the personal meaning of the accident or injury, and the secondary events which follow that have greater predictive effect on psychiatric outcome. Traumatic brain injury (TBI) accompanied by cognitive impairment is associated with a particularly high frequency of long-term psychiatric disorder and enduring personality change. There is a strong relationship between the severity of head injury and psychiatric problems. Long-term studies of World War II veterans suggest that damage to the anterior right hemisphere of the brain may be associated with greater maladjustment. TBI may also lead to serious behavioural disturbances causing major problems for families. Carers have to live with a stranger and may themselves suffer serious psychiatric morbidity.

Postconcussional syndrome is common and symptoms of memory disturbance, dysphoria, and headache are frequent long-term sequelae of even minor head injury. These symptoms are often exacerbated by compensation claims which are frequently protracted, as most authorities will wait for at least two years to judge the permanence of any disability.

Burns injuries are also associated with a particularly high long-term psychological morbidity. The pain and disfigurement associated with significant burns add an additional dimension to the suffering of patients and relatives. Burns patients and their families require particularly careful psychological management, especially in the early stages following injury. Relatives should be prepared for the sight of a disfigured patient. The infection control barrier creates a psychological barrier between a patient and relatives, and heightens the patient's sense of isolation. Each surgical intervention creates an additional crisis. Transition to the outside world must be gradual and allow for the predictable ambivalent and sometimes downright hostile public attitudes towards scarring and disfigurement. Similar problems face patients with traumatic amputations, spinal cord injury, neck, pelvic, and genital injuries, which are also associated with an increased frequency

of long-term psychiatric disorder. Psychiatric disorders after minor soft tissue injuries such as whiplash, are controversial.

Affective disorders

Depression is particularly common in the elderly following accidents and occurs more often in individuals with loss of physical function. Depression is usually of moderate severity and meets diagnostic criteria for dysthymia (persistant mild depression), adjustment disorder with depressed mood, or recurrent brief depression. The risk of developing long-term depression is increased if people close to the injured person have been killed (survivor guilt) or severely disabled during the accident. It should be borne in mind that affective symptoms (both depressive and manic) may be secondary to organic mental states.

Important facts about PTSD

- PTSD may be a lifelong disabling disorder running a chronic relapsing course
- PTSD may present with dysfunctional social behaviour such as the breakdown of previously stable relationships and antisocial behaviour
- Other psychiatric disorders such as depression, alcohol, and drug misuse are frequently associated with, and complicate the presentation of PTSD
- No single intervention effectively treats PTSD, and combinations of psychological treatments and pharmacotherapy are usually necessary
- Families become "secondary victims" and may suffer as much as the patient and should always be involved in treatment

---

Anxiety disorders

Post-traumatic stress disorder (PTSD) is the most frequent anxiety disorder seen after physical injury (see box). The full PTSD syndrome is more likely to occur following disasters and combat (Figure 16.1); isolated symptoms of PTSD ("partial PTSD") are more commonly seen after accidents and individual trauma. When PTSD does occur following civilian

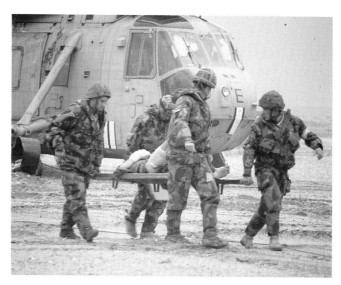

Figure 16.1 PTSD occurs in up to 50% of wounded servicemen.

accidents it is more likely when there is concomitant brain damage or premorbid personality abnormalities, predisposing for anxiety and depression. Nightmares and intrusive memories are usually related to the accident or occasionally to aspects of treatment such as ventilation. The avoidance reactions associated with PTSD are related to any stimuli associated with the accident or disaster situation. Symptoms of increased arousal such as irritability, outbursts of anger, and exaggerated startle responses are seen in about 15% of accident victims. Blanchard et al [6] demonstrated that 46% of RTA victims subsequently develop PTSD, and a further 20% have partial symptoms of the disorder. Individuals with a previous history of trauma and affective disorders appear more likely to develop PTSD following accidents. PTSD is uncommon amongst victims who have lost consciousness, suggesting that the appraisal of threat is critical for PTSD to develop. Diagnostic criteria for PTSD are listed in the box.

"Core" diagnostic criteria for post-traumatic stress disorder

- A life-threatening event outside normal human experience
- Re-experiencing the trauma
  - intrusive memories
  - dreams/nightmares
  - flashbacks (a sense of reliving the event)
  - distress at exposure to events resembling trauma
- Avoidance of stimuli associated with the trauma
- Evidence of increased arousal
  - sleep disturbance
  - irritability
  - hypervigilance
  - exaggerated startle response
- Duration > 1 month

Simple phobias may occur after physical injuries and are commonly associated with reminders of the accident (for example, a fear of driving) rather than fear of injury *per se*. Driving phobias following road traffic accidents are more likely to occur in passengers rather than the driver of the vehicle and are associated with the passenger's perceived lack of control over the situation. Fear associated with exposure to situations that symbolise the traumatic event have been found in 29% of injured adults. Some individuals may suffer from social phobia after physical injury; this occurs most frequently as a consequence of injuries causing scars or disfigurement, particularly burns.

Somatoform disorders

Physical symptoms not explained by organic pathology are the third main group of psychological reactions seen after trauma and occur in about 3% of civilian accident victims. The figure is higher in patients involved in on-going litigation or compensation. Somatoform pain disorder is probably the commonest reaction and, although it has been suggested that these disorders are more common after occupational injuries where compensation is involved, empirical evidence for this is lacking. Somatoform pain disorder is frequently aggravated by current psychosocial problems or conflicts. The diagnosis of somatoform pain disorder is often perceived by the patient as an accusation that he or she is not suffering from "real" pain and malingering. As a result of this patients may vigorously deny any current psychosocial problems and secondary gain,

thereby increasing the likelihood that such cases will be brought to court.

Whiplash injuries of the neck pose particular diagnostic and legal problems. These injuries have been reported to be the cause of chronic pain, but the aetiology is controversial and usually no demonstrable neurological findings can be found. Studies of whiplash reveal the psychological outcome is poor. Pain and headache often persist many years after the injury and are often associated with chronic depression. It is important to appreciate that pain itself may be a symptom of an underlying depressive illness.

Phantom limb pain is a particular form of pain and seen in some patients following traumatic amputation. The aetiology is unclear, but clinically is closely related to depressed mood. Rarely, patients may occasionally complain of changed appearance despite no objective evidence for this (body dysmorphic disorder).

Psychotic disorders

While acute brief reactive psychotic episodes may occur following an accident, and are often associated with delirium, the psychological impact of an injury does not increase the frequency of major mental illness such as manic-depression or schizophrenia. The presence of severe traumatic brain injury does, however, slightly increase the incidence of schizophrenia.

Psychological problems and abnormalities of mental state may have an important negative effect on physical functioning and distress. The effects of mental state on the patient's level of physical functioning should always be considered as part of any functional assessment.

Effects of trauma on others

Relatives

The effect of serious trauma on relatives cannot be underestimated. Following serious injury it is important to recognise that the patient and his relatives have widely differing perspectives and therefore very different psychological needs. These divergent perspectives often result in misunderstanding, tension, and conflict between staff, patients, and relatives. There is a reciprocal relationship between the psychological needs of patients and those of their relatives. In the emergency room, when psychological care is least important to the casualty, the needs of relatives are considerable. Intensive medical activity isolates relatives from the patient compounding their fears and distress. Information given to relatives is frequently misinterpreted and may need to be repeated several times. Relatives need time and space to assimilate what has happened and during this stage may themselves become more accident prone.

During the secondary (subacute) phase the patient may be concerned with the immediate consequences of injury while relatives are preoccupied with its long-term implications. The reaction of a family to trauma may be critical to the patient's long-term recovery; for example, a patient with a head injury may be more distressed if the family has emphasised intellectual functioning as necessary for an individual's success.

The effect of a physical injury on families and friends is particularly evident following brain injury accompanied by organic personality change, and following severe burns injuries [7,8]. Many other common long-term sequelae of trauma, such as psychosexual problems, damage relationships but go unspoken.

It is very difficult to calculate the economic cost of physical trauma. Up to 10% of relatives of the injured may be on sick leave themselves for a short period following the injury. Stress reactions and the need to care for an injured relative are given as the main reasons. In a three year follow-up study of adults injured in traffic accidents with some residual physical sequelae, a quarter of the 55 close relatives interviewed reported impaired psychological health as a consequence of the injury to their loved ones.

Trauma care staff

Serious and potentially disabling psychological and psychiatric symptoms are also well recognised in A & E personnel, rescue workers, and members of the emergency services (Figure 16.2)

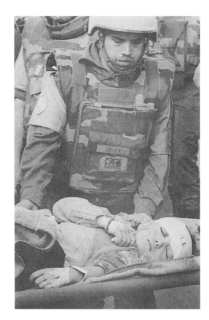

Figure 16.3 Dealing with wounded children places particular stresses on emergency workers.

which predispose to stress include a lack of adequate training, low morale, working in dangerous conditions, and a poor sense of identity and "belonging" to a close-knit cohesive team. Staff who identify with victims, for example those who handle personal effects, are particularly vulnerable. Infant deaths, victims of sexual assault, mass casualties, body handling, and identification are particularly associated with subsequent psychological morbidity and recognised as stressors that can make victims of rescuers. A system of staff support is vital in a busy department dealing with major trauma (Figure 16.4).

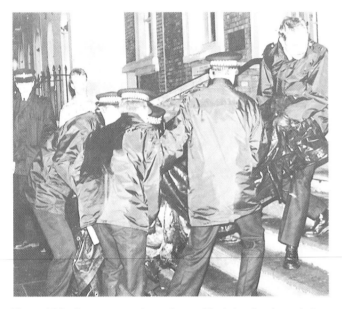

Figure 16.2 Emergency service workers and body handlers in particular often experience psychological problems.

involved in trauma care. Most A & E staff experience some features of traumatic stress following intense and distressing emergency situations. Psychological symptoms include fatigue, sadness, dysphoria and poor concentration, heightened arousal and anxiety, guilt, anger and feelings of helplessness, identification with victims, and intrusive thoughts which interfere with work. Although many of these symptoms are self-limiting, some will go on to develop more serious acute stress reactions, diverse adjustment disorders, and PTSD. The prevalence of PTSD may be as high as 30% or more in emergency workers and rescuers alike following serious accidents and disasters. Serious psychological distress may also occur in "second-line" support workers such as administrators, control room and reception staff, switchboard operators, hospital ancillary and volunteer workers, as well as the families of emergency service personnel.

Like their patients, a variety of individual and situational factors predispose staff to the effects of traumatic stress. Individual vulnerability factors include fatigue and sleep loss, poor physical health, a personal history of psychiatric disorder and a "neurotic" anxiety-prone personality, as well as a lack of supportive and confiding relationships. Adverse reactions are more likely to occur in staff subject to intense and prolonged exposure to distressing events, particularly to handling wounded children (Figure 16.3). Other situational factors

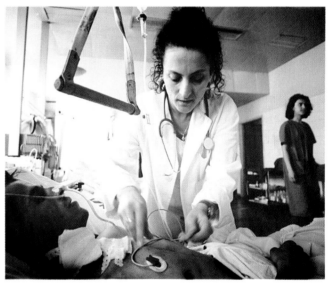

Figure 16.4 A system of staff support is vital in a busy department dealing with major trauma.

Legal aspects of psychological trauma

Compensation claims are common following trauma, and in cases that come to court a psychiatric consultation is commonly requested. A thorough evaluation must include access to previous medical records and historical information about potential vulnerability factors, including past psychiatric history, premorbid personality, previous disability, and absenteeism. Patients with pre-existing psychopathology often attribute abnormalities and distress to their injury and may claim that their mental distress and occupational instability are the direct result of trauma, despite evidence of similar problems prior to the accident. Patients may also blame inadequate medical treatment for their injuries despite obvious evidence to the contrary. These complaints often reflect neglect of psychosocial needs by helpers, and other sources of life stress must be explored before acceptance of any causal relationship between injury and psychiatric problems. Compensation claims should always be settled as quickly as possible; repeated medicolegal assessments perpetuate painful reminders of the trauma and prolong distress.

Treatment of psychological problems in the trauma unit

During the primary phase, psychological treatment of the casualty is subordinate to the treatment of physical injuries. In the immediate aftermath of trauma simple practical support to patients, and particularly to relatives, is often adequate. Relatives and staff often do not know what to say and touch alone may be appropriate and sufficient to lay the foundation of a trusting relationship that forms the cornerstone of psychological rehabilitation. With acknowledgement and the realisation of what has happened more formal counselling may be appropriate and is generally best provided by a specially trained nurse attached to the trauma unit.

Disruptive behaviour is the most common problem facing the trauma team. Firm but kind limits should be set and staff should be taught not to perceive abusive or disruptive behaviour as a personal assault. Treatment must be based on the assessment of the cause of the disturbed behaviour, and organic causes of delirium and hypoxia should always be excluded. Care must be taken to avoid a ward environment which reinforces disruptive behaviour (the more fuss and disturbed behaviour, the more attention by staff).

The treatment of delirium is always that of the underlying cause. Patients should be nursed in a well-lit room with sight of familiar objects. Wherever possible they should be nursed by the same staff. Drugs should be avoided if possible, particularly benzodiazepines, which may lead to disinhibition and worsening disruptive behaviour. If sedative medication is required, small amounts of a neuroleptic such as haloperidol or promazine should be used.

When to refer to a psychiatrist

When simple measures fail, such as the use of selective sedative medication and simple counselling, psychiatric intervention may be appropriate for some patients following trauma. Disruptive behaviour secondary to patients with substance abuse and personality disorder problems are the commonest reasons for referral.

Many authors, particularly in the United States, have advocated the routine attachment of a consultation/liaison psychiatrist as part of the trauma team to assess and manage all patients presenting with manifest psychological disturbance. Although a psychiatrist should be available to help devise policies and protocol they should not automatically be involved in the provision of psychological aftercare for victims of trauma. Not only does this unnecessarily stigmatise the patient by

turning a trauma victim into a psychiatric patient, it also potentially undermines the therapeutic relationship between the patient and the trauma team, who may feel that the patient's psychological needs are being met elsewhere. It also detracts from the skills of the general psychiatrist who should be well capable and qualified to deal with trauma patients who develop psychiatric problems without having to delegate this to a specialist colleague. In a cost conscious NHS, trauma teams will have to pay for the services of a liaison psychiatrist and against a background of increasing financial constraints it is important that these specialist services are reserved for patients in genuine need.

Patients with established psychiatric disorder should be referred to a general adult psychiatrist for assessment in the first instance. This not only enables a psychiatric diagnosis to be confirmed but facilitates access to a range of more specialist treatment services. Unlike other mental health professionals, such as the clinical psychologist, the general psychiatrist has an overview of treatment modalities both pharmacological and psychological. In addition the psychiatrist also acts as "gatekeeper", controlling access to more specialist services. Following a psychiatric assessment many trauma victims will be referred on to these specialist services for counselling and a variety of psychotherapeutic techniques as appropriate.

Prevention of long-term psychiatric disability

Efforts to minimise long-term psychiatric disability following trauma, represents a major challenge to the medical profession. The important issue facing the trauma team is what steps can be taken to minimise the incidence of subsequent serious long-term psychiatric disorder.

Communication with general practitioner

There are two broad areas in which the trauma team can influence subsequent psychiatric morbidity. Firstly, effective communication with long-term carers, particularly the patient's general practitioner, is crucial. Many patients with minor injuries are discharged directly from the A & E department and written information given to the patient to take to their GP is often discarded. Subsequent psychiatric morbidity, particularly PTSD, may not be evident and not infrequently presents months or even years later with disturbed behaviour, disrupted relationships, occupational instability, and substance misuse. A GP unaware of previous trauma may fail to recognise underlying psychopathology and treat the patient inappropriately as a consequence. Communication with general practitioners should be included in any major incident plan. Following disasters, in particular, written information should be sent directly to the GP stating that a patient has been involved in trauma, outlining the symptoms of post-traumatic stress, and briefly describing its diverse presentations.

Psychological debriefing

Psychological debriefing (PD) is the second broad area in which the trauma team can attempt to prevent or minimise morbidity following traumatic events. Calls for the routine provision of early psychological intervention for the victims of trauma have resulted in the emergence of a "disaster industry" lead by a variety of professional groups including lay counsellors, psychologists, social workers, and psychiatrists, who have all sought to establish a role for themselves following traumatic incidents. In a recent survey of senior officers of UK emergency services, 72% reported some critical incident stress provision within their local service although only 28% felt that sufficient attention was paid to this aspect of staff welfare. Early interventions are intuitively appealing and a response to perceived need, but their effectiveness is not certain.

Jeffrey Mitchell, an American psychologist, initially described "critical incident stress debriefing" (CISD) with ambulance personnel in 1983. CISD has been modified and expanded by others including Dyregrov [9] who coined the term "psychological debriefing". It is aimed at all those involved in traumatic events including victims, rescuers, emergency service workers, and the providers of psychological aftercare.

PD is a structured intervention designed to promote the emotional processing of traumatic events through the ventilation and normalisation of reactions, and preparation for possible future experiences. Although initially designed for use in groups, it has also been used with individuals, couples, and families. A typical PD takes place 48–72 hours after the trauma as a single group meeting lasting approximately two hours.

Seven stages are passed through during PD. A brief introduction stressing the focus of the intervention and its confidentiality is followed by consideration of the facts of what happened from the varied perspectives of all those attending. The expectations, thoughts, and impressions of those involved are then discussed. By this stage of the PD a detailed reconstruction of what happened will have occurred, and, at least in theory led to the open expression of associated emotions including guilt and anger. These are considered in depth and normalised as far as is reasonably possible. Group processes such as universality and peer support are mobilised during group PD which helps with the acceptance of experienced emotions. The emphasis remains on normalisation throughout and this is discussed formally towards the end of the PD. In conclusion the debriefer (s) prepares the participants for future symptoms and reactions, should they occur, and gives guidelines as to when further help should be sought and where it can be found. These points are often reinforced with written information distributed to the participants before they leave.

How does PD work?

Trauma psychology suggests that most victims of severe trauma will endure some distressing symptoms as they assimilate their experience. Horowitz's Information Processing Model predicts alternating intrusive symptoms (for example, nightmares and flashbacks) and avoidant symptoms (for example, denial and avoidance of cues). These diminish in intensity with time and form an integral part of the normal stress response. Such symptoms are only considered pathological when they become excessive in frequency, magnitude, or duration.

How effective is PD

The chaos and unpredictability of disasters and accidents alike makes research difficult and the vast majority of published data suffer from serious methodological difficulties. The commonest shortcomings are:

- Not prospective
- Small sample size
- Absence of control group
- Varying degrees of trauma
- Absence of random allocation

- Other confounding variables ignored
- Low response rates
- Sampling bias
- Lack of uniformity of PD
- Timing variance
- Questionnaire versus interview results.

Anecdotal reports supporting the effectiveness of PD are plentiful and have fuelled its increasing use. In a long-term study of the course of post-traumatic morbidity in 469 firefighters exposed to a bushfire disaster over 25 months, individuals who were not debriefed afterwards were more likely to develop an acute post-traumatic stress reaction than those who were [10]. However, the effectiveness of the debriefing process was thrown into doubt by the finding that those individuals who developed a delayed onset post-traumatic stress reaction were more likely to have attended a debriefing than individuals who had remained well throughout the follow-up period.

In another study, 60% of 172 emergency workers who had received PD following various traumatic incidents in Australia completed questionnaires two weeks after the PD [11]. The majority found the PD useful and felt it had helped to reduce their symptoms of stress. Unfortunately the absence of a control group, lack of more objective data, a short follow-up period, and low completion rate limited the value of these findings. Other studies supporting PD suffer from similar methodological problems. One study that does boast a control group is that of Bunn and Clarke [12] who assessed the use of a 20 min supportive interview with a psychologist as opposed to no intervention in the relatives of severely ill or injured patients admitted to an emergency ward. The subject group were less anxious immediately after the interview but no follow-up data were collected.

In a recent study examining the effectiveness of PD in 74 British Gulf War veterans, no demonstrable difference was found in psychological morbidity at nine months between those who had been debriefed and those who had not [13]. Similarly, a study comparing two groups of Norwegian firefighters exposed to dead bodies found no difference in psychological symptoms two weeks later between those formally debriefed and those who had talked with colleagues [14]. Both of these studies have their weaknesses but importantly do include comparison groups, which, given the lack of knowledge on the natural history of post-traumatic stress reactions, is essential.

More complex preventative interventions following traumatic events have been more convincingly shown to have a positive effect in better designed studies. However, a recently reported intervention showed no difference at one and six month follow-up between a group of road traffic accident victims who received a preventative counselling programme and those who did not [15]. Interestingly, in common with Robinson and Mitchell's findings [11], those who received the intervention said they found it useful.

PD is not without its own risks. Mandatory attendance at a PD has, not surprisingly, been associated with passive participation and resentment and it is widely accepted that debriefers themselves may become "secondary victims". Overenthusiasm for primary preventative methods might delay the diagnosis and effective treatment of those who do suffer psychological sequelae.

It is important to define clearly the limitations of the crisis intervention approach and the point at which more formal treatment is required. Many individuals with psychiatric disorders as a result of the Australian bushfires presented late because of other professionals' fears that labelling by referral to a psychiatrist would occur.

The effectiveness of PD is far from proven even though it appears to be popular with the consumer. The data available from methodologically flawed studies suggest that, at best, PD affords some protection against later sequelae and, at worst, makes no difference. It is already apparent that individuals receiving PD are not immune to subsequent psychological morbidity. Therefore, if PD is employed following traumatic events, formal follow-up to facilitate the identification of individuals who do go on to develop serious psychological sequelae is vital.

The current body of knowledge suggests that the presence or absence of other factors, for example an acute stress reaction, personality, past psychiatric history, and adequate social support, is likely to affect the psychological outcome of individuals involved in traumatic events more than the presence or absence of PD; these factors should perhaps receive greater attention when emergency service personnel are recruited. Indeed, when individuals have an adequate support network and do not have other vulnerability factors, a PD may be redundant.

Despite a lack of adequate data supporting PD, clinical experience suggests that many individuals value the opportunity to express feelings of anger and guilt and derive comfort from the realisation that these are a normal emotional response to trauma. Many of the feelings expressed during PD are intensely personal and disaster workers and victims often experience difficulty in confiding in, and tend to be suspicious of, "outsiders", especially mental health professionals. If PD is to be effective it should be a team responsibility taking place within groups of emergency workers carried out as locally and rapidly as possible. The role of mental health professionals should be directed towards educating these groups rather than trying to provide a service themselves.

Summary

Many accident and trauma victims appear to respond in a remarkably calm and controlled fashion and cope well with the effects of trauma and emerge at least as strong, if not stronger, than they were before. Severe behavioural disturbances of sufficient severity to interfere with medical care are infrequent following civilian accidents (< 5%), and when such reactions occur are often the result of predisposing factors. The psychological aftermath of disaster can, nevertheless, result in significant long-term psychiatric disability and suffering to victims, relatives, and emergency workers alike, and the psychosocial dimension of injury should be an integral part of trauma management. All trauma victims go through well-defined stages of psychological adjustment which give rise to predictable, and sometimes distressing, reactions. Recognising and helping the patient on this journey of adjustment not only helps the patient come to terms with injury and its consequences but may well reduce the incidence of subsequent long-term psychiatric morbidity, both in patients and their relatives. Simple measures taken early on can reduce the likelihood of long-term psychiatric disability. Increased psychiatric and behavioral disturbance among the patients places an additional burden on staff, and failure to provide adequate personnel and staff support results in low morale and excess sick leave because of staff burn-out.

Effective communication with relatives and the general practitioner is an important part of trauma care and this itself may influence the patient's long-term psychological well-being.

Various psychological interventions have been advocated after trauma of which psychological debriefing (PD) is the best known. If this or any other professional psychological intervention is to be made routinely available to trauma victims, considerable resources would be required. At present PD is one of many psychological interventions that requires proper evaluation with the use of prospective controlled study designs and random allocation to PD or non-intervention groups. It is not known whether PD should be routinely offered to everyone involved in traumatic events, restricted to "high risk" individuals, or abandoned. Whatever the outcome of such research, overenthusiasm for primary preventative methods must not be allowed to delay the institution of diagnosis and effective treatment for those who do suffer psychological sequelae.

Successful trauma management requires the application of the most technological aspects of modern medicine. In a busy trauma unit psychosocial considerations and a holistic approach to patient care can all too easily be neglected. Trauma care does not end with a satisfactory surgical outcome and failure to acknowledge and meet the psychological needs of patient, relatives, and staff can result in considerable distress and significant long-term morbidity for all concerned.

References

1. Whetsell LA, Patterson CM, Young DH, Schiller WR. Preinjury psychopathology in trauma patients. *J Trauma* 1989;**29**: 1158–62.
2. Malt UF. The long-term consequences of accidental injury. *Br J Psychiat* 1988;**153**:810–18.
3. Mayou R, Bryant B, Duthie R. Psychiatric consequences of road traffic accidents. *Br Med J* 1993;**307**:647–51.
4. Lishman WA. *Organic psychiatry: the psychological consequences of cerebral disorder* (2nd edn), Oxford: Blackwell, 1988.
5. Patterson DR, Carrigan L, Questad RA, Robinson R. Post-traumatic stress disorder in hospitalised patients with burn injuries. *J Burn Care Rehab* 1990;**11**:181–4.
6. Blanchard EB, Hickling EJ, Taylor AE *et al.* Psychiatric morbidity, associated with motor vehicle accidents. *J Nervous Mental Dis* 1995; **183**:495–504.
7. Livingston MG, Brookes DN, Bond MR. Three months after severe head injury: Psychiatric and social impact on relatives. *J Neurol Neurosurg Psychiat* 1985a;**48**:870–5.
8. Livingston MG, Brookes DN, Bond MR. Patient outcome in the year following severe head injury and relatives psychiatric and social functioning. *J Neurol Neurosurg Psychiat* 1985b;**48**:876–81.
9. Duregrov A. Caring for helpers in disaster situation: psychological debriefing. *Disaster Manag* 1989;**2**:25–30.
10. McFarlane AC. The longitudinal course of post-traumatic morbidity: The range of outcomes and their predictors. *J Nervous Mental Dis* 1988;**176**:30–9.
11. Robinson RC, Mitchell JT. Evaluation of psychological debriefings. *J Traumatic Stress* 1993;**6**:367–82.
12. Bunn, TA, Clarke AM. Crisis intervention: an experimental study of the effects of a brief period of counselling on the anxiety of relatives of seriously injured or ill hospital patients. *Br J Med Psychol* 1979;**52**:191–5.
13. Deahl M, Gillham AB, Thomas J *et al.* Psychological sequelae following the Gulf War; factors associated with subsequent morbidity and the effectiveness of psychological debriefing. *Br J Psychiat* 1994;**165**:60–5.
14. Hyton K, Hasle A. Fire fighters: A study of stress and coping. *Acta Psychiat Scand* 1989;**80**: (Supplementum 355).
15. Brom D, Kleber RJ, Hofman MC. Victims of traffic accidents: incidence and prevention of post-traumatic stress disorder. *J Clin Psychol* 1993;**49**:131–40.

Further reading

Bisson JI, Deahl MP. Does psychological debriefing work? *Br J Psychiat* 1994;**165**:717–20.

Black D, Newman M, Harris-Hendricks J, Mezey G (eds). Psychological trauma. A developmental approach. London: Gaskell Press, 1997.

Gibson M. *Order from chaos. Responding to traumatic events.* Birmingham: Venture Press, 1991.

Hackett TP, Cassem NH (eds). *Massachusetts General Hospital Handbook of General Hospital Psychiatry* (2nd edn), Littleton, Mass: PSG Publishing Co. Inc., 1987.

Miechenbaum D. *A Clinical handbook/practical therapist manual for assessing and treating adults with post-traumatic stress disorder (PTSD).* Ontario: Institute Press, 1994.

Raphael B. *When disaster strikes: how individuals and communities cope with catastrophe.* New York: Basic Books, 1986.

Ursano RJ, McCaughey BG, Fullerton CS (eds) *Individual and community responses to trauma and disaster.* Cambridge: Cambridge University Press, 1994.

Wilson JP, Raphael B (eds). *The international handbook of traumatic stress syndromes.* New York: Plenum Press, 1993.

17 Paediatric trauma

Jenny Walker

Consultant Paediatric Surgeon, Paediatric Surgical Unit, Sheffield Children's Hospital NHS Trust

---

OBJECTIVES

■ To be aware of the relevant differences between adults and children when affected by trauma.

■ To know how to assess the patient in a structured way, that is ABCDE, and to recognise the similarity of assessment and resuscitation between injured children and adults.

■ To be able to recognise the presentation and know the management of severe injuries in order of priority, that is ABCDE.

■ To remember the importance of the family in the management of an injured child.

Trauma is the most common cause of death in children aged 1–15 years and, even with intense effort at injury prevention, there are still over 500 deaths per year from trauma in England and Wales. Most paediatric trauma is accidental, but sadly up to 10% of trauma deaths are due to non-accidental injury. Infants (children under the age of 12 months) rarely undergo serious injury, except non-accidental injury. Road traffic accidents – involving passenger, pedestrian or cyclist – are the most common cause, and in older children sporting injuries occur. Blunt injury is much more common than penetrating injury, which is still fortunately very rare in the UK.

Anatomy and physiology

The anatomy of the child is not only smaller than that of adults, but there are also differences in proportions, and these may have effects both on the child's response to trauma and to the clinician's management of that child. Some of those relevant features which differ between children and adults are mentioned here.

Airway

The child's head is relatively large with a pronounced occiput, a relatively small face, and a short neck. This leads to neck flexion and airway obstruction in an obtunded patient and, in order to straighten the airway maximally, the infant's head must be laid in the neutral position (that is, looking straight at the ceiling) and the child's head in the sniffing position (that is, looking slightly upwards) when laid supine.

The airway can also be difficult to keep open optimally, because of the relatively large tongue and the soft tissues of the floor of the mouth; these cause the resuscitator's fingers to compress the tongue up to the roof of the mouth. To avoid this, careful positioning of the fingers on the bony edge of the jaw is needed when a mask is held on the face. Another hazard is the possibility of loose teeth and/or dental brace (Figure 17.1).

If laryngoscopy is necessary, difficulty may be encountered with:

● floppy large tongue;
● adenotonsillar hypertrophy (common in children especially of Infant School age);
● horseshoe-shaped epiglottis obstructing the view of the relatively high and anteriorly placed larynx.

Breathing

The airways are relatively small in a child, and can easily be obstructed. Children breathe faster than adults, in order to cope with their increased oxygen consumption and greater metabolic rate.

The ribs are very compliant and, consequently, crush injuries (such as from seatbelts) can produce lung contusion without visible rib fractures. If the ribs do fracture, the force must have been very high, and lung damage is even more severe.

Circulation

The circulating volume in a child is slightly higher, at 80 ml/kg, but the actual volume is small, meaning that, in small children, loss of a small volume of blood can have serious consequences. Children have a faster heart rate and a lower systolic blood pressure, but their response to hypovolaemic shock has lesser effect on the circulation parameters, until the patient is relatively more fluid depleted, when there is a sudden and possibly catastrophic or irreversible change in the vital signs. Symptoms and signs of hypovolaemic shock may not occur until 25% of the total circulating volume has been lost, and hence resuscitation volumes are in 20 ml/kg boluses (that is, 25% of the total 80 ml/kg volume). It is therefore important for a child's weight to be known, or to be "guesstimated" by using the formula:

$$\text{Weight in kg} = \text{twice (age} \pm 4)$$

or by using a Broselow tape, which relates the child's height to their weight.

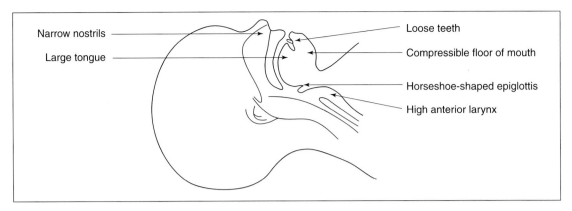

Figure 17.1 Upper airway anatomy. (From *Advanced Paediatric Life Support*, BMJ Publishing Group, 1993.)

Psychology

The psychological effect of trauma on a child can be extreme, in particular in those children who have any feeling of responsibility for the accident. As in all ill children, their "functioning" mental age decreases when they are vulnerable or feel out of control of their surroundings, and it is essential to remember that a child needs continuing support and truthful explanation. If the child is conscious, somebody must be designated to talk to him or her, to reassure, and to explain what is happening.

Initial assessment

As in any patient who has been affected by trauma, the initial assessment and management will follow the usual principles of ABCDE:

- **A**irway with cervical spine control
- **B**reathing and ventilation
- **C**irculation with haemorrhage control
- **D**isability
- **E**xposure and environment

ensuring that life-threatening problems are treated as soon as they are found, and that, on any detectable deterioration in the patient's condition, the attention returns to **A** and then **B** etc. Only on total and safe completion of this primary survey and resuscitation should the secondary survey and further investigations begin.

Airway with cervical spine control

The airway is the most important part of the initial assessment because, without a clear airway, oxygen cannot get into the lungs and hence into the patient's circulation; without good oxygenation, it is irrelevant how effective the care the child receives, the outcome will not be as good.

During the assessment and management of the airway, it is essential that the cervical spine is controlled, as any child that has been involved in an accident is presumed to have a cervical (and/or a thoracic or lumbar) spinal injury until this has been excluded. This cervical spine control consists of a semirigid collar of the correct size, with the use of sandbags or their equivalent adjacent to the head, with tape over the forehead and chin to maintain complete immobilisation in the supine position. Whenever this immobilisation needs to be removed, either partially or completely for investigations or examination or for nursing care, the cervical spine must be held in the same immobilised position by manual in-line stabilisation by a trained doctor or nurse.

If the patient is intubated, the semirigid cervical collar must remain in place until after the patient has been extubated and x-rays passed as normal, and a senior doctor with appropriate training has made a clinical assessment of the child's neck. Two thirds of cervical spine injuries occur without x-ray change (Spinal Cord Injury Without Radiological Abnormality – SCIWORA) and this is why normal x-rays are not sufficient to enable the collar and care of the cervical spine to be abandoned. As the child becomes more awake and mobile, the sandbags and tape may be removed because the child maintains his or her neck immobilised relative to the rest of the body, but the hard collar must not be removed until the child has been clinically assessed. This is particularly hard to remember some days down the line in a ventilated patient on the Intensive Care Unit.

Breathing and ventilation

Once the airway has been cleared and protected, the breathing and effectiveness of breathing is assessed by looking at the respiratory rate, effort, and symmetry of movement, and ventilatory support provided if appropriate. Oxygenation of both lungs is the aim, and both sides of the chest need to be moving with adequate bilateral air entry to achieve this. This may be prevented by the injuries received, or by dislodgement of the endotracheal tube if used, either into the oesophagus or one or other of the main bronchi – both main bronchi are equally likely in children.

Adequate oxygenation is essential, and an oxygen mask with high flow oxygen and reservoir is mandatory. Children can tire easily, and a high index of suspicion is necessary to assess whether intubation and assisted ventilation would be helpful.

Circulation with haemorrhage control

Obvious and overt bleeding must be controlled whilst the assessment of the circulation occurs.

Assessment will include the measurement of pulse, blood pressure, capillary refill time, skin colour, and (later) urine output. Knowing the different normal values in different aged children is useful (Table 17.1).

Tachycardia may be due to fright, anxiety, pain or hypovolaemia, or any combination of these. Hypotension is a very late sign of hypovolaemia in a child, and other signs should have been detected earlier.

Table 17.1 Vital signs: approximate range of normal*

Age years	Respiratory rate (breaths/min)	Systolic BP (mmHg)	Pulse (/min)
<1	30–40	70–90	110–160
2–5	25–30	80–100	95–140
5–12	20–25	90–110	80–120
>12	15–20	100–120	60–100

* From *Advanced Paediatric Life Support*, BMJ Publishing Group, 1993.

When intravenous access is obtained, this is done with two relatively large but short cannulae; blood will be sent for baseline haematology, biochemistry (including blood sugar and amylase) and cross-match. As in adults, the veins of choice are in the antecubital fossa, long saphenous vein, etc. Central venous access is difficult in children and not suitable for use in resuscitation. Peripheral venous access allows resuscitation to commence with appropriate fluids at 20 ml/kg until definitive venous access is obtained. Intra-osseous access is very useful in children in the emergency situation, especially in those of preschool age, but can be used at any age, as children have marrow present in all long bones. Continued attempts at definitive access must continue once resuscitation using the intra-osseous access has occurred, and the intra-osseous access should be removed within six hours to decrease the risk of infection.

Any inability to stabilise the child's circulation after an initial bolus of 20 ml/kg of warmed fluids (either colloid or crystalloid) must alert the resuscitating team to the possibility of continuing blood loss, and urgent telephone consultation with a paediatric surgeon in the nearest Paediatric Surgical Unit (which is likely to be a Regional Referral Centre) is essential.

After every intervention, the patient must be reassessed to ensure that good progress is being made, but if there is any sign of deterioration, the assessor must return to the Airway, and then Breathing and then Circulation, to ensure that any life threatening incidents are dealt with as they are found.

Disability

If all the cardiovascular parameters remain steady, the patient will then be assessed for disability. Even if a head injury is definite or suspected, neurological assessment before this stage is not relevant, as the effect of the head injury is not going to affect the child's outcome, if oxygenation and hypovolaemia have not been corrected. In practice, a brief initial neurological assessment will happen simultaneously with the assessment of the airway, in order to help with the prognosis; once the child is intubated and sedated and paralysed, that initial neurological assessment is impossible.

Neurological assessment is done quickly by AVPU, with assessment of response:

- **A**lert
- Responds to **V**oice
- Responds to **P**ain
- **U**nresponsive

The pupillary size and reaction is also noted.

These observations are repeated regularly. The open anterior fontanelle in a child under 12–18 months can be useful to assess the intracranial pressure directly.

In particular unequal pupils and non-reactiveness to light may indicate a serious intracranial problem which must be investigated and managed appropriately, after consultation with a neurosurgeon.

Exposure

The patient must be fully exposed in order to enable the assessors to complete a full examination. Children have a large surface area relative to their size, and consequently lose heat very quickly; it is crucial that the child's body temperature is maintained by covering the child as much as possible during the necessary exposure for examination and investigations. This will also help preserve the child's dignity, as they are very unhappy and do not react well to being naked in strange surroundings.

This examination will allow any obvious sources of external bleeding to be located, and any obvious injury that has not been already identified.

Mandatory x-rays

The essential x-rays are of the lateral cervical spine, the chest, and the pelvis.

The interpretation of lateral cervical spine x-rays are even more difficult in children than in adults, and must be referred to an experienced paediatric radiologist for a definitive report. This is because of the various epiphyseal lines and ossification centres which mimic fractures, as well as the pseudosubluxation of C2 on C3 and C3 on C4, which can occur in up to 40% of children especially before the age of 7 years.

As was mentioned earlier, chest x-rays may not reveal any fractured ribs, but pulmonary contusion can occur without rib fracture and is even more likely if rib fractures are seen. Fractures of the lower ribs increase the possibility of solid organ damage, for example in liver, spleen, or kidney.

Pelvic x-rays will reveal fractures and will raise the suspicion of bladder and urethral injuries, and give an idea of potential hidden blood loss.

Other x-rays are only taken if clinically indicated by the findings on examination during the secondary survey.

Internal examination

The usual teaching of "fingers and tubes in every orifice" in an adult must be seriously considered before application in a child. Vaginal examination is contraindicated in all girls under the age of consent (16 years).

Rectal examination is also non-contributory in children, as boys do not have a palpable prostate, and the examining finger may traumatise the small anus by an investigator who cannot interpret the findings; the examination should be left to the paediatric surgeon at the Regional Centre if it is felt that it would change the child's management, which is very rare.

Gastric tubes

Children swallow a lot of air, especially when they are crying, and so they should have a large-bore nasogastric tube (or orogastric, if a basal skull fracture is suspected, to prevent entry of the tube into the intracranial space via the fracture) passed to enable the stomach to be empty of air, and food and fluid if possible. This tube should be left on free drainage and aspirated regularly.

Urinary catheters

Catheterisation of a child should only be carried out if the child cannot pass urine spontaneously, or if very accurate hourly urine measurement is required for continued monitoring. Neither girls nor boys will accept urinary catheterisation if they are conscious, and urethral damage can occur in boys, especially if a catheter, that is not entirely silastic and is large, is used. There is usually very little need to contemplate catheterisation in a child in the first hour or two after immediate resuscitation, and it is therefore entirely reasonable to leave the question and the method of urinary drainage to the team with ongoing management responsibility, who can decide whether to catheterise the child at all, and whether it should be via the urethral or suprapubic route.

Repeated monitoring and reassessment

The patient must be reassessed regularly during the initial assessment and resuscitation phase to ensure that steady progress is being made. If there is any sign of deterioration, the assessor must return to the Airway, then Breathing, Circulation and Disability, to ensure that any newly presenting life-threatening incidents are dealt with.

Once the patient is stable, a more thorough and complete examination is made of the patient in the form of a secondary survey.

Secondary survey

This is identical to that in an adult, apart from the following features:

- *Head.* The Glasgow Coma Scale varies in children because of their inability to speak when they are young; a chart for under four-year-olds is available (Table 17.2).

- *Face.* Deciduous teeth may have been loose or absent before the accident, or may have become dislodged and can be lost in the airways during the accident.
- *Abdomen.* Internal examinations are avoided as indicated above.

Diagnostic peritoneal lavage is rarely performed in children, as a positive result will not alter the usual policy of non-operative management in a Paediatric Surgical Centre. Uncontrollable hypovolaemic shock will necessitate an urgent laparotomy without recourse to diagnostic peritoneal lavage.

Ultrasound may be readily available, but is not the investigation of choice, as solid organ damage can easily be missed. It may be useful for identifying free intraperitoneal fluid, but not necessarily the source.

A double contrast (intravenous and intragastric) abdominal CT scan is the investigation of choice, but should only be performed when the patient has been adequately resuscitated and is stable.

Specialist referrals

As the assessment progresses, it will become apparent to the doctor in charge, what underlying injuries are possible or definite.

All children that have been injured would benefit from definitive care in a Paediatric Surgical Unit. The mechanism of injury, lower rib fractures, and free intraperitoneal fluid will raise the suspicion of intra-abdominal pathology, and the management of this patient must be discussed with a paediatric surgeon. The child can then be transferred to the care of the paediatric surgeon.

The timing of this referral and transfer will depend on the severity of the injuries and the arrangements as dictated locally.

It is appropriate at this stage to contact the relevant specialists, including anaesthetists, paediatricians, and general

---

Table 17.2 Glasgow Coma Scale and Children's Coma Scale

Glasgow Coma Scale (4–15 years)		Children's Coma Scale (<4 years)		
Response	Score	Response		Score
Eyes		Eyes		
Open spontaneously	4	Open spontaneously		4
Verbal command	3	React to speech		3
Pain	2	React to pain		2
No response	1	No response		1
Best motor response		Best motor response		
Verbal command:		Spontaneous or obeys verbal		
Obeys	6	command		6
Painful stimulus:		*Painful stimulus:*		
Localises pain	5	Localises pain		5
Flexion with pain	4	Withdraws in response to pain		4
		Abnormal flexion to pain		
Flexion abnormal	3	(decorticate posture)		3
		Abnormal extension to pain		
Extension	2	(decerebrate posture)		2
No response	1	No response		1
Best verbal response		Best verbal response		
Orientated and		Smiles, orientated to sounds,		
converses	5	follows objects, interacts		5
Disorientated and		*Crying*	*Interacts*	
converses	4	Consolable	Inappropriate	4
Inappropriate words	3	Inconsistently consolable	Moaning	3
Incomprehensible sounds	2	Inconsolable	Irritable	2
No response	1	No response	No response	1

paediatric, neurosurgical, orthopaedic, plastic, ENT, ophthalmic, and maxillofacial surgeons.

In a stable patient, transfer can be well planned and timed. In a child where there is severe injury, or where the history raises a high index of suspicion, the case should be discussed with a senior paediatric surgeon in the appropriate nearest unit. This is likely to be a consultant or senior specialist registrar on call.

Transfer

A safe transfer is essential, and the principles are the same as those discussed for adults elsewhere in this book.

Specific injuries: presentation and management

Airway

Injuries to the airway are soon identified owing to the first priority being a clear and protected airway. If facial injury exists, the maxillofacial surgeons may be called early, or even the ear nose and throat surgeon, if the child needs an emergency tracheostomy.

Breathing

Internal chest injuries may have occurred with very little external bruising or sign of injury, and even the chest x-ray can be normal in a child with severe intrathoracic problems.

Chest injuries may lead to respiratory distress and may increase in the work of breathing. The diaphragm is used in breathing, which is hindered by gastric dilatation, and hence necessitates the early placement of a nasogastric or orogastric tube. Hypoxia will lead to irritability, drowsiness, or unconsciousness. The heart rate increases, the skin is pale, and bradycardia and cyanosis are both late signs.

Some injuries are life threatening and will be detected during the primary survey and treated at that time. These injuries are listed below.

Tension pneumothorax

This produces severe respiratory distress and circulatory compromise as air collects outside the lung under tension, the lung collapses, and the mediastinum is pushed over to the opposite side of the chest, which kinks the great vessels (aorta, pulmonary artery or vein, or superior or inferior vena cava), venous return to the heart is decreased, and hence cardiac output is reduced.

Signs include hypoxia and shock, with decreased air entry and hyperresonance to percussion on the side of the pneumothorax, distended neck veins, and tracheal deviation away from the side of the pneumothorax.

Emergency treatment consists of:

- high-flow oxygen administration;
- needle drainage of the tension pneumothorax in the second intercostal space in the midclavicular line;
- definitive chest drain insertion in the midaxillary line in the fourth or fifth intercostal space.

Massive haemothorax

A haemothorax will also prevent adequate oxygenation of that lung (owing to lung collapse/compression) and presents as a life-threatening respiratory emergency and, if adequate blood is lost into the haemothorax, symptoms of hypovolaemia.

Signs include hypoxia and possibly shock, with decreased air entry and hyporesonance to percussion on the side of the haemothorax.

Emergency treatment consists of:

- high-flow oxygen administration;
- vascular access and fluid resuscitation;
- definitive chest drain insertion.

Open pneumothorax

An open wound into the chest allows air into the pleural cavity outside the lung and prevents the usual flow of oxygen into that lung via the trachea, as there is more resistance, and this leads to collapse of the lung.

Signs include hypoxia, with decreased air entry and hyperresonance to percussion on the side of the pneumothorax.

Emergency treatment consists of:

- high-flow oxygen administration;
- covering of the chest wound on three sides (to prevent converting the open pneumothorax to a tension pneumothorax);
- definitive chest drain insertion.

Flail chest

This is extremely rare in childhood, owing to the compliance of the ribs. Fractured ribs can prevent adequate chest expansion from pain, as can a flail segment (when three or more adjacent ribs are fractured in two places, and this flail segment moves in the opposite direction to the chest wall during respiration, compromising ventilation and producing hypoxia).

Emergency treatment consists of:

- high-flow oxygen administration;
- adequate analgesia;
- possible intubation and ventilation (particularly when the child is exhausted, or if indicated by the arterial blood gases).

Cardiac tamponade

This is due to blood collecting in the space outside the heart, inside the fibrous pericardial sac, decreasing the space available for venous return to the heart; this leads to a progressive decrease in cardiac output.

Signs include shock, quiet heart sounds, and distended neck veins (if there is not associated hypovolaemia).

Emergency treatment consists of:

- high-flow oxygen administration;
- vascular access and fluid resuscitation;
- needle drainage of the pericardial collection.

These life-threatening injuries may have been detected during the primary survey, or they may also have a delayed presentation, and be detected in the child's assessment on the Intensive Care Unit when, again, they require immediate treatment.

Any child with even a small simple pneumothorax will run into problems if ventilated, as air will be forced out into the pleural cavity and the simple pneumothorax will become under tension.

Some chest injuries are severe but present later.

Pulmonary contusion

This is common in children as the chest wall is very mobile, and there might not be any associated rib fractures. Hypoxia is progressive, and often requires ventilation.

Rupture of a major airway (trachea or main bronchus)

This may be fatal but, if not, will present as a persistent air leak into the chest drain. Treatment is with oxygen and by open thoracic surgery.

Rupture of a great vessel (aorta, pulmonary artery or vein, or superior or inferior vena cava)

This is usually fatal at the scene of the accident. If the child reaches hospital, the rupture will have sealed itself off, and will be suspected from the mechanism of injury (acute deceleration), and from the widened upper mediastinum seen on the chest x-ray. The diagnosis is confirmed on a contrast arch aortogram, and is treated by open cardiac surgery. Disruption of the thoracic aorta is very rare in childhood.

Rupture of the diaphragm

This produces hypoxia owing to lung compression by the abdominal contents, and is diagnosed on the chest x-ray, although positive pressure ventilation may apparently reduce the abdominal contents back into the abdomen. The rupture should be repaired by a paediatric or thoracic surgeon.

The majority of severe chest injuries can be managed with oxygen, vascular access and fluid resuscitation, chest drainage, intubation and ventilation, and occasionally pericardial drainage. Only rarely is a cardiothoracic opinion needed.

Circulation

Injuries leading to hypovolaemia include those mentioned above in chest injuries (massive haemothorax and cardiac tamponade), as well as intra-abdominal bleeds (including into the retroperitoneal space), scalp lacerations in a small child, and pelvic and long bone fractures.

Signs are of hypovolaemia, and all the sites where "invisible" haemorrhage can occur must be examined.

Treatment is with vascular access, fluid resuscitation, and referral to the appropriate specialist, in order to stop any continuing haemorrhage.

Disability

Head injury is the most common single cause of death in children. The management is similar to that in an adult.

Spinal injuries are rare in children, but are seen more often in the multiply injured child. Assessment can be difficult, and significant cord damage can occur without radiological abnormality (SCIWORA – see above). Pseudosubluxation of the cervical spine can occur in up to 40% of children under 7 years, and may be difficult to assess without a senior paediatric radiologist's opinion.

Management of spinal injury is similar to that in adults, with spinal immobilisation maintained in any child who could have sustained a spinal injury, until it has been excluded, both clinically and radiologically, by senior and experienced personnel.

Abdominal injuries

Abdominal trauma that is blunt is most common in the UK, and it is important to keep reviewing the abdomen, to look for bruising, and watch abdominal movement during respiration, remembering gastric dilatation, retention of urine, and to hear complaints of pain.

Intra-abdominal injuries include solid organ rupture, for example liver, spleen or kidney, and bowel perforation. Bruises on the upper abdomen and lower chest may suggest liver and spleen injury. Bruises on the flank and lower chest may suggest renal trauma, and haematuria will increase this suspicion. A seatbelt may produce bruising in the iliac fossae and be associated with bowel perforation, and bicycle handlebars classically rupture the duodenum and/or pancreas, as these organs are fixed on the posterior abdominal wall, and the handlebars crushes them against the child's spine. A double contrast (intragastric and intravenous contrast) CT scan is the most useful investigation, although this is only performed if the child is haemodynamically stable. If either the blood white cell count or serum amylase levels are raised, this may also indicate intra-abdominal trauma.

Non-operative management of a ruptured liver or spleen is advocated, as the majority of these children will have self-limiting haemorrhage. Only if it is not possible to stabilise the child will an emergency laparotomy be performed for internal haemorrhage. The monitoring must be very precise, as must the fluid management, and there must be a readily available paediatric surgeon who can operate if it becomes necessary.

Bowel perforation, detected either clinically or seen on the CT scan as pneumoperitoneum or leaking of the intragastric contrast, requires a laparotomy for repair. Damage to the pancreas is usually treated non-operatively, although a traumatic pseudocyst may develop later, and be identified on serial ultrasounds. This may require internal drainage.

The CT scan will have identified renal trauma. The function of both kidneys can be assessed. Rupture of the kidney may have occurred, and this is also usually kept under close non-operative review. Even kidneys that have been totally fractured can fully recover, as long as the collecting system is intact enough to drain adequately; temporary percutaneous drainage may allow everything to settle. If the blood supply to the kidney has been avulsed (seen on the CT scan as an acutely non-functioning kidney), emergency repair may save that kidney, but the time available from injury to permanent renal damage is very short.

The bladder is an intra-abdominal organ in a child, (compared to an adult when it is protected in the pelvis), and may be ruptured, especially if full. This may heal on its own, if the bladder is kept on continuous drainage for a few days; it can be assessed with contrast studies. Urethral rupture in a boy should be excluded before a urethral catheter is passed. The treatment of choice of urethral rupture is by gentle catheterisation with a fine silastic catheter, in order to maintain a channel.

Limbs

It is uncommon for limb injury to be life threatening in a child, but haemorrhage can be hidden (in the pelvis and the thigh) and produce hypovolaemia; this requires urgent fluid resuscitation and fracture stabilization, usually with external fixators in the emergency situation, in order to stop the haemorrhage.

Haemorrhage can also be open (in a compound fracture) and should be controlled. Despite the fact that the limb injury is rarely life threatening, it is essential to optimise the fracture and soft tissue management, in order to optimise the child's subsequent outcome.

Management is similar to that in adults, remembering urgent surgical treatment for vascular injury and compartment syndrome.

Theatre

It is important if a child is going to theatre to remember that all the specialist doctors who could be involved should be coordinated by the team in charge of the child; this includes paediatric surgeons, anaesthetists, neurosurgeons, as well as those concerned with eyes, plastics (grazes/lacerations) and maxillofacial problems.

Analgesia and sedation

The degree of analgesia and sedation required in each patient will vary, but the range available extends from complete sedation, analgesia, and paralysis, through spontaneous breathing with various degrees of sedation and analgesia, to simple analgesia.

Analgesia must be regular to be effective; regular or continuous intravenous morphine is used, as it is very predictable in its effect. Intravenous analgesia is given by titrating the dose against response (making up the maximum dose in approximately 10 ml water, and injecting it in 1 ml aliquots, waiting between each aliquot until it can be seen that adequate analgesia and sedation has occurred). Although morphine can cause respiratory depression, this will be detected and managed; it can also increase constipation and prolong ileus, but it is still found by many Units to be the most reliable. Codeine may be used in head-injured patients who are not ventilated, as respiratory depression will be less. Less severe pain can be controlled with a combination of regular diclofenac and paracetamol.

After care

Children also need food and drink if possible, as this will help them feel comfortable; young children will like having their dummy or comforter if they have one as well as a favourite toy; they will like listening to familiar music, as well as receiving visits from their parents and other family and friends.

Monitoring

Monitoring of all trauma patients is the most important way to assess a patient and to detect improvement or deterioration at a stage when a change in management can be made

to improve the situation further, or to prevent continuing deterioration.

The precise monitoring will depend on availability and the child's injuries. This will include:

- cardiovascular;
- respiratory/oxygenation;
- temperature (peripheral/core);
- pupillary size/reaction;
- circulation distal to a limb injury;
- fluid balance
  - IN – crystalloid/medication/colloid/nutrition
  - OUT – urine/gastric aspiration/wound/cavity drainage

and so on.

Family

The family must have open access to the patient, but be aware, in the case of suspected non-accidental injury, that the injury may have been inflicted by a close family member or friend, with its consequent emotional and legal implications.

Access to the full information about the child's condition, and any new information as it becomes available, about the injuries and prognosis, must be given to the parents in a very sensitive but truthful way. Children on an ICU are usually under the care of more than one consultant/specialist, and it is essential that there is communication between the doctors and nurses in order that everybody involved can be clear and honest in their discussions with the family.

Summary

The child following trauma must be assessed and resuscitated according to the usual ABCDE protocol.

The possibility of multiple injuries in a child requires the carers to be aware of all the likely injuries, how they might present and be managed, and consequently able to detect and differentiate the mixture of information available. This ranges from the monitoring to following the progress of the various injuries, so that the carers recognise when there is a deterioration.

Definitive treatment does not differ in principle from that in adults, but respect, analgesia, and close attendance from the family, needs the carer to be fully aware of any problem.

Further reading

The Advanced Life Support Group *Advanced paediatric life support – the practical approach*, 2nd edn. London: BMJ Books, 1997.

Harris BH, Grosfeld JL eds. *Seminars in paediatric surgery 1995*, Vol. 4, No. 2: *Paediatric trauma and surgical critical care*. Philadelphia: WB Saunders Co., 1995.

18 Trauma in the elderly

Carl L. Gwinnutt
Consultant Anaesthetist, Hope Hospital, Salford

Michael A. Horan
Professor of Geriatric Medicine, Hope Hospital, Salford

Anthony McCluskey
Consultant in Anaesthesia and Intensive Care, Stepping Hill Hospital, Stockport

---

OBJECTIVES

- To understand the major physiological changes that occur with ageing.

- To outline some specific injuries sustained by the elderly.

- To be aware of the needs of the elderly trauma patient during surgery.

- To identify the problems faced on the ICU.

- To plan the care of the elderly patient on the general ward.

Few readers will be unaware of the demographic changes that have taken place in developed, industrialised countries with both a relative and absolute increase in the number of old people. This change has been brought about by two important factors: increased life expectancy and reduced birth rate. While the rate of increase of the number of old people in these developed countries has slowed, similar increases have now been demonstrated in developing countries.

Who are the elderly? This is, in fact, a rather difficult question to answer. Many published studies have been conveniently flexible about which individuals should be counted as old and hence it is difficult to generalise their results. Most people who reach retirement age are likely to enjoy good health and the functional impairments generally associated with "ageing" do not become particularly prevalent until after the age of about 75 years, but become increasingly common thereafter. Hence, there is an increasing tendency to adopt the terms used by the US Bureau of the Census: *young-old* (age 65–74), *old* (age 75–84) and *oldest-old* (age 85 +). Paradoxically, in extreme old age, average morbidity, physiological parameters, and function seem to improve, probably as a result of selective survival.

Even though injuries are much more common in young people, old people who sustain them are more likely to die as a result, regardless of injury severity; accidental injuries are recorded as the tenth commonest cause of death in old age. In industrialised countries, the death rate from accidents for people aged over 65 years is about 56/100 000 (versus 24/100 000 between the ages of 15 and 24 years). Recent figures from the USA report that 38% of all hospital bed-days for patients in whom injury was the primary cause of admission were accounted for by those older than 65 years. With 1986 costs, the hospital expenses of this group amounted to $4.4 billion. Despite the huge amount of trauma-care resources consumed by this group, most of the research has been directed towards the needs of the young.

Do older trauma victims differ much from their younger counterparts? The most obvious difference is that the older injured tend to be women while the younger injured tend to be men. Initial analysis of the results of using TRISS methodology to predict outcome after major trauma showed the elderly to be over-represented in the "unexpected deaths". This problem was overcome by the use of the MTOS (UK) database to develop age-specific coefficients to allow a more accurate calculation of probability of survival (Ps). More recently, the effect of increasing age on mortality after major trauma has been shown to reflect the presence of pre-existing medical conditions, the prevalence of which increases with age. If the elderly population with no such problems are analysed separately, they show little increase in mortality for a given injury severity compared with their younger counterparts until they reach their eighth decade. In contrast, by the age of 65 years, those with pre-existing medical conditions show significantly increased mortality (M. Woodford, MTOS (UK), personal communication). Another important difference is the occurrence of "late deaths". For example, a recent study looking at survival times of fatally injured pedestrians stratified for injury severity showed that older patients had a higher proportion of their deaths late after the injury.

Another study has shown that the elderly had a greater "physiological disturbance" (assessed by the Simplified Acute Physiology Score; SAPS) for any given injury severity score. The relative impact of physiological disturbance and chronological age on morbidity and mortality in the elderly-injured has been demonstrated in a recent validation exercise for the APACHE III methodology. Age accounted for only 3% of the variation in survival while acute physiological abnormalities accounted for 86%. Other workers have reported similar findings and have suggested that the appropriate action to improve survival is early invasive monitoring.

Table 18.1 Important age-related physiological changes

System	Change	Implications
Respiratory	↑ Chest wall rigidity ↓ Lung elasticity ↓ Area for gas exchange ↓ Mucociliary clearance ↓ Sensitivity of cough reflex	Prone to respiratory failure Prone to respiratory infection Poorly tolerate lung injuries
Cardiovascular	↓ Ventricular function ↑ Importance of atrial contraction ↑ Lability of blood pressure ↑ Reliance on the Starling mechanism	Highly vulnerable to excesses and deficits of circulating blood volume
Thermoregulatory	↓ Basal metabolic rate ↓ Ability to generate heat ↓ Perception of temperature changes	High risk of hypothermia
Renal	↓ Renal plasma flow ↓ Glomerular filtration rate ↓ Sensitivity to vasopressin Functional hypoaldosteronism	Reduced ability to secrete a water or salt load Reduced ability to retain salt Prone to hypokalaemia Reduced ability to excrete an acid load and to compensate for acid-base disturbances Reduced excretion of polar drugs

Age-related physiological changes

Advancing age is associated with many important changes in a number of body systems. Those felt to be relevant for the management of the injured older person are discussed below and summarised in Table 18.1.

Respiratory system

During ageing, the chest wall becomes increasingly rigid as a result of costochondral calcification, spinal shortening, and an increased thoracic kyphosis. All of these will reduce rib excursion and conspire to increase the likelihood of injury when external forces are applied. Combined with loss of elasticity of the lungs and increasing respiratory muscle fatigue, there is reduced respiratory endurance, particularly in expiration. The result of this is an impaired ability to cough effectively and a reduced capacity to sustain increases in ventilatory effort.

One of the most significant changes with ageing is the progressive increase in the closing capacity because of collapse of the small airways. By the age of 65, the closing capacity will have exceeded the FRC in the seated position, a situation exacerbated further by assuming the supine position. As the closing capacity exceeds the FRC, large volumes of lung are ventilated for only part of each ventilatory cycle while others remain unventilated. This clearly increases the physiological dead space to tidal volume ratio (V_D/V_T ratio), and predisposes initially to air trapping and ultimately to areas of ventilation/perfusion (V/Q) mismatch and hypoxaemia. Anatomical dead space is also increased, predominantly from an increase in the laryngeal and tracheal diameters. By the time 80 years of age is reached, the patient will have undergone about a 33% reduction in lung area available for gas exchange. The full extent of this on oxygenation can be judged by the fact that the normal arterial oxygen tension in the elderly approximates to:

$$Pa_{O_2}\,mmHg = 100 - 0.32\,(\text{age in years}).$$

Unless steps are taken to improve ventilation, the trapped air is eventually absorbed leading to the formation of areas of atelectasis which, along with the reduced mucociliary clearance and decline in protective airway reflexes, predisposes to pneumonia (often from Gram-negative organisms). There is also considerable blunting of the reflex increase in ventilation normally seen in the young in response to hypoxia and hypercarbia. The absence of this clinical sign places the elderly at considerable risk from unidentified hypoxia and hypercarbia, particularly when they occur in combination.

It is not surprising therefore that for the elderly patient, with such severe reductions in their respiratory reserve, isolated chest injuries cause roughly double the fatality rate seen in the young. Whereas a simple flail chest may be manageable in a young patient with analgesia and physiotherapy, those aged over 65 years will frequently need a period of ventilatory assistance, particularly if there is coexisting chronic lung disease or congestive cardiac failure.

The rigidity of the chest wall and loss of elasticity of the underlying lungs make the elderly particularly susceptible to pulmonary contusions. The subsequent response ultimately results in damage to the pulmonary endothelium, with increased permeability, the formation of interstitial oedema, and hypoxia. When combined with injudicious fluid therapy during and beyond the initial resuscitation phase, a potentially fatal progressive hypoxia can arise. This can only be averted by the early use of invasive respiratory and haemodynamic monitoring to optimise oxygen delivery. Consequently, these elderly trauma victims will clearly need the resources of the ICU.

Cardiovascular system

Ageing is associated with a progressively increasing rigidity of the arterial system as a result of changes in the connective tissues of the arterial walls. These changes cause a greater afterload to the left ventricle (often already fibrotic), which responds by hypertrophy and becomes even less compliant. To maintain ventricular filling and cardiac output, there is an increasing reliance on the role played by the atria during diastole. By the age of 70 years, the contribution of atrial contraction to ventricular filling has approximately doubled. Therefore, the elderly are far less tolerant of a tachycardia as this predominantly shortens diastole, thereby reducing the atrial contribution, a situation which is exacerbated if the tachycardia is not sinus in origin. A further consequence of the increasing stiffness of the arterial system is the gradual increase in systolic blood pressure with age. Diastolic pressure increases relatively little and the net effect is a widened pulse pressure. For the same reason, the blood pressure in the elderly is more labile and likely to swing between greater extremes. Interestingly, it has now been shown that the elderly who have no overt heart disease show no significant deterioration in cardiac output and are able to maintain it at adequate levels during exercise. This is achieved predominantly by increasing venous return and end-diastolic volume. Consequently, the increase in cardiac output results mainly from the Starling mechanism increasing stroke volume rather than by the tachycardia characteristic of the young.

Dysrhythmias and autonomic neuropathy are frequently seen in the elderly (see box). Up to one-third of those over 70 years of age will have demonstrable, though not necessarily symptomatic, postural hypotension.

The impairment of ventricular function makes the elderly peculiarly intolerant of even modest circulating volume depletion or expansion. These effects are all compounded by the decrease in renal function making it difficult for the elderly patient to both concentrate urine and handle excess of water. The physician responsible for the care of these patients after the resuscitation room in any situation must therefore pay particular attention to the status of the circulation. This is a further reason for using invasive haemodynamic monitoring early on in the management of these patients.

Common dysrhythmias seen in the elderly

- Atrial ectopics
- Ventricular ectopics
- Atrial fibrillation
- First-degree atrioventricular block

Thermoregulation

There is a gradual decline in the lean body mass with age and, secondary to this, a loss of the ability to generate heat with a fall of 25% in resting energy expenditure by the age of 80 years. In addition, thermoregulation is impaired in a number of ways. The sensitivity of cutaneous thermoreceptors is reduced which makes the old less able to detect changes in ambient temperature. Autonomic control of the cutaneous arteriovenous shunts diminishes, resulting in impaired vasoconstriction, which in turn results in the loss of heat directly via the skin. The onset and intensity of shivering thermogenesis is reduced as is non-shivering thermogenesis because of diminished adrenergic receptor sensitivity and lipolytic heat production. Careful monitoring of core temperature is therefore essential at all times and oral or axillary measurements are not acceptable.

If hypothermia is allowed to develop, the consequences are generally very serious. Shivering increases oxygen demand three- to eight-fold, which places increased demands on an already limited cardiopulmonary reserve. Gastric emptying is delayed (particularly after significant head injuries), predisposing to inhalational lung injury. A number of endocrine and metabolic changes arise as the core temperature falls. There is sympathetic nervous system activation, although the circulating adrenaline concentration is variable. Plasma insulin tends to vary inversely with the adrenaline concentration because adrenaline inhibits its release. There is also intense activation of the hypothalamic–pituitary–adrenal axis and the plasma cortisol concentration tends to exceed even that found in Cushing's disease, although the precise underlying mechanisms are unknown. Glycogen reserves are soon depleted and the sympathetic nervous system response mobilises substrates via lipolysis (fat becomes the favoured fuel) and release of the glucogenic amino acids (alanine and glutamine) from skeletal muscle. As core temperature falls, plasma glucose also falls as a result of uptake into peripheral tissues in excess of glucose production. At a core temperature of about 30°C, tissues become almost completely insensitive to insulin and plasma glucose concentration rapidly increases because glucogenesis is not inhibited. In the absence of ethanol intoxication (when profound, symptomatic hypoglycaemia can occur), neither hypoglycaemia nor hyperglycaemia merit treatment until the patient becomes normothermic, even in people with diabetes. The administration of insulin to hypothermic patients can lead to severe, often lethal, hypoglycaemia when the body temperature increases. Administration of glucose to "hypoglycaemic" patients can also be hazardous by increasing blood viscosity.

Patients also have a metabolic acidosis, largely as a result of lactate release from skeletal muscle, and this reduces cardiac output and increases the risk of dysrhythmias. Peripheral vasoconstriction increases the systemic vascular resistance and diminishes the venous return. Cardiac output is reduced, whilst at the same time myocardial oxygen demand is increased in the face of reduced delivery. Renal blood flow and function are reduced, further hindering the ability to excrete drugs, and finally platelet function is diminished.

Clearly, the elderly patient represents a major challenge at all stages in the attempt to maintain normothermia. The most important principle is that prevention is always better than cure.

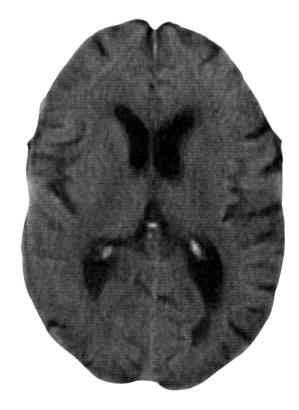

Figure 18.1 CT scan of normal elderly brain.

Central nervous system

Following completion of cerebral maturity at the age of 30 years, there is a gradual decline in brain mass, which is maximal after the sixth decade. By the eighth decade, the brain is approximately 18% smaller, from loss of neurones rather than glial cells. Radiologically, there is marked enlargement of the cerebral sulci, which may be up to 35% larger than in young adults (Figure 18.1). Cellular depletion is particularly marked in the cerebral and cerebellar cortices, thalamus, and basal ganglia. Interestingly, higher intellectual functions and long-term memory suffer little decline, with short-term memory, visual and auditory reaction times, and the ability to rapidly process information deteriorating to a greater extent. The effect of these changes is to place the elderly at greater risk of injury and difficulty in providing details of the events that took place.

Cerebral blood flow also declines with age, but parallels the decline in functioning neurones. Autoregulation and the cerebrovascular response to changes in arterial carbon dioxide tension remain intact. This almost certainly accounts for the rarity of a patient suffering an intraoperative stroke, despite the commonly perceived idea of an unreactive cerebral vasculature and precarious cerebral perfusion. However, as most elderly patients will have a degree of hypertension, the lower limit of autoregulation will be higher than in those patients who are normotensive.

Kidneys

Significant changes occur within the renal system during ageing. There is a progressive loss of the renal cortex with a reduction in the number of functioning glomeruli and consequently a reduced cortical blood flow. In the medulla, blood flow is better preserved but with shunting of blood directly from afferent to efferent vessels. As a result of these changes, in old age, renal blood flow, glomerular filtration rate, and renal concentrating ability are reduced to about half their level seen at 20 years of age. Creatinine clearance undergoes a marked progressive decline with age but the serum creatinine stays relatively unchanged, reflecting the reduced muscle mass and decreased turnover. Furthermore, there is a reduced sensitivity of the tubules to vasopressin which, along with the changes in the medulla, leads to a relative inability to concentrate urine as demonstrated by a fall in the normal urine osmolality from 400 to 280 mosmol/l. A reduced intake or increased loss (diuretics, diarrhoea) of potassium is not uncommon and, when combined with the loss of lean body mass reducing the exchangeable potassium, frequently results in hypokalaemia. This may be offset to some extent by the development of a functional hypoaldosteronism. Occasionally, the latter predominates which, in combination with the reduced GFR, leads to hyponatraemia, uraemia, and mild hyperkalaemia.

The reduced tubular function makes the aged vulnerable to both excesses and deficits of water. The administration of large volumes of hypotonic solutions in the presence of an inability to excrete free water can rapidly cause hyponatraemia, while the converse, water deprivation, in the face of an impaired ability to concentrate urine rapidly, leads to dehydration and hypernatraemia. Similar problems exist in old people's ability to handle excess sodium and acids, the latter clearly impairing compensation for either a respiratory or metabolic acidosis. These changes lead to the potential for accumulation of drugs that rely on renal function for their excretion, necessitating a reduction in dose and frequency of administration.

Gastrointestinal tract and liver

Impaired swallowing, weak cricopharyngeal and pharyngeal muscles, and delayed gastric emptying all contribute to an increased incidence of aspiration of gastric contents in the elderly. Other age-related changes tend to be minor and of little clinical consequence.

Pharmacological aspects of ageing

Therapeutic drugs commonly cause problems for old people. Many drugs cause hypotension and/or confusion in the elderly, thus predisposing to falls and consequent injuries. The reasons for such problems (usually called adverse drug reactions, ADRs) may be age-related changes in the individual that predispose to drug toxicity, or the coadministration of several drugs with the potential for interactions. The risk of ADRs increases with the number of drugs being taken. When someone takes nine or more drugs, drug-related problems are inevitable. A good rule in any situation, but especially in the critically ill elderly, is to stop all but the essential medications and to consider that any new problem could be treatment-related.

Many changes occur with ageing that alter drug handling or responsiveness. Furthermore the likely behaviour of a drug in an elderly recipient can seldom be inferred from its behaviour in a younger one. Although many age-related changes have been described in the gastrointestinal tract, they mostly have little effect on drug absorption. Changes in body composition such as a reduced body size, reduced lean body mass, and reduced total body water together with increased fat mass may significantly alter pharmacokinetics. The increased volume of distribution of lipid-soluble drugs tends to lead to prolonged elimination times (such as opioids and benzodiazepines) whilst the decrease in volume of distribution for water-soluble drugs results in increased plasma levels for a given dose (such as local anaesthetics). In addition, water-soluble drugs are excreted predominantly by the kidneys and the age-related changes already described prolong their elimination exacerbating this effect.

Many drugs bind to plasma proteins, particularly albumin, although it is generally only unbound drug that is active. Healthy ageing is not associated with significant changes in albumin concentration but sick old people are often hypoalbuminaemic. Drugs that bind extensively to albumin (such as warfarin and tolbutamide) will have much higher plasma concentrations of free drug in such patients.

Many drugs are metabolised in the liver, either by phase 1 (mainly oxidation, reduction, demethylation, and hydrolysis) or by phase 2 reactions (mainly acetylation, glucuronide formation, and sulphation). Impairments of all kinds of reactions have been described in old people but there is considerable variation between drugs as well as between individual people. Much larger impairments accompany illness, frailty, and coadministration of drugs.

As well as the pharmacokinetic changes just described, pharmacodynamic changes are also common in old age. These changes represent altered responsiveness to a drug and might occur because of age-related changes in homeostatic mechanisms such as cardiovascular reflexes or from receptor and postreceptor events. The former changes predispose to hypotension and the latter are associated with increased sensitivity to benzodiazepines, drugs with anticholinergic properties, and many anaesthetic agents.

A patient's chronological age should not be regarded as a contraindication to anaesthesia and surgery after trauma nor should it limit their access to the facilities of the ICU. In order to achieve the optimal outcome, management of the elderly trauma patient must take into account the physiological changes outlined above at all stages of their care.

Some specific injuries

Head injuries

A subdural haematoma is the commonest traumatic intracranial haematoma, particularly in the elderly. The progressive loss of brain volume in these patients leads to an increase in the space around the brain with greater potential for displacement. The bridging veins between the dura and cortex tear at the cortical surface, usually along the vertex of the skull as they drain into the saggital sinus. Blood collects between the brain and dura and expands to form a mass affecting the underlying cortex. An acute subdural haematoma is usually associated with significant underlying brain injury, and it is the extent of this which affects the overall recovery (Figure 18.2). Even if surgery is performed rapidly to evacuate

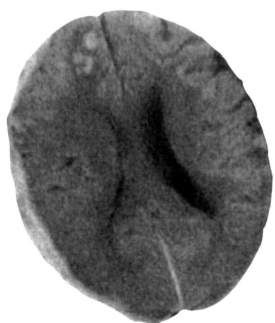

Figure 18.2 CT scan of brain showing right-sided subdural haematoma and frontal lobe contusions.

the clot, mortality approaches 50%. In contrast, as the brain ages, its dura becomes tightly adherent to the skull which makes extradural haematomas uncommon.

Even mild head injuries, particularly in patients with pre-existing cognitive impairment, may have permanent neurological sequelae. One study reported that eight of 42 elderly patients with a Glasgow Coma Scale of 13 or more had massive haematomas. If there is a skull fracture and an associated hemiparesis, a traumatic intracranial haematoma should be assumed, not a stroke. In addition to the standard recommendations for performing a CT scan, any elderly patient with confusion lasting more than 12 hours after head

injury, even without a skull fracture, or who has been unconscious for more than five minutes after a head injury, warrants a CT scan. Any deterioration demands immediate action. **Note**: A subdural haematoma evolves through an isodense phase between days 7 and 20, making it difficult to detect on unenhanced scans (Figure 18.3).

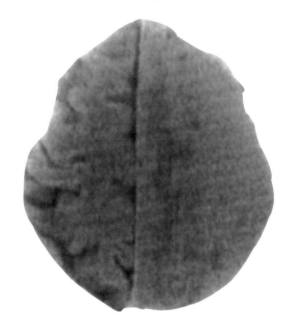

Figure 18.3 CT scan showing the appearance of an isodense subdural haematoma.

Head trauma exacts a devastating toll in the elderly; the fatality rate is around 90% for those with a Glasgow Coma Scale of 8 or less. Neurosurgical intervention is probably not warranted for those who have sustained injuries sufficiently severe to cause immediate coma that persists after correction of hypoxaemia and hypovolaemia.

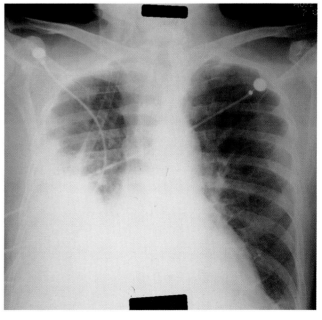

Figure 18.4 Chest x-ray showing multiple rib fractures and haemothorax.

Injuries to the chest

Insignificant falls or blows may cause rib fractures and associated haemo- or pneumothoraces in older people (Figure 18.4). Suspect rib fractures if there is ecchymosis or haematoma along with crepitation, grating, or focal tenderness when the chest wall is pressed. Such fractures heal slowly and underlying pulmonary contusions are common. These problems conspire with pain to impair ventilation. Patients must be monitored for signs of exhaustion or respiratory distress (confusion, respiratory rate > 40/min, Pa_{O_2} < 60 mmHg, and/or Pa_{CO_2} > 50 mmHg); if they develop, intubation and mechanical ventilation will be needed.

The elderly are not immune from deceleration injuries causing traumatic disruption of the aorta. As with their younger counterparts, most of those with this complication will die immediately. Those who survive should be managed as discussed in Chapter 3.

Abdominal trauma

The principles of care for old people with abdominal trauma are the same as for the young. Be aware, however, that "peritoneal signs" may be blunted or absent and the elderly tolerate emergency laparotomy badly. Therefore, assessment of older people with abdominal injuries demands a sense of urgency and high level of clinical acumen. Those with a history or clinical evidence of previous major abdominal procedures should preferably have either a CT or ultrasound scan of the abdomen rather than diagnostic peritoneal lavage.

One perplexing finding that is not uncommon in old people is a rectus sheath haematoma, often as a result of a ruptured inferior epigastric artery. It characteristically follows a bout of coughing or twisting injuries and presents as a painful fusiform mass associated with the rectus abdominis muscle. Consequently the haematoma usually becomes more prominent in supine patients when the head is elevated (Fothergill's sign). Other than that, symptomatic treatment is very rarely needed.

Fractures

Decreasing bone density with age coupled with post-menopausal osteoporosis results in the elderly sustaining fractures with the application of less force compared to the young and a greater incidence of multiple fractures. Another variation from young adults is the incidence of injuries sustained during an epileptic seizure. There is an increased risk of developing upper femoral fractures, ankle fractures, and fractures of the proximal humerus, but not wrist fractures.

In old people with multiple injuries, fractures must be stabilised to permit optimal positioning and movement, both for immediate management and later rehabilitation. The aim of treatment should be to undertake the least invasive, most definitive procedure with a view to early mobilisation as soon as other problems permit. Whilst isolated fractures of the humeral shaft are managed conservatively, there is no logic to such management in patients with leg injuries, who will need to use a walking frame or crutches for mobilisation.

Care in the operating theatre

The most important aspects of care in the operating theatre are summarised in the box. Although recent developments in anaesthesia and surgery have lead to significant declines in morbidity and mortality, several factors have been identified which place the elderly at risk, the most important of which are: emergency surgery, the site of surgery, and physical status of the patient at the time of operation.

At-risk factors

Emergency surgery

This is associated with an increase in risk of up to 10 times that for similar elective procedures. Inadequate preparation of the patient, particularly adequacy of resuscitation in terms of circulating volume, electrolytes, and oxygenation, is not uncommon. In the trauma patient, hypoxaemia, haemorrhage, and acidosis may have resulted in irreversible physiological damage to the patient, while the elderly are at increased risk of infection and sepsis subsequently. All these factors are compounded by the fact that emergency surgery is not infrequently carried out with facilities and staff at times far removed from what would be available for elective surgery.

Operative site

While peripheral and superficial surgery does not greatly increase risk in the elderly, surgery to body cavities certainly does, with abdominal surgery, particularly those procedures involving the large bowel, having a mortality approaching that seen after thoracic and major vascular procedures.

Physical status

It is the presence of concurrent diseases rather than the ageing process alone which leads to increased risk. The elderly patient is far more likely to be suffering from hypertension, ischaemic heart disease, pulmonary disease, renal or hepatic dysfunction, or diabetes. It should be noted that the majority of fatal perioperative myocardial infarcts are reinfarcts and that pulmonary complications are also more common in those patients with pre-existing disease. Perioperative morbidity and mortality are similar in fit 80-year-old patients compared to their younger counterparts when undergoing similar surgical procedures.

Care in the operating theatre

- Handle carefully to avoid further injuries
- General anaesthesia and mechanical ventilation is usually needed
- Intubation is usually easy but take care with the cervical spine
- Apply cricoid pressure during intubation
- Carefully assess "volume status", invasively if necessary
  - Watch for dysrhthmias and consider:
  - hypoxaemia
  - hypocarbia
  - hypercarbia
  - hypovolaemia
- Monitor urine output via an indwelling catheter
- Prevent hypothermia
- Prevent nerve compression/traction
- Prevent pressure sores

General or regional anaesthesia?

General anaesthesia with tracheal intubation is commonly used because the presence of multiple injuries makes the use of a regional anaesthetic technique difficult. In addition there is the attendant risk of profound hypotension in the face of uncorrected hypovolaemia. However, regional anaesthetic techniques are widely used for isolated limb injuries, the classical example being the use of spinal anaesthesia (or more correctly, central neural blockade) for a patient undergoing surgery for a fractured femoral neck. Despite the claims of the superiority of this technique, many studies have failed to demonstrate any significant difference in the long-term outcome between regional or general anaesthesia.

Airway

Tracheal intubation is usually easier in the elderly owing to the resorption of the mandible and the frequent absence of teeth. However, the possibility of the presence of degenerative disease of the cervical spine and risk of instability must be borne in mind. Consequently, the lateral cervical spine radiograph should be examined carefully before intubation, and extremes of neck movement avoided (Figure 18.5). Head flexion must

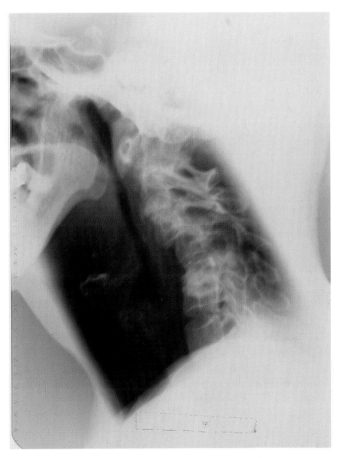

Figure 18.5 Lateral cervical spine x-ray showing severe degenerative disease.

be prevented because it can disrupt the cervical spine, whilst head extension may impair cerebral blood flow via the vertebrobasilar system. This latter point is important because some old people have bilateral internal carotid artery occlusions and rely totally on an intact circle of Willis and blood flow through the posterior cerebral circulation.

The trauma patient requiring surgery is likely to have a full stomach and therefore cricoid pressure (Sellick's manoeuvre) should always be used to reduce the risk of regurgitation and aspiration of gastric contents (see Chapter 2). This risk is greater in old people because of the increased incidence of a hiatus hernia reducing the competence of the gastro-oesophageal junction. Awake intubation under local anaesthesia is another technique which should be considered in those patients who are likely to be difficult to intubate, especially where there is obvious deformity or rigidity of the cervical spine or temperomandibular joints.

Respiratory system

Mechanical ventilation is widely used in these circumstances to help overcome the tendency to hypoxaemia secondary to the reduced compliance and increased closing capacity and Vd/Vt ratio. Care needs to be taken to avoid excessive minute volumes and consequent hypocarbia which may reduce cerebral and coronary blood flow. Furthermore, peripheral vasoconstriction will increase myocardial workload and oxygen demand at the very time when oxygen delivery is compromised. The resultant alkalosis also has the effect of shifting the oxyhaemoglobin dissociation curve to the left, increasing the affinity of haemoglobin for oxygen, and thereby reducing availability at the tissues. All of these effects are less well tolerated by the elderly.

The presence of chronic lung disease will cause further reductions in compliance and increase in airway resistance, leading to higher inflation pressures and the need for relatively longer inspiratory and/or expiratory times to ensure adequate ventilation. The effect of this will be to increase the mean intrathoracic pressure, impeding venous return and reducing cardiac output, an effect exacerbated in the presence of any degree of hypovolaemia. It will also predispose to pulmonary barotrauma and rupture of any emphysematous bullae.

Cardiovascular system

Owing to very limited tolerance of either hypovolaemia or fluid overload, the adequacy of the circulating volume must be frequently assessed. The jugular venous pulse and the fullness of peripheral veins can be extremely difficult to assess in the elderly and should not usually be relied on. The ability to raise heart rate is reduced and bradycardia occurs with depletion of the circulating volume. Hypotension therefore tends to occur with a loss of a smaller percentage of the patient's circulating volume. Invasive monitoring should be considered early, initially by trends in the central venous pressure, although this can be misleading in those with significant heart disease. In prolonged cases, those where there are large fluid losses (surgical, evaporative, and into a "third space"), or in complex cases where the infusion of fluids needs to be accurately assessed (head injury, high spinal cord injury, pulmonary contusion, heart failure), the insertion of a pulmonary artery flotation catheter must be considered. A non-invasive technique that shows promise but has not yet been adopted in clinical practice is Doppler aortovelography, although anatomical changes common in the aged can make this difficult to perform.

Dysrhythmias are common in the elderly. Care must be taken to avoid precipitating a tachycardia because of the deleterious effect on ventricular filling and cardiac output, while at the same time the tachycardia increases oxygen demand. Before resort is made to pharmacological means of treating dysrhythmias, care must be taken to ensure that hypoxaemia, hypo/hypercarbia, hypovolaemia, and hypotension have all been eliminated as the cause. If antiarrhythmic agents are needed, the dose must be adjusted appropriately for the patient's age and weight and administered slowly as almost all have profound negative inotropic actions.

Catheterisation of the urinary bladder is essential in all but the shortest procedures, with a meticulous aseptic technique to prevent infection. This will generally have been done in the resuscitation room. In fit old men, catheterisation can be difficult because of prostatic hypertrophy. As with all patients with multiple injuries, a rectal examination must always be done before a catheter is passed. The appearance of blood at the urethral meatus, or a displaced or boggy prostate, indicates the need for a retrograde urethrogram before an attempt should be made to pass a urinary catheter. If the catheter cannot be easily passed atraumatically, then expert help should be sought rather than persisting (see Chapter 12). Catheterisation prevents distention of the bladder, as the crystalloids and colloids administered during resuscitation are excreted, gross incontinence, or overflow soiling the operative site; lying on a damp surface increases heat loss and the risk of pressure sores. Furthermore, the catheter allows the urine output to be monitored and used as an indicator of the adequacy of the circulating volume. However, it is not as reliable as in the younger patient owing to the limited ability of the kidney to concentrate urine in the face of reduced renal perfusion. This can lead to a reassuringly good urine output in the face of relative hypovolaemia.

Thermoregulation

During anaesthesia and surgery, shivering is abolished and body heat can only be generated by non-shivering thermogenesis, mediated by catecholamines, a mechanism impaired in the elderly owing to reduced beta-adrenergic receptor sensitivity. Consequently in the operating theatre, elderly patients cool rapidly unless great care is taken to prevent heat loss. The ambient temperature is often only around 18–20°C for the comfort of the surgical team, with frequent exchanges of warmed air for cold. Large areas of the patient are exposed, and then covered with cold skin prep, which is usually left to evaporate; thus the patient is quickly robbed of body heat. Finally, large areas of tissue are exposed or body cavities opened allowing further evaporative losses.

Anaesthesia not only stops shivering, but also lowers the thermoregulatory set point by up to 2.5°C, thereby delaying the onset of heat production. Further radiative heat losses occur as a result of inhalational agents preventing vasoconstriction of cutaneous arteriovenous shunts. If regional anaesthesia is used radiative losses will be exacerbated by the loss of sympathetic vasoconstrictor activity, leading to widespread vasodilatation. All of these, combined with the administration of large volumes of intravenous fluids and blood at below body temperature, and the use of cold, dry respiratory gases result in hypothermia being the rule rather than the exception in the elderly trauma patient who requires emergency surgery.

If cooling is allowed to go unchecked, it is accompanied by a variety of sequelae that can be devastating for the elderly patient. Ultimately vasoconstriction occurs, reducing the intravascular volume, venous return, and cardiac output at a time when myocardial oxygen demand is increased. Coupled with a left shift of the oxyhaemoglobin dissociation curve, the increased affinity of haemoglobin for oxygen predisposes to the development of a metabolic acidosis with all the attendant consequences. Hypothermia reduces renal and hepatic blood flow, thereby reducing the excretion and metabolism of drugs and prolonging their effects. Finally, there is an increase in

blood viscosity and numbers of platelets which may place the patient at greater risk of venous thrombosis.

It is essential that core temperature is monitored in all elderly patients and vigorous attempts made to minimise heat loss during surgery. Ideally oesophageal temperature is measured with a thermistor passed either orally or nasally. However, a pulmonary artery catheter provides the most accurate assessment of the core temperature. Although tympanic membrane temperature may be a suitable alternative, the older type probes can be traumatic and the more modern infrared devices require a scrupulous technique. Even this can mislead when the auditory meatus is impacted with wax (so common in the elderly). As a last resort, rectal temperature can be measured if the facilities for the other sites are unavailable. Axillary temperature measurements should never be relied on.

A number of steps can and should be undertaken to prevent heat loss. The operating theatre temperature should be raised, but the comfort of the staff should also be borne in mind. Exposure of the patient should be kept to the minimum necessary for safe preparation and surgical access. Use warm skin preparation solutions and dry excess fluid with swabs rather than waiting for it to evaporate. The patient should be placed on a warming blanket (warm water or air filled) and, if available, a device used to blow warm air over the remaining areas (such as Bair Hugger) (Figure 18.6). **All intravenous**

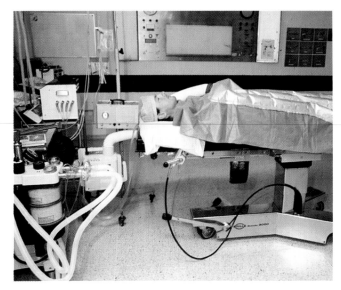

Figure 18.6 Devices for keeping patients warm in the operating theatre: patient lying on warming mattress, covered by warm air blanket, water bath for intravenous fluids, circle system for anaesthesia.

fluids must be warmed to 37°C (particularly blood) with the use of one of the many commercially available devices. The gases used for ventilation should also be warmed and humidified. This can be achieved by the use of humidifiers or the simple placement of a heat and moisture exchanger (HME) adjacent to the patient in the anaesthetic system. Alternatively a circle system with a soda lime absorber can be used; as carbon dioxide is absorbed there is an exothermic reaction and liberation of water which results in the respiratory gases passing through the absorber being heated and humidified.

Despite the best efforts, many elderly patients are still cold by the time they reach the recovery room (or ICU) after surgery. As their thermoregulatory set point returns to normal, they are faced with a large thermal deficit to correct, usually by shivering, (which can increase oxygen consumption three to eight fold). This can clearly place significant demands on both respiratory and cardiovascular reserves which are already limited in such patients. In addition there may be an element of hypoxaemia as a result of hypoventilation secondary to the use of opioids, pain, V/Q mismatch, and pre-existing pulmonary disease. Consequently oxygen must be administered to all patients to minimise hypoxaemia. The efficacy of this may be monitored by the use of a pulse oximeter, but if shivering is excessive then this may interfere with the signal.

As a cold postoperative patient starts to rewarm, the accompanying vasodilatation may unmask occult hypovolaemia. It is essential therefore that monitoring of the cardiovascular system is continued into the recovery period so that appropriate volumes of intravenous fluids can be administered. For the same reason, postoperative analgesia should not be administered intramuscularly as it will not be absorbed from the poorly perfused, often thin, muscles. This will be ineffective and if further doses are given, they will be absorbed simultaneously with the potential for overdose and respiratory depression, at a time when the patient may no longer be under close supervision.

If at the end of surgery the patient's core temperature is less than 35°C, and ICU is not merited, then it is probably safer to keep the patient anaesthetised and ventilated with warm humidified gases and use surface warming along with warmed intravenous fluids to compensate for the increasing vascular space while the core temperature is restored. Care must be taken with active surface rewarming as, paradoxically, the reduced cutaneous circulation cannot dissipate heat, thereby increasing the risk of burns. It is also crucial to employ an adequate strategy for the prevention of pressure sores; note that the use of pressure-dissipating surfaces does not remove the need for a repositioning schedule.

With little doubt, hypothermia can be one of the greatest risks for the elderly trauma patient requiring surgery; however, it is far easier and safer to prevent than to treat. Recently it has also been shown that in patients whose body temperature is maintained during major abdominal surgery, protein catabolism in the postoperative period is reduced. If the same is true for the trauma patient, recovery might be enhanced.

Musculoskeletal

Ageing is associated with reduced bone mass in both sexes and women bear the additional burden of postmenopausal bone loss. These changes reduce the breaking strength of bone and make older people particularly vulnerable to careless handling. Likewise, some degree of degenerative joint disease is universal and, in some, it is severe. Other arthritides (such as rheumatoid disease) are also common in old age and treatment with glucocorticoids may have led to even greater bone loss. Thus, the utmost care must be taken when older people are handled to avoid iatrogenic injuries, particularly to the cervical spine during tracheal intubation and while they are being positioned to facilitate surgical access. Arthritis of the temporomandibular joints may demand fibreoptic intubation (Figure 18.7). It is also important to note that peripheral nerves need protection at sites where they pass over bony prominences since compression or traction neuropathies are not uncommon and will complicate rehabilitation. The peroneal and radial nerves are particularly vulnerable to compression, and the brachial plexus to traction (if an arm is left dangling for a prolonged period).

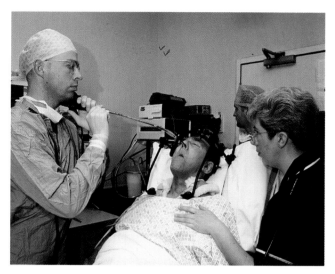

Figure 18.7 Fibreoptic nasotracheal intubation.

Skin

The skin becomes thin during ageing, particularly at sites of sun exposure. This predisposes to fissuring and lacerations from rough handling or even from the careless removal of adhesive tape used to secure cannulae or tracheal tubes. The rate of wound healing is moderately impaired in the elderly, although paradoxically, the cosmetic quality of the healed wounds tends to be better than in the young. Undernutrition and infection are the main causes of impaired wound healing.

In anaesthetised patients and the seriously ill, the skin overlying bony prominences is extremely vulnerable, especially in the haemodynamically unstable and/or malnourished patient. This should be borne in mind from the moment a patient presents to the hospital and throughout the course of hospital stay. Pressure sores are almost entirely avoidable with the use of pressure dispersing surfaces and regular changes in position. The development of pressure sores will markedly prolong the duration of hospital stay, will lead to untold misery for the patient and may well be the cause of subsequent litigation.

Finally, the widespread use of surgical diathermy requires the application of an indifferent (earth) plate or electrode to the patient's skin. Ideally this is placed with good contact over an area with a good blood supply, usually muscle, to aid dispersion of any heat generated. In the elderly, frail, shocked patient this may prove to be difficult and poor application may easily cause significant burns. A popular site for application is under the buttock, but care must be taken to ensure that the site remains dry as this area easily becomes wet with urine if the patient is not catheterised and is incontinent.

Intensive care

Treatment on the ICU requires a greater input of resources, is more expensive and is associated with a higher mortality than elsewhere in the hospital. Patients admitted to the ICU, whatever their age, should have acute, severe but potentially reversible illnesses. Although age does influence both hospital and ICU mortality, more important predictors of outcome are the previous health and physical status of the patient and the severity of the acute illness. Many old people who have required ICU care have returned to a good, self-perceived, quality of life. Thus, age *per se* should not determine whether admission to the ICU is appropriate. The important aspects of management in the ICU are summarised in the box.

Care in the intensive care unit

- Age is a good indicator, but a poor determinant of outcome. Comorbidity is a more important determinant
- The endocrine/metabolic response to injury is triggered normally but the elderly may not be able to sustain a high metabolic rate. Some aspects of the response persist for a very long time (for example, cortisol secretion, insulin resistance)
- Understand the special problems of ventilating old people
- Monitor cardiovascular parameters very carefully
- Prevent hypothermia
- Prevent pressure sores
- Think twice about the need for any drug
- Use sedatives and hypnotics sparingly
- Proper nutritional support is essential
- Delirium is a symptom and not a diagnosis. Always seek the cause

---

Metabolic and neuroendocrine response in the elderly

The normal metabolic response to major trauma is classically described as comprising an early (initial 12 hours) ebb phase during which the metabolic rate, oxygen consumption, and body temperature are depressed, followed by a later, sustained (days, weeks, or months) catabolic flow phase. Both phases are driven by characteristic endocrine changes. During the flow phase, there is an increase in the metabolic rate and oxygen consumption of up to 50%, and in severe burns this may rise to 100%. In order to "fuel the furnace" of repair and recovery, energy is obtained by two primary metabolic pathways:

- production of ketone bodies via lipolysis;
- increased gluconeogenesis from amino acids derived from skeletal muscle and other proteins.

Lipolysis is unimpaired in the injured elderly but the mobilisation of amino acids from skeletal muscle is poorly tolerated and a disproportionate negative nitrogen balance ensues, the consequences of which include poor wound healing, impaired immunocompetence, and severe muscle wasting. The cortisol response, which is associated with insulin resistance, is unimpaired in the old and may continue for considerably longer than occurs in young people, thus possibly contributing to sustained muscle wasting, immunosuppression, and impaired wound healing. Furthermore, this will mean that people with diabetes must be carefully monitored for many weeks after their injuries since their insulin requirements will be expected to fall over time.

Respiratory system

The elderly have a diminished respiratory reserve and are more likely to suffer from respiratory diseases such as chronic bronchitis, emphysema, or asthma. Consequently, it is often necessary to institute IPPV at an earlier stage than in a younger, fitter patient. However, elderly patients are more at risk of developing a "ventilator pneumonia" because of impaired local, cellular, and humoral defence mechanisms. Furthermore the elderly patient is also more difficult to "wean" from the ventilator because of weakness and wasting of skeletal muscle. However, the intensivist has to use different criteria for weaning, such as accepting relatively poor arterial blood gases because of the normal decline in Pa_{O_2} with aging. Thus the decision to ventilate mechanically such patients must be carefully considered. Although it is preferable to avoid mechanical ventilation or to limit its duration, it often must be continued for days or weeks. As a result there is an increase in the frequency of the problems and complications over those seen in younger patients.

Cardiovascular system

Significant ischaemic heart disease is present in 10–20% of all elderly patients. Furthermore the most frequent causes of death on the ICU following major trauma are cardiac and/or sepsis related. If mortality is to be minimised, it is essential to monitor cardiorespiratory indices closely in the same manner as in the young patient, and to avoid hypotension, hypoperfusion, and hypoxaemia. It is often necessary to provide pharmacological support for the cardiovascular system to maintain adequate perfusion of vital organs, including the "virtual" organ comprising the damaged tissues. Inotropic drugs are used to augment cardiac index and oxygen delivery to the supranormal levels associated with recovery. In addition vasopressors may be required to counteract the vasodilating effects of toxic mediators released following major trauma.

Although the principles of treatment are the same for all ages, there are particular problems associated with the elderly. The physiological reserve of the left ventricle and the cardiovascular homeostatic reflexes may both be impaired. If significant coronary artery disease is present, ischaemia, infarction, left ventricular failure, and acute dysrhythmias (usually tachycardias) may all result from attempts to drive the heart with inotropes. The circulating volume must therefore be kept at a level shown by invasive haemodynamic monitoring to be optimal in terms of myocardial performance. However, there is less margin for error when compared with younger patients. Hypovolaemia may rapidly cause hypotension and organ hypoperfusion, whereas volume overload may precipitate LVF, pulmonary oedema, and hypoxaemia.

Measurement of haemodynamic indices with a pulmonary artery catheter together with analysis of arterial and mixed venous blood gases is currently the best method for achieving optimal fluid loading, cardiac index, and oxygen delivery to the tissues. It should, therefore, be considered early, particularly in the critically ill elderly patient. Inotropic therapy may be relatively ineffective in the elderly heart. There is often coexisting disease and a relatively fixed cardiac output, unresponsive to even high doses of inotropes, which only serve to produce tachydysrhythmias. The outlook for such patients is poor as they are unable to fuel the catabolic flow phase because of inadequate oxygen delivery to the tissues.

Renal function

There are important implications for the dosage regimens of many drugs used on the ICU because renal performance declines with age. A dose reduction is required for renally excreted drugs, such as digoxin, many antibiotics (aminoglycosides, amphotericin, cephalosporins), milrinone, and morphine. Other drugs should be considered very carefully before use, especially ACE inhibitors and oral hypoglycaemic drugs. Non-steroidal anti-inflammatory drugs should not be used in other than exceptional circumstances (for example, acute gout). Very careful attention must be directed towards maintaining fluid and electrolyte balance. Many elderly patients are prone to hypokalaemia and/or hyponatraemia owing to diuretic therapy and nutritional deficiency.

Acute renal failure supervenes more frequently and at an earlier stage in the elderly, requiring extracorporeal renal support, usually by continuous haemofiltration. Although the decision to institute such support needs to be carefully considered if the result is not merely to delay the death of a patient, there is evidence that the survival rates of elderly patients with multiple organ failure who require haemofiltration are comparable with younger patients with similar disease severity defined by APACHE II and organ failure scores.

Thermoregulation

Elevation of the ambient temperature into the thermoneutral zone (30–32°C) is valuable in reducing metabolic requirements towards a level that the elderly patient is capable of sustaining. Although such uncomfortable (for the staff) temperatures are often found on specialised burns units, they are seldom achieved on a general ICU. However, a local thermoneutral environment can be produced around the patient using one of the various types of warming blankets available.

Nutrition

It is essential that the nutritional requirements of elderly trauma victims are met as they are more likely to have a poorer underlying standard of general nutrition. In the absence of appropriate nutritional support, the catabolic flow phase must be fuelled entirely by the consumption of endogenous fat and protein. Although it is not usually possible to prevent a negative nitrogen balance, it can be limited by a suitable nutritional regimen. There are several equations to estimate the amount of energy needed to maintain body weight but, in practice, around 2000 calories will be needed for a 60–70 kg old woman. In addition, it is important to supplement the protein, carbohydrate, and fat components of the regimen with trace elements and water- and fat-soluble vitamins as these may be deficient.

Feeding should be commenced as early as possible, and in practice this usually means within 24–48 h. The enteral route is the best as it is cheaper, simpler, and associated with fewer complications and deficiencies of vitamins and minerals. However, a percutaneous endoscopic gastrostomy (PEG) will be needed if tube feeding is difficult or likely to be prolonged (Figure 18.8). Patients with head injuries often have lower oesophageal sphincter dysfunction and any feeding tube is best sited in the jejunum. Total parenteral nutrition (TPN) is best kept for those cases in whom gut function is compromised, which prevents enteral feeding.

Psychological aspects

The elderly patient is very prone to develop acute confusional states (delirium) during any significant illness or injury. These are usually easily recognised when associated with arousal and agitation but more difficult to detect when these features are absent. It is very important that the cause of delirium is found and, if possible, corrected. Those with pre-existing brain damage are particularly susceptible to delirium. The most likely causes are persistent and unrecognised hypoxaemia, metabolic disturbance, infections, and drugs. Benzodiazepine or alcohol withdrawal may also cause delirium in those already dependent on them. A pulmonary embolus should always be considered in an acutely confused patient.

Delirium is not only distressing to the patient, relatives, and staff, but may also be dangerous in so far as accidental extubation or disconnection from vital drug infusions may occur. Agitation also stresses myocardial reserve unnecessarily and may precipitate acute tachydysrhythmias or myocardial ischaemia. Nevertheless, it is most important to titrate the

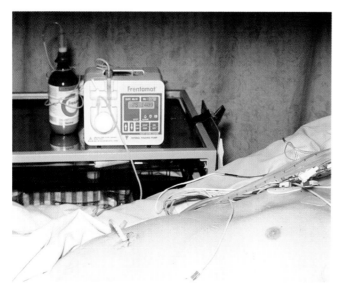

Figure 18.8 Percutaneous gastrostomy (PEG) feeding system.

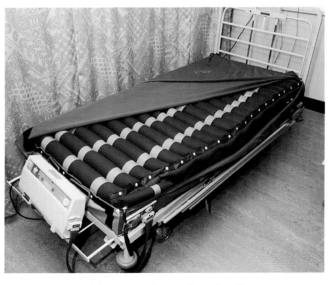

Figure 18.9 Mattress to reduce the formation of pressure sores.

dose of sedative and analgesic drugs carefully and precisely so that the patient is calm, cooperative and in contact with reality. This not only facilitates recovery, in particular successful weaning from mechanical ventilation, but also reduces the degree of immunosuppression associated with deep sedation.

Wound care and hygiene

As previously mentioned, scrupulous attention must be paid to the prevention of ischaemic pressure sores. Good nursing practice (that is, sufficient numbers of experienced ICU trained nurses) is the most important factor in preventing their occurrence. The patient must be turned regularly and where this is not feasible because of cardiorespiratory instability or injuries, specialised devices such as beds with ripple or water mattresses must be used (Figure 18.9). However, these devices are adjuncts to and do not remove the need for repositioning. The development of pressure sores adds considerably to the cost and duration of the subsequent hospital stay, retards rehabilitation, and will be the cause of much misery. Their development may also be grounds for legal action for negligence!

The elderly are at special risk for nosocomial infections (ventilator pneumonia, catheter sepsis, and wound infections). Scrupulous hygiene is therefore essential. Invasive monitoring devices, particularly those which breach the body's local defence mechanisms, must be monitored regularly for early evidence of inflammation/infection. In general, however, there is little that can be done specifically with regard to the elderly that does not apply equally to younger patients in the ICU.

The general ward

Transfer to a general ward can, paradoxically, be a peculiarly hazardous time for the multiply injured elderly, both for those whose injuries are not severe enough to warrant admission to the ICU and for those transferred from it. Unlike younger patients, older patients will frequently have co-morbid conditions that complicate management on return from the operating theatre. The most important of these will generally have been detected and stabilised before surgery takes place. Thus, for most of these patients, medical as well as surgical input will be required. In fact, for those patients whose medical problems overshadow their surgical ones, admission to an acute medical or geriatrics ward rather than to a trauma ward, may be the best management option. For other patients, all but the fittest will require collaborative management and eventual transfer to a rehabilitation ward in preparation for discharge from hospital. In our own hospital, a geriatrician shares management from the time of hospital admission and is present on the trauma wards every day.

Postoperative assessment

Important aspects of the assessment of patients transferred to a general ward are summarised in the box.

The assessment on the general ward

- Always summarise the main events that have gone before
- Record gaps in knowledge and arrange to get the missing information
- Note previous medications, health, and function: these help when setting goals
- Look specifically for depression and cognitive impairment
- Take steps to overcome barriers to communication (see next box)
- Reassure, explain what happens now, and answer any questions the patient may have
- Review the need for parenteral fluids
- Review medications and stop all but the essential
- Restart essential drugs that might have been stopped (for example, drugs for Parkinson's disease)
- Never label someone as demented without an expert opinion. Surgeons often misdiagnose dysphasia as dementia
- Always perform a full examination (see text)
- Always assess function as well as impairments

Case notes review

The first step is to summarise what has gone before and to highlight what information is missing and still needs to be elucidated. A clear description of the events leading up to the injuries is always required so that potentially modifiable factors can be identified and suitable management instituted. This will also be very useful if litigation ensues. An eye-witness account can be invaluable. If the injuries resulted from a fall, did the patient lose consciousness? If so, was the patient white, limp and possibly sweating (suggesting a Stokes–Adams attack) or was the patient rigid, blue, and possibly exhibiting jerking movements (suggesting epilepsy)? Is alcohol abuse a possible contributing factor?

The management of the patient should be summarised with careful note made of all procedures undertaken (surgical operations, ventilatory support, nutritional support). Any known complications should be recorded and whether these represent ongoing problems (for example, episodes of heart failure, pulmonary emboli, and respiratory infections, etc.). Laboratory test results should be reviewed to detect abnormalities that may have been overlooked and/or may still be ongoing problems; the most commonly overlooked test results are hyponatraemia, hypokalaemia, and anaemia. The drug history must be reviewed, with particular attention paid to any drugs that might have been stopped (such as anti-Parkinson's disease medication, benzodiazepines, and oral hypoglycaemic drugs) and need to be re-started, and any drugs that have been prescribed during this admission which may no longer be needed (such as antibiotics and sedatives).

Any previous hospital notes should be scrutinised so that any significant co-morbid conditions can be identified, particularly those that may impinge on further management and recovery. Frequently, particularly for patients already known to the Geriatrics Service, information about existing functional impairments and continence can be found.

Talking with the patient

The first contact should not be an ordeal for the patient but rather, a reassuring experience and a means to establish effective communication. Common barriers to communication are summarised in the box below. The interview should start with a general discussion during which it should be possible to detect any disorders of arousal (suggesting delirium), memory and cognition (suggesting delirium or dementia), and mood. Disorders of vision and hearing are usually easily detectable at this time. The opportunity should be taken to ensure that the patient understands what has already been done and why, and, in general terms, what will happen next. For those doctors unfamiliar with assessing affect and cognition, questionnaires such as the mini-mental state examination (MMSE) should be used along with the brief Carroll depression rating scale (BCDRS). If other scales are preferred, care should be taken to select a depression screening instrument that has been validated for patients with somatic disorders.

Patients should be asked about anything that is worrying them now. Follow-up questions can be asked to elucidate these problems, to highlight things that may need to be addressed further in the physical examination or those pieces of information that may need to be sought elsewhere (such as: Who is looking after the cat? Does my husband know where I am? Is the house properly secured? etc.). Specific questions must be asked about other significant medical conditions, particularly those that may complicate recovery (for example, stroke, Parkinson's disease, or arthritides) and any medications

---

Barriers to communication

- Comprehension
  - dysphasia
  - foreign language
  - dialect
  - deafness
- Attention
  - anxiety
  - delirium
  - dementia
- Memory
  - delirium
  - dementia
- Expression
  - dysphasia
  - dysarthria
- Circumstance
  - lack of privacy
  - irritable doctor
  - background noise
  - frequent interruptions
- Concealment
  - fear of loss of control
  - fear of reprisals (especially in cases of "elder abuse")
  - litigation may be likely
- Interpretation
  - doctor's knowledge and skills
  - patient's understanding of the situation

---

habitually taken. These aspects can also be checked or confirmed by contacting the patient's GP. It is also essential to gather information about the patient's previous level of function and social support and to check this information with a witness account whenever possible. A patient who was already wheelchair-bound and living in a nursing home will not be rehabilitated to a degree that discharge to an independent lifestyle will be feasible. Finally, if it has not emerged in the discussion, the doctor needs to ask about the adequacy of pain control and whether the patient is constipated.

Physical examination

This should commence with attention to any sites of injury and immediately surrounding areas. Any wounds should be inspected for evidence of infection and delayed healing. The skin must be inspected, particularly at "pressure sites" and around any cannulae. Thereafter, a reasonably comprehensive examination can be undertaken. In addition to recording the pulse (rate and character) and blood pressure, it is wise to also note the respiratory rate without the patient being aware that you are doing this. A raised respiratory rate is a useful indicator of occult respiratory infection or pulmonary embolism. The lung fields should be examined: look for signs of respiratory infection or heart failure, remembering that physical signs in the lung fields of pulmonary embolism are rare.

The jugular venous pressure should be assessed with the patient correctly positioned at approximately 45°. This item of physical examination can be very difficult for inexperienced doctors. In practice, if the external jugular vein is compressed at the root of the neck and the vein fills and then empties when the pressure is removed, it is safe to conclude that the jugular venous pressure is not raised. However, it is still possible that the jugular venous pressure is abnormally low, such as may occur with hypovolaemia.

The heart should be examined for enlargement, added sounds, and murmurs. The significance of any peripheral oedema is often wrongly interpreted. It occurs in conditions of volume overload such as liver, heart, and renal failure, in which case, treatment with diuretics is appropriate. However, oedema also occurs commonly in patients with normal blood volume (for example, hypoalbuminaemia and stasis oedema). The administration of diuretics in this case leads to blood volume contraction, a feeling of malaise and possibly postural hypotension. The axiom is therefore: "Only give diuretics to patients with an expanded blood volume!"

The breasts should always be examined in older female patients who will seldom undertake self-examinations. During examination of the abdomen, evidence of faecal loading and urinary retention should be sought. Urinary retention is common, even in women, following injuries of or around the pelvis. A rectal examination is probably not needed unless other symptoms or signs point to an abnormality.

A detailed neurological examination is also generally unhelpful unless the circumstances indicate it is needed. Nevertheless, all four limbs need to be assessed for strength. The hands should be assessed for fine movements (hand function is an important predictor of overall function) and whether there is any evidence of a radial nerve palsy or traction injury to the brachial plexus. The legs should be examined for peroneal nerve palsies, and evidence of peripheral neuropathy should be sought, especially in diabetics. The feet should also be examined for other problems that may limit walking, such as corns, bunions, and untended toenails.

Provided there is no contraindication, the ability of the patient to sit unsupported should be assessed. The patient should then be stood and any lightheadedness or balance impairment recorded. Either of these will require elucidation later. If the patient can sit and stand safely, the ability to walk must also be assessed ensuring that assistance is always at hand.

Initial management plan

The formulation of an initial management plan is summarised in the box. The first task is to make decisions about medications. All drugs should be reviewed and should only be continued if there is a clear need. Any drugs that were stopped before transfer to the ward should also be reviewed. For example, if the patient was taking drugs for Parkinson's disease, these will need to be restarted. Furthermore, if the patient has been on benzodiazepine hypnotics for a long time, these should also be written-up. Hypnotics and sedatives should not be prescribed routinely. Rendering a patient stuporous is not the solution to a noisy nocturnal ward environment! If a patient needs a hypnotic, try to avoid benzodiazepines since they tend to be continued even on discharge and thus, the patient will have acquired a new problem: benzodiazepine dependence. Chloral hydrate and dichloralphenazone are more suitable hypnotics.

Analgesic medication should also be reviewed. There is a wide choice of effective drugs and there is really no excuse for inadequate pain relief. However, certain analgesics are so often poorly tolerated by the elderly that they are probably best avoided (pethidine, buprenorphine, and non-steroidal anti-inflammatory drugs). Reasonably safe and effective drugs for moderate pain include nefopam and tramadol. Try to avoid intramuscular injections: they are painful and drug absorption is unpredictable.

Prophylaxis against deep venous thrombosis (usually subcutaneous, low-dose heparin) should be continued until the patient can achieve a reasonable level of activity. The need

for parenteral fluids should also be reviewed. If the patient can tolerate reasonable volumes of fluids orally, then parenteral fluids should be stopped. If they must be continued and no intravenous drugs need to be given, subcutaneous administration of fluid (with daily hyaluronidase) is a safer but rarely used alternative.

If the patient has an indwelling urinary catheter, its removal should be considered. However, it should remain in place if urine output needs to be measured because this is notoriously inaccurate when assessed in spontaneously voiding patients.

All but the fittest patients with trivial injuries will not take in sufficient food for their daily requirements and dietary supplementation should be the rule rather than the exception. A daily intake of at least 1500 calories must be ensured. Hospital food is so often monotonous and unattractive that it is not surprising that so many patients do not eat it. In these circumstances, "healthy eating" should be forgotten and energy-rich foods such as chocolate, cream cakes, fish and chips can all be encouraged. Even these may not be eaten when edentulous patients do not have their dentures. If, as is so often the case, they have been left at home, they need to be retrieved and replaced if lost or damaged in the original accident.

The nurses and physiotherapists need to be given specific instructions about the types and level of activity that are permissible and patients should be encouraged to undertake them. They will not be able to do so without adequate, supportive footwear and dignified clothes, and this is a good time to have them brought into hospital. Few people will be keen to walk up and down the ward wearing a night-dress or theatre gown secured behind by tapes, leaving them almost completely exposed, and wearing temporary plastic foam "slippers" which give no support or protection, impair sensation in the feet and absorb any liquid that has been spilt on the floor. If such temporary, cheap footwear serves any purpose at all, it is only decorative. When the patient is capable of a modest level of activity, the occupational therapist should also be involved and informed of the likely permanent impairments so that suitable aids can be considered.

Ongoing management

Patients on parenteral fluids, those needing regular analgesics, those with a catheter *in situ*, and those with ongoing problems need to be reviewed daily. Stable patients with adequate pain control need not be reviewed so often by the medical staff, but always be vigilant for the development of depression or delirium. There should be a weekly review of progress with the patient, nurses, therapy staff, and social worker. By this time, it should be clear what the patient will need to be able to do for themselves before discharge is possible and what prosthetic services (such as home-helps and meals on wheels) or treatment services (such as domiciliary physiotherapy and home nursing) will be needed to support them. The timescale of any likely discharge date should be estimated and arrangements should be started. In a number of places, schemes for accelerated discharge have been set up with the aim of achieving rapid discharge from hospital by the provision of intensive nursing, physiotherapy, occupational therapy, and domestic support in patients' homes. These schemes seem very attractive to hospitals and patients alike, but their effectiveness remains undetermined and they are probably more costly than the standard hospital regimen. No more such schemes should be instituted until existing ones have been properly evaluated and demonstrated to be cost-effective.

Initial management on the general ward

- Do not prescribe hypnotics and sedatives routinely. Stupor is not the answer to a noisy and disturbing environment.

- Ensure adequate analgesia. Avoid pethidine and buprenorphine. Nefopam and tramadol are better tolerated alternatives.

- Continue prophylaxis against DVT until an adequate activity level is reached.

- Continue pressure sore prophylaxis.

- Review nutrition. Hospital food is notoriously unpalatable and often uneaten. Don't forget the dentures!

- Give instructions about permitted activities and weight-bearing.

- Ensure dignity and privacy for the patients. Patients will be unlikely to want to walk wearing a hospital gown exposing their rear to all.

- Proper shoes will be needed. Temporary footwear provided by the hospital usually has no more than a cosmetic function.

- Ensure provision of any aids and orthoses (such as ankle–foot orthosis for foot drop).

- Involve the Geriatrician in all but the most straightforward cases.

If discharge planning seems unrealistic, the patient will almost certainly need to be transferred to a rehabilitation unit unless it seems inevitable that the degree of likely recovery will be insufficient for independent living. However, any potentially irrevocable decisions about institutional care should not be made without an independent review by a Geriatrician. Likewise, no patient should be labelled as "demented" unless there has been a similar review. Many surgeons seem unable to distinguish fluent dysphasia from dementia with potentially disastrous consequences. In fact, a trauma service that does not have the routine involvement of a Geriatrician is probably operating to an unacceptably low standard.

The regular reviews should also seek to detect any barriers to rehabilitation and any complications that may have arisen (see box). The nurses must be asked about pressure areas and, if there is any doubt, patients should be checked by the doctor. Depression may arise insidiously and go undetected unless specifically sought. The adequacy of nutrition and pain relief should also be re-assessed and the patient asked if there are any other problems requiring attention.

Common complications and barriers to rehabilitation

- Depression
- Delirium
- Inadequate pain control
- Hyponatraemia (usually iatrogenic; incompetent fluid regimens)
- Depressed consciousness (may be sign of delirium, often due to medication)
- Myocardial infarction
- Venous thrombosis/thromboembolism
- Pressure sores
- Infections (wound, elsewhere)
- Malnutrition
- Constipation
- Urinary retention (may also occur in women – see text)
- Physical deconditioning
- Communication problem (learn how to replace a hearing aid battery)
- Failure to provide appropriate aids/appliances

Discharge from hospital

All hospitals will have formal schedules to ensure that proper discharge arrangements have been instituted and that proper support services are in place. This is important information to be reported to the GP in the discharge letter. It is also important to record functional status at the time of hospital discharge and to list all important impairments and complications. A list of the patient's discharge drugs with the reason for their prescription and planned duration needs to be included. Any arrangements for out-patient review must also be recorded.

Summary

In this chapter, we have tried to give a practical account of the management of older trauma victims. We have needed to rely on our own experiences of the management of such patients owing to the dearth of published evidence. However, where possible, we have tried to reflect what is actually known, and, elsewhere, we have given what we consider to be reasonable advice with which few would be likely to disagree. We hope that we have conveyed the idea that the old can benefit immensely from the very best management but that they tolerate suboptimal and incompetent management badly.

Further reading

Chelluri L, Grenvik A, Silverman M. Intensive care for critically ill elderly: mortality, costs and quality of life. *Arch Intern Med* 1995;**155**: 1013–22.

Gunnarsson L, Tokics L, Brismar B, Hedenstierna G. Influence of age on circulation and arterial blood gases in man. *Acta Anaesthesiol Scand* 1996;**40**:237–43.

Horan MA, Barton RN, Little RA. Ageing and the response to injury, in *Advanced geriatric medicine 7* (JG Evans & FI Caird, eds). Bristol: Wright. 1988, pp. 101–35.

Horan MA, Roberts NA, Barton RN, Little RA. Injury responses in old age, in *Oxford textbook of geriatric medicine* (JG Evans & TF Williams, eds). Oxford: Oxford University Press, 1992, pp. 88–93.

Kong LB, Lekawa M, Navarro RA *et al.* Pedestrian-motor vehicle trauma: an analysis of injury profiles by age. *J Am Coll Surg* 1996; **182**:17–23.

Levy DB, Hanlon DP, Townsend RN. Geriatric trauma. *Clin Geriatr Med (US)* 1993;**9**:601–20.

McKenzie PJ, Wishart HY, Smith G. Longterm outcome after repair of fractured neck of femur. Comparison of subarachnoid and general anaesthesia. *Br J Anaesth* 1984;**56**:581–4.

Munn J, Willatts SM, Tooley MA. Health and activity after intensive care. *Anaesthesia* 1995;**50**:1017–21.

Oh TE. *Intensive care manual*, 3rd edn. London: Butterworths, 1990.

Perls TT. The oldest old. *Sci Am* 1995 (Jan):50–5.

Rockwood KR, Noseworthy TW, Gibney RTN *et al.* One-year outcome of elderly and young patients admitted to intensive care units. *Crit Care Med* 1993;**21**:687–91.

Santora TA, Schinco MA, Trooskin SZ. Management of trauma in the elderly patient. *Surg Clin N Amer* 1994;**74**:163–86.

Shabot MM, Johnson CL. Outcome from critical care in the "oldest old" trauma patients. *J Trauma* 1995;**39**:254–9.

Thomas DR, Ritchie CS. Preoperative assessment of older adults. *J Am Geriatr Soc* 1995;**43**:411–21.

Watters JM, Moulton SB, Clancey SM *et al.* Aging exaggerates glucose intolerance following injury. *J Trauma* 1994;**37**:786–91.

Williams-Russo P, Sharrock NE, Mattis S *et al.* Cognitive effects after epidural vs general anaesthesia: a randomized controlled trial. *J Am Med Ass* 1995;**274**:44–50.

Zietlow SP, Capizzi PJ, Bannon MP, Furnell MB. Multisystem geriatric trauma. *J Trauma* 1994;**37**:985–8.

19 Thermal injury

Keith Judkins
Medical Director for Burn Care, Consultant in Anaesthesia and Intensive Care, Yorkshire Regional Burn Centre, Pinderfields Hospital, Wakefield

Alan Phipps
Consultant Burns and Plastic Surgeon, Yorkshire Regional Burn Centre, Pinderfields Hospital, Wakefield

OBJECTIVES

- To understand the many manifestations of thermal injury.

- To understand the basic pathophysiology of burn injury.

- To give basic knowledge of the principal complications of burn injury.

- To give knowledge of the differences between burn shock and other manifestations of shock.

- To give a summary of basic principles in the initial management of a burn.

- To clarify which patients need what clinical expertise following a burn.

- To give knowledge of which clinicians it is relevant to involve, and when.

- To give knowledge of the appropriate routes for onward referral of the burned patient.

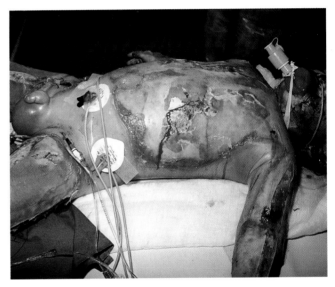

Figure 19.1 A child with 70% body surface burns and smoke inhalation. Severe facial burns complicate this injury.

The term "thermal injury" encompasses scalds, contact burns, cold and electrical injury, and flame burns, and is therefore preferred to "burns". Most injuries are trivial. Many are self-treated, sometimes with bizarre remedies – butter, bicarbonate of soda, or toothpaste. Others are ably managed as outpatients by general practitioners or emergency department staff with dressings.

Deeper or larger burns are treated in hospital. Prompt, appropriate surgical management may be needed to minimise disfigurement or disability, but life is seldom at risk in burns covering less than 10% of the skin surface.

At the other extreme, a small proportion of thermally injured patients each year includes those who have suffered a massive or complicated life-threatening burn (Figure 19.1). In between is a significant number of moderate injuries which, although usually straightforward, may become complicated or lethal if inadequately assessed or treated incorrectly. Referral to an appropriate burn care facility, where all aspects of the injury can be managed by experienced staff, is essential in both cases.

Mechanisms of injury

A high proportion of patients are either children or elderly. Scalds account for the majority of child injuries, whereas adults are more often injured by flame. Electrical, chemical, and similar injuries are also commoner in adults as a result of industrial or domestic accident.

Scalds

Water

Domestic hot water, commonly at 65–100°C, has a high specific heat so can cause serious injury. Immediate cooling of the wound with running cold water for up to 15 minutes minimises the injury, but carries a risk of hypothermia if the injury is extensive. Wrapping the patient up to keep warm during transfer to hospital will reduce this risk.

Scalds account for 85% of all paediatric burn admissions in children under 3 years of age [1]. Part of every doctor's responsibility is to increase public awareness of simple safety precautions in the home: care with hot drinks; care with kettles and saucepans; safety devices such as coiled kettle flexes.

Very rarely, neck scalds in infants may stimulate oedema formation in the trachea sufficient to cause respiratory obstruction. Scalds colonised with *Staphylococcus aureus* may cause toxic shock syndrome [2] in small children that in rare cases may prove fatal. A minor scald is therefore not always a safe scald.

The elderly may get into a bath that is too hot, and because of infirmity or dementia may respond too slowly to the excessive temperature. Installation of thermostatic mixers on bath taps would help prevent this kind of accident; bath handles may enable escape if something does go wrong. Spillage of hot liquids can cause injury in this age group also.

Scalds in any age group may be the consequence of disability, an epileptic fit, myocardial infarction, diabetic crisis or hypoglycaemia, cerebrovascular accident, or other medical emergency including alcohol or drug intoxication.

Other hot liquids

In the kitchen, fat from deep fat fryers causes injuries which are usually deep, as are those caused by tar and molten metal. Treatment is as for other burns, but their severity should not be underestimated.

Flame burns

Flame burns result from combustion in a house fire or road traffic accident, or clothes may catch fire. Petrol is sometimes involved, owing to accident, self-immolation, or assault. Bystanders may be injured. The elderly are again vulnerable, particularly those who indulge in smoking in bed. Intoxication by drugs or alcohol, or sudden illness, may be a factor in the causation of a flame burn, and will certainly impede the ability to escape, as will pre-existing disability.

Cooling of the burn with water may minimise injury once the flames are extinguished, but benefit must be weighed against the risk of hypothermia which may be significant if the burn is large; whether or not cooling has been used, the victim should be wrapped up and the ambulance heated well for transfer to hospital. Once the patient arrives in the Emergency Department, further cooling is inappropriate and may cause hypothermia.

Flame burns are often complicated by smoke inhalation. In addition, there may be other injuries, for instance following a road traffic accident or an explosion. A history from the firemen is important: has there been a roof collapse, for example, or has the patient escaped by jumping?

Explosions

House fires feature explosions more often than is commonly realised, a phenomenon known in some quarters as the Chatham Mattress Effect: at high temperatures some flammable materials may vaporise before burning, forming an explosive mixture in air. Explosions featuring liquid petroleum gas (LPG, butane, propane) are not uncommon in boats, caravans, and some residences. Carbon monoxide poisoning should be excluded following domestic gas explosions; a gas leak resulting in an explosion may have gone unnoticed for some time by an intoxicated or sleeping person, or a suicide attempt may have gone wrong.

Contact burns

Contact burns occur when part of the body comes in contact with a hot object. The burn may be small or extensive, superficial or deep, depending on the nature and temperature of the heat source and the duration of contact. So a deep injury will be sustained by a child touching a cooker ring momentarily, or by an ill elderly person lying against a radiator for several hours.

Chemical burns

Chemicals can cause skin damage indistinguishable from a burn. They are fortunately rare, the result of industrial accidents, domestic violence, or deliberate assault. Four types of chemical injury need specific mention:

- *Phosphorus burns:* Phosphorus ignites spontaneously and burns fiercely, even in the presence of water. Small, deep burns occur which may nevertheless be numerous and cover a substantial total area which is difficult to assess accurately (see box).
- *Phenol burns* [3]: Phenol rarely causes full thickness skin loss, but may be absorbed through the skin to give systemic toxicity including renal failure (see box overleaf).
- *Hydrofluoric acid burns* [4,5]: Widely used in glass manufacture, in electronics and for cleaning purposes in industry, hydrofluoric acid causes intensely painful burns with progressive skin colliquation and inexorable systemic absorption causing ionised calcium depletion. Even small (< 2.5% body surface area burned [bsab]) injuries are often fatal (see box).
- *Cement burns:* Cement is a weak alkali and may cause a burn on prolonged contact. These injuries are rarely large, but are an important cause of full-thickness shin and knee burns in building site labourers, requiring skin grafting.

Management of chemical injuries is broadly the same as for thermal injury, bearing in mind the caveats contained in the box below.

Electrical burns [6]

These can be divided into low- and high-tension injuries. *Low-tension injuries* often cause a small deep burn at each entry and exit point. Other effects depend on the path of the current and the time for which it flows. Cardiac dysrhythmias may occur, but routine ECG monitoring is not necessary unless there has been a cardiac arrest or admission 12-lead ECG shows a dysrhythmia.

High-tension injury is rare but much more sinister. The current may arc, causing a flash burn. Entry and exit burns may be small or large. Microvascular coagulation in the capillary circulation causes extensive ischaemic damage to soft tissues with deceptively intact peripheral pulses. Spinal cord and other nerve damage may cause paralysis, whilst myoglobin and other products of tissue destruction pose a serious threat to renal function; fluid loss into tissues may cause hypovolaemia.

Specific treatment notes: chemical burns

- *General*
  - Always protect yourself – wear rubber gloves and other protection as appropriate.
  - Except as indicated below, first aid includes copious irrigation with running water.
  - Antidotes (sodium bicarbonate for acids and weak vinegar for alkalis) must be used with caution as some reactions are exothermic; a phosphate buffer solution is safer but water is most readily available.
- *Phosphorus*
  - First aid by water irrigation does not stop the burning while the phosphorus remains in the wound. The phosphorus must therefore be picked out with forceps, a process helped by the use of 1% copper sulphate solution which turns the phosphorus particles black. But beware: this may cause systemic copper toxicity if used on a large area.
- *Phenol*
  - Irrigation with copious running water will help remove the phenol, but **water/saline soaks applied to the wound are contraindicated** because this may enhance absorption of the phenol through the skin. Polyethylene glycol soaks may assist removal of phenol from skin. Ingestion should not be treated by drinking water, which will enhance absorption by dilution – activated charcoal is preferred.
- *Hydrofluoric acid*
  - Treatment includes immediate irrigation with cold water and removal of finger or toe nails if the acid has penetrated beneath. Calcium gluconate gel must be rubbed in continuously until pain is relieved; very large quantities may be needed.
  - Intra-arterial injection of calcium gluconate 10% relieves pain and may preserve the part if the injury is peripheral to the area supplied by the artery, for example radial artery injection for hand exposure to hydrofluoric acid.
  - Infiltration of 10% calcium gluconate under the wound is advocated, but may be discouragingly ineffective.
  - Serum calcium levels may become dangerously low; they must be measured frequently.
  - Once the hydrofluoric acid has penetrated the superficial layers of the skin, the only way to remove it may be immediate excision of the wound. The advice of the Burn Centre should be sought.
- **Avoid secondary injury** by making sure all care personnel are protected from contact with the chemical on the patient.

Other complications including disseminated intravascular coagulation may occur.

The next box contains some pointers to problems that may be encountered in managing a high-tension electrical injury.

Specific treatment notes: high-tension electrical injuries

- Vigilance is essential as signs of soft tissue damage may be insidious. There should be a high index of suspicion based on the history.
- Monitoring must include neurological examination, frequent soft tissue inspection, electrocardiogram and, when indicated, invasive monitoring – considerable, unpredictable fluid resuscitation may be required.
- Emergency surgery consists of fasciotomy and ruthless debridement of all devitalised tissue, several times if necessary.
- Amputation is common and varying degrees of physical disability may result, including paraplegia or quadriplegia if the spinal cord is injured.

Non-accidental injury

Burns are just as likely as any other method of physical abuse to feature in patterns of non-accidental injury (NAI). It may be that injury by burning represents a particularly vicious form of NAI since it often indicates a high level of premeditation or cruelty, as distinct from fractures which may more readily be attributed to loss of control. In the United Kingdom NAI is most often seen in children, but it should not be forgotten in adults (such as spouse abuse).

Some injury patterns are very clearly due to abuse. Cigarette burns, pattern burns due to holding a child on a hot grill, buttock and foot pad sparing, and absence of splash injury in bath scalds, for example, should all be regarded with a high level of suspicion. However, in most cases, NAI is suspected only because of an inconsistency in the history, and confirmed only by careful investigation and the revelation of, for instance, old, healed fractures.

Most scalds in children occur because of poor social circumstances, momentary carelessness, ignorance of risk, or a combination; many, however, are the result of inadequate or neglectful parenting. In these latter cases, the full child protection machinery must be brought to bear, but they do not warrant the pejorative label, NAI. Distinguishing between neglect and NAI can be very difficult and requires multidisciplinary investigation by experienced people. A paediatrician must be consulted early if it is thought neglect or NAI may have occurred; the most the emergency doctor can usually do is raise the suspicion: it is for the burn care team and their liaison paediatricians to follow this up in accordance with well-established protocols.

Pathophysiology of thermal injury [7]

There are two components to a thermal injury:

- the cutaneous burn;
- its systemic consequences.

Respiratory tract injury adds a further dimension; smoke inhalation is a whole-patient, not merely a lung, injury.

Pathophysiological process

The primary pathophysiology is an inflammatory response proportional to the area of skin burned. The reader is referred to other sources for a full account of this process, which is summarised in Figure 19.2. It is a normal physiological process,

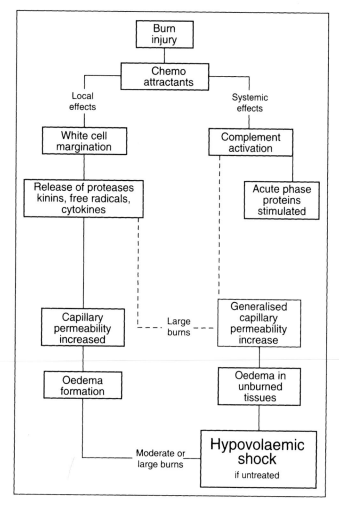

Figure 19.2 The inflammatory response in burns and scalds (simplified).

the function of which is to set the scene for healing but the effects are damaging when injury is extensive.

Oedema forms around and beneath the burned tissue. In superficial burns, where the eschar (dead skin) is thin, blisters form. The oedema contains water, electrolytes, and plasma proteins, and in larger burns causes a reduced circulating volume which threatens organ, particularly kidney, function.

In large burns, inflammatory mediators cause oedema in unburned tissues. A so-called burn toxin and myocardial depressant factor are described by some; it remains unclear whether these are real substances produced in tissues by combustion, or whether these authors were merely describing some of the clinical manifestations of the more recently identified inflammatory mediators.

Three sizes of thermal injury may be described:

- *Small injuries*: These seldom cause significant physiological disturbance. The pathophysiological process is confined locally and the clinical challenge they present is to minimise future disability or disfigurement.

- *Moderate injuries*: These are under about 40% bsab (but see below) and greater than 15% bsab (10% bsab in children and the elderly, who are more vulnerable). If uncomplicated, they threaten life infrequently, except perhaps in the elderly or very young. Transcapillary fluid loss will cause hypovolaemic shock if left untreated, so intravenous fluid replacement is always necessary. However, the exact percentage surface area dividing moderate from severe injuries depends on other factors including the depth of the injury, as well as the area. It is wise therefore to monitor *all* injuries requiring fluid resuscitation carefully; wide discrepancies between predicted and actual fluid requirements will unmask burns with a significant systemic response.

- *Large burns*: In these patients, the pathophysiological process is sufficient to cause oedema in unburned tissues. Cardiac output may be low owing to intravascular fluid loss, depressed by inflammatory mediators (plus the effects of carbon monoxide and cyanide, if smoke has been inhaled), or increased by catecholamine release in response to injury. These changes may vary with the time since burning. Disseminated intravascular coagulation or respiratory distress syndrome may be triggered and multisystem organ failure may ensue. Delayed resuscitation results in tissues being underperfused, which in turn leads to overproduction of toxic free radicals when flow is restored, a classic reperfusion injury; this inevitably exacerbates the inflammatory response and extends the depth of the burn.

As already indicated, a high-tension electrical burn should be regarded as a *major injury* until proved otherwise. The presence of airway obstruction or smoke inhalation also converts any size burn into a major injury.

The burn wound

Thermal injury causes a thin layer of dead or dying tissue over a proportion of the body surface area. The microcirculation below the wound is disturbed, owing to margination and microaggregation of white cells. The resultant zone of stasis may, but does not always, enjoy renewed flow when the inflammatory response subsides, so this zone may become an addition to the initial depth of the burn. Burns that look as though they should heal spontaneously therefore do not always do so. Inadequate resuscitation further reduces the chance of recovery of the zone of stasis. On the other hand, overzealous resuscitation increases the oedema.

Coagulation of blood in the subcutaneous capillary beds accompanies a full thickness injury, giving red cell destruction proportional to burn size. This makes no contribution to the hypovolaemic shock of thermal injury, however, which is caused by the body's reaction to the burn and is more insidious than hypovolaemia due to haemorrhage.

Heat loss and thermoregulation

All thermal injuries cause an upward resetting of thermoregulation so that, especially in children, a steady pyrexia (37.5°C in adults, up to 38.5°C in children) occurs within hours of injury [8]. Therefore pyrexia does not necessarily signify infection in burn injury.

On the other hand, some patients with major or complex burns are unable to maintain their body temperature adequately [9]. This may be due to impaired thermoregulation, or heat loss by evaporation from an extensive wound, or a combination of both. It is therefore vital to keep burned patients warm, a need that is not assisted by first aid using cold water or by exposure for wound area assessment. The need for warmth may override the need for first aid in large burns.

Respiratory tract injury [10]

The respiratory tract may be damaged by one of two mechanisms, often by both. Heat may injure the upper airway causing *pharyngeal and laryngeal oedema*, but heat damage below the trachea is unusual. Because the glottic tissues are loose and elastic, the oedema once started will rapidly occlude the airway. Early signs or symptoms suggesting obstruction therefore require urgent intervention. Promptly treated, the prognosis is good unless smoke inhalation is also present, as it all too frequently is.

Products of combustion vary enormously from fire to fire [11], depending on the materials burned, the temperature, and the availability of oxygen. Carbon dioxide, carbon monoxide, and cyanide are usually present, unlike oxygen which has been exhausted to support combustion. Other effluents include a range of aromatic compounds, oxides of nitrogen and sulphur, strong acids such as hydrochloric acid, and many more.

In high concentrations *carbon dioxide* causes mental paralysis inhibiting flight to safety; it also stimulates respiration. Initially, the glottis closes in response to smoke. Oxygen lack eventually stimulates a deep breath, which inhales smoke and more carbon dioxide. Hypercarbia causes hyperventilation, increasing the amount of smoke inhaled.

Carbon monoxide (CO) competes with oxygen for haemoglobin, to which it binds more firmly, with a half-life of about 4 hours in air and 40 minutes in 100% oxygen. It also shifts the oxygen dissociation curve to the left, impairing deposition of oxygen in tissues. In the tissues it competes with oxygen for myoglobin, having a half-life of about 24 hours at this level. Lastly it impairs the activity of cytochrome oxidase.

Cyanide causes mitochondrial poisoning and cytochrome oxidase inhibition, exacerbating the effects of CO. The effect of these two toxins is therefore threefold:

- reduced oxygen carriage by the blood;
- reduced oxygen transfer to the tissues;
- impaired use of oxygen in the energy production cycle

. . . in other words, a high risk of global hypoxia.

Other components of smoke cause chemical injury to the tracheobronchial tree. This in turn sets up an inflammatory response (see Figure 19.2), the consequences of which for the lung are very different from those for the skin [12].

Interstitial pulmonary oedema develops, increasing the diffusion gradient for gas exchange. There is progressive deterioration in the alveolar–arteriolar oxygen gradient and a sharp increase in extravascular lung water. Interstitial oedema increases the mass of the lung tissue which increases the mass effect on intrathoracic pressure, especially in dependent parts of the lung. Small airway closure occurs earlier in the respiratory cycle, or throughout it for some lung components. Atelectasis is inevitable, predisposing to the respiratory distress syndrome.

In the larger airways, mucus production increases and commonly becomes viscid. Mixed with soot and debris (migrant leucocytes, fibrin, and damaged mucosal cells), these secretions have the consistency of thick black glue. Mucosal slough begins to separate and "casts" are formed; these may block the airway (Figure 19.3). Bronchospasm is caused by

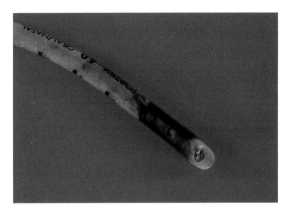

Figure 19.3 Mucus, soot, and cellular debris in a child's tracheal tube.

inflammatory mediators, particularly arachidonic acid precursors such as thromboxane A_2 which are potent smooth muscle constrictors.

The patient, who has already suffered acute hypoxia at the fire, is now at risk for upper airway obstruction, severe bronchial narrowing and bronchospasm, lung damage with impaired gas exchange, reduced oxygen delivery to the tissues, and diminished oxygen uptake and utilisation at tissue level. An inhalation injury thus becomes a whole-body insult.

The inflammatory response from the lung injury will add significantly to the effects of the cutaneous burn. A respiratory injury therefore increases the mortality from a burn, and it is no surprise that the mortality from major burns with smoke inhalation exceeds 50% in most published series.

Assessment and management

Priorities

Airway, breathing and circulation (**ABC**) are the first priorities for assessment, accompanied by examination to determine the extent of the burn, whether there are any other injuries, and whether there are any acute or pre-existing illnesses. Because the patient's ability to maintain body temperature may be impaired, it is vital that this assessment is carried out in a very warm environment; a thermal ceiling is helpful if available.

Small injuries: < 15% bsab (10% bsab in children and elderly)

The crucial requirement for minor burns is to ensure prompt, appropriate treatment. Dressings may be all that is needed for very small or superficial burns; skin grafting should otherwise be considered, usually under the care of a plastic surgeon; rehabilitation services and psychological help may also need to be involved.

Moderate injuries: 15% (10% in children and elderly) to 40%, uncomplicated

Unless the burn is superficial, the goal after resuscitation is to excise it at the earliest opportunity. Intravenous fluid resuscitation is needed to prevent shock. A good drip should be inserted and the patient resuscitated, initially according to an appropriate formula.

It has been traditional in the UK to recommend colloid resuscitation for burns. However, ATLS training advocates crystalloid based on US practice, so harmony with this before transfer avoids confusion for ATLS-trained staff inexperienced in burns. A recent meta-analysis suggesting an increased mortality using albumin for resuscitation [13] generated much public concern about this practice. Only three of the 32 cited papers studied burned patients and only one looked at a protocol in common use so the relevance of this study in burns is questionable. However, in its light, prudence dictates caution in the use of albumin which should usually be left to the Burn Centre to initiate. Moreover, both the ATLS course and the recently introduced Emergency Management of Severe Burns (EMSB) course advocate crystalloid resuscitation in the first instance. The traditional Muir & Barclay formula is however given in the Box below for completeness; it can be invoked if single-donor plasma is available but synthetic colloids should *not* be used. Because albumin can sequester in the interstitial tissues of the lung, causing persistent changes after resuscitation is complete [14] albumin is not normally recommended in the early stages in patients with smoke inhalation.

Fluid resuscitation formulae

- **Baxter (Parkland) Formula** (using crystalloid)
  - Lactated Ringer's (Hartmann's) solution 4 ml/kg/% bsab in first 24 hours
    - *half* to be given in the *first 8 hours from time of injury*, or to simplify, 0.25 ml/kg/% bsab *per hour from time of injury*
  - Children will need additional metabolic water as dextrose 5% 1–3 ml/kg/h depending on age.
- **Original Muir & Barclay (Mount Vernon) Formula** (using colloid)
  - 0.5 ml/kg/% bsab of colloid (HAS 4.5% or single-donor plasma) in *first 4 hours, from time of injury*.
  - Metabolic water is needed in addition, as dextrose 5% 1–4 ml/kg/hr depending on age.

Note: Synthetic colloids (gelatines; etherified starches) are hypertonic with respect to plasma, and should therefore not be used in substitute for natural colloids in the Mount Vernon Formula. If single-donor plasma is unavailable, it is preferable to use Ringer's Lactate according to the Baxter Formula.

Invasive monitoring is rarely needed unless there is smoke inhalation. The wound should be covered (see below), the patient should be kept warm, and transfer should be arranged to the Burn Unit as soon as possible.

Major or complex burns

In these patients, the need for speedy transfer to a Burn Centre is even greater but appropriate stabilisation must be achieved first. The standard ABC approach is best, and should involve other disciplines from an early stage – an anaesthetist if respiratory injury is suspected, or the appropriate discipline if the history suggests the presence of other injuries or illnesses.

The upper airway

Impending **A**irway obstruction may not be immediately apparent so frequent reassessment is needed when any of the indicators in Figure 19.4 is positive. If intubation is not required immediately, frequent reassessment by an anaesthetist is essential. However, even minimal laryngeal oedema requires

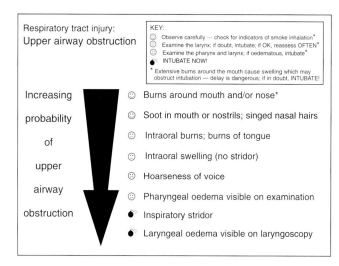

Figure 19.4 Indicators of respiratory obstruction in respiratory tract injury.

intubation as it will always get worse. If no smoke has been inhaled, ventilation is not needed once the intubating relaxant has worn off; continuous positive airway pressure (CPAP) is sufficient pressure support.

Smoke inhalation [15]

Breathing may initially be normal, but when *any two* of the signs in the box below so indicate, investigation for smoke inhalation is required:

- Arterial blood gas analysis.
- Carboxyhaemoglobin estimation – if this test cannot be done in the Emergency Department, a heparin or EDTA sample should be taken, labelled for time, and sent with the patient to the Burn Centre.
- Cyanide measurement – in practice, this test is rarely available, but cyanide can be assumed if carbon monoxide levels exceed 10% with an accompanying metabolic acidosis [16].

If smoke inhalation is diagnosed or if there is respiratory distress, the patient should be ventilated; delay increases the risk of decline into respiratory distress syndrome. Again, as for airway assessment, early help from an anaesthetist should be sought. Frequent reassessment including serial blood gases will help clarify the diagnosis.

Respiratory tract injury: indicators for smoke inhalation

Two or more risk factors present = smoke inhalation.
- History of fire in enclosed space or of rescue from smoke
- Any signs indicating upper airway injury (see Figure 19.4)
- Altered level of consciousness
- Symptoms/signs of respiratory dysfunction developing in first few days
- Carbon particles or mucosal casts in sputum
- Carboxyhaemoglobin > 10%
- Low Pa_{O_2} or increasing $(A–a)O_2$ gradient
- Mucosal changes and/or soot seen on bronchoscopy

Note: In mild smoke inhalation, signs may develop over a day or two; even a severe injury may not become apparent immediately.

100% oxygen should be given by ventilation for up to 12 hours or while metabolic acidosis persists, to maximise displacement of carbon monoxide from tissues; mask oxygen is inappropriate for this purpose. Thiosulphate administration may be of benefit if cyanide intoxication is suspected. The pulse oximeter is misleading for monitoring in the presence of carbon monoxide because it cannot distinguish between oxyhaemoglobin and carboxyhaemoglobin.

Hyperbaric oxygen [17] is usually unavailable. If access to a hyperbaric chamber is to hand, it is tempting to divert the smoke-injured patient to it, especially as there is some evidence that it may also improve the recovery of the zone of stasis under the burn wound. However, in these patients, delay in instituting active intensive therapy and appropriate wound care may more than offset any benefit. Hyperbaric oxygen should therefore only be used if it can be made available in the Burn Centre, or if members of the burn care team can be spared to treat the patient while undergoing hyperbaric therapy. This must therefore be a decision for the Burn Centre team.

Breathing may be restricted by circumferential chest burns, requiring release by incision until the wound edges pull apart (escharotomy) in a chequerboard pattern. Similar problems may arise in the limbs, impairing the **C**irculation; longitudinal escharotomy may be needed, a decision that can be guided by flow measurement using a Doppler probe. For further comment on the timing of escharotomy, see the section on *The burn wound*, below.

Fluid resuscitation

Circulating volume must be maintained. Good intravenous access (two drips if possible) is essential, through the burn if necessary. Appropriate fluid replacement depends on accurate burn area assessment using the Rule of Nines or, preferably, a Lund and Browder Chart (Figure 19.5). A further guide is the patient's hand, which equates to 1% of body surface. A simple check of accuracy is possible by assessing the *un*burned area also, subtracting this figure from 100%, and comparing with the first calculation. Fluid requirements should be calculated *from the time of injury*, and initial therapy given according to formula (see the section *Moderate injuries* above, and also the box on fluid resuscitation formulae, p. 244).

It is common to over- or underestimate the wound size by inclusion of erythema or exclusion of superficial injury mistaken for erythema. A useful test for doubtful areas is to apply a gentle sheer stress with a (sterile-gloved) thumb: erythema will not be affected; the surface of a superficial burn will break because it is weakened by oedema.

Catheterisation and hourly urine volume measurement are needed for all burns greater than about 25% bsab. Standard monitoring is non-invasive: pulse, blood pressure, central and peripheral temperatures, haematocrit, urine flow, and renal tubular function (osmolality, *not specific gravity*). Invasive monitoring is only occasionally needed, in massive or complex burns or when non-invasive monitoring shows fluid requirements to be much greater than the formula used predicts. Central venous pressure (CVP) or pulmonary artery catheter (PAC) measurements may be helpful in these cases to guide fluid replacement or to monitor cardiac function made unpredictable by pre-existing disease, carbon monoxide, cyanide, "burn toxin", inflammatory mediators, and catecholamines. Even in these patients, *it is seldom necessary to delay transfer simply because invasive monitoring is not yet in place, unless the transfer journey will be prolonged or the patient's condition is seriously unstable.*

The burn wound

Following assessment of wound area, the wound should be covered in a sterile manner and the patient kept warm or actively rewarmed if hypothermic. All intravenous fluids should be warmed and ventilation gases should be warm-humidified, although this may not always be possible during ambulance transfer.

Suitable wound coverings include *dry* sterile cotton cloths or plastic food wrap (e.g. Cling Film®). Saline-soaked coverings promote hypothermia by evaporation, so should be avoided. Antibacterial creams such as Flamazine® should be avoided initially. This is because they may interfere with assessment of wound depth by the burn care team, whose priority is to plan early wound excision – accurate area and depth estimations are essential for this purpose.

Escharotomy

Unless transfer is delayed or respiratory excursion is embarrassed, escharotomies may usually be left to the burn care team, but ask their advice and follow their guidance.

Antibiotics

The burn wound is sterilised by heat so antibiotics are unnecessary in the early hours. Subsequent prophylaxis is usually reserved for at-risk patients or those with smoke inhalation. Narrow spectrum agents against known population commensals are usually chosen.

Pain relief [18]

It is very easy to be so engrossed in the management priorities described above that the patient's pain is forgotten. A major,

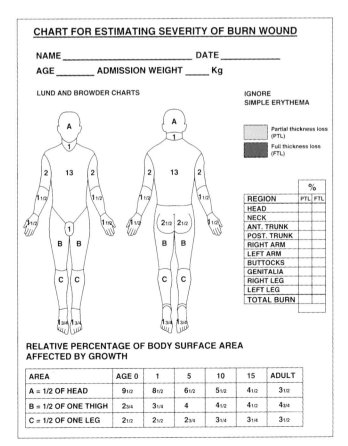

Figure 19.5 Lund and Browder burn area assessment chart.

full-thickness burn may not be very painful of itself, and the patient may be more distressed by the horror of what has happened than by physical pain; nevertheless, although the nerve endings in a full thickness burn are damaged, the wound edges are still innervated and even subcutaneous tissues carry pain fibres. In contrast, partial thickness and especially superficial burns can be very painful. Attention should therefore be given as soon as possible to high quality analgesia and relief of distress.

In major burns, circulation to peripheral tissues may be dubious, intramuscular injections are unreliable, and pain relief must be immediate. For these reasons, the intravenous route is preferred. Small increments of diluted (1 mg/ml) morphine or diamorphine are best, titrated until comfort is achieved. This requires a little time and patience, but it is well worthwhile. In patients who are intubated and ventilated, opiates by infusion should form a major component of the sedation regimen, guided by an anaesthetist.

Non-steroidal anti-inflammatory drugs (NSAIDs), such as ibuprofen, will enhance the analgesic benefit of opiates synergistically and are thought by some to have a beneficial effect on the extent of the inflammatory response. There is therefore nothing to be lost, and possibly much to be gained, by adding NSAIDs to the analgesia regimen from the start.

Relief of distress may require a last resort to benzodiazepines, but the human approach of the calm, reassuring professional who keeps the patient informed, answers questions, and responds to anxieties expressed, produces by far the best results in this regard.

Criteria for referral to a Burn Centre

Remember: All Burn Centres are happy to give telephone advice to a doctor who is uncertain about managing a particular thermal injury.

- Extensive burns, including scalds, assessed as:
  - >10% of TBSA* in patients younger than 12 or older than 60
  - >15% of TBSA* in patients aged 12–60
- Full thickness burns >5% TBSA*, all ages
- Deep circumferential burns of an extremity or the chest
- Burns of the face, hands, feet, perineum, or across joints
- Electrical burns incl. lightning, high tension, low tension
- Chemical burns, fat burns, industrial injuries
- Inhalation injury, suspected or actual, associated with a burn
- Burn patients with associated trauma or pre-existing illness
- Other causes of extensive skin loss such as toxic epidermal necrolysis
- Any burn of any size about which you are unhappy

* TBSA = total body surface area.
Local policies may exist for referring small and moderate burns to a local Plastic Surgery service. These protocols should be followed.

Communication with other appropriate professionals

General guidance

Important considerations guiding onward referral of a thermally injured patient are summarised in the box. These general principles are amplified below.

Minor burns

Refer these to a Plastic Surgeon if they involve the face, perineum, feet or hands, if they are across joints, or if there is any doubt about management such as the need for skin grafting. Emergency department doctors should make themselves aware of local procedures for referral of these patients.

Moderate burns

Burns > 15% bsab (10% in children and the elderly) should usually be transferred to the nearest Burn Centre. In some regions, the Burn Unit takes all comers, including minor burns. In other regions, local plastic surgery departments are comfortable managing burns below about 25–30% bsab in their wards or in a small, designated burn care facility. Therefore local policies should be clearly stated in staff protocols, and followed carefully.

Major burns

Major and complex injuries should ideally be treated in a Burn Centre capable of providing care for every possible contingency, including renal support and on-site intensive care. This is currently not available everywhere, so referral must be to the nearest Burn Unit. They will advise the most appropriate destination, which will be either the Burn Unit or the Intensive Therapy Unit of the Burn Unit's hospital, depending on complexity.

A telephone call to the Regional Burn Unit as early as possible after admission to the Emergency Department will allow the emergency doctor to confirm the treatment he or she should give and help plan the optimum future management of the patient. It also enables the burn care team to prepare appropriately to receive the patient. Essential information includes the items in Figure 19.6, a version of which may be helpful to send with the patient. Any information given by the Fire Brigade or by ambulance staff is vital to send on; the time and cause of injury and any known past medical history are especially important items of information.

Call an anaesthetist

If respiratory injury is a possibility or if intravenous access is difficult, the help of an anaesthetist should be sought early, as already indicated. It is wise to avoid unnecessary intubation, especially in children. However, patients at risk of airway damage should usually be intubated and *must* be accompanied by an anaesthetist. Intubation before transfer is indicated if there is stridor or visible oedema of the pharynx or larynx. Golden rule: if in doubt, ask for help from an anaesthetist!

TRANSFER INFORMATION CHART
Contact your Regional Burn Unit, for advice
Insert telephone number: ....

TIME OF ARRIVAL IN A & E:

HOW ACCIDENT HAPPENED:

CLOTHING WORN (material):

FIRST AID GIVEN:

HOW LONG FOR?   mins

I.V. CANNULA SIZE:

SITE OF INSERTION:

CATHETER PASSED? Yes/No

CATHETER SIZE:

URINE VOIDED: ml.

Time measured:

Analgesia/ Antiemetics:

Drug & Dose	Route	Time

TETANUS TOXOID (please tick)

Up to date □   Given □

COMMENTS:

FLUID REQUIREMENT CALCULATION:

WEIGHT OF PATIENT: kg

ESTIMATED BURN AREA: %bsab

Wt (kg) x % burn x 0.5   ml
= HAS 4.5% solution first 4 hours from injury

OR: Wt (kg) x % burn x 2:   ml

= Hartmann's infusion first 8 hours
        (0.25 ml/kg/% bsab/h) from injury
REMEMBER: Metabolic water needed as well
(1.5 to 4 ml/kg/h depending on age)

FLUID GIVEN - FIRST 4 HOURS AFTER INJURY:

HOUR	FLUID	AMOUNT
1		
2		
3		
4		

RESPIRATORY INJURY:

SUSPECTED?   Yes/No

SOOT IN NOSE/THROAT?   Yes/No

INTUBATION REQUIRED?   Yes/No

Tube size   mm

BLOOD GASES:

Fi O_2 =   Pa O_2 =   Pa CO_2 =

pH = HCO_3 =

CARBOXYHAEMOGLOBIN:
Sample as soon as possible after injury; note time.

If you cannot assay HbCO, send heparinised or EDTA
sample to Burn Centre with the patient.

TIME of sample: HbCO =   %

Figure 19.6 Transfer information chart.

Transfer

Transfer the patient as soon as the airway is secure, appropriate respiratory support is under way, and i.v. therapy has been commenced in accordance with the formula (see box on fluid resuscitation formulae, page 244). Transfer typically gets the patient to specialised treatment within the first two to three hours after injury. Unnecessary delay magnifies errors caused by inexperience in wound area calculation. Seriously burned patients should be accompanied by a doctor, and additionally by an anaesthetist if the patient is intubated and/or ventilated, or at risk for respiratory obstruction.

Patients with unusual burns

Management of chemical or electrical injuries requires attention to some specific considerations, and these have already been described in the section on *Mechanisms of injury* (see boxes on chemical burns and high-tension electrical injuries). As these will be encountered infrequently, it is even more important to involve the staff of the Burn Centre by telephone at a very early stage.

Patients with other injuries

If other injuries are severe, they should take priority initially. However, good advice should be obtained promptly from experienced burn care staff about managing the burn wound. The resuscitation requirement will include the demands of the burn but should be guided by invasive monitoring. Emergency surgery may include escharotomies, but otherwise surgery to the burn can be deferred until other injuries are stable. Unnecessary delay thereafter increases the risk of infective complications. The burn care team *must* be involved from the outset, to plan burn surgery alongside other needs and to supervise wound care and dressings.

Summary

Major burns comprise just a small proportion of all thermal injuries, but can be frightening for the inexperienced. The key to success is to access accurately, start treatment promptly and transfer expeditiously. Changes occur more slowly and predictably than in other trauma, so the goal is to stabilise quickly then transfer to specialised burn care. Unnecessary delay compromises care. Small injuries also require accurate assessment and often the expertise of a plastic surgeon, whose advice should be sought early.

References

1. Smith RW, O'Neill TJ. An analysis into childhood burns. *Burns* 1984;**11**:117–24.
2. Childs C, Edwards-Jones V, Heathcote DM, Dawson M, Davenport PJ. Patterns of *Staphylococcus aureus* colonization, toxin production, immunity and illness in burned children. *Burns* 1994;**20**: 514–21.
3. Horch R, Spijker G, Stark GB. Phenol burns and intoxications. *Burns* 1994;**20**:45–50.
4. Kirkpatrick JJR, Enion DS, Burd DAR. Hydrofluoric acid burns: a review. *Burns* 1995;**21**:483–93.
5. Kirkpatrick JJR, Burd DAR. An algorithmic approach to the treatment of hydrofluoric acid burns. *Burns* 1995;**21**:495–99.
6. Haberal M. Electrical burns: a five-year experience – 1985 Evans Lecture. *J Trauma* 1986;**26**:103–9.
7. Dziewulski P. Burn wound healing: James Elsworth Laing Memorial Essay for 1991. *Burns* 1992;**18**:466–78.
8. Childs C. Temperature regulation in burned patients. *Br J Intens Care* 1995; **4**:129–34.
9. Platt AJ, Aslam S, Judkins K, Phipps AR, Smith GL, Temperature profiles during resuscitation predict survival following burns complicated by smoke inhalation injury. *Burns* 1997;**23**:250–5.
10. Kinsella J. Smoke inhalation. *Burns* 1988;**14**:269.
11. Prien T, Traber DL. Toxic smoke compounds and inhalation injury – a review. *Burns* 1988;**14**:451.
12. Traber DL, Linares HA, Herndon DN. The pathophysiology of inhalation injury – a review. *Burns* 1988;**14**:357.
13. Cochrane Injuries Group albumin reviewers (Roberts I, *et al*). Human albumin administration in critically ill patients: systematic review of randomised controlled trials. *Br Med J* 1998; **317**, 235–40; editorial pp. 223–4.
14. Goodwin CW, Dorethy J, Lam V, Pruitt BA Jr. Randomized trial of the efficacy of crystalloid and colloid resuscitation on hemodynamic response and lung water following thermal injury. *Ann Surg* 1983; **197**(5); 520–29; discussion 529–31.
15. Pruitt BA, Cioffi WG, Shimazu T, Ikeuchi H, Mason AD. Evaluation and management of patients with inhalation injury. *J Trauma* 1990;**30**(Suppl):S63.
16. Baud FJ, Barriot P, Toffis V *et al*. Elevated blood cyanide concentrations in victims of smoke inhalation. *New Engl J Med* 1991; **325**:1761.
17. James PB. Hyperbaric oxygen in the treatment of carbon monoxide poisoning and smoke inhalation injury: a review. *Intens Care World* 1989;**6**:135.
18. Laterjet J, Choinière M. Pain in burn patients. *Burns* 1995;**21**: 344–8.

Further reading

The following are cited as excellent further reading on aspects of burn injury and management. They are not referenced to the text, because to do so would detract from their broader applicability and usefulness.

Clarke JA. *A colour atlas of burn injuries*. London: Chapman & Hall Medical, 1992.
Driscoll PA, Gwinnutt CL, Jimmerson C LeDuc, Goodall O (eds). *Trauma resuscitation – the team approach*. London: MacMillan, 1993, (Ch. 12).
Herndon DN (ed.). *Total burn care*. Philadelphia: WB Saunders Co. Ltd, 1997.
Settle JAD (ed.) *Principles and practice of burn management*. London: Churchill Livingstone, 1997.

20 Drowning and near drowning

Anthony D. Simcock

Consultant Anaesthetist, Royal Cornwall Hospitals, Truro, Cornwall

OBJECTIVES

- ■ To relieve hypoxia.
- ■ To restore cardiovascular stability.
- ■ To assess apparently dead carefully.
- ■ To maintain CPR until rewarmed.

Medical conditions predisposing to drowning

- ● Stroke
- ● Epilepsy
- ● Myocardial infarction
- ● Acute hypoglycaemia
- ● Alcohol/drug intoxication
- ● Muscular diseases
- ● Suicide

Death from drowning is the third commonest cause of accidental death in the United Kingdom and United States [1,2]. It is the second commonest cause of accidental death in children and a recent UK survey reported over 150 deaths per annum in children over a 2-year period [3]. Population studies consistently estimate deaths in the population as a whole in excess of 500 per annum. It is difficult to give accurate figures for immersion accidents overall but it is estimated that near drowning incidents are eight to nine times more common. Traditional terminology has defined drowning as "death as a result of suffocation by submersion in water". Near drowning is a term reserved for the initial survival of an individual after suffocation by immersion in water.

Much attention has been given to accident prevention in recent years and there is no doubt that fencing or covering of domestic pools and the supervision of water leisure areas by trained staff will lead to a reduction, particularly in childhood accidents.

Pathophysiology

In post mortems of drowning victims, the lungs are found to show no evidence of aspiration in 7–10% of cases and these deaths may be due to intense glottic spasm resulting from hypoxia, or cardiac arrest induced by sudden exposure of the body to cold water. This is hypothesis and deaths from so-called "dry drowning" are still an ill-understood phenomenon.

Anyone who is unconscious when entering the water will have an unprotected airway and water will enter the lungs on inspiration leading to increasing hypoxia and rapid death. Such occurrence may be due to trauma causing the patient to lose consciousness and enter the water, or may be as a result of striking the head against solid objects, for example inappropriate diving in shallow water. Unconsciousness or diminished consciousness may also occur from a variety of medical conditions and these are shown in the box.

By and large the above list leads to either reduced consciousness or incapacity and an inability to maintain the airway above the water. Epilepsy is perhaps the most common problem and certainly epileptics should be closely supervised when taking part in water activities. The physiological effects of cold water immersion can produce profound rises in peripheral resistance and the elderly, in particular, may be prone to stroke or myocardial infarction as a result. Alcohol-related incidents are particularly common in young males, and suicide by drowning seems to have a very patchy geographical distribution.

Those who are unable to swim and are out of their depth will make every effort to inhale only when they have their airway above the water. This leads to the swallowing of large quantities of water and frantic beating of the arms to try and maintain the head-up position. If rescue is not at hand it is inevitable that eventually the victim is forced to take a breath under water. It is thought that the downward spiral of events is for the first inspiration to produce profound glottic spasm with little aspiration but loss of the control of breathing. There is then repeated inspiration under the water with increasing aspiration and hypoxia until the victim becomes unconscious which may take several minutes.

In swimmers exposed to cold water there will be the inevitable onset of hypothermia if the swimmer is not insulated from the cold environment. Above 35°C there is normal cerebral function and co-ordination of breathing and arm and leg movements. The first signs of hypothermic problems occur below 35°C with a period of amnesia, confusion, and disorientation. Swimmers filmed at this stage exhibit a swimming pattern akin to "dog paddling". The arms produce an ineffective paddle movement, the legs remain at 45° producing little forward propulsion and the head rolls from side to side. Anyone seen exhibiting these signs should be rescued immediately as, if left, hypothermia will gradually reduce conscious levels and the ability to keep the airway above the water. Unconsciousness starts to occur at 33°C and few remain conscious once the central temperature has fallen to 30°C [4]. These people then die from drowning but the reason they drown is that they have become hypothermic.

The pathophysiological effect of aspiration of water into the lungs is to produce profound ventilation/perfusion mismatch, with subsequent right-to-left shunt and hypoxaemia. *In vitro* experiments have shown that there are different physiological results between the aspiration of fresh water and sea water. In animal experiments hypotonic fresh water can be shown to be absorbed into the pulmonary circulation and, conversely, hypertonic sea water may cause fluid from the pulmonary circulation to move into the alveoli [5]. However, in clinical practice the immediate and intensive care management of these patients is identical and such considerations are of theoretical rather than practical importance.

Although the role of hypothermia in producing diminished consciousness and death in swimmers has already been alluded to, it is undoubtedly a reason why there have been some remarkable survivors after prolonged submersion. The drowning process exposes initially the body surface area to cold water, but later the upper gastrointestinal tract and eventually the lungs to hypothermia. It is thought that this leads to increasing hypothermia of the venous return and, as long as the heart remains in sinus rhythm, progressively colder blood is pumped to the brain. It has long been accepted that normal oxygen requirements are reduced in hypothermia and it is estimated that there is a 30% reduction at 30°C [6] and 66% at 20°C [7]. It is thought that the cerebral sparing effects of hypothermia are the reason why resuscitation and cerebrally intact survival is possible after prolonged periods of submersion. Normal cerebral recovery after hypothermic cardiac arrest has been reported after prolonged cardiopulmonary resuscitation lasting up to three hours [5]. Hypothermia is usually accompanied by metabolic acidosis and pH levels of < 7.0 can be recorded with central temperatures below 30°C.

Assessment and immediate care

The early assessment, relief of hypoxia and immediate care are vital not only for successful resuscitation but also for achieving cerebrally normal survival. Vigorous efforts of the intensive care team will be unlikely to reverse any delays or mistakes made at the accident site. Ideally an assessment and initial treatment of the drowned or near-drowned victim should take place in the water as soon as the accident is discovered. In practice this is only feasible in calm water with trained personnel. In such circumstances it may be possible to detect apnoea or cardiac arrest. In most cases, however, assessment can only take place once the victim has been rescued. The problems of rescue are immense and can only briefly be alluded to in this chapter.

Wherever possible the rescuers should endeavour to remove the victim from the water (Figure 20.1) in the horizontal position [8] and supporting the airway. The possibility of cervical spine injury should always be recognised in drowning caused by trauma or shallow water diving accidents.

The initial assessment consists of the identification and relief of *hypoxia*. The interval between the airway slipping below the water with ensuing hypoxia and this being relieved is referred to as the "hypoxic gap", and it is reducing the hypoxic gap to a minimum which is the object of immediate care [9]. The fundamental question for a rescuer is to consider the patient's ventilatory status [10]. The two primary questions therefore are:

1. Is this patient breathing? If the answer is yes, then:

2. Is this patient breathing adequately?

Apnoea should be treated with airway clearance and immediate ventilation (Figure 20.2). This may initially have to

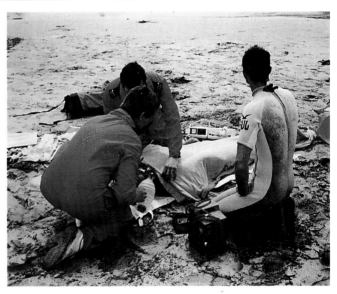

Figure 20.2   First-class immediate care is vital.

take the form of expired air resuscitation but as soon as possible should consist of ventilation with 100% oxygen via Guedel airway, laryngeal mask, or preferably endotracheal tube. Apnoea from near drowning leads to cardiac standstill. If there is clinical evidence of cardiac arrest then all authorities on the subject are now agreed that external cardiac massage should commence along standard UK Resuscitation Council guidelines. Once commenced, resuscitation should continue throughout the period of transport to hospital. Even in those patients whose ventilation is preserved there is still a significant

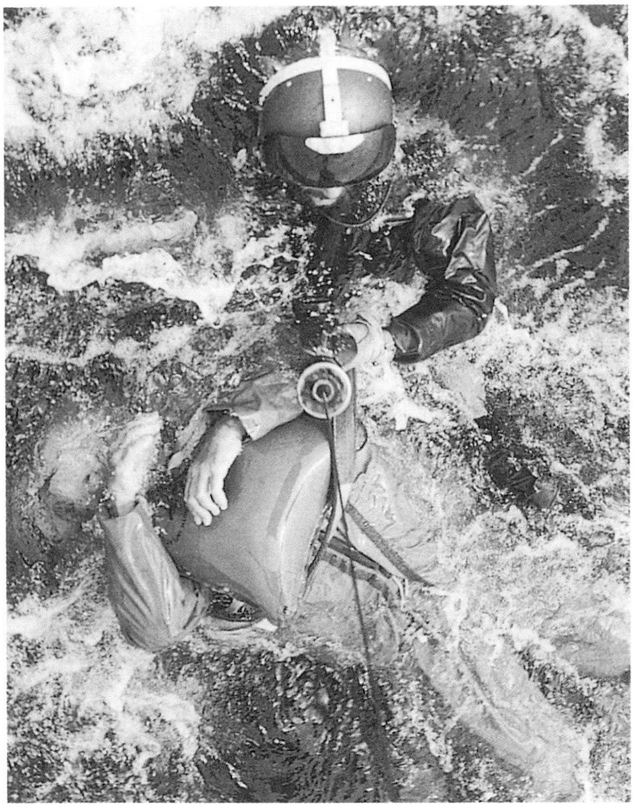

Figure 20.1   Rescue of unconscious heavy male in rough water.

risk of hypoxia. Wherever this is suspected the patient should be given high-flow oxygen therapy by mask and moved to hospital with the utmost speed. In the unconscious, drainage of the nasopharynx is difficult and time-consuming in adults, but there may still be a place for simple drainage in the head-down, lateral position in small children. The Heimlich manoeuvre has been largely abandoned. The vast majority of people rescued from an immersion incident will be hypothermic to a greater or lesser extent and insulation with warm dry clothing or blankets is simple and effective during the immediate care phase. The use of foil insulation sheets (the so-called space blankets) is less effective than warm dry woollen equivalents. Once airway management and adequate ventilation have been established at the accident site, the patient should be transported as rapidly as possible in the horizontal position to a well-equipped hospital with accident and intensive care facilities. Where the patient is unconscious or has suffered cardiac arrest, prior notification to the hospital should be made wherever possible and the victim met on arrival by a resuscitation team.

Hospital/intensive care management

Anyone who has had to be rescued from difficulties in the water should be brought to a well-equipped resuscitation bay of an A & E department. Initial hospital management is really an extension of the immediate care phase. Wherever possible the patient should be assessed immediately on arrival by A & E and intensive care staff. There will be many patients who have had to be rescued who, by the time they reach hospital, appear to have fully recovered. They are conscious with no clinical or radiological evidence of inhalation. The incidence of deterioration in these patients – so-called *secondary drowning* [11], is of the order of 2–3%. Secondary drowning is essentially acute respiratory failure occurring as a result of hypoxic damage to the lung parenchyma at the time of the accident. It is wise, therefore, to admit such patients to hospital overnight for careful nursing observation and monitoring of oxygen saturations (Sa_{O_2}) by pulse oximetry. A falling Sa_{O_2} accompanied by rising respiratory rate and the onset of cough with white frothy sputum should be regarded as an urgent indication to transfer from ward to intensive care unit. Late onset cerebral oedema has been recorded but is extremely rare and if deterioration is going to occur it will usually occur in the first 12 hours after the accident.

The conscious patient

Anyone who has inhaled water but is still conscious and breathing at an adequate rate and depth should be given high-inspired oxygen therapy by mask in the resuscitation room and then moved to an intensive care unit for further management. There, treatment should be aimed at restoring cardio-respiratory normality in the shortest possible time [12]. Oxygen therapy should be continued by mask and determination of Sa_{O_2} by pulse oximetry should commence. If the peripheral circulation is shut down by either a hypovolaemic-like picture or cold peripheral vasoconstriction, then an arterial line should be inserted under local anaesthetic as a matter or priority. The patient's progress should then be monitored by either Sa_{O_2} or arterial partial pressure (Pa_{O_2}). If normal oxygenation is not rapidly restored by giving up to 60% oxygen by mask then the use of constant positive airway pressure (CPAP) or elective intubation and ventilation should be considered. CPAP

circuits have been used in the United States with excellent results and can certainly prevent the necessity for ventilation in those patients whose oxygenation is borderline. Modern circuits are quiet, comfortable, and allow oxygen percentages of up to 100% to be used in the inspired mixture. The overriding principle, however, is not to let the patient become or remain hypoxic, and intubation and ventilation may be necessary to prevent this. In the majority of patients, this aggressive early treatment leads to improvement and both blood gas pictures and chest x-rays will return to normal in the next 48 hours.

The question of fluid shifts in the acute near-drowning scenario is ill-understood. Both salt and fresh water drownings exhibit a picture akin to hypovolaemia. An intravenous line should be established and any hypotension treated with an initial rapid infusion of 10 ml/kg of warmed crystalloid solution given over 30 minutes. This is normally sufficient to restore circulatory normality. The choice of fluid is probably not important but normal saline is the usual replacement after fresh water and 5% dextrose after sea water incidents. If cardiovascular instability persists then further fluid therapy should be titrated against central venous pressure (CVP) measurements. Hypothermia and accompanying metabolic acidosis are usually mild in this group and a central temperature of 34°C or above should be expected. Blood gas analysis will normally show a pH > 7.2 and both hypothermia and metabolic acidosis are self correcting as the patient recovers.

Further investigations should include chest x-ray, blood glucose, urea/electrolytes, and examination of the blood film. Significant electrolyte abnormalities or haemolysis would not be expected but the chest x-ray often shows a widespread diffuse white infiltration. This is not a problem with the left ventricle and there is no place for diuretic therapy in the early management of near drowning. The x-ray appearances are due to aspirated water and will rapidly improve as long as cardiovascular normality is maintained. Certainly the chest x-ray and blood gas picture should be expected to revert to normal and any late deterioration in oxygenation or chest x-ray appearance may herald the onset of adult respiratory distress syndrome although this is rare.

There is no place now for the prophylactic use of steroids as they have never been shown to improve outcome [13]. Antibiotic therapy should be withheld until the result of cultures from tracheal aspirates are known unless the patient has fallen into obviously polluted water or has aspirated vomit. In these circumstances after the initial tracheal aspirate has been taken it is reasonable to start an intravenous broad spectrum antibiotic, such as co-amoxiclav, whilst the results of culture are awaited. Regular physiotherapy in the immediate period is helpful not only in producing specimens for culture but also in assisting a patient to control their breathing which is usually associated with repeated coughing bouts and quite distressing retrosternal pain. It should be expected that amounts of sputum actually expectorated in these circumstances are, however, small. Given careful observation and management most patients in this category will recover within 48 hours and can be discharged to the ward when they have a normal x-ray and blood oxygenation breathing room air.

The unconscious patient

The patient who remains unconscious after rescue following an immersion incident is one of the main reasons why a member of the intensive care staff, practised in airway management, intubation, and ventilation, should be present when such a patient arrives in the resuscitation room. The immediate management of the airway and prevention of cardiac arrest makes a significant difference not only in results but to cerebrally normal survival. Cervical spine damage should always be considered after shallow water accidents. The unconscious patient is usually shut down, cyanosed, with gasping diaphragmatic respiration accompanied by the exhalation of small amounts of inhaled water. Vomiting and aspiration may have occurred in up to 40% of these patients. Airway clearance, intubation, and ventilation should be achieved before transfer to the intensive care unit. Usually depressant drugs are not necessary for these manoeuvres. Positive pressure ventilation by hand using 100% oxygen will not normally be resisted by the patient but initial ventilation is usually accompanied by regurgitation of aspirated fluid from the large airways and this will need to be repeatedly cleared with endobronchial suction catheters. When continuous ventilation without frequent need for suction has been achieved, the patient can then be transferred to the intensive care unit and mechanical ventilation commenced. An inspired oxygen percentage of 100% should be employed initially and it is to be expected that compliance will be poor with high inspiratory pressures of up to 50 cm of water. This is, of course, the pressure in the large airways and there is little risk of pneumothorax. A ventilator with provision for fixed volume cycling is probably the mode of choice in the first instance.

As peripheral circulation will almost certainly be poor, pulse oximetry may be inaccurate, and arterial cannulation with subsequent serial measurements of arterial oxygenation and carbon dioxide will be required. The priority is to obtain a Pa_{O_2} of > 60 mm of mercury with normocapnea as soon as possible. If high-inspired oxygen concentration continues to be necessary after resuscitation of the cardiovascular system, then the use of positive end expiratory pressure (PEEP) should be considered. This may be increased in 2.5 cm of water increments but only after restoration of adequate circulating blood volume and in the presence of invasive cardiovascular monitoring. Further intensive care management includes the passage of a nasogastric tube after the airway is secure. Large volumes of water may subsequently be removed and it is neither necessary nor desirable to commence nasogastric feeding early in treatment. An H_2 antagonist or barrier should be used according to the unit's normal policy.

Restoration of an adequate circulating blood volume will almost certainly be necessary in all unconscious patients. An initial intravenous rapid infusion of 10 ml/kg of warmed colloid solution should be undertaken as a priority. Any conventional plasma volume expander can be employed and in the past albumin solutions and warm blood have been used with good effect. Further fluid therapy should be titrated against central venous pressure in children or against pulmonary capillary wedge pressure (PCWP) in adults [14]. It may be that in the future transoesophageal echocardiography may prove useful in monitoring cardiac output.

The danger of fluid overload is greatest in the middle-aged, elderly, and those with pre-existing cardiovascular disease. Any rapid rise in wedge pressure in these patients is an indication to restrict fluid therapy to basic requirements and consider the use of inotropes [15]. Inotrope therapy regimens usually combined dobutamine 5–15 µg/kg/min and dopamine 2–5 µg/kg/min. However, this should only be instituted in the presence of invasive cardiovascular monitoring enabling regular measurement of cardiac output, oxygen delivery, oxygen consumption, and systemic vascular resistance.

Hypothermia and metabolic acidosis

The treatment of hypothermia and metabolic acidosis remains somewhat controversial. The expected range of central temperature after admission would be 30–33°C. As long as there is cardiovascular stability and resuscitation is progressing satisfactorily then the hypothermia will be self-correcting with the patient's general improvement. Active rewarming (Figure 20.3) is not necessary in these circumstances. Hypothermia is

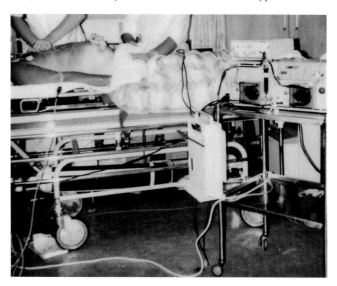

Figure 20.3 Active rewarming in an ICU.

usually accompanied by quite profound metabolic acidosis and pH levels < 7.0 are frequently recorded. Although there is controversy surrounding the use of sodium bicarbonate, there is little doubt that such marked acidosis has a negative inotropic effect on myocardial function [13]. It is still advocated that the pH be raised to 7.2 by the use of $NaHCO_3$, 1 mEqv/kg, followed by repeat blood gas estimations [16]. Further correction above pH 7.2 is unnecessary and would only lead to an overswing into metabolic alkalosis as the patient recovered. Temperatures below 30°C are often accompanied by cardiac instability, and simple measures available in all major hospitals to correct hypothermia include warming the room temperature, warm woollen blankets, and heating humidifiers and intravenous fluids to 37°C.

Monitoring

Passage of a urinary catheter is extremely useful in all except small children to help monitor not only hourly urinary output but as a further guide to cardiovascular stability. Serial arterial blood gas sampling will be necessary and an arterial line is an essential piece of invasive monitoring. Continuous respiratory observation can be made by means of a CO_2 monitor and, when the peripheral circulation is restored to normal, by the use of pulse oximetry. A portable chest x-ray should be taken as soon as convenient. This will show not only the degree of infiltration of the lung fields but also the position of any central lines. It should be anticipated that the initial x-ray will show extensive pulmonary infiltration from aspirated water. Given the restoration of blood pressure and normal oxygenation, subsequent x-rays should show rapid improvement.

Biochemical investigation of blood sugar, urea, electrolytes, as well as a full blood count and film should be undertaken. Both haemolysis and electrolyte disturbances are rare and transient. If any serious and sustained biochemical abnormality occurs, the simplest way of correction is either by peritoneal dialysis with isotonic solutions or by haemofiltration. Although haemofiltration may lead to a more rapid normalisation of blood electrolyte concentrations, its use in near drowning is extremely limited and it has the potential drawback of being a source of further heat loss. On the other hand, warmed peritoneal dialysis solutions can aid in rewarming if necessary.

Further care

It may be necessary to employ sedative respiratory depressant drugs to enable ventilation to continue after initial resuscitation but it is important to continue ventilation until blood gas analysis, chest x-ray, and cardiovascular normality have been restored and maintained with an inspired oxygen concentration of < 40%. Sedative drugs can then be discontinued and on commencement of spontaneous ventilation weaning can commence. In young people, free from previous cardio-respiratory disease, this is usually a rapid process and extubation can take place when consciousness and the cough reflex have returned. Difficulty or prolonged weaning may occur in those in whom return of consciousness is delayed, those with pre-existing cardiorespiratory disease, or in those who develop chest infections. It is in these circumstances that the use of pressure support or CPAP modes of ventilation can be extremely useful. After extubation, oxygen by mask or CPAP delivering around 40% inspired oxygen concentration may be necessary at least initially. Discharge to a ward can take place when the patient is conscious, able to cough, and has satisfactory oxygenation on room air or with minimal supportive oxygen therapy.

Treatment of cardiac arrest

The cerebral protection afforded by hypothermia has already been discussed earlier in this chapter. There are many records of successful resuscitation after prolonged periods of submersion and cardiopulmonary resuscitation. Most, but not all, of these cases have involved children whose relatively large surface area to weight ratio leads to more rapid cooling than in adults. Furthermore, survivors have usually been submersed in water of < 10°C. Severe hypothermia can cause a clinical picture akin to cardiac arrest but an ECG may show the presence of slow sinus rhythm and such cases are eminently survivable given careful management. An apparently lifeless body taken from the water should not be declared dead without careful assessment of the circumstances. The box shows the criteria for the assessment of the apparently dead after an acute immersion incident.

Assessment of the apparently dead after an acute immersion incident

- What is the estimated period of submersion?
- What is the known or estimated water temperature?
- What is the patient's central temperature recording?
- What does an ECG show?

The decision to resuscitate or not may have to be taken on estimates of the first two of these questions and thermometers and portable ECGs are only rarely available at the rescue site. The longest recorded survivor is a child of $2\frac{1}{2}$ years of age submersed for 66 minutes at 5°C [16]. Certainly any submersion incident of this order of time or shorter should be considered a case for resuscitation if the incident has occurred

in cold water. Resuscitation once commenced should continue until further assessment can be made in an intensive care unit.

All authorities now agree that standard resuscitation procedures are applicable in drowning. The ABC of recognised resuscitation protocols should be followed. On arrival in hospital central temperature and ECG monitoring is essential from the outset. The question of defibrillation in the presence of hypothermia is controversial but successful defibrillation has been reported in children at temperatures below 30°C [17]. It is certainly worthwhile attempting a single cardioversion for ventricular fibrillation even in the presence of hypothermia. Repeated attempts, should be avoided, however, as they can lead to direct damage to the skin and chest wall as well as the myocardium. If the heart can be restarted and an effective cardiac output restored then management should follow the lines previously outlined. The major difficulty occurs if cardiopulmonary resuscitation is in progress and the heart cannot be restarted. **It is now well accepted that resuscitation should not be abandoned until the central temperature has been raised to 32°C.**

The majority of these patients will be profoundly hypothermic and temperatures of less than 28°C are not uncommon. Active rewarming is therefore essential from the outset and in practice this can be extremely difficult without the availability of extracorporeal rewarming. Surface rewarming with heated water blankets and the use of intragastric or intravesical warmed fluids seem to be of little help. A double lumen oesophageal rewarming tube connected to a heated water circulator has been helpful in severe hypothermia where there is still an intact circulation [18] but its usefulness post cardiac arrest is unknown. The use of a heated haemodiafiltration circuit has also been extremely disappointing. If facilities for right heart bypass are not available then the inspired gases of the ventilator should be warmed to 42°C, all i.v. fluids should be warmed to 37°C, and consideration should be given to commencing peritoneal dialysis with isotonic fluid warmed to 37°C. Extracorporeal rewarming is far more certain and, where facilities are available, this can be achieved by sternotomy, and arterial and venous cannulation, or even via femoral arterial/venous lines [19]. As well as a membrane oxygenator, the circuit must include a heat exchanger with the temperature of the perfusate set at 10°C above the known body temperature. Even with these efforts, rewarming will be erratic but it is important to continue resuscitation until a central temperature of 32°C has been reached when a decision on whether to discontinue further resuscitative efforts can be made. Certainly there have been reports of successful cerebral recovery after periods of CPR of up to three hours [4]. Where resuscitation results in the restoration of cardiac output, consideration must be given to cerebral protection. Intracranial pressure monitoring has been used in several centres but has not so far been shown to alter outcome. The use of mannitol is still reasonable practice for sudden increases in intracranial pressure but the use of profound hyperventilation, induced hypothermia, barbiturate coma, and diuretics has largely been abandoned [13].

Complications

With prompt immediate care and transfer to hospital, followed by the realisation of the importance of cardiorespiratory normalisation, complications of near-drowning incidents should be rare. The most worrying complication, that of cerebral damage, is fortunately relatively uncommon and will be discussed later. Other complications are listed in the box.

Complications of near drowning
● Respiratory distress syndrome
● Diffuse intravascular coagulation
● Haemolysis
● Renal failure
● Chronic pulmonary infection
● Epilepsy
● Cerebral damage

Summary

The future lies in the prevention of accidents through fencing of danger areas and supervision of those taking part in water sports by personnel trained in rescue and cardiopulmonary resuscitation. However, once an immersion accident occurs it is the reduction in hypoxia which will govern the survival of the patient and the level of cerebral damage. The role of intensive care staff is to appreciate the importance of restoring the cardiorespiratory system to a state which provides and maintains adequate cerebral oxygenation. There is no place for delay in management as the results of studies worldwide have shown.

Results and prognosis

The importance of immediate care at the accident site and on arrival in hospital cannot be overemphasised. Where basic life support is given at the waterside, 70% of children will survive, whereas if this is delayed until arrival at hospital the overall survival figure is 40%. Studies agree that in those who do not suffer cardiac arrest the prognosis not only for survival but cerebrally normal survival is excellent. In the UK, the Cornwall Drowning Study reported 198 normal survivors out of 201 patients who were treated prior to cardiac arrest [9]. A UK paediatric survey reported 100% normal survival in 125 children who received resuscitation at the accident site and were conscious by the time they reached hospital [3]. The same study reported 61 survivors out of 64 who reached hospital with an impaired level of consciousness. A Canadian paediatric study gave similar figures and reported that even those who remained comatose had a 47.7% chance of normal recovery [20]. Some remarkable survivals have occurred after cardiac arrest; the Cornwall Drowning Study reported 31 patients treated after cardiac arrest in whom there were five survivors but two of these had a degree of cerebral damage [9]. Overall the incidence of cerebrally damaged survivors is in the order of 5%. Poor prognostic indicators are listed in the box.

Poor prognostic indicators after near drowning
● Prolonged submersion
● Delayed CPR
● Asystole on ECG
● Glasgow coma score of < 5
● Fixed dilated pupils
● Resuscitation required for > 25 minutes
● First spontaneous breath delayed > 40 minutes
● Arterial pH < 7.0
● Fitting after resuscitation

References

1. Office of Population Censuses and Surveys. *Registrations of deaths by cause*. London: OPCS, 1988–90.
2. Baker SP (ed.). *Drowning*. Injury Fact Book, Lexington, MASS: DC Heath & Co., 1984.
3. Kemp AM, Sibert JR. Outcome in children who nearly drown: a British Isles Study. 1991 *BMJ*, **302**:931–3.
4. Golden FStC, Hervey GR, Tipton M *et al*. Circum rescue collapse. *J Royal Navy Med Service* 1991;**77**:139.
5. Orlowski JP. Drowning, near drowning and ice-water submersion. *Paediat Clin N Amer* 1987;**30**:75–92.
6. Stern WE, Good RG. Studies on the effect of hypothermia on CSF oxygen tension and carotid blood flow. *Surgery* 1960;**48**:13–30.
7. Wong KC. Physiology and pharmacology of hypothermia. *West J Med* 1983;**138**:227–32.
8. Golden FStC. The management of rescued shipwreck survivors. *J Royal Naval Med Service* 1980;**66**:107–13.
9. Simcock AD. The treatment of immersion victims. *Care Crit Ill* 1991;**7**:177–81.
10. Simcock AD. The treatment of immersion victims – a review of 130 cases. *Anaesthesia* 1986;**41**:643–8.
11. Pearn JH. Secondary drowning involving children. *BMJ* 1980; **281**:1103–5.
12. Simcock AD. The resuscitation of immersion victims. *Appl Cardio-pulm Pathophysiol* 1989;**2**:293–8.
13. Modell JH. Drowning. *New Engl J Med* 1993;**328**:253–6.
14. Edwards ND, Timmins AC. Randalls B, Morgan GAR, Simcock AD. Survival in adults after cardiac arrest due to drowning. *Intens Care Med* 1990;**16**:336–7.
15. Hildebrand CA, Hartman AG, Arcinue EL, Gomez RJ, Bing RJ. Cardiac performance in paediatric near drowning. *Crit Care Med* 1988;**16**:331–5.
16. Botte RG, Black PG, Bowers RS, Kent-Thorne J, Conelli HM. The use of extracorporeal rewarming in a child submerged for 66 minutes. *J Am Med Ass* 1988;**260**:377–9.
17. Simcock AD, Morgan GAR. The treatment of immersion victims. *Curr Anaesth Intens Care* 1990;**1**:181–5;**3**:327–32.
18. Kristensen G, Gravesen M, Benveniste D, Jordening H. An oeso-phageal thermal tube for rewarming in hypothermia. *Acta Anaesth Scand* 1985;**29**:846–8.
19. Gentillelo LM, Cobean RA, Jurcovitch GJ, Soderberg RW, Offner PJ. CAVR – a new technique for treating hypothermia. *J Trauma* 1991;**31**:151–4.
20. Conn AW, Barker GA. Freshwater drowning and near drowning an update. *Can Anaesth Soc J* 1984;**31**:538–44.

21 Radiation

Robin Wood
UKAEA, Harwell, Didcot, Oxon

Julie Nancarrow
Royal Preston Hospital, Fulwood, Preston

OBJECTIVES

- To give an understanding of the difference between external radiation exposure and contamination with radioactive materials.

- To put the radiation hazard into perspective.

- To give principles of contamination control and decontamination of patients.

- To outline the special arrangements for receipt and management of contaminated patients.

- To consider their monitoring, dose assessment, and continuing care.

- To summarise the long-term effects of radiation exposure.

Accidents involving radiation may give rise to patients with:

- conventional injuries;
- external or internal contamination with radioactive materials;
- external radiation exposure to the whole body or part of the body;
- any combination of these.

Suitable radiation monitoring equipment and the assistance of an experienced health physicist will be required in handling radiation casualties.

- Treatment of serious, conventional injuries *always* takes priority because even life-threatening radiation exposures are unlikely to produce symptoms within an hour or two of the exposure taking place and do not have the same urgency as Airway, Breathing and Circulatory emergencies.
- External contamination is best managed as part of the immediate care. In some rare accidents, such as Chernobyl, the radioactivity of external contamination can be so high that doses to skin and body are potentially life-threatening. Only in these rare circumstances must external decontamination be performed with urgency. Usually the radioactivity of external contamination will be low and present no risk of radiation burns to the skin or acute radiation effects to either the casualty or attendants. It

should never delay assessment or management of life-threatening problems, including CPR and essential i.v. access. It is best controlled early, if the patient's condition allows, in order to avoid cross-contamination of staff, equipment, or buildings.

- Assessment of whole body radiation exposure should be made as soon as possible after an incident and preferably within a few hours. In those cases where patients have received high whole body doses, this assessment will influence decisions on patient management which may need to be made within a few hours or days, but can extend to several weeks.
- Assessment of part body exposures and internal contamination should also be made within a few hours, if possible.

This chapter will address the management of a radiation incident at the scene, in the emergency department, and as part of the patient's long-term care.

Prehospital care

A summary of prehospital care is given in the box.

Summary of prehospital care

- Ensure scene safety
- Triage if multiple casualties (on basis of conventional injuries) (see Chapter 23)
- Resuscitate and treat immediately life-threatening injuries
- Alert hospital early
- Monitor external contamination
- Remove contaminated clothing
- Arrange appropriate transport to hospital
- Decontaminate staff and equipment

Scene assessment

Emergency staff attending incidents involving radioactivity must ensure their own safety. In addition to other conventional risks, they should attempt to establish from emergency services control:

- whether they are entering an external radiation field and, if so, whether or not dose rates are high enough to impose a time limit on entry;
- whether or not there is surface or airborne contamination with radioactive materials and, if so, what protective clothing and respiratory protective equipment is necessary for safe entry;
- whether or not release of radioactive iodine is involved; if so prophylactic stable potassium iodate should be taken.

These features can usually be determined readily by Emergency Services personnel using simple monitoring. It should not therefore delay the provision of medical care to casualties. Where incidents have occurred in a nuclear factory or a workplace where radioactive materials are used, management should be able to advise on conditions and provide guides for rescuers.

External radiation field

Where scene assessment suggests that there has been no release of radioactive materials to environment and the hazard is external radiation from a sealed source, management is extremely straightforward.

Casualties will have received external radiation exposure but will not themselves be radioactive. They do not pose any hazard to their attendants and require no special arrangements for their transportation or receipt at hospital.

Staff should wear radiation dosimeters, if possible, but not be deterred if these are unavailable. They should be aware that they can reduce radiation doses to themselves and to patients by:

- reducing *time* spent in a radiation field;
- keeping the maximum *distance* between themselves and a radiation source;
- arranging for shielding (any dense material) to be placed between themselves and a radiation source; however, this is often impossible at the accident scene.

In practice, radiation fields are unlikely to be high enough to carry a risk of acute health effects, and the clinical condition of the casualties will determine the priority and speed with which they are removed from the scene. It will rarely, if ever, be justified to risk further injury to casualties by removing them from the scene without proper assessment and stabilisation, as may be justified for some hostile environments (see Chapter 23). Nevertheless, attendants should not loiter or leave patients unnecessarily in a radiation field. If they do not have dosimeters they should take some notice of the time they spend in proximity to the source; this will allow an assessment of their dose to be made later.

External contamination

Where scene assessment suggests that there has been a release of radioactive materials to environment it is possible that wounds, exposed skin, and outer clothing of casualties may be contaminated. Internal contamination through wounds, inhalation, or more rarely ingestion, may also have occurred. The surfaces of any objects, including roads, vehicles, and debris could also be contaminated.

Contamination control

A summary of contamination control is given in the box.

> **Summary of contamination control**
>
> - Prevent personal contamination of attendants
> - Prevent cross-contamination between casualties
> - Avoid spreading contamination from the scene

Control of personal contamination is by use of protective clothing. This need not be elaborate. Waterproof jacket and trousers would certainly suffice, but even a light coverall will be effective in keeping contamination away from the clothing and skin. A pair of surgeon's gloves should be worn at least, and preferably a second pair, which can be changed frequently, thereby controlling cross-contamination. It is most unlikely that airborne contamination, if present, will be at levels requiring respiratory protection. Nevertheless a surgeon's mask should be worn to prevent inadvertent transfer of contamination from hands to nose and mouth.

It is important to ask if radioactive iodine has been released in the accident in every case; this occurs mostly after accidents and incidents involving irradiated nuclear fuel. Stable iodine preparations taken prophylactically in such circumstances will saturate the thyroid and minimise uptake of the radioactive isotope which would otherwise irradiate the gland (see later).

Suitable radiation monitoring equipment must be available to the emergency team and they must know how to use it. Emergency teams should wear dosimeters if available. If sufficient numbers of attendants are available, it is best to divide them into "clean" teams, who remain on the uncontaminated side of the forward control, and wait for "dirty" teams, who enter the contaminated area, to bring the casualties to them.

Spread of contaminated material from the incident scene should be prevented by leaving contaminated outer clothing and equipment at the scene, which can be recovered later when resources are available for monitoring and decontamination of equipment.

For all seriously injured casualties, airway, breathing and circulatory emergencies take priority, and the presence of contamination should not delay their assessment and management, including CPR and i.v. access; i.v. access should not be set up routinely, but if necessary, it should not be achieved through heavily contaminated skin if a suitable uncontaminated site is available. An adhesive dressing, such as Opsite is useful in controlling contamination if i.v. access must be achieved through or close to a contaminated area.

Decontamination of casualties

Uninjured or "walking wounded" casualties should be mustered at the forward control for monitoring. Contaminated outer clothing can be removed here and left on the contaminated side of the line – this is usually all that is necessary or feasible at the scene.

Casualties should be monitored for external contamination as an early part of the secondary survey. At this point it is only necessary to establish whether or not contamination is present. Identification of the type of contamination and measurement of the amount is not essential at this stage.

For transportation, the "dirty" teams must transfer the casualty to the forward control. Here they are met by the "clean" team who have the ambulance stretcher spread with a sheet of polythene. The casualty is placed on this and the edges of the polythene are wrapped around the casualty to minimise contamination of the ambulance or its equipment (Figure 21.1).

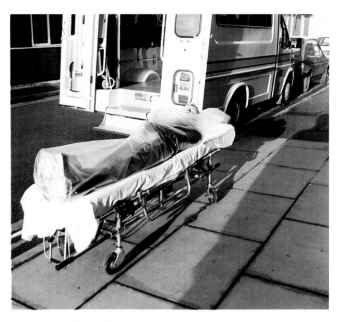

Figure 21.1 Externally contaminated patient prepared for transportation.

If human resources are scarce, and members of the "dirty" team must accompany the casualty, they should leave contaminated gloves and coveralls at the scene and put on clean gloves. Members of the "dirty" team must themselves be monitored by a health physics monitor at the scene or on returning to hospital, or preferably both.

Members of the clean team, the ambulance, and its equipment must also be monitored and decontaminated if necessary after delivering the casualty but before returning to service.

Uninjured attendants have lower priority for monitoring than casualties and may have to wait until monitoring resources are available. They must not eat, drink, or smoke until they have been monitored clear of contamination.

As soon as it is confirmed that contaminated casualties are involved, the receiving A & E department staff must be informed. They will need as much notice as possible (at least 20 minutes) to prepare their department to receive them, as described in the following paragraphs. Information about the nature of the contamination may be available from labels, signs, hazard warnings, inventories, or responsible persons, and this must be passed together with the usual information about numbers and types of casualties.

Emergency room receipt of radiation casualties

A summary of emergency department care is given in the box.

Summary of emergency department care

- Prepare department before arrival of patient
- Triage if multiple casualties (on basis of conventional injury)
- Resuscitate and treat immediately life-threatening injuries
- Monitor external contamination
- Externally decontaminate patient
- Decontaminate and treat wounds
- Decontaminate staff and equipment

External radiation exposure

Casualties who have received exposures from a sealed source of radiation, and are not contaminated with radioactive materials, do not require any special arrangements for their receipt at hospital. They can be admitted through the usual entrance. They are not radioactive and they constitute no hazard to their attendants.

In addition to standard assessment and treatment, the hospital Health Physicist must be notified. He will coordinate attempts to determine the whole body dose received by the casualty; this information may be important to subsequent surgical and medical management.

The contaminated casualty

Management of a contaminated casualty involves the usual assessment, stabilisation, and treatment of serious injuries, but is complicated by the need to practise contamination control. This control involves:

- Decontamination of the casualty. The objectives of decontamination are:
  - to reduce skin and whole body doses by removing the radioactive contamination from the skin, hair, nose, mouth, and wounds;
  - to minimise internal contamination by using techniques which prevent the contaminant from entering the casualty's body.
- Staff should achieve decontamination without, in the process, contaminating their department, equipment, or themselves, apart from contact contamination with their protective clothing, which is inevitable.
- Staff need to ensure that contamination is not spreading beyond their department to the rest of the hospital and that all contaminated materials are safely bagged for analysis, if necessary, and eventual safe disposal.

No team can hope to achieve these goals unless it has prepared and practised beforehand and has the services of an experienced Health Physicist with suitable radiation monitoring equipment.

Planning

Contaminated casualties cannot be admitted through the usual entrance. If they are, and they contaminate it, other users may inadvertently spread contamination to the whole of the department and beyond.

A special entrance must be designated which gives access to an area where casualties can be received, assessed, and monitored.

In use, this area will be cordoned off and patients, staff, samples, and equipment will not be allowed to leave it until they have been monitored clear of contamination.

When it is confirmed that contaminated casualties are on route to the department, the following steps must be taken:

Notification of the duty health physics team

They will prepare and calibrate radiation monitoring equipment, prepare dosimeters for use by A & E staff, and put on caps, masks, gowns, boots, and surgeons' gloves. They should be given any available information about the type of contamination.

Preparation of the department

This involves removing non-essential equipment and furniture from the receiving area and covering non-essential equipment which cannot be removed with polythene sheets. If the floor is impervious it should *not* be covered with polythene because such coverings may cause staff to trip or slip. Carpeted floors will have to be covered as they are usually impossible to decontaminate. If emergency floor coverings are used they must be securely taped down. A suitable trolley or table, on which the casualty will be placed, can then be brought in and covered with polythene or other waterproof covering. Waste bins lined with polythene bags should also be available in the receiving area.

Air conditioning must be switched off to avoid the possibility of spreading airborne contamination by this means. The receiving area will be cordoned off and once inside nothing will be allowed to leave it until monitored clear of contamination by the Health Physicist.

Preparation of staff

A "dirty" team who will enter the controlled area should dress in caps, masks, gowns, and boots. In addition the team needs polythene aprons and two pairs of gloves. The inner pair must be taped to the cuff of the gown and the outer pair can be changed as often as necessary if they become contaminated.

A "clean" team, who will service the "dirty" team needs to wear standard theatre clothing – caps, masks, gloves, and overshoes.

Receipt of casualties

If there are several contaminated casualties, an assessment of their condition should be made in the ambulance. Triage should be on the basis of severity of injury and not on level of contamination. Any information about the nature of the contamination must be passed to the Health Physicist.

Assessment of contamination

The casualty's clothing is removed and bagged in the receiving area. Assessment of clinical condition has priority, but in

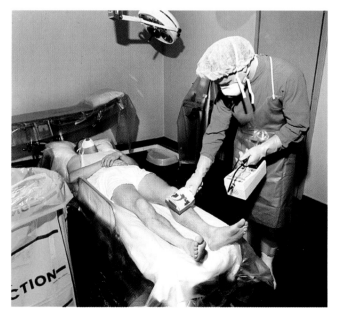

Figure 21.2 Monitoring for external contamination.

addition the Health Physicist must monitor the surface of the body (Figure 21.2), including skin folds, back and front of the patient, wounds, hair, and face.

People with trivial or no injuries at all, for example bystanders, firemen, or medical staff, may be sent to hospital for decontamination. There is a temptation to simply put them under a shower and wash until clean, but this is not adequate management. Swabs should be taken from the lips, teeth, and tongue, and swabs should be taken from inside the nostrils or a nose blow sample provided. Areas of contamination and the amount of activity can then be recorded on an anatomical diagram (Figure 21.3).

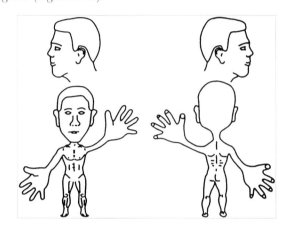

Figure 21.3 Anatomical diagram to help with contamination assessment.

Decontamination of the skin

Intact skin is an effective barrier which will keep most radioactive materials out of the body. It is essential therefore not to apply vigorous techniques that make the skin sore or breach its surface. Washing with soap and water, or a mild detergent such as cetrimide, is usually all that is required to decontaminate intact skin, although repeated washing is often necessary.

It is usually recommended to wash from the periphery to the centre of a contaminated area. Other techniques sometimes recommended include gentle scrubbing with mild abrasives such as sugar or corn starch. Water spreads contamination and is difficult to contain so its use should be as sparing as possible. Swabbing and sponging is preferred to sluicing.

An effective technique used in the nuclear industry for fixed contamination on the skin of the hands and forearms is to paint the skin with a saturated solution of potassium permanganate and, after leaving this to dry for a few minutes, removing the coloration with a 2.5% solution of sodium metabisulphite (Figure 21.4). This technique achieves slight desquamation and is very effective. It has the additional advantage that the colour changes of the skin involved in the operation allow visual confirmation that no part of the contaminated area has been missed. Showering is allowed from the neck downwards, but to avoid incorporation of contamination, the head should be dealt with by other means. Head hair must be back washed (Figure 21.5). Head and facial hair can be clipped, if necessary. Shaving is not recommended because of the danger of cutting the skin. Swabs and trimmed hair must be kept for monitoring.

Unless the Health Physicist indicates the rare danger of radiation burns, it is better to put a dressing over persistently fixed contamination, and to try to decontaminate the next

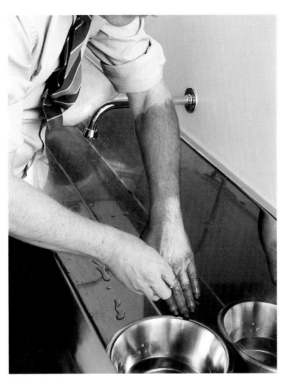

Figure 21.4 Decontamination of forearm with potassium permanganate and sodium metabisulphate solutions.

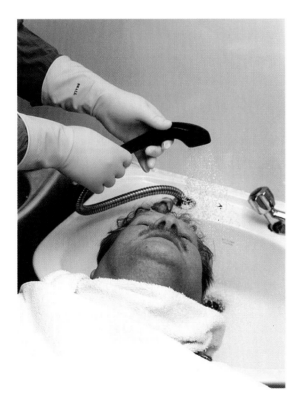

Figure 21.5 Back washing contaminated hair to avoid incorporation of contamination.

day, rather than to risk damaging the skin. If the contaminant is in a corrosive chemical form, the management becomes that appropriate for a chemical burn (see Chapter 19). After each decontamination attempt, the area should be remonitored, and the new (reduced) activity level noted.

Wounds

Serious wounds must be dealt with as their severity requires, but if they are contaminated, foreign material should be removed from the wound and excised tissue, swabs, and washings must be bagged for monitoring as must surgical instruments. Less severe wounds are best covered with a waterproof dressing until intact skin has been decontaminated.

This sequence assures the operator that any contamination remaining is indeed *in* the wound and not simply close to it. Position and level of contamination should be recorded on an anatomical diagram.

Contamination in a wound, if not removed, may be incorporated locally at the wound site or be mobilised from the wound to other tissues. The physical and chemical characteristics of the contaminant will determine its behaviour.

Wound decontamination is a form of surgical toilet. Visible foreign material can be removed by forceps, swabbing, or irrigation, but materials removed from the wound, including debrided tissue, must be bagged for monitoring. The wound should be remonitored periodically during decontamination and the level of activity recorded (Figure 21.6).

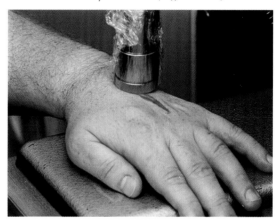

Figure 21.6 Wound monitoring with a "Harwell" wound probe.

Irrigation with water or saline should be continued for as long as monitoring indicates that the level of contamination is being progressively reduced. If, after repeated irrigation, activity remains in the wound, excision of contaminated tissue may be considered, but the likely benefit of any such wound excision must be judged to outweigh any risks, such as damage to important structures.

Following the assessment, stabilisation, decontamination, and basic wound management described above, consideration can be given to continuing care.

Continuing care

A summary of continuing care is given in the box.

Continuing care
● Dosimetry assessment
● Baseline full blood count
● Monitor symptoms and ensure they are not due to trauma
● Complete initial and reparative surgery within 48 hours
● Continue wound decontamination
● Monitor and treat internal contamination
● Counsel patients

The initial emergency room response should be directed towards identifying and treating life-threatening conditions, effect of trauma, and thermal and chemical burns in a conventional way with conventional priority. Contamination control needs to be carried out in handling affected individuals and decontamination performed as far as possible. Patients who have not been fully decontaminated in the emergency department may need urgent surgery. In these cases the operating theatre must be prepared in the same way as the emergency department, ideally a theatre within the emergency department if available. Non-essential equipment should be removed; the floor may be covered as previously described. Air conditioning must be switched off to avoid spreading airborne contamination by this means. All medical staff should wear surgeons' gowns, caps, masks, and double gloves. All waste materials and fluids must be collected, bagged, labelled "radioactive", and be disposed of appropriately. The theatre must be cordoned off and only essential staff given access. All staff must be monitored clear before leaving the area, and equipment and the theatre must be decontaminated before it is used again. Similar precautions must be taken in any area where a patient who is not fully decontaminated is cared for. If possible, all contaminated patients must be treated in the same area until full decontamination has been achieved.

When the casualty's condition has been stabilised, attention can be given to possible radiation injury.

A dosimetry assessment must be performed in order to estimate whole body, local, and internal doses using:

- results from any dosimeters worn;
- information and monitoring results from the incident scene;
- the history of the incident from the casualty, responsible informants and rescuers;
- results of monitoring the casualty in the emergency room;
- full blood count results;
- the development of symptoms in the casualty;
- result of biological monitoring and whole body monitoring, if appropriate;
- other investigations in special cases.

Health physics advice is essential.

Whole body dose

The acute effects of high dose body radiation result from damage to radiosensitive tissues such as the bone marrow, gastrointestinal tract, blood vessels, and nerves. The acute radiation syndromes, which result from damage to these tissues, have some important characteristics.

- There is a *threshold* of dose below which they will not occur. It is important to realise that the vast majority of incidents involving whole body radiation exposure will not exceed the threshold for these deterministic effects or even begin to approach them. The whole body dose assessments will therefore usually be profoundly reassuring to both patient and doctor. Assessments are subject to a margin of error and this will be greatest initially. Caution and uncertainty are also likely to produce assessments which overestimate dose.
- If the threshold is exceeded the effects will occur *soon* after exposure but not at once. First symptoms may develop in hours with other effects in days or weeks. Radiation injury therefore never requires the same urgent treatment that serious conventional trauma may.
- If the threshold is exceeded the severity of injury will be proportional to the dose received as will the type and

severity of the symptoms and the speed with which they develop.

Circumstances which may give rise to higher whole body doses include reactor accidents, incidents involving irradiated nuclear fuel or waste arising from reprocessing, and accidents involving highly active sealed sources such as are used in radiotherapy and industrial radiography. Criticality excursions (arising from chain reactions in critical masses of fissile material) may also give rise to very high whole body doses.

A & E consultants must be aware of any facilities with these potential hazards in their catchment areas.

With whole body absorbed doses exceeding 2 Gy symptoms are likely and with doses exceeding 4 Gy serious effects are certain and may become life-threatening within weeks. It is prudent, therefore, to call in the advice of consultants in clinical haematology and radiotherapy if initial assessments of whole body dose exceed 2 Gy or for any patient in whom symptoms occur. These experts will be able to advise on both the treatment of acute symptoms and long-term management of the radiation injury.

Timing of surgery in combined trauma and radiation injuries

Limited human data and more extensive animal data indicate that combined problems of delayed wound healing and increased susceptibility of infection will complicate surgical intervention in radiation casualties [1] whose whole body dose is high enough to cause bone marrow damage. In such cases it is desirable to complete initial and reparative surgery within 48 hours of the radiation exposure and then to avoid further surgical intervention for the next two months, by which time recovery from survivable radiation damage should have occurred.

Three steps in particular can be taken by A & E department staff which are invaluable in achieving the earliest possible assessment of whole body dose. These are:

- Taking a careful history of the accident, making an early symptomatic enquiry, and establishing baseline vital signs, including temperature.
- Taking a blood sample *as soon as possible* for full blood count. Early, short-lived neutrophilia followed by neutropenia, immediate progressive fall in lymphocyte count, and a quickly following fall in platelet count should enable confirmation of a dose exceeding 2 Gray within two or three days, but the earlier the baseline sample is obtained the better.
- Careful recording of symptoms possibly attributable to acute radiation syndromes and especially the time after exposure at which they occur.
  - Transient erythema, occurring within two to three hours and then disappearing, headache, nausea and vomiting, diarrhoea, and elevated temperature are the most important symptoms to observe in this respect and will help the specialist to assess dose.
  - Where there is significant trauma co-existing with radiation exposure it would be a serious mistake to miss alternative treatable causes of these symptoms, especially head injury.

Where bone marrow damage is confirmed, specialist advice will be needed for longer term management, including possible use of antibiotics, whole blood or blood products, combination cytokine therapy, and marrow transplantation.

External contamination

The extent and level of activity of any areas of skin contamination will have been recorded on an anatomical diagram during initial management in the emergency room. The results of decontamination attempts will also have been recorded.

It is quite possible that decontamination will have been completely successful with no activity above background remaining detectable. It is equally possible that decontamination will be incomplete and that further attempts must be made on areas where contamination was fixed and had been covered with a dressing.

After 24 hours dressings can be removed and both skin and dressing monitored. If the skin condition allows, further attempts at decontamination can be made using the same techniques as used in the emergency room. Contamination on healthy, intact skin will come off eventually, so it is more important to keep the skin healthy and decontaminate in stages over several days if necessary, rather than to risk damaging the skin by being too vigorous.

Areas of minor skin damage, such as grazing, can be dealt with in a similar way and, if such wounds are dressed from day to day, activity is likely to transfer from wound to dressing as the wounds heal. Sometimes this transfer occurs quite suddenly, for example when scabs fall off.

Localised exposures

In radiation accidents, even if whole body exposure has occurred, it is most unlikely to have been completely uniform. In other accidents, for example those involving malfunctioning industrial x-ray equipment, very high doses can occur to parts of the body even though no whole body dose has been received.

Where local exposures have occurred either from penetrating radiation or from skin contact with unsealed radioactive materials or sealed sources, it is important to have health physicists calculate skin doses. These will indicate whether or not hair loss or radiation burns are likely to develop. Burns develop usually within a week of exposure as painful redness which, depending on the dose received, may progress to blistering and ulceration. The severity of the skin lesions that do occur can itself be used to assess skin doses, while if none occurs the exposure must obviously have been below the thresholds for such effects.

Rarely, skin burns may be the presenting sign of a previously concealed or unknown accidental radiation exposure. Unexplained, persistent, painful redness of the fingers or hands of an industrial radiographer should be regarded as a radiation burn until proved otherwise.

In management, analgesia may be necessary and the opinion of a dermatologist should be obtained. If ulceration occurs healing may be delayed and infection may be a problem.

Health physicists will attempt to estimate other tissue or organ-specific doses if necessary.

Internal contamination

When radioactive materials are released to the environment in an accident, it is possible that internal contamination of casualties can occur. Inhalation of airborne contamination

(Figure 21.7) or absorption through contaminated wounds are the most common routes of entry. Ingestion is also possible.

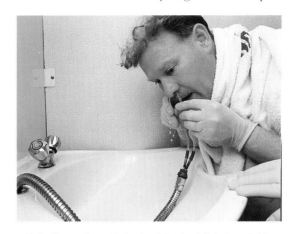

Figure 21.7 Forward nasal irrigation following inhalation of airborne activity.

External contamination of the face should be removed in such a way that incorporation is minimised. However, it should be assumed that internal contamination may have occurred if wounds have been contaminated, positive swabs have been taken from the lips, teeth, mouth, or nose, or if a positive nose blow sample has been provided.

Identification of the isotopic, chemical, and physical nature of the contaminant is essential as it will determine what further monitoring should be done and what treatment options are available.

Monitoring and dose assessment

When internal contaminants give out energetic gamma rays they can be detected easily by equipment outside of the body and depending on the contaminant, monitoring over the thyroid, chest, or whole body may be appropriate (Figure 21.8). Note, however, that all external contamination must be

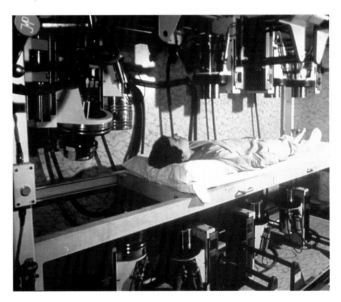

Figure 21.8 Whole body monitoring for internal contamination.

removed before such monitoring can be performed. The monitoring equipment cannot distinguish between the signals from internal and external contamination, consequently intake will be overestimated unless external decontamination has been completed.

It might be difficult or impossible to detect intakes of materials that give only weak gamma or x-ray signals by external monitoring techniques. For these materials biological monitoring must be used.

Urine and faecal samples should be kept for radiochemical assay unless the Health Physicist advises that it is unnecessary to do so. Because some inhaled material is cleared from the airway by cilliary action and then swallowed, faecal samples can be of value even when inhalation is the portal of entry.

Incorporated nuclides will continue to irradiate tissues for as long as they remain in the body and in this respect differ from external exposure which ceases as soon as the source is removed.

The actual dose to tissues, organs, and the body as a whole will depend on the nature of the contaminating materials, route of entry, mobilisation from this site, distribution through the body, and effective half-life. In any case, for as long as the radioactive material remains in the body the patient will be committed to receiving a dose from it. This committed dose should be estimated and decisions about treatment made from an understanding of the likely health effects of the committed dose.

Treatment

The most important treatment option is the administration of stable iodine to patients who have received intakes of radio-active iodine. The stable material competes with the radio-active isotope for take-up by the thyroid gland thereby reducing the dose to the organ. In practice, potassium iodate should be given as soon as possible to people who have been exposed to radioiodine and will be effective in reducing uptake to some extent even if given several hours after exposure. It is said to have a reduced effect if more than 12 hours have elapsed following exposure [2,3].

Tablets of potassium iodate (85 mg) each containing 50 mg of iodine are available. The recommended dosage is as follows [4]:

adult	170 mg	(2 × 85 mg tablets)
3–12 years	85 mg	(1 × 85 mg tablet)
1 month–3 years	42.5 mg	($\frac{1}{2}$ × 85 mg tablet)
birth–1 month	21.25 mg	(liquid preparation advised)

Contraindications to the use of this treatment are:

- known iodine sensitivity
- hypocomplementaemic vasculitis
- dermatitis herpetiformis.

Other treatment options range from wound and gastric lavage and the use of absorbents, antacids, and laxatives, through the use of chelating agents, to dramatic options such as lung lavage. It is essential to be sure that any expected benefits of treatment outweigh the likely disadvantages, and specialist texts should be consulted for available techniques for each contaminant.

Long-term effects of radiation exposure

Patients who have received accidental exposures to radiation will be worried about possible long-term effects. Concern will certainly include the increased risks of developing cancer and for younger people may now include worry about increased risks of disease developing in their children.

It is, of course, always wrong to give bland reassurances but two facts can be used to reassure as much as possible as early as possible.

- Acute (deterministic) effects have a threshold, and if whole body doses are below this threshold the effects will not occur.
- Long-term (stochastic) effects which are due to genetic damage are also dose-dependent. They include both the risk of an individual developing cancer and transgenerational effects.

These occur after a variable period of latency and with stochastic effects it is the probability that they will occur at all which is proportional to dose. If whole body doses are small the associated risks are therefore proportionately small. Worried patients should be referred for professional counselling when appropriate, but a good estimate of dose, both received and/or committed, will be necessary if sound advice is to be given.

Summary

Health care professionals can safely manage patients who have been involved in radiation accidents. They should distinguish between those who have simply received external radiation exposure and who therefore need no special arrangements for their management, and those who are contaminated with radioactive materials.

External contamination is best managed as part of the immediate care by simple control measures.

Treatment of serious, conventional injuries always takes priority.

References

1. Conklin JJ, Walker RJ. *The medical basis for radiation accident preparedness II* (eds RC Ricks, SA Fry.), New York: Elsevier, 1990.
2. ICRP 40. *Protection of the public in the event of a major radiation accident* Oxford: Pergamon Press, 1984.
3. Kevari M. *Radiol Protection* 1994;**14**:131–46
4. PL/CMO [93]. *Potassium iodate (stable iodine) prophylaxis in the event of a nuclear accident.*

Further reading

Crosbie WA, Gittus JH. *Medical response to effects of ionising radiation* London: Elsevier Science Publications, 1989.

Gonber GB, Thomas RG eds. *Radiation protection dosmetry. Guidebook for the treatment of accidental internal radionuclide contamination of workers.* Ashford, Kent: Nuclear Technology Publishing, 1992.

IAEA. *Assessment and treatment of external and internal radionuclide contamination.* Vienna: IAEA, TECDOC-869, 1996.

IAEA. *Manual on early medical treatment of possible radiation injury.* Vienna: IAEA, 1978.

IAEA. *What the GP should know about medical handling of overexposed individuals.* Vienna: IAEA, TECDOC 366.

National Council on Radiation Protection and Measurement. *Management of persons accidentally contaminated with radionuclides*, Report No. 65. Washington DC: NCRP, 1980.

National Radiological Protection Board. *Handbook on the national arrangements for incidents involving radioactivity.* Revised edn, Oxford: NRPB, 1995.

22 Gunshot and blast injury

Jim Ryan
Leonard Cheshire Professor of Conflict Recovery, University College, London

Tim Hodgetts
Consultant in Accident and Emergency Medicine, Frimley Park Hospital NHS Trust, Frimley, Camberley, Surrey

---

OBJECTIVES

- To indicate the epidemiology of gunshot and blast injury.
- To describe the mechanisms of injury.
- To describe the process of resuscitation in the emergency room.
- To give guidelines on indications, assessment, and rules for immediate surgery.
- To describe the postoperative care needed.
- To discuss definitive surgery required in different types of injury.

GUNSHOT INJURIES

Epidemiology

Gunshot injury, whether malicious or accidental, is a significant cause of trauma in the developed world. In the United States firearms cause 22% of the deaths from violence or accidental trauma, a ratio of 1:1.5 to road accidents, which are the commonest cause [1]. The United Kingdom and Australia share a similar trauma profile, with blunt trauma being far more prevalent than penetrating trauma: in Australia in 1993, 1941 died on the roads [2], whereas around 600 died of gunshot wounds [3], a ratio of 1:3.2 road accident deaths. Even in these countries where gun violence is relatively uncommon there are occasional multiple shootings. On 19 August 1987 in Hungerford, a small town in southern England, Michael Ryan shot and killed 16, and injured a further 16 before shooting himself; on 17 August 1991 in Strathfield Plaza shopping centre, a suburb of Sydney, Wade Frankum shot and killed seven (and stabbed one other to death) and injured a further seven before also shooting himself. An even more terrible shooting incident occurred in Dunblane, Scotland, where a disgruntled gun enthusiast killed one teacher and 16 children in a primary school.

AIDS has been described as a modern epidemic. Deaths resulting from gunshot wounds in the United States equal or exceed deaths from AIDS in all age groups, even in the most AIDS-prevalent group of 25–34 years. In Australia there are 25% more deaths from gunshot than from AIDS. The United States has a murder rate almost nine times that of the United Kingdom, and over four times that of Australia: 61% of the murders in the United States are a result of firearms. (Although many more people are assaulted with sharp weapons than with guns, death from a gunshot is five times more likely.) Only 14% of the firearms deaths in Australia are a result of murder; 81% are from suicides.

Prevention of gun violence must be a high priority. The availability of handguns has been shown to be responsible for a seven-fold difference in the murder rate in Vancouver, Canada, and Seattle, United States [4], and has contributed to recent changes in United States gun laws. The murder rate in the United States by those under 18 years rose by 61% between 1980 and 1991 [5]. Factors such as television and video violence have been blamed, but so far only an association with increased aggression rather than a direct causal link has been proven [6].

Mechanism of injury

A bullet, or any other missile, produces injury when it transfers its energy into the body. The degree of injury will depend on how much energy is transferred, which in turn is dependent upon how much energy the missile has to start, and how much the missile is retarded by the body's tissues.

The energy of a missile is a product of its mass, and the square of its velocity:

$$\text{kinetic energy (KE)} = \tfrac{1}{2}mv^2$$

where m is the mass of the missile, and v its velocity. It follows that if the mass is doubled the energy is doubled, but if the velocity is doubled then the available energy increases four times. A low mass–high velocity bullet is therefore more potentially destructive.

The retardation of a missile by the body is influenced by the tissue's density and elasticity, and by the size and stability of the missile. The densest tissue, bone, will usually greatly retard the missile with resultant high energy transfer: the bone typically shatters and the bullet may fragment or deform but this is not always the case and a low energy transfer wound may be seen [7]. The wounding potential can be represented mathematically as follows [8]:

$$\text{wounding potential} = \text{energy transfer} \times$$
$$\frac{1}{\text{period of transfer}} \times \frac{1}{\text{area}} \times \frac{1}{\text{tissue factors}}$$

All missiles produce injury by crushing and laceration along their direct path through the body. This wound track is known as the *permanent cavity*. The size of the permanent cavity will depend upon the size of the missile, whose frontal area may increase on impact with the body – a feature of "hollow-point" or "soft-nosed" bullets. Military rifle rounds are "jacketed", that is they have a rigid alloy coating around the softer lead, and are generally intended to retain their shape on impact.

> All missiles produce injury by laceration and crushing along the missile's path. This is the permanent cavity.

The larger the area the missile presents, the more energy will be transferred. Rifle bullets are inherently unstable (Figure 22.1).

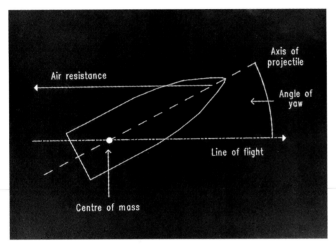

Figure 22.1 Yawing. Deviation of the long axis of the bullet from its line of flight.

The centre of mass lies behind the point of air resistance and thus any deviation of the long axis from line of flight (angle of yaw) will tend to increase until the bullet is induced to tumble end over end. Rifling the weapon barrel, causing the bullet to spin, improves stability and greatly reduces the yaw tendency – modern rifle bullets in flight typically possess very small angles of yaw (2/3°). However, this small degree of instability becomes significant when bullets strike human tissue – the high forces on the initial small angle of yaw may now initiate tumbling of the bullet within the wound. Wedge-shaped bullets are particularly unstable and have a tendency to tumble in flight, therefore presenting a variable profile with maximal tissue damage when the bullet is 90° to its short axis.

If a missile breaks into fragments then the presenting area is also effectively increased. Bullets designed to fragment on impact are outlawed for military use by the Geneva Convention of 1949 (and indeed many earlier Conventions), and include bullets that are scored, have soft noses, are partially jacketed (semijacketed), or have hollow points. The term "dum-dum" refers to the soft bullet manufactured by the British in 1897 in an Indian munitions factory of the same name, that would increase in size on impact. A "semijacketed" bullet has some of the soft lead core exposed, and the jacket may shed along the wound resulting in multiple diverging lacerations within the wound. Hollow-point bullets may be filled with shot

("Glaser safety slug"), or explosive powder in an attempt to increase tissue damage, or with mercury to produce poisoning if the bullet fails to kill. These fragments derived from the missile are known as *primary* fragments: *secondary* fragments of dense tissue, such as bone, may be generated and produce additional injury (Figure 22.2).

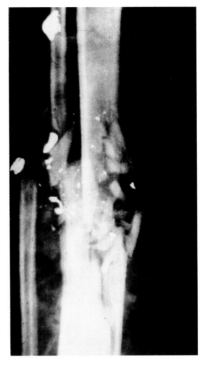

Figure 22.2 Open, comminuted fracture of tibia and fibula caused by a high energy rifle bullet. Primary fragments from the bullet and secondary bone fragments are shown.

It has been traditional to subdivide all missiles as "low velocity" or "high velocity", with the arbitrary cut off being the speed of sound. The importance of this is in recognising that high velocity missiles have a greater *available* kinetic energy to transfer to the wound. However, velocity is merely one of the criteria involved in energy transfer and wound severity, and attempts to describe missile wounds in terms of velocity alone have been recently abandoned in favour of the more descriptive "low energy transfer" and "high energy transfer" wound terminology. High velocity missiles have the potential to produce a *temporary* cavity in addition to a permanent cavity, but this may also occur with lower velocity missiles that are greatly retarded. It is the temporary cavity that has the potential to produce severe tissue disruption remote from the wound track.

> Where there is high energy transfer to the wound a temporary cavity may be formed.

A temporary cavity forms as a consequence of substantial energy transfer to soft tissue. The cavity forms behind the missile and results from the acceleration of tissue radial to the path of the missile and reaches its maximum volume within 2–3 milliseconds (ms) by which time a perforating missile will have passed, and it may reach up to 14 times the diameter of the permanent cavity [10] (Figure 22.3).

As the cavity forms it creates a vacuum, sucking in clothing, dirt, and skin flora, and disseminating these widely, which produces a highly contaminated wound (particularly with *Clostridium tetani* and *C. welchii*). The cavity begins to collapse

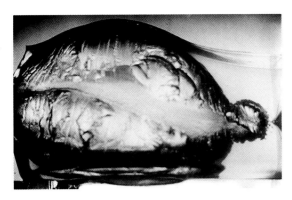

Figure 22.3 A temporary cavity demonstrated in 20% gelatin caused by a high available energy military rifle bullet.

after a few milliseconds – this is a process of repetitive collapse and re-expansion of reducing magnitude.

A common misconception is that the formation of a temporary cavity is an "all or none" phenomenon. Cavities vary widely in size, shape and effect. Some tissues are more susceptible to temporary cavitation; inelastic tissues of high density such as bone, liver, and spleen fare particularly badly – total disruption may occur. Other structures such as muscle and lung form cavities but with little resultant tissue injury. However, tissue planes may be widely stripped exposing otherwise uninjured structures to widespread contamination by foreign material and mixed bacterial species. Normal clinical judgement will guide a surgeon in decision-making concerning tissue viability following exposure to cavitation. Judgement on the extent of soft tissue excision may sometimes be difficult in the immediate period after injury as there is a period of microvascular instability with some tissues irreversibly damaged but with other apparently devascularised areas capable of recovery [11].

When a gun is fired at "point blank" range there will be tattooing and burns around the entrance wound from the propellant, and if the muzzle is touching the skin it may leave an imprint. Gases discharged from the barrel can enter and exacerbate the wound. Bullets travelling at high velocity generate a *sonic shock wave* which precedes their passage through the tissues; but the wounding potential of this shock wave is not thought to be significant.

Shotguns

A shotgun fired at short range (< 5 m) will behave as a high energy fragmenting missile. On impact the multiple lead shot balls act as a single mass with a wide presented area that may further extend when the lead shot deforms. However, the shot spreads out in a conical fashion as individual fragments produce injury by permanent and temporary cavitation. The mortality from such an injury approaches 90% [9]. At distances of 5–15 m the shot will behave as individual low energy missiles, that may penetrate beyond deep fascia.

Inside the cartridge the lead shot is packed in a plastic cylinder, or "unitising wad", which is also expelled from the barrel and opens out to release the shot: with wounds sustained from a short range the unitising wad together with filler wadding (cardboard) may be found in the victim's clothes or in the superficial part of the wound. Shotguns can also fire a single rifled lead slug, and may also be used to propel "plastic" or "rubber bullets". At close range these missiles have a high mass and high velocity, and cause devastating injury.

Airguns

Airguns are common, and their wounding potential should not be underestimated. Deaths are reported, often from brain penetration via the orbit. Wounds are usually low energy transfer, but the available energy can be increased by "piggy-backing" (sitting a pellet on top of another) and "dieselling" (oiling the barrel just before firing to produce an explosion). Venous embolisation is reported, where the pellet has entered the peripheral circulation and lodged in the lungs.

Resuscitation

The first consideration in the emergency department (ED) must be safety. Is this an innocent victim, or was there a two-way exchange of gunfire? One would want to avoid a hypoxic, aggressive casualty producing his own gun in the resuscitation room. Personal safety also extends to all team members having suitable protection against blood contamination.

The priorities for resuscitation are the same as those for blunt trauma, namely Airway, Breathing, and Circulation, but in general the decisions in the ED are simpler. Gunshot wounds usually require surgical exploration under a general anaesthetic. Consequently immediate surgery should not be delayed where it is difficult to gain haemodynamic stability. *Surgery is part of resuscitation, it does not follow resuscitation.*

The emergency physician has the potential to destroy forensic evidence during resuscitation. Clothing may have been cut off at the scene by ambulance staff, or is removed at hospital – the temptation to cut through the gunshot holes should be avoided. The clothing should be placed in a paper bag, labelled, and handed directly to the police (nursing staff have the authority to release forensic items): the more people who handle it, the harder it is for the police to establish a continuity of evidence. The entrance wound is usually small and circumscribed in civilian practice. Before it is cleaned and excised, it should be documented. In the ED this may be most easily done with a polaroid camera, with a ruler or biro adjacent to the wound to assist in scaling. If propellant or a missile fragment is recovered or falls from the wound, it must be handed to the police in a plastic bag with the patient's documentation details.

A search should always be made for a second wound: a patient lying supine may exsanguinate from a missed wound on the back. The exit wound is bigger than the entrance wound in 60% of cases [10] and often ragged, as the missile pushes out through unsupported skin (it can be small if clothing is tight or if the victim is against a firm surface). The site of these wounds gives some clues as to the organs that may be damaged, but the path can be unpredictable. If there is no exit wound then all the missile's energy has been expended in the body and consequently there is potential for greater damage.

As gunshot wounds are contaminated, tetanus prophylaxis (toxoid and human immunoglobulin) should be given where immune status is not known. Penicillin should also be presribed to cover *C. welchii* but local policy will dictate the antibiotics for regional injuries such as the head or abdomen.

Immediate surgery

In United Kingdom practice, surgical intervention following penetrating missile injury is considered mandatory by most surgeons. The authors recognise the emerging trend towards conservatism in some trauma centres in the United States and South Africa [12]. In these centres, there is considerable expertise allowing a conservative approach for certain clearly defined categories of patient, typically stable with low energy transfer wounds. They are managed according to agreed guidelines by clinicians expert in missile wound care. In our practice, missile injuries are still uncommon (however, the trend is upwards) and few clinicians have expertise in management.

Indications for surgery

It is safe practice to intervene surgically in all cases, even for wounds that may appear trivial. In some modest wounds involving soft tissues only (modern peppering type wounds caused by new military preformed fragments for example), initial exploration under local anaesthetic may be appropriate.

Usually, the presence of a penetrating missile wound will be obvious. A history will be available, the diagnosis will be confirmed by clinical assessment and, if time permits, appropriate investigations. Very occasionally, an unconscious or incapacitated patient may present with a wound in an occult site, typically on the back. In these circumstances resuscitation proceeds as described earlier and may even lead on to surgical resuscitation before the diagnosis is clear. This need not cause anxiety provided the patient is being managed according to a well-tried trauma system, ATLS for example [13].

In most instances, the presence of missile injury will be known, resuscitation successful, appropriate investigations possible, and surgical intervention planned. In cases involving gunshot wounds in a civilian setting, the timing, duration, and extent of intervention can be predicted with some accuracy. Wounds are usually single, although a number of body systems may be involved. A single or multistaged approach, or a synchronous combined operation by, for example, orthopaedic and plastic surgeons, may be indicated.

Provided the receiving hospital is working to a trauma system, patients who are transiant or minimal responders should be readily identified and surgically resuscitated. The problem will invariably be ongoing haemorrhage in the chest or abdomen, the response to aggressive fluid resuscitation will be minimal or transient, and an urgent laparotomy or thoracotomy becomes necessary to control haemorrhage; this is discussed later (page 268). Surgical intervention as part of haemorrhage control is now a well-described and accepted part of missile wound management, particularly in war and conflict settings where multiple casualties are likely, and medical resources may be modest and overstretched.

Rules for "war" surgery

Perusal of contemporary literature reveals varying views on surgical management for missile injury [14,15]. In centres where missile injury is a daily event and experience considerable, surgical management is individual and tailored to need. Treatment ranges from non-operative intervention for some to full exploration with wide surgical excision and multiple procedures for others. This approach is undoubtedly successful in expert hands but leaves the non-expert with little guidance.

The problem for the inexperienced lies in wound assessment and how much or how little to do. While it is impossible to formulate a single management doctrine to meet all eventualities it is possible to define certain principles and to outline safe management guidelines. These principles and guidelines are derived from accumulated military experience in wars of this century. They have evolved over time and are based on knowledge of wound ballistic science and hard learned lessons of military surgeons. The principles and guidelines combine to form what may be termed the rules for the surgery of war or conflict [14–17] and are based upon a number of assumptions.

- All missile wounds are associated with wound contamination by bacteria and foreign bodies.
- Wound infection remains the principle threat to life and limb in those who survive their initial injury (that is, those successfully resuscitated).
- Antibiotics are of secondary importance to adequate surgery in preventing wound infection.
- Most patients will be managed by surgeons inexperienced in managing missile wounds.
- Postoperatively, most patients require evacuation or transfer.

Assessment of immediate priorities

This has been largely covered in Chapter 1 and involves the assessment and resuscitation of patients. However, some points need emphasis. A history with timings is vital. Delay beyond six hours before antibiotic administration and wound exploration is associated with significant incidence of wound infection and systemic sepsis. Knowledge of the wounding agent(s) while not vital does give some general indicators. For example, injury caused by fragments result in more severe contamination and infection. In addition, wounds caused by fragments are typically multiple [16,17].

Pain relief

Acute anxiety is universal and, coupled with pain, may lead to extreme distress. Incremental intravenous boluses of an opiate are particularly helpful.

Antibiotics

The overriding problem associated with missile injury is primary wound infection caused by clostridial species and beta haemolytic streptococcus. Infection by other species tends to supervene later and often postoperatively. Appropriate agents in adequate dosage, administered sytemically, and commenced as soon as possible after wounding are the key issues.

Preoperative investigations

These are possible only in stable patients. Very little is required prior to first surgical intervention. Limb wound x-rays may localise missiles; biplanar views may assist in outlining the missile track. Other general investigations not specific to missile injury and appropriate to all injured patients may be undertaken if time permits.

Planning

Some attempt should be made to plan the timing, sequence of activities (which cavity or structure first), and the nature and extent of surgery. This may involve anaesthetists, surgeons of different specialities, as well as radiology and laboratory staff. In most instances, a two-staged approach would be used,

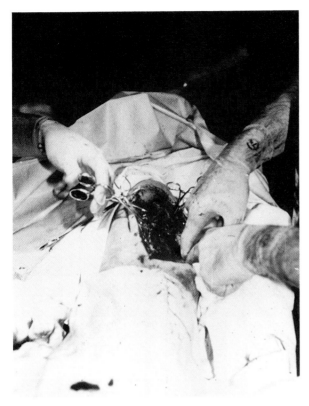

(a)

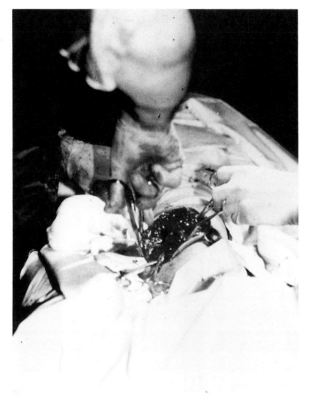

(b)

Figure 22.4 Through-and-through gunshot wound to lower femur. Note the extent of the skin incisions over both entry (a) and exit (b) wound sites. (Photograph taken at Ajax Bay field hospital during the Falklands War, 1982.)

the first being concerned with wound exploration, haemorrhage control, wound excision, and repair of vital structures. The second stage should deal with overall definitive repair and delayed primary wound closure.

Surgical technique

In a chapter of this nature it will not be possible to give detailed guidance on technique – this may be found elsewhere [18]. We are concerned here with principles. These are:

1. Wound cleansing and preparation must be over a sufficiently large area so as to allow extended access in any direction.

2. Skin incision should be generous (Figure 22.4) and counter (over the exit wound) incisions may be required. In contrast, skin *excision* should be kept to a minimum.

3. Fasciotomy is critical. Tension in the depths of missile wounds leads to necrosis and wound infection. Wide fasciotomy results in unbridling of a wound. This is the true meaning of the term *debridement*.

4. Haemorrhage may be life-threatening on the one hand or merely a nuisance interfering with wound assessment on the other. Full haemostastis should be achieved quickly.

5. Wound irrigation with copious fluids should follow haemostasis.

6. It is now appropriate to assess the wound fully; it should be widely exposed, unbridled, and irrigated. In the case of limb wounds, a decision must be made on the extent of soft tissue excision required.

> In injuries to body cavities the approach may be quite different. A full cavity exploration, laparotomy or thoracotomy, may be required to achieve haemostasis or to deal with faecal spillage. This will take precedence over attention to the primary missile wound.

Wound care, dressing, and splintage are areas of special importance. With certain exceptions, missile wounds are left open following surgery. Surgeons should not be frightened to leave wounds open because, provided they are carefully dressed (not packed) and splinted, open wounds come to no harm. Wounds left open drain well, wound infection rates are reduced, and postoperative pain is rarely a problem. There are exceptions to leaving wounds open:

- head wounds;
- face and neck;
- hands and feet – exposed tendons and neurovascular structures should be covered;
- joints – capsule and synovium should be covered.

Laparotomy and thoracotomy are formally closed in most instances – there are exceptions and these are discussed in a later section (page 268).

Operative records are of importance, particularly if multiple teams are involved and staged procedures planned. Notes of the first procedure are of the utmost importance. Clear descriptions of injury and procedures performed will guide subsequent operators – diagrams and clinical photos are particularly useful.

Life- and limb-saving surgery

All surgery following missile injury has as its purpose the saving of life and limb. In many instances, surgical procedures following missile injury may be planned and performed on patients who have been well resuscitated. However, on occasion rapid surgical intervention is demanded and may constitute part of the initial resuscitation phase. Typically, a patient, shot in the abdomen or chest, may present with ongoing bleeding from a solid organ or major vessel (Figure 22.5).

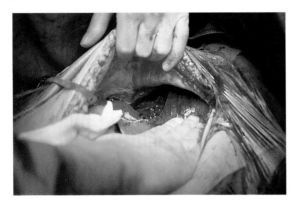

Figure 22.5 Fragment wound to liver. Laparotomy was required to control haemorrhage. (From the archives of the Department of Military Surgery.)

Response to resuscitation will be minimal or transient and immediate cavity exploration is required to arrest haemorrhage. In such instances wide exposure is needed and, in the case of the abdomen, a full-length midline abdominal incision is most useful. Rapid aspiration of blood using multiple wide-bore suckers is the first requirement followed by removal of the bowel from the peritoneal cavity to optimise visualisation. Once a bleeding site has been found, the safest approach is to pack and apply direct pressure. Having achieved control of haemorhage, effective fluid resuscitation now takes precedence. The surgeon has a number of options – proceed to definitive haemorrhage control and repair, or seek help. In the austere circumstances of war or conflict or in the face of multiple casualties, it may be possible to leave the packs in place, pack or towel clip close the laparotomy incision and return the patient to an intensive care facility for on-going resuscitation and further investigation prior to embarking on a planned definitive procedure some hours later. This approach has been recently described in the literature and has been termed

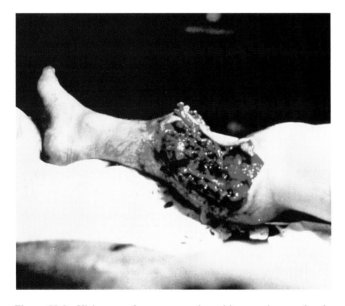

Figure 22.6 High energy fragment wound requiring tourniquet and early surgical intervention to control haemorrhage.

"damage control" surgery by Mattox in the United States [19].

It may also be necessary to intervene rapidly following extremity injury (Figure 22.6).

The aim will be haemorrhage control and limb salvage. Wide exposure is again the rule – bleeding is controlled initially by direct pressure and later by direct vessel control. Temporary revascularisation by on-table external shunting is particularly suitable if extensive orthopaedic procedures are required. Definitive vascular repair is best deferred until bony injury has been fully dealt with. In many instances, wide fasciotomy of all lower limb compartments is required, particularly after revascularisation following prolonged ischaemia. It should be noted that internal bony fixation devices are best avoided following missile injury – wounds are invariably contaminated and the risk of sepsis considerable. External fixators are particularly appropriate under these conditions.

Postoperative care

Intensive care is necessary for those requiring respiratory and/or cardiovascular support, or invasive monitoring after surgery.

Wound infection is commonplace if missile wounds are treated by primary suture or closure, which may be the temptation in units unfamiliar with their management. The patient should return to the operating theatre after four to seven days and, if the wound is clean, then the wound is closed ("delayed primary closure/suture). Postoperative antibiotics will be continued in wounds that were highly contaminated at operation, or where a large amount of necrotic tissue was excised.

Continuing surgical care

Surgical care for the victims of missile injury is at least a two-stage enterprise – the first procedure, as we have shown, is life- or limb-saving, and in most situations further definitive procedures are required. At its most basic, a second procedure will involve delayed primary or secondary closure of skin, typically between four and seven days. Much more may be required and the list of procedures below is far from exhaustive:

- delayed primary closure by suture ± skin grafting or flap;
- operative fixation of fractures;
- nerve repair – early or late;
- closure of colostomy/ileostomy;
- definitive cover for extensive soft tissue/bone loss.

The planning and timing of definitive procedures is a multidisciplinary problem and requires early consultation with those specialists likely to be involved. In some instances a synchronous combined approach by general and orthopaedic, or orthopaedic and plastic teams may be appropriate but requires early consultation, investigation, and planning. Following definitive procedures many patients may need to embark on a prolonged phase of rehabilitation, and this may include psychological support.

BLAST INJURY

Epidemiology

The causes of blast injury are listed in the box. Most of the experience outside the theatre of war stems from terrorist bombs. The first Irish terrorist bomb in Britain was on 13 December 1867 when there was an attempt to spring Fenian prisoners from the Clerkenwell detention house in London [20]. At the height of the civil unrest in Northern Ireland in 1972 there were 1500 bomb explosions with 5000 injuries [21].

The causes of blast injury

- Terrorist bomb
- Industrial (mining; munitions or fireworks factory)
- Domestic (gas)
- Military

In a meta-analysis of the published results of 220 bombings from across the world between 1969 and 1983, Frykberg and Tepas found that bombs involve multiple casualties with a mean of 15.3 (range 4.5–34.6); one-eighth die at the scene; and of those who survive, 30% require inpatient treatment [22].

The terrorist bomb is difficult to detect. Modern "plastic" explosives are odourless (munitions manufacturers have opposed the addition of a distinctive odour as this would jeopordise clandestine operations in war), relatively radiolucent, and malleable to almost any shape.

Mechanism of injury

A bomb injures in six ways (see box). The degree of injury depends on the *type* and the *amount of explosive*. The three principal types of explosive are:

- chemical
- mechanical
- nuclear.

Chemical explosives can be divided into low explosive or "deflagrating", such as gunpowder or petrol contained in a barrel or tanker; and high explosive or "detonating", such as TNT or Semtex. Some "unstable" high explosives may detonate spontaneously; however, most require chemical decomposition. Detonation, for example, may be triggered by percussion or horizontal movement (mercury tilt switch).

The mechanisms of blast injury

- Blast wave
- Blast wind
- Fragmentation
- Flash burns
- Crush
- Psychological

Blast wave

The blast wave is a spherical front of overpressure expanding rapidly away from the point of explosion. The magnitude of this wave falls very rapidly as the distance increases:

$$\text{overpressure} \propto \frac{1}{\text{distance}^3}$$

Attempts have been made to increase the area of influence of

the blast wave by spreading the explosive "fuel" as a gas or vapour cloud before detonation: these are known as "fuel-air" weapons or explosives. The effect of the blast wave is attenuated in water, and is increased on reflection from a solid surface when it overlaps with the incident wave: the solid surface may be a wall, ceiling, or internal viscera.

The blast wave causes injury in four ways:

- compression
- spalling
- implosion
- shearing.

Initially the blast will surround individuals and compress them, resulting in underlying solid organ contusion, although the exact clinical significance of this contusion injury is still the subject of debate. As the wave passes through the body it produces "spalling" at tissue interfaces of varying density, and particularly at air–water interfaces. Spalling can be likened to the plume of water at the surface of a pond into which a grenade is thrown. The result in the lungs is intra-alveolar haemorrhage and alveolar disruption – clinically manifested as "blast lung". *Blast lung* is a common post-mortem finding in those who die at the scene, but occurs in < 1% of those admitted to hospital when its development may be delayed for up to 48 hours. Alveolar disruption may produce pneumothorax and haemothorax, and may further allow air into the pulmonary circulation which embolises to the cororary arteries leading to sudden "unexplained death". Death without evidence of external injury has been noted for centuries (Pierre Jars in 1758 first correctly linked this to the question of gases following the explosion) and animal experimentation has confirmed this to be due to coronary artery or cerebral air embolisation.

Gas trapped in organs or structures is momentarily compressed and superheated: on re-expansion there may be perforation of bowel, lung, or tympanic membrane (which may also be affected by the incident pressure wave). Shearing stresses also occur at the interfaces of tissue planes and may produce subserosal or submucus haemorrhage. The healthy tympanic membrane ruptures at a lower overpressure than that required to produce blast lung (about 100 kPa compared to 175 kPa), and a perforated ear drum is therefore a suggestive sign that a victim has been exposed to a significant blast load. An intact ear drum does not, however, exclude this as the incident angle of the blast wave appears to be important – in other words the victim's ear must be correctly orientated to the incident pressure for damage to occur.

Blast wind

The blast wind is the rush of displaced air that follows the blast wave. This may be sufficiently forceful to cause whole body displacement, torso disruption, and avulsive amputations in those close to the point of the explosion. The victim may be carried by the wind and thrown against a solid surface, with resultant impact and deceleration injuries. Environmental fragments of glass, wood, and stone will also be carried by the wind and act as missiles.

Fragmentation and missiles

The vast majority of injuries following a bomb blast result from penetrating missiles and the number and severity varies depending on the device and environment. *Primary* missiles come from the bomb itself and are termed natural (parts of the bomb casing) or *preformed* (ball bearings, nails, nuts, and bolts packed around the explosive). Military munitions (grenades, shells, and bombs) (Figure 22.7) are manufactured to

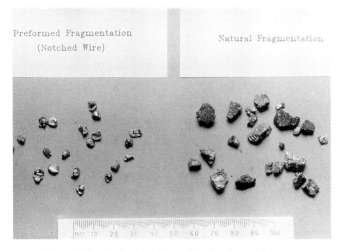

Figure 22.7 A selection of natural and preformed fragments.

fragment consistently in the same manner, and have a predictable radius of injury; terrorist bombs are completely unpredictable in the pattern of missile injuries they will produce. *Secondary* missiles are those environmental fragments carried by the blast wind.

Missiles injuries can be blunt or penetrating. The potential injury from a penetrating bomb fragment, like a bullet, will depend on its available energy: most fragments will have a kinetic energy less than that of a handgun bullet.

Flash burns

Burns following a bomb blast are usually superficial and restricted to exposed parts of the skin, namely the hands and feet. However, only those victims close to the point of the explosion will be affected by the brief burst of thermal radiation, and other more serious injuries from the blast wave, blast wind, and fragmentation should be anticipated.

More severe burns and smoke inhalation may result from the secondary fires started by the explosion.

Crush injury

An explosion inside a building may trap the victim in the rubble for several hours. If a limb has been crushed and hypoperfused for more than 30–60 minutes and the circulation is suddenly restored, death may follow immediately from hyperkalaemia. Later deaths ensue from acute renal failure from renal tubule blockage by myoglobin and cytochrome C. In prolonged entrapment a decision may be made to amputate at the site or use a high tourniquet prior to amputation in hospital rather than release a severely damaged limb. Profound shock of complex aetiology is another feature of crush injury and adequate fluid resuscitation is necessary to maintain perfusion to vital organs such as the brain, myocardium, and kidneys.

Psychological sequelae

The primary objective of a terrorist is not to injure or kill but to induce a change in behaviour through fear. As terrorist bombs are unpredictable in where they are placed and indiscriminate in whom they injure, few people (including the carers) will be prepared for the psychological effects that will follow (see Chapter 23). After a bomb explosion many more people than are physically injured can be expected to have psychological symptoms.

Resuscitation

Medical personnel called to the scene of an explosion should follow the principles applicable to any major incident scene (see Chapter 23). In particular medical staff should be aware that *secondary devices* are common and often intended to harm emergency service personnel: they should not enter an area which has not been searched for such devices, and should not use a radio until this is declared safe to do so by the police (in case the secondary device is radio-controlled). The scene of a bomb explosion is a scene of crime and should be disturbed as little as possible by those involved in the casualty rescue.

Resuscitation priorities are the same as those for any serious injury – Airway, Breathing, Circulation, and Dysfunction of the CNS. A casualty with flash burns to the face is at risk of upper airway obstruction: this should be closely monitored. Signs of inhalational burn may prompt elective intubation to protect the airway.

With casualties who have features of blast lung there may be a difficult theoretical balance of providing adequate ventilation against a risk of air embolism if positive pressure is used.

Clinically, it appears that air embolism is an early phenomenon, often immediate or within the first hour of injury. CPAP in the spontaneously breathing patient, intermittent positive pressure ventilation, with additional PEEP in those requiring formal ventilation, is therefore almost certainly safe, will improve arterial oxygen concentration, and will limit the alveolar transudation. Positive pressure also increases the risk of pneumothorax. It may not be necessary to consider prophylactic chest drains if this risk is appreciated and the patient is carefully observed.

Limbs that have been avulsed may be brought to the ED with the patient, but unlike guillotine amputations these are generally not amenable to reimplantation. Missile wounds are treated in the same way as gunshot wounds.

Immediate surgery

The vast majority of patients surviving an explosion whether military, terrorist, or industrial will have fragment wounds, often multiple, and involving multiple body systems [23]. Many will have combined injury, that is to say they will have pulmonary complications either as a result of blast exposure or as a consequence of toxic inhalation or lung burn. Equally, many will have surface burns, particularly flash burns to exposed parts.

The management of the penetrating missile wounds is in no way different from that described in the first part of this chapter. It should be noted that missile wounds caused by primary terrorist fragments (such as vehicle parts or bomb casing) and secondary fragments from the environment result in multiple, severe wounds, invariably highly contaminated. It is particularly important under these circumstances to obey the rules of war or conflict surgery. A policy of primary wound closure or inadequate surgery for these wounds may be catastrophic.

Secondary injuries as a consequence of blast winds may be devastating with partial dismemberment and traumatic amputations being notable features. In managing traumatic amputations it is good practice in most instances *not* to attempt the construction of a definitive amputation at a site of election. Infection rates are extremely high and will likely result in reamputation at a higher level.

Burn injuries should be managed in the normal way accepting that planned surgical procedures must take account of other injuries and procedures such as wound excision, revascularisation, fracture stabilisation, or colostomy, to name but a few possibilities. Plainly, a planned, multidisciplinary disciplinary approach is vital.

Postoperative care

Intensive therapy and invasive monitoring will again be necessary for those requiring respiratory or circulatory support postoperatively. Careful monitoring of fluid balance is important when there is alveolar damage, as excessive intravenous fluid, and particularly crystalloid, will exacerbate pulmonary oedema: such monitoring would be best provided by a pulmonary artery catheter. A prolonged period of ventilation is commonly needed in patients with blast lung, although improvement is often seen within 24 hours in those who eventually recover. Steroids have no proven value in its treatment.

As stated, the features of blast lung may be delayed and this should be considered in a patient who suffers a deterioration in respiratory function on day two. However, other conditions should be excluded, including pulmonary contusion (from blunt trauma), aspiration pneumonitis, multiple blood transfusions with unfiltered blood, and fat embolism. A chest x-ray may help distinguish between contusions, aspirations, and blast lung; fat embolism may be inferred from a purpuric skin rash. Oxygen toxicity has been implicated as a cause of worsening respiratory function with existent alveolar damage, a result of intra-alveolar fibrosis. This is unlikely to be important if the inspired oxygen concentration is kept to the minimum required to maintain an adequate arterial oxygen tension.

Many people will attend the ED following a bomb blast with what is popularly known as "shock", and will be identified as suffering from critical incident stress and in need of post-incident psychological counselling. But this is easy to forget in those admitted to hospital where the management of their physical injuries is paramount. Adequate counselling is an important element of the patient's recovery (see Chapter 16).

Continuing surgical care

The approach is as for missile injury patients. Notably, injury is more severe following a blast, and multiple definitive procedures, typically involving plastic and orthopaedic teams, are the norm. Limb loss victims may face multistaged procedures to achieve a useful stump. The presence of burn injury may influence or delay certain definitive procedures, insertion of internal fixation devices for example. Rehabilitation may be prolonged and complex, particularly if patients have suffered loss of limbs or sight.

Summary

Penetrating ballistic and blast injury is no longer confined to the battlefield. Civilian doctors are therefore obliged to understand the principles of injury and be able to institute early and effective management. Victims do not suffer and die in some esoteric or unusual way. The basic rules for the surgery of trauma still apply. It is important to recognise important factors such as the likelihood of multiple wounds and multisystem injury. All ballistic wounds are highly contaminated and the risk of postoperative wound infection (which may be lethal) is high. This has implications for surgery which have been emphasised. The prevalence of multisystem penetrating injury with widespread contamination following blast exposure is not often appreciated nor is the relative rarity of blast lung injury among survivors.

In approaching the victims of gunshot and blast injury, remember that the rules of resuscitation and early management are those for any victim of trauma – namely ABC!

References

1. McSwain NE (ed.). *Pre-hospital trauma life support* (3rd edn). Illinois: Mosby-Year Book Inc., 1994.
2. Federal Office of Road Safety. *Road fatalities Australia: 1992 statistical summary*. Canberra: FORS, 1994.
3. Chapman S. Gun control. *BMJ* 1995;**310**:284.
4. Sloan JH, Kellerman AL, Reay DT *et al*. Handgun regulations, crime, asaults and homicide. *New Engl J Med* 1988;**319**:1256–62.
5. Shepherd JP, Farrington DP. Preventing crime and violence. *BMJ* 1995;**310**:271–2.
6. Black D, Newman M. Television violence and children. *BMJ* 1995; **310**:273–4.
7. Clasper JC, Hodgetts TJ. High velocity gunshot wound through bone with low energy transfer. *Injury* 1994;**25**:264–6.
8. Presswalla FB. The pathophysics and pathomechanics of trauma. *Med Sci Law* 1978;**18**:239–46.
9. Ordog GJ (ed.). *Management of gunshot wounds*. New York: Elsevier, 1988.
10. Parr MJ, Grande CM. Mechanisms of trauma, in (Grande CM, ed.) *Textbook of trauma anaesthesia and critical care*. St Louis: Mosby; 1993.
11. Hodgetts TJ, Haywood I, Skinner D, Ryan JM, Blast and gunshot injuries, in (Skinner D *et al*., eds) *ABC of major trauma* (2nd edn). London: BMJ Publishing, 1995.
12. Marcus NA, Blair WF, Shuck JM, Omer CE. Low-velocity gunshot wounds to extremities. *J Trauma* 1980;**20**:1061–4.
13. Committee on Trauma, American College of Surgeons. *Advanced trauma life support manual*. Chicago: ACS, 1993.
14. Cooper GJ, Ryan JM. Interaction of penetrating missiles with tissues: some common misapprehensions and implications for wound management. *Br J Surg* 1990;**77**:606–10.
15. Bowyer GW, Cooper GJ, Rice P. Management of small fragment wounds in war: current research. *Ann Roy Coll Surgeons Engl* 1995; **77**:131–4.
16. Spalding TJW, Stewart MPM, Tulloch DN, Stepehens KM. Penetrating missile injuries in the Gulf war 1991. *Br J Surg* 1991;**78**: 1102–4.
17. Ryan JM, Cooper GJ, Haywood IR *et al*. Field surgery on a future conventional battlefield: strategy and wound management. *Ann Roy Coll Surgeons Engl* 1991;**73**:13.
18. Kirby NG, Blackburn G. *Field surgery pocket book*. London: HMSO, 1981.
19. Hirshberg A, Mattox KL. "Damage control" in trauma surgery – leading article. *Br J Surg* 1993;**80**:1501–2.
20. Neal W. *With disastrous consequences: London disasters 1830–1917*. Enfield Lock: Hisarlik Press, 1992.
21. Clarke RS. Northern Ireland, in (Grande CM, ed.) *Textbook of anaesthesia and critical care*. St Louis: Mosby, 1993.
22. Frykerg ER, Tepas JJ. Terrorist bombings. Lessons learned from Belfast to Beirut. *Ann Surg* 1988;**208**:569–76.
23. Maynard RL, Cooper GJ, Scott R. Mechanisms of injury in bomb blast and explosions, in (Westaby S, ed.) *Trauma – pathogenesis & treatment*. Oxford: Heinemann, 1989, pp. 30–41.

23 Major incidents

Tim Hodgetts
Consultant in Accident and Emergency Medicine, Frimley Park Hospital NHS Trust, Frimley, Camberley, Surrey

David V. Skinner
Consultant and Clinical Director, Accident and Emergency Department, Radcliffe Hospital, Oxford

---

OBJECTIVES

To answer the following questions:

- What is a major incident?
- How can you prepare for a major incident?
- What is the immediate and continuing response to the scene?
- What is the immediate and continuing response in hospital?
- What are the long-term effects of a major incident?

Major incident definition

A major incident in medical terms is an incident where the number, severity, or type of *live* casualties, or because of its remote location, requires extraordinary arrangements by the health services. Incidents can be subclassified as natural or man-made, simple or compound, and compensated or uncompensated. A *natural* incident is the result of a hurricane, flood, volcano, earthquake, or tsunami (seismic tidal wave) – or any other natural phenomenon. A *man-made* incident is the result of human intervention or technology, such as a road, rail, or air transport accident, or a bomb. A *compound* incident involves disruption of the infrastructure of a community (such as in an earthquake), and specifically disruption of transport and communications systems, or the hospital itself; a *simple* incident does not. If resources mobilised during the major incident response can cope with the casualties then the incident is *compensated*. A failure to cope is recognised in some definitions as a "major disaster", which is synonymous with an *uncompensated* major incident.

Preparing for a major incident

Adequate preparation for a major incident will involve a combination of planning, acquiring equipment, and training.

Planning

Major incidents are fortunately rare, but may occur virtually at any place, any time. No healthcare system can consider itself immune from the need to plan for a major incident.

To fail to plan for a major incident, is to plan to fail with the response on the day.

Every hospital that provides a 24-hour service for casualties through an A & E department (in England these are termed "listed" hospitals, which also assumes a capability to provide a medical team) needs a major incident plan. This plan must be consistent with the regional health authority plan, which in turn should follow the guidelines of the state or national plan. For example the Department of Health of New South Wales, Australia, publishes a state plan ("MEDPLAN") for the medical response to a major incident or disaster [1]. Metropolitan Sydney, the capital of the state, is divided into a number of health authorities which have developed their own area plans. Each hospital within a given authority will have its own hospital major incident plan. In England it is unusual to find an area plan, but the hospital plan will follow the national Department of Health recently updated guidelines layed down in *Emergency Planning in the NHS* [2].

Like the history of war throughout the centuries, the pattern of major incidents is repetitive: major incidents are not necessarily unpredictable, and are certainly frequently avoidable. The first objective of major incident planning must be to identify a particular hazard and to take steps to prevent the incident from occurring. Some hazards are obvious, such as a chemical or nuclear installation; some are less obvious, with perhaps even a reluctance to acknowledge a potential problem. There have been two major incidents involving the crowd at Burnden Park football stadium, Bolton, this century, and three at Ibrox football stadium, Glasgow. Numerous other sporadic incidents have occurred in football stadia across Europe (Moscow 1982; Bradford 1985; Brussels 1985; Sheffield 1989) and the rest of the world (Peru 1964; Kathmandu 1988; Orkney, South Africa 1991). The Taylor report, which followed the Hillsborough stadium tragedy in Sheffield, is an example of how legislation may prevent future incidents in the UK by imposing all-seater stadia and recommending minimum standards of medical support at football matches.

Medical plans require an *all hazard* approach. This means that the broad principles of response must be the same for all incidents. A systematic approach to major incident management can only improve the quality of the medical response: such an approach to the management of the scene is given in the box. Major incident national, state, or regional

Systematic approach to major incident scene management
● Command
● Safety
● Communication
● Assessment
● Triage
● Treatment
● Transport

plans must encompass an *all agency* approach, and detail the specific roles of the individual emergency services.

In the recovery phase of the incident, local major incident plans will be reappraised and altered in the light of practical experience. These lessons should be widely publicised, so that others may plan to prevent a similar incident, or act to improve their response. Major incident planning is therefore continuous and follows the cyclical process of *prevention, preparation, response,* and *recovery.*

Equipment

Equipment can be considered in terms of personal clothing and medical equipment. Personal clothing must be visible, durable, and comfortable: protection of the individual is the primary concern. It can be difficult to persuade a hospital to provide quality clothing, which may only be rarely used in major incident exercises. Overalls have been the traditional clothing for medical team personnel, but a single layer of cotton provides little protection against cold, rain, glass, or jagged metal. Overalls are available which are fire-retardant, and which have knee and elbow pads. In temperate climates, waterproof, high-visibility jackets should also be available. Overalls and jackets should be clearly marked "DOCTOR" or "NURSE". National guidelines for uniform colours are required to ensure that medical personnel are easily identified at the scene. In the UK guidelines are provided by the British Association for Immediate Care, who recommend the same colour jackets (green and yellow) as the Ambulance Service – although medical personnel are identified by a different colour helmet (medical, green; ambulance, white).

Helmets serve to identify and protect. They identify the service, and may display rank (through colour, banding, or writing). Kevlar-composite material provides the best protection. A secure chinstrap similar to a climbing helmet is essential, as personnel will often discard a loose helmet. A light source can be fitted to the helmet, which leaves both hands free, as can a visor and ear defenders. Wellington boots are popular footwear, but not very versatile over difficult terrain. Heavy duty gloves are recommended when personnel are moving about the scene, and latex gloves are needed for patient handling. Medical personnel who are inappropriately dressed are a hazard to themselves and can be denied access to the scene.

Medical equipment needs to encompass triage, basic life support, and advanced life support. Table 23.1 lists the categories of equipment a hospital medical team should carry.

Equipment will be shared at the scene between hospital teams, and between medical and ambulance staff. Standardisation of equipment, and how it is packed, will improve the effectiveness of individuals providing care and facilitate resupply. This is exemplified by the national standardisation of major incident medical equipment in France. Medical equipment should supplement rather than duplicate Ambulance Service equipment, and reflect the additional skills of the Mobile Medical Team, although there will be some overlap. Packaging can be in boxes or rucksacks. Rucksacks are robust and easy to carry, leaving hands free, and are useful as the first response bag. They can carry, for example, enough disposables (airways, cannulae, fluids) to treat two casualties and a single set of non-disposable items (stethoscope, laryngoscope, sphygmomanometer). Large secure boxes are ideal for resupplying further disposable items. Surgical equipment is rarely required at the scene, and should be stored in a separate bag at the hospital: it will be brought by a Mobile Medical Team with surgical capability if needed.

Training

Education is learning from other people's mistakes: experience is learning from your own.

Anon

Post-incident reports show the same rudimentary mistakes are made in incidents across the UK, and in similar incidents across the world. Common criticisms are inadequate equipment, poor communication between the emergency services, and a lack of training for the Medical Incident Officer at the scene [3,4]. This stems from a failure to appreciate the need to train for the medical response to a major incident. Training has time and cost implications, and this favours the attitude, "Why train as it will never happen to us?" This is no defence for being inadequately prepared.

The most pressing need is to provide training for those in medical command roles at the scene, and particularly the Medical Incident Officer (MIO). Of secondary importance is a need to train all members of the medical team in prehospital care and major incident principles. It is unlikely that an individual health authority would provide funds to train a large number of doctors for the MIO role, nor is it necessary: a small number of individuals on an MIO roster held at Ambulance Control can provide cover for the area. The background of the doctor is less important than the fact that they are appropriately trained. Consequently the doctor may be drawn from hospital or general practice.

In the UK doctors support the Ambulance Service on a daily basis, particularly at road traffic accident entrapments. Many are members of BASICS (the British Association for Immediate Care) and notably will have their own safety

Table 23.1 Categories of medical equipment

Category	Equipment
Triage	Triage labels Waterproof marker pen
Documentation	Pens/pencils, notebooks
Basic life support	Simple airway adjuncts Control of external haemorrhage
Advanced life support	Rigid cervical immobilisation Endotracheal intubation Intercostal catheterisation Intravenous access and infusion Intraosseous access*
Drugs	Analgesia Anaesthesia (general and regional) Medical emergencies

* For children <6 years when repeated peripheral access fails.

clothing, transport, and communications, as well as being familiar with the operation of the other emergency services. In areas where a BASICS scheme exists, these doctors are a valuable resource for command and treatment roles at the scene, although the statutory responsibility of the local "listed" hospitals to provide staff remains. Some hospitals will identify a "non-essential" doctor to take the MIO role – for example, a gynaecologist or ophthalmologist who is unlikely to be central to the internal hospital response; additional training in prehospital care and attendance at regional planning meetings would be important for such doctors. When an MIO comes from outside the immediate area, the first immediate care doctor or medical team leader would have to assume this role temporarily.

MIMMS (*Major Incident Medical Management and Support*) is a three-day course which teaches a systematic "all hazard" approach to scene medical management for medical staff from team member through to Medical Incident Officer. In a similar way to the established Advanced Trauma Life Support course (Early Management of Severe Trauma, Australia), it can offer a consistency of training nationally. In Australia a five-day course for Medical Commanders (the equivalent of the MIO) is held by Emergency Management Australia in their national training centre at Mount Macedon, Victoria. A higher level of accreditation in major incident management is available by examination in the Diploma of Immediate Medical Care from the Royal College of Surgeons of Edinburgh, and by obtaining a Master of Science degree in Civil Emergency Planning from the University of Hertfordshire. The Society of Apothecaries of London have recently introduced a Diploma in Military and Civil Catastrophes. The minimum suggested training requirements for Mobile Medical Team members are given in the box.

Minimum training requirements

- *Doctors*
  - MIMMS*
  - ATLS or PHTLS or PHEC
- *Nurses*
  - MIMMS*
  - ATNC or TNCC or PHTLS or PHEC

* or equivalent
ATLS, Advanced Trauma Life Support; PHTLS, Prehospital Trauma Life Support; PHEC, Prehospital Emergency Care; ATNC, Advanced Trauma Nursing Course; TNCC, Trauma Nursing Core Course

---

An individual aspect of major incident management can be highlighted during continuing hospital training. Most doctors and nurses will not be comfortable with using a radio, which is the principal communication tool at the scene. Radio voice procedure, including message construction and the use of key words and phrases, can be taught in practical communication exercises. Triage exercises may be performed on paper, using lollipop sticks to represent casualties, or on simulated live casualty models. A table-top exercise teaches an understanding of the command roles of individual emergency services, and is most beneficial when all emergency services are involved in the discussion. A workshop on personal equipment and medical equipment will familiarise staff with the layout and contents of equipment, which may otherwise lie ignored in the hospital's major incident store. Command skills are learned on a Practical Exercise Without Casualties (PEWC). This is really a table-top exercise on a grand scale where participants are able to

pace out the sites for key areas (Casualty Clearing Station; Ambulance Parking Point; Ambulance Loading Point; Incident Control Point) on the ground. The complete response can be practised in a joint service exercise with simulated casualties.

Scene response: the first few hours

Immediate response

The immediate response to the scene will depend on the quality of the initial information. It is vital that a "major incident" is declared as soon as it is evident, although this can be delayed through fear of criticism. The content of the initial message can be remembered as "ETHANE" (see box). The ambulance service will often despatch a single vehicle until multiple casualties have been confirmed. The attendant of the first ambulance on the scene will assess the scene and communicate with Ambulance Control, then coordinate the deployment of subsequent ambulance personnel until the arrival of the designated Ambulance Incident Officer. The first ambulance crew *must not* involve themselves in casualty treatment.

Initial information from the scene

Your name or call sign
"Major incident declared at ... hours"

- **E**xact location
- **T**ype of incident
- **H**azards, present and potential
- **A**ccess to the scene
- **N**umber, severity, and type of casualties
- **E**mergency services present and required

"Acknowledge major incident declared at ... hours"

Command and control

Each emergency service at the scene will have a commander, or Incident Officer, but the overall control of the incident is a police responsibility. Command therefore operates vertically within a service, whereas control is horizontal across the services. Within each service there are three important tiers of command – bronze, silver, and gold. *Silver* (tactical) command represents the Incident Officers; *bronze* (operational) command is the Forward Incident Officers in charge of each service at the "coalface"; *gold* (strategic) command is the senior emergency service officers operating from a coordination centre remote from the scene. In the case of fire or chemical hazard, the Fire Service will control the incident at bronze level. There can be any number of bronze *sectors* within the incident.

In the United Kingdom the senior doctor is usually the Medical Incident Officer at silver command; very few ambulance services involve a doctor at gold level. Together with the Ambulance Incident Officer this doctor has to coordinate treatment at the scene, collate availability of beds in surrounding receiving hospitals, and decide on the flow of casualties to each hospital. Adequate communications between the MIO at the scene and the receiving hospitals are therefore essential, as is a knowledge of the resources and capabilities of each hospital. In Australia the system allows for much of this burden to be removed from the MIO by appointing a

Medical Controller (gold doctor) who is located at a Disaster Medical Control Centre (DMCC) with the Ambulance Controller: bed availability and casualty disposal is coordinated from this DMCC. Direct communication by hospitals with the scene is discouraged, and the Medical Controller can talk to the Medical Commander on a medical command radio network (Quebec Disaster Radio Network in metropolitan Sydney).

Incident officers are recognised by chequered tabards which are marked with their appointment (Ambulance and Medical, green and white; Police, blue and white; Fire, red and white). Other key officers may have their appointment on a tabard. Each service has a different rank structure, and ideally equivalent ranks should carry the same epaulette markings (as in New South Wales). Clinical seniority does not dictate precedence at the scene: medical staff will take orders from the appointed MIO irrespective of his specialty or grade. The first vehicles on the scene become the Forward Control Units and a marshalling point for each service. The Forward Control Units should be the *only* vehicles that do not extinguish their rotating beacons. Each service will send a mobile command and communications vehicle, the Emergency Control Vehicle (ECV): this vehicle may display a static green beacon or have a green and white chequered dome. Medical personnel will report to the Ambulance ECV if present, otherwise the Forward Control Unit.

Safety

Safety can be thought of in terms of:

1. personal safety
2. scene safety
3. casualty safety.

This is the *1–2–3 of safety*. Personal safety always comes first, and is ensured by correct protective clothing. A scene should not be approached unless it has been declared safe by the police or fire service: some examples of hazards are given in Table 23.2.

Table 23.2 Incident hazards and actions

Incident	Hazards	Action
Rail crash	Electricity (overhead cables; third rail); diesel trains on electrified track; hazardous load	Ensure power off; signals at rear to red; red flags at rear; detonators on track to warn approaching drivers
Bomb	Unexploded primary device; secondary devices	Stay out of line of sight of primary device; wait for police to complete sweep for secondary devices
Chemical incident	Fire; chemical contamination	Wait for Fire Service to declare safe to approach

The scene will be secured by the Police, who establish an outer cordon. This is a physical cordon and may be a vehicle parked to block the road, plastic tape, or portable metal crowd barriers: it acts to protect those approaching the scene from entering a hazardous area. The inner cordon surrounds the bronze area, and may not be a physical barrier unless personnel movements need to be controlled. The safety of casualties should sensibly follow these precautions, but heroic efforts are often recorded at the expense of personal safety.

Communications

Poor communications are the commonest failing at a major incident, both between services and along individual service chains of command. Commanders at all levels must talk regularly to their counterparts in other services. The Medical and Ambulance Incident Officers should remain close together, as many decisions are made jointly.

The most important communication tool is the radio. All health services' messages should be passed through the Ambulance Emergency Control Vehicle (ECV). UHF radios with a short range will be issued by the Ambulance Service for use on the scene. The existing VHF radios (with a longer range) allow the ECV to communicate with Ambulance Control and the receiving hospitals on the "Emergency Reserve Channel"; normal ambulance work will continue to be controlled on the daily operations channels.

Mobile telephones are an attractive alternative to a radio. Awkward radio voice procedure is avoided, and communications are not restricted to a predetermined net. However, if messages are not logged with the ECV that is coordinating the scene response, then efforts may be duplicated, or requested resources may fail to materialise. Cellular systems also have a finite capacity, and in metropolitan areas they may be rapidly saturated by the media. "Access Overload Control" is a system of protected cells, but telephones must be individually registered via the Cabinet Office: "Powerfail" is a similar system in Australia.

The radio net will be very busy and there are alternatives for communicating around the scene. Runners are reliable, and volunteers from the Red Cross or St John Ambulance may be willing message carriers: a written message is advisable (at the Moorgate Underground Railway crash in 1975 a verbal request for "Entonox" manifested as an "empty box"). A whistle or loud hailer may be useful to a commander.

Assessment

The first assessment of casualty numbers and severity does not have to be accurate. Its purpose is to mobilise enough resources to the scene and to allow receiving hospitals to make adequate preparations. It can be refined later. The type of casualties is important: a large number of injured children, or multiple specific injuries such as burns, may alter the casualty distribution.

Triage

Triage is the sorting of casualties into priorities for treatment. A *primary triage officer* (ambulance) will place a colour coded label on all the casualties where they are found; treatment officers will then direct their attention to the "immediate" priorities first.

Those with minor injuries will quickly start to self-evacuate. The first ambulance officer on the scene will identify an area to set up the Casualty Clearing Station, where the early evacuees can gather. The triage priorities are shown in Table 23.3.

Table 23.3 Triage priorities

Priority	Colour code	Injury example
Immediate	Red	Obstructed airway; tension pneumothorax
Urgent	Yellow*	Fractured femur; simple pneumothorax
Delayed	Green	Colles' fracture; sprained ankle
Expectant	Green endorsed "expectant", or blue	Witnessed cardiac arrest; open head injury with GCS 3
Dead	White or black	

* May use orange, for example in Australia.

Some casualties are unsalvageable, and to treat them would divert resources from those who can be saved. These are termed "expectant", but this category will only be rarely instituted at the MIO's discretion. Triage is dynamic: it is repeated at all steps of the evacuation chain, and priorities change. The labelling system must allow for this. Single colour label systems can cause a number of problems. If the label is changed, the earlier information is lost and the patient may also change identity (if there are individual numbers on each label); if labels are added the current status can be difficult to determine. The cruciform folding label system is recommended as a dynamic, easily interchangeable label, with adequate space for patient information.

A rapid, safe, and reproducible system is needed for the initial triage. This is the *triage sieve* (see box). A more detailed patient assessment, the *triage sort*, can be made at the Casualty

Clearing Station: this is a physiological score based on the Triage Revised Trauma Score (TRTS), but anatomical injury should be taken into account. The TRTS codes systolic blood pressure, Glasgow Coma Score, and respiratory rate from zero to four – the maximum score is 12, and the minimum zero (dead). Table 23.4 shows the triage priorities corresponding to the TRTS.

Table 23.4 Triage priority with corresponding TRTS score

Priority	TRTS score
DELAYED	12
URGENT	11
IMMEDIATE	1–10
DEAD	0

NOTE: if the expectant category is used, this would correspond to a score of 1–3.

Treatment

The skills of individual ambulance, medical, and nursing officers should be identified so that personnel are used appropriately. Most treatment is concentrated in the Casualty Clearing Station (CCS). Procedures such as cannulation should not be performed under difficult lighting or position if the casualty can be easily moved to the CCS.

The CCS should be on firm, flat ground as close to the site as is safe, and must be accessible to ambulances. Tents, groundsheets, or a triage label tied to a stick in the ground can be used to identify the treatment areas for each priority. All casualties should enter through a triage point, coordinated by the *secondary triage officer* (a doctor, nurse, or ambulance officer). Once treated, casualties will move through the treatment area and await transport in an evacuation area. Problems to anticipate in the CCS are:

● Tents are commonly overcrowded, prohibiting treatment.
● Casualties are carried in through the rear of the CCS, miss triage, and are placed in inappropriate areas.
● Casualties are not moved into an evacuation area once treated, leaving no room for new casualties.
● Casualties wait a long time in evacuation area, so need medical supervision.

Treatment is based on "ABC" principles and ranges from first-aid (police, fire service, volunteer organisations), through ambulance-aid, to advanced life support (paramedics, doctors). Medical resources will be concentrated in the CCS. Individual doctors or medical teams will only be allowed forward with the express permission of the MIO or deputy, and must then return to the CCS for retasking.

Transport

The Ambulance Incident Officer is responsible for organising the most appropriate transport, and for deciding the receiving hospitals. Casualties should be sent in pulses to a number of hospitals, to prevent any one being overwhelmed. Road ambulances are the standard form of transport, but alternatives should be considered. "Delayed" priority casualties may be evacuated *en masse* by coach or train away from the main receiving hospitals: they can be moved straight through the CCS and treatment provided *en route* by first-aiders.

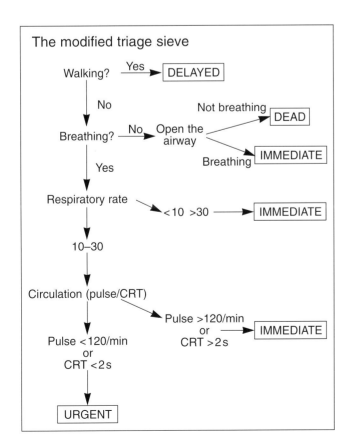

Helicopters have three main uses at a major incident:

- transport of key personnel, including medical teams, to the scene;
- aerial reconnaissance;
- casualty transport.

Helicopters have limited capacity, offer little opportunity to treat the casualty in flight, are cold, noisy, and vibrate; additionally, changes in altitude may adversely affect the patient's condition. They can, however, access remote places and cover large distances in a short time. Helicopters should generally be reserved for the transport of specific injuries to a distant specialist centre (see Chapter 24).

When the best form of transport is being considered, it is useful to think of "CASMOVE" (see box).

Factors to consider when transporting a casualty	
● Capacity	How many patients can it carry?
● Availability	Can I get hold of one?
● Suitability	Is it suitable for this patient, for this terrain, and for the distance of journey?
● Move	Move directly to appropriate hospital (avoid secondary transfer)
● Observe	What observations are needed during transport?
● Verify	Verify treatment before transport: enough O_2, fluids, analgesia?
● Escort	Does the patient need a paramedic, nurse or doctor escort?

Hospital response: the first few hours

Initial response

In December 1988 a rail crash at Clapham, London, killed 35 and injured 115. The main receiving hospital was not prepared for the influx of casualties because of confusion with a colour-coded major incident alert given to the hospital switchboard. Major incident warnings are now standardised nationally (see box).

National major incident alerting procedure
● **Major incident: standby**
● major incident not confirmed
● inform key staff only
● do not activate hospital plan
● **Major incident declared: activate plan**
● major incident is confirmed
● hospital major incident procedure to be instituted
● **Major incident: cancelled**
● overrides previous activation
● hospital to return to normal daily activity status

Warning may be through the hospital switchboard, who will then contact Ambulance Control to confirm, or directly to the A & E department, who must immediately instruct switchboard to notify key staff. The switchboard cannot call every member of staff, and a cascade system is often used: one member of staff will notify the next, and so on. On arrival staff should go to the medical and nursing reporting points, from where they will be assigned to a treatment, transfer, or operating team.

Command and control

The hospital's response is controlled by the Medical Coordinator, a senior clinician (often a physician), who heads the Hospital Coordination Team (see box).

Hospital coordination team at the hospital control room
● Medical Co-ordinator
● Chief Triage Officer
● Senior Nurse Manager
● Senior Hospital Manager

The Hospital Coordination Team will operate from the Hospital Control Room. Action cards should be made available for all those with key roles in the hospital's response, together with an identifying tabard. Immediate priorities for the hospital are to ensure a Mobile Medical Team is ready if requested, to prepare casualty reception areas, to prepare the operating theatres, and to clear postoperative beds (low dependency patients may be sent home, and surgical patients moved to medical wards). The composition of the Mobile Medical Team is not standardised, but would typically be two doctors and two to four nurses: emergency physicians and nurses are probably the best equipped to function in this environment, because of the least deviation from normal working practice.

The A & E department must still be prepared to provide an emergency service for the rest of the community, but those waiting for attention with minor ailments should be advised to attend their general practitioner or a remote hospital. A sign should be posted outside the A & E department advising that the hospital's major incident plan is in operation.

Safety

The senior hospital manager will place security guards at main entrances to check staff identity. The safety of hospital staff, other than standard precautions against contamination with a patient's blood, is not usually a great concern unless the casualties are contaminated with chemical or radioactive dust/liquid. In these circumstances staff must decontaminate patients (remove clothes; wash thoroughly) before treatment, and those performing decontamination must be adequately protected (see Chapter 21).

Communications

The Ambulance Service is responsible for providing the hospital with communications between central Ambulance Control, and the Ambulance Emergency Control Vehicle (ECV) at the scene. An Ambulance Liaison Officer will assist with radio communications and set up a VHF radio, if one is not fitted in the A & E department. Attempts to contact the Medical Incident Officer directly by radio or mobile telephone should be discouraged: detailed casualty information is not required, only casualty numbers, triage priorities, and estimated arrival times, which can be obtained through the Ambulance ECV via central Control. The hospital administration is responsible for providing adequate internal communications. Additional external and internal lines must be available for the Control Room, together with a dedicated facsimile. The Police Hospital Documentation Team will require a room with telephone and facsimile facilities: they will relay information on all those treated (admitted or discharged) to the Police Casualty Bureau. The hospital's plan should include guidelines on how to request an emergency radio or local television broadcast to alert staff.

Triage

All casualties will be retriaged on arrival at hospital. This is coordinated by the Chief Triage Officer (senior emergency physician). Documentation will now start in hospital notes, which should have a characteristic series of numbers. It is important that all surgical decisions are accurate and consistent: the duty consultant surgeon will therefore act as the Surgical Triage Officer and make all triage decisions on priorities for emergency surgery. He will liaise closely with the senior surgeons in charge of the operating teams. Medical problems are also common following a major incident. The duty consultant physician or intensivist will act as the Medical Triage Officer, and determine the treatment priorities of the non-surgical patients. A surgical triage registrar and medical triage registrar will be delegated to determine treatment priorities in the "delayed" treatment area.

Treatment

The first casualties to arrive at hospital will often be the minor injured who have transported themselves. Each hospital plan will identify the immediate, urgent, and delayed treatment areas. The dead will not be brought to the A & E department, but taken directly to the temporary mortuary. Resuscitation follows standard "ABC" principles. The Team Coordinator in the A & E department will be sent staff to assign to treatment or transfer teams. As there will be many staff in the A & E department who are unfamiliar with its layout, regular A & E nursing staff should be identified by a coloured tabard or armband, as they can quickly locate specific items. These staff will be most usefully employed in the "immediate" and "urgent" treatment areas.

Unlike normal practice surgery must be limited to life-saving procedures only. The Medical Coordinator must recognise the need to rotate and refresh the surgical teams, which may continue to work long after the A & E department response has finished. Additional surgical teams can be requested from neighbouring hospitals.

Transport

Some patients will require secondary transfer. Ideally, those with isolated specific injuries such as a spinal injury, closed head injury, or burns will be transported from the scene directly to a specialist centre, but this will not always be the case. Furthermore, the need for intensive care may be initially underestimated, or a patient may deteriorate who requires intensive care when all the resources are used. If the hospital accepting the patient is not a main receiving hospital for the incident, then a medical retrieval team and ambulance should be sent from the accepting hospital. In the UK there is no medical appointment to coordinate interhospital transfers. As an example in New South Wales, a Medical Retrieval

Consultant works with the Medical Controller in the Disaster Medical Control Centre. This doctor continually assesses the bed state of the receiving hospitals and coordinates staff and transport for interhospital transfers.

Continuing scene management

Areas of responsibility

Police

The police retain overall control. The identity of all health care personnel will be checked on arrival: without identification admission may be refused. A Survivor Reception Centre is set up inside the "silver" area, where uninjured survivors can be documented. Those requiring temporary accommodation are moved to a Rest Centre (outside the "silver" area); a Relatives' Reception Centre can be co-located with this, where the survivors are reunited with family who come to the scene. A Casualty Bureau is established to collate and distribute information on the injured and dead. The police will gather the media at a media liaison point, and appoint a media liaison officer to provide them with regular statements and key personnel to interview: failure to do this will encourage the media to take their own initiative. The police are responsible for all volunteers on the scene.

Ambulance and medical

Command roles must be filled at the scene at the expense of providing treatment officers. Table 23.5 shows the ambulance and medical command appointments.

Table 23.5 Ambulance and medical command appointments

Ambulance	Medical
Ambulance Incident Officer	Medical Incident Officer
Ambulance Parking Officer	
Ambulance Loading Officer	
Ambulance Communications Officer	
Primary Triage Officer	Secondary Triage Officer
Casualty Clearing Officer	Casualty Clearing Station Doctor in charge
Forward Ambulance Incident Officer	Forward Medical Incident Officer
Ambulance Safety Officer	

An ambulance and medical presence will be maintained at the scene until it is declared closed by the police. If medical teams are surplus at the scene, the MIO should return them to their base hospitals or redeploy them to assist with resuscitation at the receiving hospitals. Additional surgical teams may be valuable at the receiving hospitals, but as there is usually no "gold" Medical Controller to coordinate such requests in the UK, the teams would have to be negotiated between individual hospitals.

Fire Service

Rescue is the province of the Fire Service in the UK. No other service carries rescue equipment. In contrast, in New South Wales rescue can be performed by any service unit accredited with the State Rescue and Emergency Services

Board. In a particular area this may be provided by a professional unit (Police Rescue Squad; Fire Service; [Ambulance] Special Casualty Access Team) or a volunteer organisation (State Emergency Services; Volunteer Rescue Association). Amputation is rarely necessary to assist extrication, but should this be necessary a Mobile Surgical Team is called from the hospital to perform the procedure. The Fire Service are highly resourceful and will assist with additional lighting and makeshift shelters, and will facilitate easy movement around difficult terrain. When the hazards are secured the Fire Incident Officer may release personnel to assist with first-aid and stretcher-bearing.

Casualty treatment and distribution

The Medical and Ambulance Incident Officers will continually reassess the incident to ensure an adequate health services response. Hospitals from an increasingly greater distance may be alerted to receive casualties, or provide a medical team; adjacent ambulance services may be asked to provide personnel, vehicles, or equipment. The St John Ambulance (or St Andrew in Scotland) and Red Cross can provide patient transport vehicles or personnel to assist with first-aid and stretcher-bearing, and drivers. In Australia the State Emergency Service and Volunteer Rescue Association (New South Wales only) are also a resource trained in advanced first aid.

The dead

The police are responsible for identifying the dead through the Police Identification Commission, and for moving the bodies to the *temporary mortuary* for pathological examination. The temporary mortuary is usually remote from the scene, and bodies are transferred from a *body holding area* at the scene. The dead should only be moved prior to authorisation by the police Scenes of Crime Officer (SOCO) when the body is preventing access to the living or is in imminent danger of being destroyed by fire or corrosive chemical. A doctor must pronounce death, and should do so in the presence of a police officer. A white or black triage label can then be attached to each victim.

Team welfare

The MIO has an overall responsibility for the welfare of medical and nursing personnel. Stress amongst staff is inevitable during a major incident and preparation involving exercises, an understanding of the normal psychological response to an abnormal situation, and a realistic expectation of task performance will help to reduce this. A team member's performance will be enhanced if he is briefed and rebriefed, priorities are clearly stated, if he communicates with his team mates, and if his physical needs are met (food, drink, sleep). At a simple compensated incident (such as a rail crash) it would be usual to relieve staff every four hours with a new team; at a protracted or uncompensated incident (such as a flood or earthquake) it may be necessary to rotate limited staff every four hours.

Individuals who are showing signs of "critical incident stress" should be withdrawn, but debriefed before they leave the scene. Professional counsellors can be part of the medical response to the scene and provide psychological debriefing to all participants at the incident site, as well as coordinating the post-incident counselling (see Chapter 16). This system is in operation in New South Wales where the area health service

Director of Disaster Counselling is mobilised by the Medical Controller.

Humans function as low-capacity single-channel information processors. Specifically, performance of one task will reduce the performance of another simultaneous task. For example, if the MIO is monitoring the radio or watching the development of the incident through binoculars, he will not hear what the Ambulance Incident Officer says. Performance can be increased by regular practice, so that initial actions are performed as a drill, leaving more capacity to make decisions; an aide memoire may also assist in structuring priorities, and reduce unnecessary thinking – an example is the *Management Master* [5].

Support services

Local authority

The local authority can provide heavy plant equipment, such as bulldozers and cranes, and portable toilets or prefabricated buildings in protracted incidents. Accommodation and catering will be given to the temporarily homeless, together with social services support. In the recovery phase the local authority will clear debris and support the community in its slow return to normality.

Volunteer organisations

The Voluntary Aid Societies and BASICS have already been mentioned. Catering can be provided by the Salvation Army or the Women's Royal Voluntary Service (or Country Women's Association in rural Australia). Alternative communication systems are offered by the Radio Amateurs Network (RAYNET), but care must be taken to monitor all transmissions to maintain control; in New South Wales the Wireless Institute Civil Emergency Network (WICEN) provides HF, VHF and UHF bands and the Citizens' Radio Emergency Service Teams (CREST) provides CB bands; both are part of the Volunteer Rescue Association. The Australian Red Cross operates a disaster blood transfusion service, assists the police with survivor registration at the Survivor Reception Centre, and provides volunteers for the State Disaster Inquiry Centre (the equivalent of the Casualty Bureau).

Communication companies

British Telecom or Telecom Australia can provide additional mobile telephones, a field telephone system, or lay supplementary landlines – the latter requiring about one day. Payphones can be converted into "no charge" telephones.

Military

Multiple disciplined personnel, field canteens, tentage, engineering (such as bridging), medical resources, and vehicles are some of the ways the military can assist at a major incident. Military help is requested through the Police Incident Officer.

Continuing hospital management

A major incident can disturb the working of a hospital for weeks or months. Routine surgical lists will be cancelled to allow definitive general surgical, orthopaedic, and plastic surgery procedures for the injured. Outpatient clinics may continue to follow these patients for years.

Hospital information centre

Information on all casualties admitted, or treated and discharged from the accident and emergency department, is centralised and regularly updated in the hospital information centre. All enquiries from relatives, friends, or other agencies are directed to this centre.

Media

A nominated area for the media is advisable, with telephone and refreshment facilities. Regular bulletins from the media liaison officer, and interviews with key personnel, should be timed to coincide with editorial and broadcast deadlines (for example, half an hour before the lunchtime news). It is important to avoid suppositions of cause, or apportioning of blame, as this may influence subsequent judicial hearings. A prepared statement is the safest. VIP visits should also be anticipated. Briefings should be positive: there will be plenty of people who will offer criticism of your best efforts.

Transfusion service

Blood and blood product stores will rapidly be depleted within the hospital. Should cross-matched blood not be used (if, for example, the patient dies) inform the blood bank immediately so that the units may be made available for someone else. The public will often attend their local hospital to give blood when they hear of an incident; the National Blood Transfusion Service can send a mobile unit to the hospital or to the scene, which not only provides a blood harvesting service but also a resource for equipment and fluids for intravenous resuscitation.

The aftermath

A major incident will have psychological effects on the helpers, and the victims.

Helpers

Support will be required for all emergency service personnel. Common symptoms of "critical incident stress" are physical, cognitive, emotional, behavioural, and perceptual (see box).

Symptoms of critical incident stress	
● Physical	Nausea, diarrhoea, tachycardia, sweating, dizziness, headache, fatigue
● Cognitive	Poor concentration, difficulty making decisions or naming familiar people/objects, intrusive thoughts (Why me? What if? If only . . .)
● Emotional	Disbelief, fear of loss of control, a need for information or understanding
● Behavioural	Restlessness, irritability, insomnia, hyperstartle
● Perceptual	World looks more dangerous, daily issues seem trivial, hallucinations

The event is often re-experienced in flashbacks or nightmares. These symptoms are also referred to as post-traumatic stress disorder (PTSD) (see Chapter 16).

Debriefing is important in reducing the impact of critical incident stress and is made in stages:

- Support during the incident.
- Each medical team debriefed by the Medical Team Leader.
- All medical teams debriefed by the Medical Incident Officer before leaving the site.
- Formal debriefing of medical team members at 24–72 hours.
- Continued support for individuals.

Support during the incident may be from professional counsellors, or given as "tea and sympathy" from the Salvation Army, Red Cross, or Women's Royal Voluntary Service. Some team members may miss the site debriefing if they have accompanied patients to hospital; the site debrief must be very short as people will be eager to get home.

Tactical debriefings will occur within each emergency service, between emergency services, at the hospital, and at the regional health authority. Lessons from the incident should be incorporated as changes in the regional and hospital plans.

Victims

There are usually more psychological injuries than physical injuries following a major incident. Those delivering the support require specific training in disaster counselling. Initial support will be given in the Survivor Reception Centre: this can be information, or physical, financial, and spiritual support, as well as psychological help. The emphasis with psychological support lies in making the individual understand they are not "crazy", but their feelings are a normal response to an abnormal situation. A support centre set up in a local community may stay open for months or years, but the psychological problems are not confined to the local community: survivors of a rail disaster in London may be in Cardiff or Edinburgh the following day. Registration information should be used to inform local support agencies (general practitioner, counselling services).

Injured victims treated at hospital will have critical incident stress and this aspect of their hospital treatment should not be ignored.

References

1. Department of Health New South Wales. *New South Wales Multiple Casualty, Emergency and Disaster Medical Response Plan (MEDPLAN)*. Sydney: Department of Health, 1990.
2. NHS Executive. *Emergency planning in the NHS: Health Services arrangements for dealing with major incidents*, vol. 1. London: Department of Health, 1996.
3. Fennell D. *Investigation into the King's Cross Underground fire*. London: HMSO, 1988.
4. New B. *Too many cooks? The response of the health-related services to major incidents in London*. London: King's Fund Institute, 1992.
5. Hodgetts TJ, McNeil I, Cooke MW. *The pre-hospital emergency Management Master*. London: British Medical Journal Publishing, 1995.

Further reading

Hodgetts TJ, Mackway-Jones K (eds). *Major incident medical management and support: the practical approach*. London: British Medical Journal Publishing, 1995.

24 Stabilisation and transport

Richard J. Fairhurst
Past Chairman British Association for Immediate Care, Consultant In Accident and Emergency Medicine, Chorley and South Ribble District General Hospital

Jim Ryan
Leonard Cheshire Professor of Conflict Recovery, University College London

OBJECTIVES

- To analyse the patients needs.

- To discuss points of consultation between senior referral and receiving doctors over the most appropriate place to treat the patient.

- To analyse the risks versus the benefits of transfer.

- To help select the most appropriate mode of transport.

- To help plan the schedule carefully.

- To list equipment and drugs needed.

- To describe stabilisation and packaging of the patient for transport.

- To discuss monitoring and interventions during transport.

- To list handovers and documentation.

Following the initial management in the resuscitation room, trauma victims must be moved to the next stage in the treatment process. This entails stabilisation and transportation. It is vital that the same care and attention used in the initial resuscitation is given to these processes, whether the patient is going to the next door operating theatre or is flown way round the world.

Patient's needs

During the primary and secondary survey the immediate life-threatening injuries will have been identified and treated, and other injuries identified and documented. There should then follow a consultation between the team leader and the senior hospital staff on both the priorities for further investigation and intervention. This must include a frank appraisal of the capabilities of the individual practitioners and those of the hospital and its nursing, paramedical and rehabilitation staff. It may be that the patient can be managed entirely in the original receiving unit, or needs transfer at an appropriate stage for reconstructive surgery or rehabilitation. Nevertheless, at whatever stage it is decided to transfer the patient, it must be done without further damage. In multisystem trauma, priorities for treatment are vital. The massively deformed limb is not the priority when the patient has a major abdominal haemorrhage from a ruptured liver. In these circumstances the team leader must not be swayed by the seniority or the assertiveness of the surgeons present. Therefore, throughout the process, the patient must be reassessed and any deterioration re-evaluated from the point of view of ABCDE.

Consultation over the appropriate place for treatment

Ideally every patient should be treated in the hospital capable of delivering the highest levels of care. Unfortunately not all hospitals have all the major treatment or indeed investigative facilities for a patient with multisystem trauma. It is a historical accident in the United Kingdom that many specialised units – neurosurgery, cardiothoracic surgery, or spinal injury – are in single specialty hospitals, where patients with multisystem needs may be at major risk. In these circumstances consultation is vital, and should never be delegated to junior staff. The sending of appropriate imaging to the receiving consultant should always be considered. **If, following discussion, doubt remains, consider transferring the surgeon, rather than the patient**.

Not only the appropriate place for treatment should be considered, but also the appropriate timing. For example, the optimal time for severely burnt patients is 24–48 hours after resuscitation, before any of the metabolic or infective problems increase.

The reasons for transfer are not only strictly medical. A whole range of economic, social, and ethical factors come into play. Consequently, the consultation may involve relatives, purchasers of care, and even third parties. Various factors can be considered.

- If a patient is in hospital many miles from home or relatives, then this is one indication for patient transfer at a suitable time to the home town so that relatives and friends may play their proper part in treatment and rehabilitation. There are strong reasons for transporting a patient who is in a foreign country with different styles of health care, different social mores, and a language unknown to the patient or relatives, for example soldiers and UN personnel injured in Bosnia transferred to the UK for treatment.

- If the patient is terminally ill or injured it may be a kindness to request a transfer near to, or indeed, home.
- In these days of contracts, pressure may be applied by purchasers to move a patient to a particular hospital. This is already happening in the United States where health insurance providers will move a patient from one hospital to another simply to save costs. In Europe travel insurers have tried to insist on moving seriously ill patients from excellent but expensive hospitals in North America to Europe, simply to save a claims cost.
- A patient may be transported for transplant reasons. The transport of the potential recipient approximates to the usual medical needs evaluation. The transport of the potential donor, however, can raise ethical problems unless there is an agreed local policy.

Analysis of the risks versus the benefits of transport

Primary receiving hospitals have variable resources, thus the risk to the patient remaining in the primary receiving hospital is variable; furthermore, it is not possible to quantify risk related to any physiological or anatomical scoring system except in the crudest of ways. However, if the patient is at risk of certain death in his current location, and transport and intervention would result in good quality survival, then a higher level of risk can be accepted than where the gains from treatment are equivocal, or where there is no prospect of survival. When economic factors are put into this equation the risk is not only to the patient, but to the transporting, referring, and receiving doctors. To transfer a patient who has major medical needs to another hospital is a medical decision: if the doctors do not take that decision in the best medical interests of the patient, but simply in the financial interests of a third party, they are placing themselves at severe risk of litigation in the event of an untoward incident [1].

Selection of the most appropriate mode of transport

The overriding principles are that risk is proportional to the duration of transport, and that no harm must be done. It follows then that transport time must be kept to a minimum. Transport time is defined as the time elapsed between leaving one hospital bed to arriving in another, and not simply the time spent in an ambulance or a helicopter. Each mode of transport has its own advantages and disadvantages.

Hospital trolleys

Trolleys must have a stable platform, hard base for cardiopulmonary resuscitation, cot sides, large wheels with good castor action, variable height, possibility of tipping, oxygen with flow meter and high pressure outlets, suction, and an infusion pole. The transport team should not also be the motive power. The route should be preplanned to take the minimum time. Lifts must be held along the route prior to departing and major changes in surfaces avoided. They may be used for a distance of up to a kilometre and for multiple storeys in elevators.

Road ambulances

There are many types of conversions of commercially available vehicles, but those based on estate cars should be avoided because of lack of space. The typical light van conversion has a central self-loading trolley and access to both sides of the patient and the head (Figure 24.1). There must be communication between the patient area and the driver and with

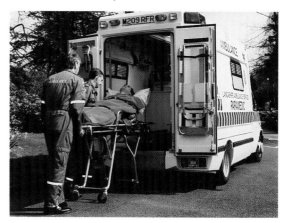

Figure 24.1 Paramedic ambulance.

both referring and receiving hospital. In some areas "mobile intensive care units" are available: these tend to be larger vehicles with more storage space for equipment, working space for the transport team, and a more dramatic painting scheme (Figure 24.2). The wide differences in types makes close enquiry

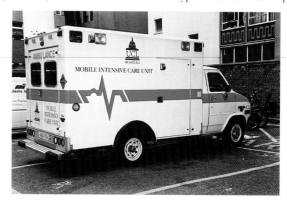

Figure 24.2 Mobile intensive care unit.

when requesting a road ambulance mandatory. Particular attention needs to be paid to volume of oxygen available, flowmeter, high pressure or both, exact specification of connectors, compatibility of defibrillator monitor systems, electrical power outputs, voltages, amperage, and plug types. Road ambulances may be the best means of transport for up to 100 km in good conditions, but are very dependent on traffic density. In central London the speed of a blue light ambulance may only be 25 kph. The vehicle driver should never be part of the patient care team but should instead concentrate on providing a smooth ride. The driver can change routes and destinations with ease if the patient's condition changes. Forces acting on the patient may be higher than in an aircraft, particularly deceleration on braking and vertical acceleration on hitting a pot hole [2]. Although a tradition has grown up in the ambulance service of transporting spinal injury patients at walking speed, this is an error and the ride is smoothest at the design speed of the suspension, that is 50–80 kph. Police escorts can be used to smooth out the progress rather than to increase speeds.

Helicopters

The few dedicated purpose-built helicopters available in the UK are normally tasked for primary rescue. They may not therefore be ideal in terms of space and equipment for secondary transport (Figure 24.3). Commercial helicopters

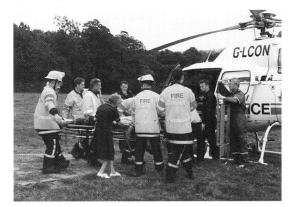

Figure 24.3   Twin Squirrel performing secondary transport.

chartered on the *ad hoc* market can be very small, have only a basic stretcher and no power supplies or oxygen. Military helicopters used for interhospital transfers are large and expensive. However, their advantages in carrying several stretchers are not significant in peace time. In Germany experiments are proceeding with dedicated large helicopters for secondary transport, although the costs involved are likely to preclude further development [3]. Helicopters are the most costly aircraft in terms of fuel used per kilometre of transport as they consume energy to produce an airfoil. In level cruise, a Beechcraft King Air 200 fixed wing consumes 225 kg fuel whilst it covers 483 km in one hour. In contrast an Aerospatiale Dauphin 2 helicopter (Figure 24.4) consumes 260 kg fuel/h

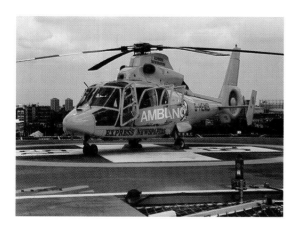

Figure 24.4   Dauphine 2 primary response helicopter.

while it covers 241 km Although these helicopters are able to operate from unmade sites, these sites have to be clear of obstructions. There are also limitations owing to weather, although these may not be so severe as perceived. In the four years between 1 March 1991 and 2 February 1995, only 21 days were lost by HEMS in London to adverse weather. Operations are, however, limited to daylight hours except in certain clearly defined situations. As helicopters operate at relatively low altitude, considerations of oxygen partial pressure and dysbarism are not relevant unless they are operating in mountainous terrain (Figure 24.5). Noise and vibration can

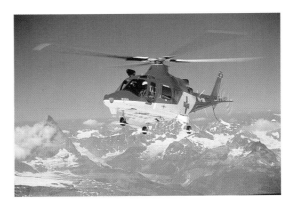

Figure 24.5   Augusta 108.

be uncomfortable, and both the transport team and the patient should wear headsets to protect their hearing and for communication. The rotor blades produce low cycle flicker which may be an epileptiform stimulus.

Fixed wing air ambulances

Very few dedicated air ambulances exist. The most sophisticated are operated by REGA from Zurich. They have a Challenger 601 with intercontinental range, capable of carrying two high dependency and two stretcher patients at the same time (Figure 24.6). The equipment is sophisticated and

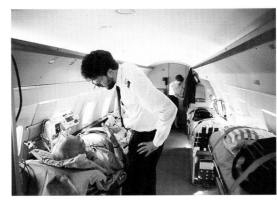

Figure 24.6   Canadair CL601. Large interior with two intensive care places, piped gases, and 240 V electrics.

includes on-board oxygen generation and special loading systems. The same organisation also operates British Aerospace 125–800 series (Figure 24.7). Scottish Ambulance Service operate dedicated Beechcraft King Air 200 s (Figure 24.8) and

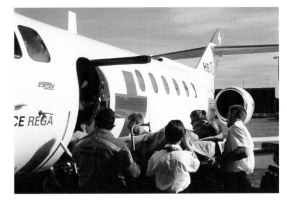

Figure 24.7   British Aerospace 125–800. Note the cantilever loading crane and electric hoist.

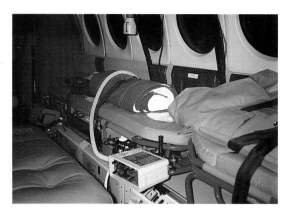

Figure 24.8 B200 King Air, showing the Life Port loading system. Note the "Transpac" ventilator, piped oxygen, and 240 V power via inverters.

Brittain Norman Islanders (Figure 24.9). All other aircraft are

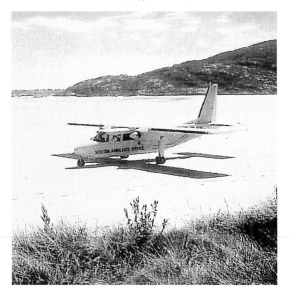

Figure 24.9 Brittain Norman Islander.

on *ad hoc* charter and modified for the air ambulance role. Great care must therefore be exercised to check exactly what facilities will be supplied. Air ambulances need fixed airfields and their use will almost always require relay with land ambulances at either end of the flight. From a medical point of view the big variables are speed, weather, and whether the aircraft is capable of pressurisation. Speed is only a factor on flights of more than 500 km. Below this the problems of approach, climb out, and air traffic mean that an aircraft with a cruising speed of 550 kph will not complete the journey any

faster than one with a cruising speed of 300 kph (Table 24.1). This is illustrated by the fact that the scheduled flight time between London and Paris was shorter in 1950 than in 1995! Unpressurised aircraft are limited to a height of 10 000 ft unless all the passengers are breathing oxygen, and are thus much more at the mercy of the weather than a pressurised aircraft, which can maintain a cabin altitude of 8000 ft up to 41 000 ft or 55 000 ft in the case of Concorde. Thus with a pressurised aircraft it is possible to transport the patients with a sea-level cabin altitude by choosing a lower flight level. Reputable air ambulance companies operate to the standards published in the *Journal of the Royal Society of Medicine* [4].

Airlines

Over very long distances airlines can provide the most comfortable means of transferring the patient; however, their use requires careful planning. The schedules are fixed and routes may require relays with road ambulances or air ambulances. The key to success is careful planning and cooperation with the airline medical department. The airline may decline carriage not for reasons of patient safety, but because of the acceptability of the patient to the rest of their fare-paying passengers. At small airports there may not be the loading facilities to lift stretcher patients safely onto a wide-bodied aircraft. Once on the aircraft the stretcher is rigged above the seats separated from the other passengers by a curtain (Figure 24.10). Lufthansa are currently experimenting with a patient transfer module, but logistic considerations make its use impractical.

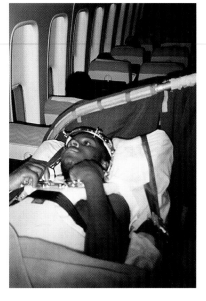

Figure 24.10 B747 with stretcher rigged. Note the minimal privacy curtains and close proximity of other passengers.

Boats

Marine transport is still used in areas such as the Channel Islands (Figure 24.11) and Venice. They are clearly susceptible to weather and tides, and loading can be hazardous. The main problems are the small dimensions of hatches and doors and the steepness of steps. The patient must be secured on a rigid platform which can be tipped and, although there are many newer devices, the Neils Robertson stretcher is still preferred by the Royal National Lifeboat Institution.

Table 24.1 Useful ranges of various types of aircraft used for rescue

Type	Altitude (feet)	Speed (mph)	Maximum flight time (hours)	Destination (from London)
Helicopter (unpressurised)	2 000	150	1.00	Birmingham
Piston engine (unpressurised)	8 000	200	2.00	Edinburgh
Turboprop (pressurised)	24 000	300	3.00	Madrid
Jet (pressurised)	36 000	550	2.75 +	Gibraltar

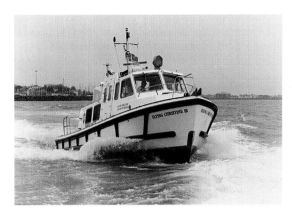

Figure 24.11 "Flying Christine" ambulance launch in the Channel Isles.

Trains

Hospital trains have a distinguished history and it is only in the last two years that the British Army Hospital trains in Germany have been withdrawn. In France the SAMU has used trains for burn and limb injury transport, but the introduction of open plan rolling stock has now made this form of transport difficult.

Planning the schedule

When an urgent transfer is agreed the temptation is to undertake the mission as soon as possible. Whilst with simple transfers in land ambulances this may be possible, due regard must be paid to factors such as traffic, time of day (patients transferred in the early hours have an increased morbidity [5]), and the time that the bed will be available at the receiving hospital. The principle is that any sources of delay are anticipated and planned for. The patient will then be moved in a smooth and continuous way into the new bed. If aircraft are to be used the weather and daylight become crucial to the safety of the patient. It is unacceptable to take any risks with minimum flight criteria.

If relays of modes of transfer are to be used then the minimum number of lifts from trolley to trolley must be used. At these times of loading and unloading, the patient is very vulnerable, and the simple unnoticed detachment of a lead or a hose can be fatal.

When long-distance transport by airline is used, scheduling is very difficult. The benefits of rests in hospital at intermediate stops has to be weighed against the desire to complete the transfer. Often the flight crew and the medical crew is changed, but the patient who is even more susceptible to fatigue goes the whole way.

The planning must include the return of the team and their equipment to base and the return of any equipment supplied by the referring hospital. This may be difficult in long-distance transfers involving much complex scheduling. Airlines which may have been very happy to carry several tons of equipment with the patient may take a totally different view when the same equipment is being returned to base, and excess baggage charges may seem like a ransom. Road ambulances may be unable to wait for handovers, or be retasked. Arrangements need to be made for taxi retrieval, and remember that a team and its equipment may need several vehicles.

The transfer team

The dangerous practice of junior staff from the referring hospital accompanying patients no longer has a place. These patients must be transferred with a minimum of two escorts, one of whom should be fully trained in any of the patient's medical requirements. Inevitably this means that most of the escorts are anaesthetists or intensive care physicians. In the United Kingdom the second team member is traditionally a nurse, though ODAs and ambulance paramedics can be used.

In France it was recognised that the problems of transport required specialist knowledge and training and in the 1960s SAMU introduced specialised transport teams [6]. This approach is particularly valuable if aircraft are used when specific knowledge of the aviation environment and how it affects sick patients is required. The other advantage of specialised teams is the regular teamwork, not just of the medical crew, but also the pilots, ambulance drivers, and controllers.

There are very specific conditions when highly specialised transport teams must be used, for example for neonates, paediatrics, extracorporeal membrane oxygenation, and transfer under hyperbaric pressure.

It is vital that the transfer team accompanies the patient from hospital bed to hospital bed. The team members should prepare and stabilise the patient on the transfer equipment before leaving the hospital. They should also receive the handover and collect the notes, handing them personally to the receiving doctors. It may be that a relative has been intimately involved with the patient in the referring hospital and consideration should be given to transferring them with the patient.

Equipment

All equipment used must be:

- portable, small, lightweight with full relevant facilities, and a display visible in a varying background light level;
- rugged, resistant to impact and vibration, have no fragile protruding parts, and be able to operate in a wide range of pressure, temperature, and humidity;
- reliable – it will be used infrequently, at short notice, far from spares or servicing;
- restrainable – it must be capable of restraint, so there is no risk of movement on acceleration;
- independent – it must have adequate power supplies for the projected length of transport, including a safe reserve. (In general batteries are used but these require careful maintenance to operate at maximum efficiency. It may be possible to use power from land ambulances or aircraft, but beware of unusual voltages (12 volt dc/28 volt dc/115 volt ac) and unusual frequencies (400 hz));
- compatible. Movement artifact on monitors is common. Pulse oximeter probes are very susceptible to varying light levels. Mercury is banned in aircraft as are unsealed lead acid batteries. Electromechanical incompatibility is a more potential problem in aircraft particularly with the advent of "fly by wire" technology. All electrical equipment for use on aircraft must be cleared before starting the transfer.

Individual major items

Ventilators

Gas drive fluid logic machines such as the Pneupack Transpack, Air Liquide Osiris and Dager Oxylog are commonly used. Their drive power is compressed oxygen, and oxygen consumption is a vital consideration (Figure 24.12). Ventures

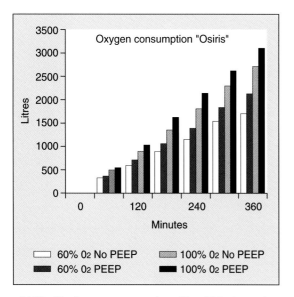

Figure 24.12 Ventilator gas consumption with a tidal volume of 700 ml and a frequency of 10 cycles per minute.

are usually fitted to entrain air, reducing oxygen consumption and giving an $F_{i_{O_2}}$ of 40%. Electrically driven ventilators such as the Bear 33 do not need compressed oxygen, but their relative complexity raises questions of reliability and safety during transport. All ventilators should always be backed up with a self-inflating bag. Disconnect alarms (which must be audible as well as visible) are advisable as is a spirometer. The trend is to monitor the patient rather than the ventilator, thus pulse oximetry and end-tidal CO_2 monitors increase safety. Oxygen monitors cause problems on aircraft because they measure oxygen partial pressure but display this as a percentage assuming normal atmospheric pressure. In flight the displays should be interpreted with the help of an altimeter.

Monitors

New generation monitors, such as the Propac, provide many functions in one machine with a liquid crystal display. It is convenient to display ECG, temperature, oxygen saturation, end-tidal carbon dioxide, and invasive pressure all on one machine that also stores a five-hour trend. However, there is only one battery, and spare power must be available. It is worth noting here that non-invasive blood pressure monitoring and LCD lights are very heavy consumers of battery power. The Propac 106 can operate for 30 hours in power-save mode; this is reduced to 6.5 hours if the back light is on and non-invasive blood pressure is used every 15 minutes [7].

Oxygen

Oxygen is normally carried in compressed cylinders and these must be restrained; all high pressure fittings must be compatible. Recently, liquid oxygen has been used but its limited availability and its slow evaporation are likely to restrict its wider application. This is unfortunate in view of its advantages in terms of weight and volume.

Suction

Gas-powered suction should be avoided. Electric suction should be backed up with a manual pump.

Infusion devices

Syringe pumps work well as do volumetric devices, but care is needed to avoid syphoning and, in view of the latest warnings about interference from cellular telephones, there must be assumed to be a risk from all radio transmissions.

Communications

Cellular radios allow direct communication between the transport team and hospitals. Road ambulances should allow talk through to hospitals via their radio system. With the introduction of digital cellular networks they can be used during international transfers. However, it must be remembered that it is illegal, a breach of the air navigation orders, and potentially dangerous to use a cellular telephone in any type of aircraft. HF radio with Selcall allows patch-through via Portishead, Berna, or Stockholm radio from aircraft.

Stretcher systems

Ideally the patient and his equipment should be loaded onto a stretcher at the referring hospital and remain on it until the receiving hospital. This is achieved with a secondary device such as a scoop stretcher or lightweight aluminium stretcher covered with either a vacuum mattress or a highloft mattress.

The equipment is mounted on a bridge attached to the stretcher, and only high pressure oxygen lines should be trailing. This ensures that compact package of patient and equipment can be safely lifted.

A recent development is the Life Port (see Figure 24.8) loading system which allows easy loading of stretchers onto suitably fitted small aircraft. The use of such devices is to be commended.

Ancillary equipment and drugs

The boxes (overleaf) show equipment and drug lists for an intensive care transport.

Stabilisation and packaging

Prior to transport the patient should have been resuscitated and any life-threatening problems dealt with and documented. Procedures may have been as simple as using an oropharyngeal airway, or as problematical as a laparotomy with packing of the liver and closure of the abdomen with towel clips. Whatever the procedure, it must have been carefully documented, so that the receiving hospital can confidently proceed with investigation and treatment. The transport team should reassess the patient according to ABCDE principles and repeat any relevant investigations, in particular blood gases. This reassessment must include an appreciation of transport risks. Motion sickness is a real risk and some of the commonly used antiemetics, metoclopramide or phenothiazines, are ineffective. Hyoscine or antihistamines are preferred [8]. If there is any doubt about the security of the airway or the efficiency of breathing the patient should be electively anaesthetised and ventilated. The patient should be on the safest mode of ventilation, that is continuous mandatory ventilation. None of the weaning or support modes should be used for transport. All hoses and lines must be secured as must any orthopaedic splintage. The patient transport system should consist of a secondary stretcher with a bridge and a vacuum mattress so that the patient and his equipment may be lifted as a single unit (this must be small enough to fit the loading aperture of any vehicle used). The airport is a dangerous place for trying to repackage the patient to fit the aircraft door.

Some specific points should be considered:

- Nasogastric tubes must be well secured to the patient's face and terminated in a drainage bag. This must be anchored to the secondary stretcher and not allowed to dangle.
- Oropharyngeal or nasopharyngeal tubes must be firmly anchored with tape around the patient's neck.
- Endotracheal tubes must have their placement checked and then be securely anchored. All push-fit low pressure connections should be taped and the ventilator must be attached to the secondary stretcher. There must be no possibility of any traction between the patient and the ventilator. Cuff pressures must be checked and, if air transport is being used, inflated with fluid to avoid the pressure changes. Humidification with a Swedish nose should be arranged, but in no circumstances should water reservoir devices be used, owing to the risk of water being syphoned into the patient's lungs or into the ventilator.
- Tracheostomy tubes should be cleaned, suctioned, and checked for adequacy of size, and the cuffs dealt with as above.
- Chest drains must have a waterless valve system, such as the Portex bag or Heimlich valve.
- The placement of central lines must be checked and the giving set secured. The risk of air embolism from open central venous pressure manometers is great and transducers are preferable. All peripheral lines must be secured and fixed to the giving sets. Infusion devices should be fixed to the secondary stretcher and fluid bags must be stabilised to poles at the bottom as well as the top. With all lines there is a major risk of unnoticed haemorrhage should they become detached. This is especially so with arterial lines.
- Electrocardiograph cables must not produce artifact on movement.
- Drains and stoma must be cleaned and drained and wounds dressed with adequate padding.
- New bags must be put onto urinary catheters.
- The spine and limbs must be straightened and immobilised. Weight traction should be avoided. Traction splints work well for legs and with imagination can be used for other

limbs. Spinal injuries can be transported safely in traction with the aid of such devices as the Edgerton Turning frame (Figure 24.13) or the Povey frame.

Finally, the patient must be packaged and well secured with straps (Figure 24.14). During transport the patient may

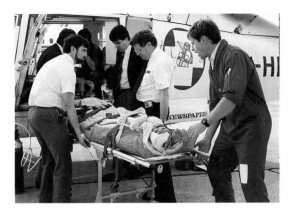

Figure 24.14 A well-packaged patient. Note the vacuum mattress, restraints holding the patient and equipment ("Propac"), long high pressure lead from the oxygen cylinder to the ventilator, and self-inflating bag in case of ventilator failure.

be lifted several times and will feel insecure and exposed if not properly restrained. The vacuum mattress is an excellent device provided that the patient is not lying in any holes in the material, and that it adequately encloses the trauma victim. If it is used in air transport it must be evacuated to the desired pressure and a correction made for the reduction of cabin pressure in flight. Do not forget to wrap the patient up well with blankets: even in summer the transport environment can be cold and wet.

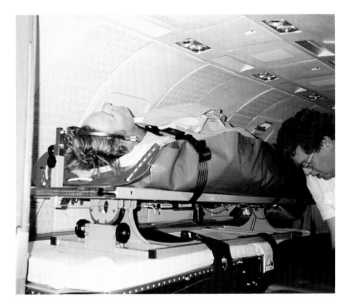

Figure 24.13 Lear Jet 36B. Note the Gardner Wells tongs, spring traction under frame, worm gear to tile the bed 40° to relieve pressure, restraint systems, and lack of space.

Equipment list (1)
- Nursing bag
- Bedding bag
- Vacuum mattress + foot pump
- Spenco mattress
- Scoop stretcher
- Electric suction
- A/A box set
- Infusion pump + bag
- Oxygen
- Pulse oximeter
- Propaq
- LifePak 12
- Spare battery
- Medical bag
- Psychiatric bag
- Burns bag 1 & 2
- Paed nurse's bag 0–1 year
- Paed nurse's bag 1 year up
- Paed Dr bag + i.v. fluid bag
- Paed paddles
- Donway splint

Equipment list (2)

- Sharps box
- i.v. giving set × 2
- Buretrol giving set × 1
- Haemaccel 500 ml × 2
- Sodium chloride 0.9% 500 ml × 2
- Glucose 5% 500 ml × 2
- Glucostix
- Elastoplast roll
- Syringes 20 ml × 2; 10 ml × 5; 5 ml × 5; 2 ml × 5; 1 ml × 2
- Insulin syringe × 2
- Needles 21 g × 2; 23 g × 2; 25 g × 2
- Venflons size 14 × 1; size 17 × 1; size 18 × 1, size 20 × 1; size 22 × 1
- Catheter extension with 3-way tap × 2
- i.v. dressings × 2
- Scissors
- Gauze bandage
- Transpore tape
- Sterile gauze squares
- Tourniquet
- Mediswabs
- Ampoule files
- Elastoplasts
- Tip caps
- Injec Lock
- String for i.v. fluids

Drugs list

- Adenosine 3 mg/ml × 7
- Adrenaline 1:1000 ml × 6
- Aminophylline 250 mg/10 ml × 2
- Amiodarone 50 mg/3 ml × 6
- Atropine 600 μg/ml × 10
- Calcium chloride 13.4% 10 ml × 2
- Chlorpheniramine 10 mg/ml × 2
- Diclofenac sodium 75 mg/3 ml × 2
- Digoxin 500 μg/2 ml × 2
- Dobutamine 250 mg/20 ml × 1
- Doxapram 20 mg/5 ml × 2
- Frusemide 20 mg/2 ml × 5
- Glyceryl trinitrate 25 mg/5 ml × 2
- Hydrocortisone 100 mg × 2
- Isoprenaline 2 mg/2 ml × 2
- Labetalol 100 mg/20 ml × 2
- Lignocaine 1% 10 ml × 2
- Lignocaine 2% 5 ml × 2
- Metoprolol 5 mg/5 ml × 2
- Midazolam 10 mg/2 ml × 10
- Nalbuphine 10 mg/ml × 10
- Naloxone 400 μg/ml × 6

Drugs list–*contd*

- Prochlorperazine 12.5 mg/1 ml × 3
- Propofol 200 mg/20 ml × 3
- Salbutamol 0.25 mg/5 ml × 2
- Sodium chloride 0.9% 10 ml × 7
- Sodium heparin (Hep-Flush) 2 ml × 2
- Suxamethonium 100 mg/2 ml × 3
- Vecuronium 10 mg + water for injection 5 ml × 5

- Glyceryl trinitrate spray × 1
- Glyceryl trinitrate patches 5 mg × 4
- Glucose 50% 50 ml × 1
- Salbutamol inhaler × 1
- Salbutamol respirator solution 20 ml × 1
- Water for injections 10 ml × 10
- Disposable razor × 1
- Adrenaline 1 mg/10 ml Mini-Jet × 1
- Atropine 1 mg/10 ml Mini-Jet × 1
- Chlorhexidine sachets 25 ml × 2

Monitoring and intervention

Once transport is commenced interventions are kept to the minimum and only performed to save life. Monitoring, however, must be continuous and comprehensive. Direct access to the patient is difficult if he is properly packaged; thus the significance of any monitoring must be well appreciated by the transport team who must be particularly aware of movement artifacts. Mouth toilet and pressure areas are important and so is talking to the patient and explaining what you are doing. All changes must be recorded and acted upon. The driver/pilot should be kept informed of the patient's condition, so that the vehicle environment can be changed to suit the patient's needs. In a road ambulance the vehicle should be stopped for patient intervention.

Handover and documentation

The transfer team must go from hospital bed to hospital bed. They must be briefed by the referring doctor and collect all the patient's notes and investigations. The original x-rays, pathology reports, and trauma sheets are much more valuable than summaries, however well written, and in these days of photocopiers this should not be a problem. A well-designed transfer form is a useful aide memoir, and gives all the transport monitoring in a logical manner. Demographic data are just as important as clinical data and are most easily forgotten (Figure 24.15).

At the receiving hospital the handover should be to the senior doctor treating the patient. The aim is to keep the chain of communication as short as possible.

Whilst it is easy to change ventilators and monitors for the return of equipment with the team, such items as external fixators or traction tongs should be left with the patient. Arrangements can be made to recover them later.

Finally there must be feedback of patient information to both the referring hospital and the transfer team, and all transfers should be subject to active clinical audit.

LOGISTICS

Date [ ][ ][ ]   File No [ ]   Doctor _____   Nurse _____

Patient _____ Forename _____ Title _____ D.O.B. [ ][ ][ ] Male [ ] Female [ ]

Address _____

General Practitioner _____

Referring Hospital _____   Receiving Hospital _____

Ward _____   Ward _____

Town _____   Town _____

Country _____   Country _____

Referring Doctor _____   Receiving Doctor _____

From _____   To _____

Departure Time [ ][ ]   Arrival Time [ ][ ] Transport Time [ ] Hr [ ] Min

Air Ambulance:- Jet [ ]   Turboprop [ ]   Piston [ ]   Helicopter [ ]   Type _____

Airline [ ]   1st [ ]   Business [ ]   Tourist [ ]   Cabin Altitude [ ]

Stretcher [ ]   Seated [ ]   Extra Seats [ ]

Road Ambulance [ ]   Type _____   Special Conditions _____

Route _____

Logistical Problems _____

Accompanied by _____   Relationship _____

HISTORY AND PROGRESS

Referral Diagnosis _____

History _____
_____
_____
_____
_____

Previous History _____
_____

Allergies _____

Social _____   Flying Experience _____

Investigations/Operations/Progress _____
_____
_____
_____
_____

CURRENT MEDICATION

Drug	Dose	Frequency	Last Dose	Drug	Dose	Frequency	Last Dose

PRE-FLIGHT ASSESSMENT

B/P [ ]   Pulse [ ]   Respiration [ ]   Coma Scale [ ]   Hb [ ]   Bowels [ ]   Micturition [ ]   Skin [ ]

CVS _____

Resp _____

CNS _____

GI _____

GU _____

MS _____

CURRENT PROBLEMS _____

TRANSPORT PLAN _____

Figure 24.15   Patient transport report. (Courtesy of The Green Flag Travellers Medical Service, Leeds, Yorkshire.)

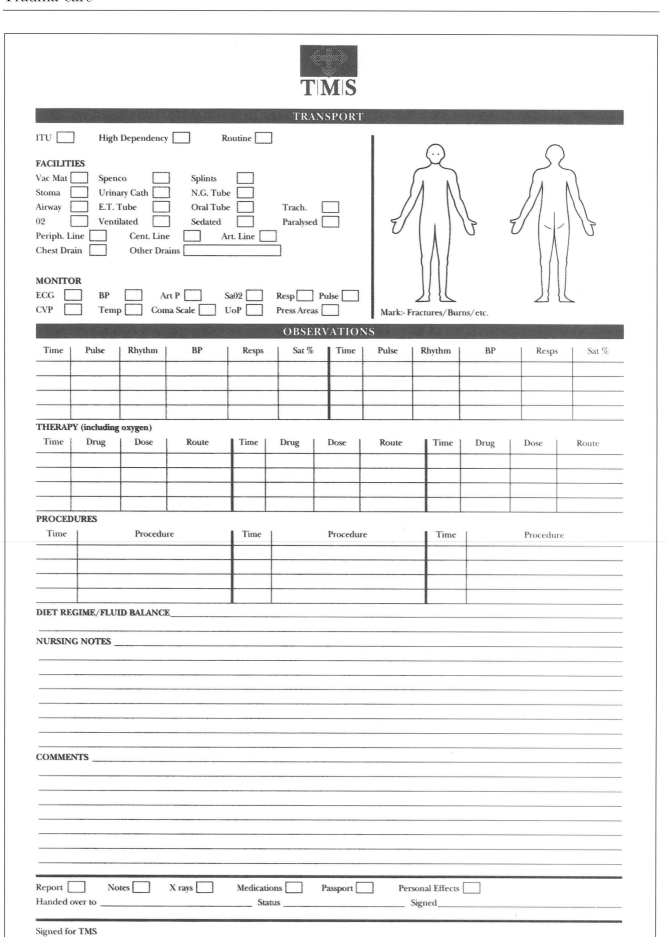

T|M|S

TRANSPORT

ITU ☐   High Dependency ☐   Routine ☐

FACILITIES

Vac Mat ☐	Spenco ☐	Splints ☐		
Stoma ☐	Urinary Cath ☐	N.G. Tube ☐		
Airway ☐	E.T. Tube ☐	Oral Tube ☐	Trach. ☐	
02 ☐	Ventilated ☐	Sedated ☐	Paralysed ☐	

Periph. Line ☐   Cent. Line ☐   Art. Line ☐

Chest Drain ☐   Other Drains ☐

MONITOR

ECG ☐   BP ☐   Art P ☐   Sa02 ☐   Resp ☐   Pulse ☐

CVP ☐   Temp ☐   Coma Scale ☐   UoP ☐   Press Areas ☐

Mark:- Fractures/Burns/etc.

OBSERVATIONS

Time	Pulse	Rhythm	BP	Resps	Sat %	Time	Pulse	Rhythm	BP	Resps	Sat %

THERAPY (including oxygen)

Time	Drug	Dose	Route	Time	Drug	Dose	Route	Time	Drug	Dose	Route

PROCEDURES

Time	Procedure	Time	Procedure	Time	Procedure

DIET REGIME/FLUID BALANCE _____

NURSING NOTES _____

_____
_____
_____
_____
_____
_____
_____

COMMENTS _____

_____
_____
_____
_____
_____
_____
_____
_____

Report ☐   Notes ☐   X rays ☐   Medications ☐   Passport ☐   Personal Effects ☐

Handed over to _____   Status _____   Signed _____

Signed for TMS

Doctor _____   Nurse _____

Figure 24.15 *contd.*

References

1. Alsop K. Personal communication.
2. De Temmerman P. Ambulance helicopters: constraints and medical applications. Abstract. *1st International Congress on Airborne Emergency Assistance*, Lyon, France, 1983.
3. Stolpe E, Lackner C. Modern concepts of E.M.S. Helicopters for different purposes: primary rescue and interhospital transport, in *Proceedings of the 4th Conference of the International Society of Aeromedical Services*, 1993.
4. Working Party Report. Recommended standards for UK fixed wing medical air transport systems and patient management during transfer by fixed wing aicraft. *J Roy Soc Med* 1992;**85**:767–71.
5. Nicholson AN, Pascoe RA, Spencer MB *et al.* Sleep after transmeridian flights. *Lancet* 1986;**2**:1205–8.
6. Cara M. Historique de secours ariens medicaux: importance de la contribution français. *Convergences Med* 1983;**2**:377–89.
7. Protocol Systems Inc. *Propac 106 Operating Manual*, 1996.
8. British National Formulary, 1996;**31**:181.

25 Medical problems in major trauma patients

Terry D. Wardle

Consultant Physician, Countess of Chester Health Park, Chester

OBJECTIVES

- To give details of the ABC in the primary survey.
- To list the AMPLE history details needed in the secondary survey.
- To discuss the physical examination.

There are four key determinants of survival following major trauma:

- pre-injury health;
- magnitude of injury;
- time to definitive care;
- quality of care.

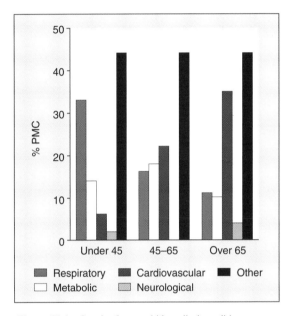

Figure 25.1 Graph of premorbid medical conditions vs age.

The last three topics are considered elsewhere in this book.

The significance and impact of coexisting medical problems are all too frequently overlooked. They may not only precipitate trauma but also affect or exacerbate the clinical picture as well as influencing the trauma patient's response to treatment. It is therefore mandatory to take an accurate AMPLE history (see page 301) so that relevant medical information is obtained, reducing the risk of inappropriate treatment. Furthermore, failure of a patient to respond to appropriate treatment can be explained by coexistent medical problems provided that potential life-threatening conditions that may have resulted from trauma have been treated or excluded. For this reason it is mandatory that the ABCDE system is adhered to.

Only recently has attention been focused on the number and type of premorbid conditions as well as their effect on patient outcome [1–7]. The incidence of premorbid conditions ranges from 4.8 to 16% in the United States. In contrast, one study in the United Kingdom, utilising data from the Major Trauma Outcome Study, has found premorbid conditions were present in 39% of major trauma patients. Furthermore, premorbid medical conditions occur in all age groups and not surprisingly their incidence increases with age (Figure 25.1).

All stages of resuscitation may be influenced by medical problems, therefore, they will be considered under the ubiquitous ABCDE system.

Primary survey

A – Airway control/cervical spine immobilisation

Airway control

Airway integrity may be compromised by pseudobulbar or bulbar palsy. These commonly result from a stroke. However,

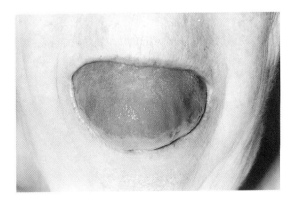

Figure 25.2 Macroglossia.

295

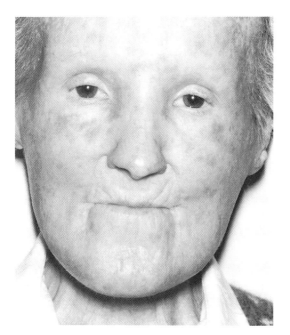

Figure 25.3 Progressive systemic sclerosis.

pseudobulbar palsy may result from disseminated sclerosis whilst bulbar muscle weakness occurs in motor neurone disease and myasthenia gravis. Therefore all of these patients have an increased risk of aspiration. The airway may also be compromised either by macroglossia associated with, for example, amyloid and acromegaly, or by the constricted, small, bird-like mouth of progressive systemic sclerosis (Figure 25.2, 25.3). Although these conditions influence airway management, in particular with simple adjuncts, they do not usually cause problems with endotracheal intubation. In contrast, difficulties may arise if the temporomandibular joints are affected by rheumatoid disease. In severe cases it may be

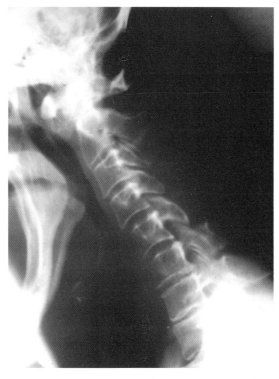

Figure 25.4 Atlantoaxial subluxation in rheumatoid disease. Note the lack of cervical lordosis and associated changes in C5, C6.

impossible to open the mouth wide enough to allow intubation. Thus, other methods of securing the airway should be considered according to the expertise of the doctor and the urgency of the situation.

Cervical spine

Patients with rheumatoid disease may have cervical spine involvement with the potential for instability and hence cervical cord injury (Figure 25.4). Ankylosing spondylitis is another inflammatory polyarthropathy that can be associated with an increased incidence of cervical spine injury (Figure 25.5).

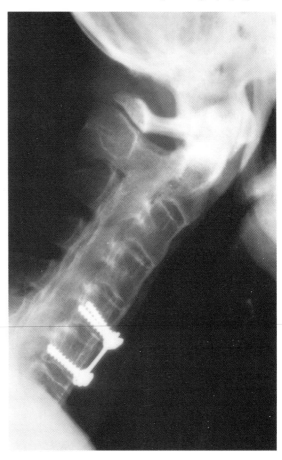

Figure 25.5 Lateral C-spine demonstrating fixed fracture in ankylosing spondylitis.

Although this condition classically produces a "rigid spine", cervical spine involvement is not infrequent. Paradoxically this does not exempt patients from, but actually increases their propensity to, a cervical spine injury. Furthermore, the amount of force required can be quite minor. More recently, the potential for cervical spine injury, in particular atlantotaxial subluxation, in Down's syndrome has been discussed [8]. **This will not create any problems providing that cervical spine injury is assumed to be present and in-line immobilisation is maintained until injury is excluded both clinically and radiologically**. It is, however, a trap for the unwary and care should be taken when clearing and securing the airway.

B – Breathing

Respiratory diseases are common, thus it is not surprising that many trauma victims present with coexistent pulmonary pathology. Many respiratory conditions may not be apparent on initial assessment, especially when the patient has sustained a chest injury. This can cause diagnostic difficulties but clues may be gained from the history, clinical examination, treatment response, arterial blood gases, and chest x-ray.

The common respiratory problems that can cause diagnostic difficulty will be considered.

Chronic bronchitis and/or emphysema

These are common causes of pulmonary dysfunction and subsequent respiratory failure. They may cause diagnostic confusion, especially in patients who are cyanosed. As some of these patients rely upon their hypoxic, rather than their hypercapnoeic, drive, concern is often expressed about the concentration of supplemental oxygen that should be given. Hypoxia, especially in the major trauma situation, is a cause of morbidity and mortality. Therefore these patients require a fractional inspired oxygen of at least 0.85. This can subsequently be titrated according to arterial blood gas results.

> The presence of chronic pulmonary disease should be regarded as an early indication for ventilation.

Bronchospasm

This can indicate inhalation of noxious compounds, asthma, chronic airflow limitation, or pulmonary oedema. It is important to remember that asthmatics have an increased risk of developing a pneumothorax and that severe bronchospasm can be associated with hypotension. An AMPLE history will facilitate the correct diagnosis. High flow oxygen, nebulised/intravenous bronchodilators, along with intravenous steroids should be administered according to the clinical situation.

Pulmonary oedema

This may indicate inhalation of noxious substances, pulmonary parenchymal injury, adult respiratory distress syndrome, neurological injury, or myocardial trauma. However, in the western world it is a common sequel to ischaemic heart disease and to a lesser extent mitral/aortic valve disease. If pulmonary oedema is clinically present when the patient arrives in the A & E Department (providing their transfer has not been delayed) then it is likely to be due to pre-existing cardiac disease. These patients will benefit from early endotracheal intubation, ventilation, and direct and indirect measurement of right and left heart pressures respectively, with a pulmonary artery catheter. Only in this way can the correct fluid resuscitation be achieved. Do not blindly treat these patients with diuretics or vasodilators as they may precipitate or exacerbate tissue hypoxia.

Pleural effusion

Many medical conditions, including left ventricular failure, pleuropulmonary malignancy, rheumatoid disease, and progressive systemic sclerosis may present with pleural effusions.

Even if they are known to exist, a chest drain is still the correct management of choice. This not only reduces pulmonary embarrassment but will also ensure that coexistent trauma is not present.

Pulmonary emboli

Following skeletal injury, in particular multiple fractures, fat emboli may occur. Clinical features include tachypnoea, petechial rash, and a spectrum of neurological manifestations. It is of interest to note that fat globules are able to traverse the pulmonary capillaries by moulding to their shape and hence gain access to the systemic circulation. This may be responsible, in part, for the neurological symptoms along with hypoxia and/or humoral and cellular factors released from bone [4].

In contrast, pulmonary embolism (PE) may follow deep vein thromboses, particularly in vehicle drivers following a long journey. Irrespective of the many potential causes of pulmonary embolism (Figure 25.6), it is likely under these

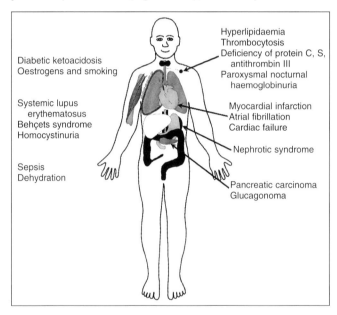

Figure 25.6 Causes for pulmonary embolism (pre-injury)

circumstances that a massive PE will present as electro-mechanical dissociation. Thrombolysis would be precluded on the grounds of prolonged resuscitation and the presence of multiple injuries. The management would entail early administration of oxygen and resuscitation according to European guidelines.

In many of the multisystem diseases (Figure 25.7) there are coexistent pulmonary problems.

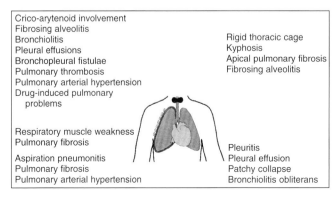

Figure 25.7 Respiratory problems in multisystem disease

C – Circulation and haemorrhage control

Hypotension

Hypotension in major trauma patients is always assumed to be due to blood loss. If the patient fails to respond to fluid administration then occult blood loss into a body cavity or soft tissues is the likely cause. However, if this is not evident then it is important to consider other medical conditions (Figure 25.8). To facilitate diagnosis the clinician will require,

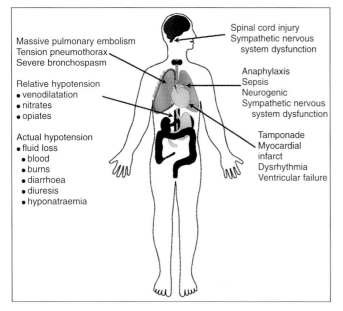

Figure 25.8 Causes of hypotension

as a minimum, a comprehensive history and examination, a 12-lead electrocardiogram, full blood count, electrolytes, arterial blood gases, and chest x-ray.

The presence of distended internal jugular veins may indicate cardiac tamponade, pulmonary embolus, or right ventricular failure (from whatever cause). Electromechanical dissociation will help in this differential diagnosis, as will pericardiocentesis.

Occult blood loss may occur in the gastrointestinal tract secondary to trauma. It may, however, reflect pre-existing peptic ulcer disease or inflammation. These may be exacerbated by stress ulceration, in particular related to burns (Curling's ulcers) or neurological injury (Cushing's ulcers).

During initial assessment it is unusual to diagnose septic shock in the trauma patient unless there has been a prolonged delay in extrication or transfer. Although these patients initially have hypotension they have warm, well-perfused peripheries. This is a useful physical sign in this differential diagnosis.

Hypotension is an important sequel to adrenal and to a lesser extent pituitary insufficiency. Glucocorticoid therapy is employed for a variety of conditions **but** even if the steroids have been withdrawn gradually adrenal function may still be suboptimal. Thus any acute stress, for example trauma, can precipitate an Addisonian crisis. This may be manifested by hypotension unresponsive to treatment or following initial stabilisation, recurrent hypotension, confusion, or even coma. Classical electrolyte changes are not always present. If this condition is suspected then the patient should be given 300 mg hydrocortisone intravenously. This should be repeated daily until it is convenient to perform a short Synacthen test. Some indication as to the presence of the disease may be gained from a random

serum cortisol and ACTH which should be taken before hydrocortisone is administered.

Ischaemic heart disease

This is the most prevalent disease in the western world and it may be exacerbated by blood loss, hypoxia, hypovolaemia, or hypotension. If the patient is unconscious, a myocardial infarction may not be apparent. In these patients, ECG monitoring is essential. The presence of an arrhythmia may be the only clue to myocardial damage which may have been either precipitated or exacerbated by the traumatic insult.

Arrhythmias

It is important to realise that arrhythmias may also reflect hypoxia, electrolyte disturbance, increased intracranial pressure, and coexistent drug therapy. They may in turn precipitate or exacerbate hypotension, cardiac failure, hypoxia, and loss of consciousness. Tachydysrhythmias are usually treated by pharmacological means, especially when the patient is haemodynamically stable with no evidence of cardiac failure or impaired consciousness. It is important to remember that these drugs can not only treat, but also cause arrhythmias, as well as depress myocardial function. In the presence of cardiac failure a tachydysrhythmia should be treated with appropriate cardioversion.

A particularly difficult problem is the trauma patient who has ischaemic heart disease and hypotension. Following major trauma the commonest cause of hypotension is blood loss – but this not be the entire answer. It may be the product of blood loss and cardiac dysfunction (arrhythmia, cardiac failure). Thus it is essential that under these circumstances fluid replacement is titrated against accurate invasive monitoring especially as correction of hypovolaemia, in particular in atrial fibrillation, can restore sinus rhythm. Furthermore, loss of consciousness may be independent of the tachydysrhythmia. Therefore, if the patient fails to respond to a fluid challenge (2 litres Ringer's lactate) then cardioversion is recommended, as the dysrhythmia can only exacerbate the clinical situation.

Valvular disease

Valvular disease, particularly affecting the aortic valve, is on the increase, especially in the elderly population. This may result in a narrow pulse pressure which may be misdiagnosed as an indicator of hypovolaemia. In this situation excessive fluid administration can result in left, or biventricular, failure. Cardiac decompensation may also occur because of ischaemic heart disease or myocardial trauma.

Patients with valvular disease should be given prophylactic antibiotics as soon as is convenient providing there are no contraindications: ampicillin 1 g and gentamicin 80 mg followed by ampicillin 500 mg after 12 h is standard practice. The presence of a metal prosthetic valve can induce haemolysis which initially can be confused with blood transfusion problems.

Cardiac pacemakers

These can profoundly influence the clinical picture following major trauma. Potential problems with pacemakers are listed in the box.

Potential pacemaker problems

- Damage to:
  - pacemaker
  - wire
- Pacemaker failure
- Inappropriate function
- Masking myocardial damage/bradycardia
- Inappropriate response to:
  - shock
  - fluid resuscitation
  - (especially of fixed rate)

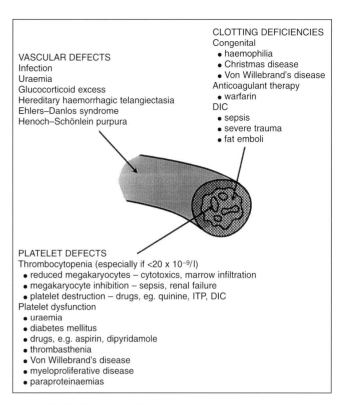

VASCULAR DEFECTS
Infection
Uraemia
Glucocorticoid excess
Hereditary haemorrhagic telangiectasia
Ehlers–Danlos syndrome
Henoch–Schönlein purpura

CLOTTING DEFICIENCIES
Congenital
- haemophilia
- Christmas disease
- Von Willebrand's disease
Anticoagulant therapy
- warfarin
DIC
- sepsis
- severe trauma
- fat emboli

PLATELET DEFECTS
Thrombocytopenia (especially if <20 x 10^{-9}/l)
- reduced megakaryocytes – cytotoxics, marrow infiltration
- megakaryocyte inhibition – sepsis, renal failure
- platelet destruction – drugs, eg. quinine, ITP, DIC
Platelet dysfunction
- uraemia
- diabetes mellitus
- drugs, e.g. aspirin, dipyridamole
- thrombasthenia
- Von Willebrand's disease
- myeloproliferative disease
- paraproteinaemias

Figure 25.10 Coagulation disorders

Hypertension

This is always a concern. The history and physical examination are important, enabling the differentiation between acute and chronic hypertension. Acute hypertension may reflect increased intracranial pressure but other circulatory signs are usually present, in particular bradycardia. Persistent or variable hypertension can indicate the presence of phaeochromocytoma. Whilst this is a rare condition it does present problems for the unwary. Acute hypertension needs careful controlled reduction and the patient will require invasive monitoring and the intravenous administration of both alpha and beta blockers.

Chronic anaemia

Anaemia is a common condition (Figure 25.9). Information as to the presence and type of anaemia may not be available from the initial haemoglobin estimation. Therefore patients should be transfused according to their haemodynamic parameters rather than their haemoglobin concentration/packed cell volume.

Haemoglobinopathies

Sickle-cell disease, in particular, may precipitate or be precipitated by major trauma. Furthermore, acute pain, in particular abdominal pain, may reflect a sickle crisis rather than intraperitoneal injury. Tenderness is not uncommon and under these circumstances diagnostic peritoneal lavage or CT scan is recommended.

Coagulopathy

A bleeding diathesis or a procoagulant disease, can profoundly influence the patient's response to both trauma and resuscitation. If a history is not available and clinical features, in particular chronic liver disease, are not obvious, then this problem will only come to light during resuscitation. The potential causes are listed in Figure 25.10. If there is any suspicion of coagulopathy then it is advisable to check both the activated partial thromboplastin and prothrombin times. These should be corrected appropriately.

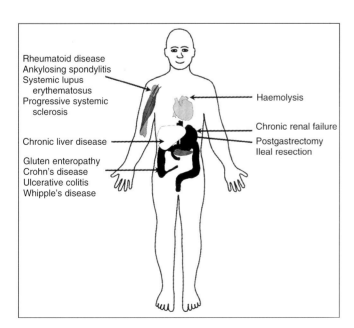

Rheumatoid disease
Ankylosing spondylitis
Systemic lupus erythematosus
Progressive systemic sclerosis

Chronic liver disease

Gluten enteropathy
Crohn's disease
Ulcerative colitis
Whipple's disease

Haemolysis

Chronic renal failure
Postgastrectomy
Ileal resection

Figure 25.9 Causes of chronic anaemia

Figure 25.11 Petechial rash: fat emboli.

Pericardial effusion

Patients with left ventricular failure, uraemia, progressive systemic sclerosis, or rheumatoid disease may already have pericardial effusion before the injury. If there is clinical evidence of a pericardial effusion then pericardiocentesis should be performed, not only to improve cardiac function but also to exclude associated pericardial or myocardial trauma.

Cardiac transplants

These are not infrequent. The type of transplant will govern whether the myocardium is able to respond either directly to neural or sympathetic simulation, or indirectly to circulating catecholamines.

Disability

With the increasing numbers of aged patients there is a coexisting increase in cerebrovascular disease. However, hypoglycaemia has many neurological manifestations. Therefore, it is mandatory that all patients have a serum glucose estimation as hypoglycaemia is easy to treat but potentially lethal and easy to miss.

Many neurological problems will be identified when airway, breathing, and circulation are assessed.

Fits or coma

These are usually ascribed to intracerebral injury; however, in the presence of a normal CT scan other conditions need to be considered (Figure 25.12). Hyponatraemia or hypocalcaemia may be precipitated by rapid volume expansion,

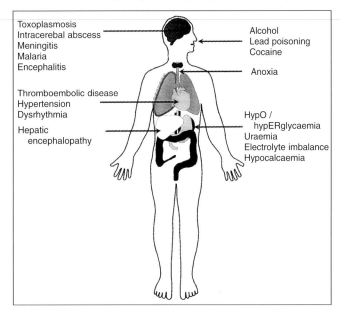

Figure 25.12 Causes of fits/coma

whereas hypernatraemia may be precipitated or exacerbated by dehydration and result in cerebral oedema (for example, in association with excessive burns).

Chronic neurological disease

Many of the chronic neurological diseases, especially stroke or demyelination, may present with lateralising signs. These may mimic or mask occult intracerebral trauma. If no history is available then the presence of these physical signs necessitates

a CT scan. It is best to exclude pathology rather than to ignore it.

Autonomic dysfunction

This not only masks the patient's response to trauma and fluid resuscitation but also mimics spinal cord injury. With the exception of diabetes mellitus the majority of causes of autonomic dysfunction are rare. Ideally one should treat patients as though they have an acute spinal injury. Cautious fluid resuscitation is therefore mandatory, inotropic agents should be considered, and invasive monitioring is essential.

Malignant hyperpyrexia/neuroleptic malignant syndrome

These are potentially fatal disorders that may not be evident during the primary survey. Often they are only diagnosed during or following anaesthesia. These conditions necessitate prompt treatment with dantrolene and measures to maintain an appropriate core temperature.

Exposure/hypothermia

Hypothermia can precipitate or be the result of either major trauma or resuscitation. Potential causes should be sought in the secondary survey. Prevention of hypothermia in the resuscitation room is important. Appropriate means must be taken to maintain the body temperature, including administration of warmed intravenous fluids and overhead heating. The treatment of hypothermia has been described in Chapter 20. Do not forget that hypothermia not attributed to exposure should alert the physician to the presence of occult pathology, in particular sepsis, pancreatitis, hypothyroidism, and phenothiazine overdose.

Investigations

Results from investigations done in the primary survey will yield additional information. Interpretation of chest radiographs is covered in Chapter 3. Furthermore, for a comprehensive review of the diagnosis and treatment of cardiac arrhythmias, the reader is referred to references 10–12.

Arterial blood gas results provide invaluable information in the resuscitation room, but they must be interpreted in the light of the clinical situation; for example, the presence of respiratory alkalosis, if the patient is ventilated, is likely to reflect inappropriate excessive ventilation. In contrast, if the patient is not ventilated, then compensatory hyperventilation may have resulted as a consequence of hypoxia, sepsis, pulmonary emboli, or anxiety.

Metabolic acidosis, however, in particular with an increased anion gap, may reflect hypoperfusion and lactic acid accumulation. If the patient fails to respond to appropriate treatment, then it is important to exclude other potential causes (see box). Many of these problems may not be apparent on initial assessment. A clue to their presence may be obtained from the history, clinical examination, failure to respond to treatment, arterial blood gases, and chest x-ray.

An electrolyte imbalance is not an infrequent finding especially in patients taking diuretics. The relevant clinical features associated with a disturbance of sodium and calcium homeostasis have been described earlier in this chapter. In

Metabolic acidosis

- *Normal anion gap**
  - renal tubular acidosis
  - acetozolamide
  - diarrhoea
  - ureterosigmoidostomy
  - small bowel fistula
- *Increased anion gap*
  - methanol
  - uraemia
  - diabetic ketoacidosis
  - salicylates
  - lactate
  - ethanol
  - ethylene glycol
  - paraldehyde

* Anion gap $= (Na^+ + K^+) - (Cl^- + HCO_3^-)$; normal range $= 14$–18 mmol/l

contrast, hyperkalaemia is likely to be the most important electrolyte problem in the acute situation. This should not be ascribed to a haemolysed sample, because patients can have coexisting renal dysfunction, metabolic acidosis in association with shock, diabetic ketoacidosis, or even tissue (especially muscular) necrosis. This is important, particularly in patients who have acute/chronic renal failure, where underperfusion may exacerbate the situation and warrant early dialysis/ intervention by nephrologist.

Secondary survey

AMPLE history

Many medical problems, beyond the scope of this chapter, will be identified in trauma patients providing that an AMPLE history has been obtained, either from the patient, police or paramedical staff. Further information may be sought from hospital records, the patient's relatives and general practitioner, as well as any witnesses. With regards to a medical problem, relevant information from an AMPLE history should include:

A *Allergies* are unlikely to be present in the trauma patient unless they either precipitated the traumatic event or resulted from medical therapy. Many of the consequent clinical features require minimal medical intervention; however, anaphylaxis – the most sinister manifestation – may mimic, mask, or coexist with shock. Its presence mandates intravenous adrenalin.

M Many patients are taking *medication* and these drugs may not be known at the time of resuscitation. Beta blockers, calcium channel antagonists, ACE inhibitors, and, to a lesser extent, nitrates are important because they modify the cardiovascular response to both trauma and resuscitation. The use of oral steroid preparations, as alluded to earlier, is common and an addisonian crisis can be precipitated if this drug is omitted. The use of recreational drugs may precipitate or modify the patient's response to trauma [13].

The link between alcohol consumption and major trauma, in particular road traffic accidents, is well established [14]. Alcohol can influence the presentation,

treatment, and outcome following trauma. It is important to realise that alcohol can produce a variety of clinical manifestations as can withdrawal from the same. In the presence of chronic alcohol consumption, adequate thiamine should be administered and careful control of withdrawal symptoms with chlordiazepoxide is mandatory. Remember that if intravenous dextrose is required it **must** be preceded by thiamine. Thus the possibility of Wernicke's encephalopathy, in susceptible individuals will be avoided.

P *Past medical history* is extremely important as this will alert the physician to potential factors that may influence the clinical presentation or response to treatment.

L *Last meal*, in the context of medical problems, may explain the cause of hypoglycaemia.

E *Events/environment* in which the trauma victim was involved or found provides important information as to the potential cause/s of hypothermia. Always consider occult pathology.

Physical examination

During the "head-to-toe" assessment of the patient, other medical problems may be identified. Their treatment will have to be viewed in the context of the patient's injuries and history, and prioritised accordingly. Regular re-assessment is mandatory especially in the light of new clinical information. Many medical conditions affect multiple systems and it is advisable to review the patient as a "whole", just in case the significance of episcleritis, for example, is not immediately apparent. Furthermore, it is important to remember that treatment can result in a deterioration in the patient's condition, for example opioids causing respiratory depression and neurological deterioration.

Summary

Medical problems occur frequently in trauma patients. They may either precipitate the trauma or arise as a consequence of the injury or its subsequent treatment. They can have a tremendous impact on resuscitation. Despite the numerous problems discussed we advocate that the approach and treatment of the major trauma patient follows the ABCDE system. If the patient fails to respond to treatment in the expected way then consider an underlying medical problem. An AMPLE history is invaluable, especially when supplemented by information by the general practitioner (if known). The physician has an important role to play in the management of major trauma patients and therefore should be included in the trauma team.

References

1. Morris JA, Averbach PS, Bleuth R, Trunkey DD. Pre-injury health: Determinant of survival in trauma patients. *J Trauma* 1986;**26**:680 (Abstract).
2. Mackenzie EJ, Morris JA, Edelstein SL. Effect of pre-existing disease on length of stay in trauma patients. *J Trauma* 1989;**29**: 757–65.
3. Whetsell LA, Patterson CM, Young DH, Schiller WR. Preinjury psychopathology in trauma patients. *J Trauma* 1989;**28**:1158–62.
4. Morris JA, Mackenzie EJ, Edelstein SL. The effect of preexisting conditions on mortality in trauma patients. *J Am Med Assoc* 1990; **263**:1942–6.

5. Morris JA, Mackenzie EJ, Diamiano AM, Bass SM. Mortality in trauma patients; The interaction between host factors and severity. *J Trauma* 1990;**30**:1476–82.
6. Milzman DP, Boulanger BR, Rodriguez A, Soderstrom CA, Mitchell KA, Magmant CM. Pre-existing disease in trauma patients; a predictor of fate independent of age and injury severity score. *J Trauma* 1992;**31**:236–44.
7. Wardle TD, Driscoll, P Woodford M. Medical problems in major trauma. *Injury* 1995;**26**:137.
8. Cervical spine instability in people with Down's syndrome. *CMO Update* 1995; **7** (Oct.).
9. Fulde G, Harrison P. Fat embolism, a review. *Arch Emerg Med* 1991;**8**:233–9.
10. Schamroth L. *Introduction to electrocardiography*. Oxford: Blackwell Scientific, 1990.
11. Rowlands DJ. *Understanding the electrocardiogram*. Imperial Chemical Industries PLC, 1987.
12. Advanced Life Support Group. *Advanced cardiac life support: the practical approach*. London: Chapman & Hall, 1992.
13. Clark RF, Harchelroad F. Toxicology screening of the trauma patient: A changing profile. *Ann Emerg Med* 1991;**20**:151–3.
14. Orsay EM, Doan-Wiggins L, Lewis R, Lucke R, RamaKrishnan V. The impaired driver: Hospital and police detection of alcohol and other drugs of abuse in motor vehicle crashes. *Ann Emerg Med* 1994;**24**:51–5.

Index

Index

Index